Comprehensive Endocrinology

Comprehensive Endocrinology

Editor-in-Chief: Luciano Martini

Comprehensive Endocrinology

The Endocrine Functions of the Brain

Editor

Marcella Motta, Ph.D.
Professor of Physiology
Department of Endocrinology
University of Milan
Milan, Italy

Raven Press ■ New York

Raven Press, 1140 Avenue of the Americas, New York, New York 10036

Made in the United States of America

Great care has been taken to maintain the accuracy of the information contained in the volume. However, Raven Press cannot be held responsible for errors or for any consequences arising from the use of the information contained herein.

Library of Congress Cataloging in Publication Data

Main entry under title:

The Endocrine functions of the brain.

(Comprehensive endocrinology)
Includes bibliographical references and index.
1. Neuroendocrinology. 2. Brain. I. Motta, Marcella. II. Series.
QP356.4.E52   612'.82   77-84553
ISBN 0-89004-343-4

Preface

The participation of the brain in the control of endocrine processes has been one of the most active and profitable areas of investigation in the last decades. The discovery of the hypothalamic hypophysiotropic hormones (TRH, LHRH, somatostatin) has opened new lines of research as well as new approaches in clinical practice. More recently, other peptides (e.g., neurotensin, vasoactive intestinal peptide, substance P, etc.), which are common to the brain and surprisingly to the gastrointestinal tract, have been identified and shown to play a major role in neuroendocrine integration. Spectacular results have been obtained in the area of the opioid peptides (endorphins, enkephalins, etc.), which appear to be formed independently in peptidergic neurons and in the pituitary gland. Extensive investigations have clarified the role of the central nervous system receptors for peripheral and anterior pituitary hormones in the control of endocrine functions and in the modulation of behavioral phenomena. Because of these impressive developments, the time has probably come to consider the brain as a real "endocrine" organ.

This volume, which is part of the "Comprehensive Endocrinology" set, explores in detail the ways through which the brain regulates the endocrines as well as the mechanisms underlying hormonal effects on central nervous system functions. It provides information on the anatomical and electrophysiological aspects of the "endocrine" brain. Other topics dealt with are the distribution, the localization, and the mechanism of action of steroid and peptide hormones. The presence and the significance of the peptides with opioid-like activities and of other active peptides are reviewed. Some chapters are devoted to the participation of extrahypothalamic centers in neuroendocrine processes, and to the interaction of the central neurotransmitters with hormone-producing or hormone-sensitive cells. The control of neurohypophysial hormones and the role of neurophysins are also discussed in detail. A clinical section deals with the hypothalamic dysfunctions in humans and provides valuable information on the diagnostic tests available for the evaluation of neuroendocrine disturbances.

This volume is intended to meet the needs of a variety of readers. It is designed as an important source of references for a wide range of investigators engaged in the study of neuroscientific disciplines as well as for clinicians; the volume will be especially valuable to advanced medical students.

Marcella Motta, Ph.D.

Acknowledgment

The contributors are all internationally recognized authorities within their respective fields. The editor is very grateful to all of them for having devoted time and effort to the preparation of their outstanding chapters.

Contents

Contributors

Nicholas Barden
Medical Research Council
Group in Molecular Endocrinology
Le Centre Hospitalier de
* l'Université Laval*
Quebec, Quebec G1V 4G2, Canada

Michèle Beaulieu
Medical Research Council
Group in Molecular Endocrinology
Le Centre Hospitalier de
* l'Université Laval*
Quebec, Quebec G1V 4G2, Canada

Carol Bennett-Clarke
Department of Anatomy
University of Rochester
School of Medicine and Dentristry
Rochester, New York 14642

Pierre Borgeat
Medical Research Council
Group in Molecular Endocrinology
Le Centre Hospitalier de
* l'Université Laval*
Quebec, Quebec G1V 4G2, Canada

Roger Boucher
Clinical Research Institute of
* Montreal*
Montreal, Quebec H2W 1R7, Canada

Michael J. Brownstein
Laboratory of Clinical Science
National Institute of Mental Health
National Institutes of Health
Bethesda, Maryland 20205

Barbara Burchanowski
Department of Anatomy
University of Rochester
School of Medicine and Dentristry
Rochester, New York 14642

Jean-Louis Charli
Neuroendocrine Program
Departments of Psychiatry and
* Biochemistry*
University of Pittsburgh
School of Medicine
Western Psychiatric Institute and
* Clinic*
Pittsburgh, Pennsylvania 15213

Pier Giorgio Chiodini
Divisione di Endocrinologia
Ente Ospedaliero di Niguarda
20162 Milano, Italy

Renato Cozzi
Divisione di Endocrinologia
Ente Ospedaliero di Niguarda
20162 Milano, Italy

Lionel Cusan
Medical Research Council
Group in Molecular Endocrinology
Le Centre Hospitalier de
* l'Université Laval*
Quebec, Quebec G1V 4G2, Canada

Francine Denizeau
Medical Research Council
Group in Molecular Endocrinology
Le Centre Hospitalier de
* l'Université Laval*
Quebec, Quebec G1V 4G2, Canada

Bernard T. Donovan
Department of Physiology
Institute of Psychiatry
London SE5 8AF, England

Jacques Drouin
Medical Research Council
Group in Molecular Endocrinology
Le Centre Hospitalier de
l'Université Laval
Quebec, Quebec G1V 4G2, Canada

André Dupont
Medical Research Council
Group in Molecular Endocrinology
Le Centre Hospitalier de
l'Université Laval
Quebec, Quebec G1V 4G2, Canada

Franz Ellendorff
Institut für Tierzucht und
Tierverhalten,
FAL
Mariensee
3057 Neustadt 1, Federal Republic of
Germany

Louise Ferland
Medical Research Council
Group in Molecular Endocrinology
Le Centre Hospitalier de
l'Université Laval
Quebec, Quebec G1V 4G2, Canada

Robert C. A. Frederickson
Lilly Research Laboratories
Eli Lilly and Company
Indianapolis, Indiana 46206

Lawrence A. Frohman
Division of Endocrinology and
Metabolism
Michael Reese Medical Center and
Department of Medicine
University of Chicago
Chicago, Illinois 60616

Jacques Genest
Clinical Research Institute of
Montreal
Montreal, Quebec H2W 1R7, Canada

Martin Godbout
Medical Research Council
Group in Molecular Endocrinology
Le Centre Hospitalier de
l'Université Laval
Quebec, Quebec G1V 4G2, Canada

James N. Hayward
Departments of Neurology and
Medicine
Neurobiology Program
University of North Carolina
Chapel Hill, North Carolina 27514

Shirley A. Joseph
Department of Anatomy
University of Rochester
School of Medicine and Dentristry
Rochester, New York 14642

Patricia Joseph-Bravo
Neuroendocrine Program
Departments of Psychiatry and
Biochemistry
University of Pittsburgh
School of Medicine
Western Psychiatric Institute
and Clinic
Pittsburgh, Pennsylvania 15213

Pierre Jouan
Laboratoire de Neurobiologie
Moléculaire
ERA—C.N.R.S.
Centre Régional de Recherche en
Endocrinologie
35042 Rennes CEDEX, France

David C. Klein
Section on Neuroendocrinology
Laboratory of Developmental
Neurobiology
National Institute of Child Health
and Human Development
National Institutes of Health
Bethesda, Maryland 20205

Karl M. Knigge
Department of Anatomy
University of Rochester
School of Medicine and Dentristry
Rochester, New York 14642

Fernard Labrie
Medical Research Council
Group in Molecular Endocrinology
Le Centre Hospitalier de
l'Université Laval
Quebec, Quebec G1V 4G2, Canada

Lisette Lagacé
Medical Research Council
Group in Molecular Endocrinology
Le Centre Hospitalier de
l'Université Laval
Quebec, Quebec G1V 4G2, Canada

André Lemay
Medical Research Council
Group in Molecular Endocrinology
Le Centre Hospitalier de
l'Université Laval
Quebec, Quebec G1V 4G2, Canada

Jérome Lépine
Medical Research Council
Group in Molecular Endocrinology
Le Centre Hospitalier de
l'Université Laval
Quebec, Quebec G1V 4G2, Canada

Jean-Claude Lissitzky
Medical Research Council
Group in Molecular Endocrinology
Le Centre Hospitalier de
l'Université Laval
Quebec, Quebec G1V 4G2, Canada

Antonio Liuzzi
Divisione di Endocrinologia
Ente Ospedaliero di Niguarda
20162 Milano, Italy

Catherine Loudes
Neuroendocrine Program
Departments of Psychiatry and Bio-
chemistry
University of Pittsburgh
School of Medicine
Western Psychiatric Institute and
Clinic
Pittsburgh, Pennsylvania 15213

Jocelyne Massicotte
Medical Research Council
Group in Molecular Endocrinology
Le Centre Hospitalier de
l'Université Laval
Quebec, Quebec G1V 4G2, Canada

Jeffrey F. McKelvy
Neuroendocrine Program
Departments of Psychiatry and
Biochemistry
University of Pittsburgh
School of Medicine
Western Psychiatric Institute
and Clinic
Pittsburgh, Pennsylvania 15213

Thomas G. Muldoon
Department of Endocrinology
Medical College of Georgia
Augusta, Georgia 30902

Giuseppe Oppizzi
Divisione di Endocrinologia
Ente Ospedaliero di Niguarda
20162 Milano, Italy

Miklós Palkovits
First Department of Anatomy
Semmelweis University Medical
School
1450 Budapest, Hungary

Nahid Parvizi
Institut für Tierzucht und
Tierverhalten
FAL
Mariensee
3057 Neustadt 1, Federal Republic of
Germany

Georges Pelletier
Medical Research Council
Group in Molecular Endocrinology
Le Centre Hospitalier de
l'Université Laval
Quebec, Quebec G1V 4G2,
Canada

Vincent Raymond
Medical Research Council
Group in Molecular Endocrinology
Le Centre Hospitalier de
l'Université Laval
Quebec, Quebec G1V 4G2,
Canada

Troy A. Reaves, Jr.
Departments of Neurology and
Medicine
Neurobiology Program
University of North Carolina
Chapel Hill, North Carolina 27514

Steven M. Reppert
Section on Neuroendocrinology
Laboratory of Developmental
Neurobiology
National Institute of Child Health
and Human Development
National Institutes of Health
Bethesda, Maryland 20205

Mary A. Romagnano
Department of Anatomy
University of Rochester
School of Medicine and
Dentistry
Rochester, New York 14642

Suzanne Samperez
Laboratoire de Neurobiologie
MoléculaireRA—C.N.R.S.
Centre Régional de Recherche en
Endocrinologie
35042 Rennes CEDEX, France

Thomas Sherman
Neuroendocrine Program
Departments of Psychiatry and
Biochemistry
University of Pittsburgh School of
Medicine
Western Psychiatric Institute and
Clinic
Pittsburgh, Pennsylvania 15213

Ludwig A. Sternberger
Department of Anatomy
University of Rochester
School of Medicine and
Dentistry
Rochester, New York 14642

Walter E. Stumpf
Departments of Anatomy and
 Pharmacology
University of North Carolina
Chapel Hill, North Carolina
 27514

Guy Valiquette
Istituto di Endocrinologia
Università di Milano
20129 Milano, Italy

Raymond Veilleux
Medical Research Council
Group in Molecular Endocrinology
Le Centre Hospitalier de
 l'Université Laval
Quebec, Quebec G1V 4G2, Canada

Giorgio Verde
Divisione di Endocrinologia
Ente Ospedaliero di Niguarda
20162 Milano, Italy

The Endocrine Functions of the Brain,
edited by Marcella Motta.
Raven Press, New York © 1980

1

Functional Anatomy of the "Endocrine" Brain

Miklós Palkovits

First Department of Anatomy, Semmelweis University Medical School, Budapest, Hungary

Several peptides are produced by central nervous system (CNS) neurons and exert actions outside the CNS via the blood circulation. This is consistent with their denomination as hormones or, more precisely, as neurohormones. The system of hormone-producing cells was termed the "endocrine" brain to distinguish these cells from brain centers participating solely in neural control. This distinction appears to be reasonable from the didactic aspect, but there are two relevant points requiring attention.

First, neurohormones are not exclusively hormonal in nature. When they are transported by the bloodstream to target regions or organs distant from their site of production, their action can readily be regarded as hormonal (Fig. 1A). It is also possible that the same substances are liberated at the axon terminals of the producing neuron and affect the function of another neuron. This is an effect characteristic of a neurotransmitter (Fig. 1B). However, it cannot be ruled out that a substance produced by a neuron is released into both pericapillary space and synaptic cleft. Thus depending on the site of its action, it may be either a neurotransmitter or a neurohormone (Fig. 1C). One single CNS neuron may possess several hundreds or thousands of nerve terminals, serving as a structural basis of the above assumption.

Second, the topographical distinction between the "neural" and the "endocrine" brain seems not to be fully justified. Until recently the hypothalamus was regarded as the center of the neuroendocrine system following the assumption that this area was the exclusive site of production of neurohormones. This view became outdated after the demonstration of extrahypothalamic hormone-producing neurons that have no direct vascular link with the pituitary gland and after the recognition of routes other than the pituitary portal system through which neurohormones may leave the CNS.

Based on the above, the "endocrine" brain can be defined as a diffuse system of neurons that produce neurohormones. Neurohormonal systems widely distributed throughout the CNS have now been visualized by immunohistochemical techniques and characterized quantitatively by radioimmunoassays.

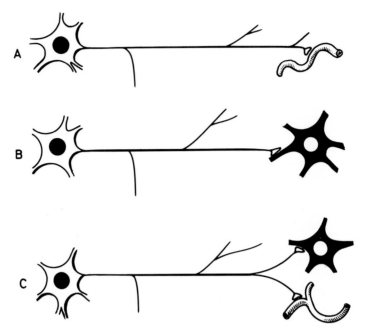

FIG. 1. Model for neurohormonal cells **(A)**, neurotransmitter cells **(B)**, and their combined **(C)** actions.

When the results of these studies are surveyed, it becomes evident that neurohormones are present in practically all brain areas (9,17,22,23,37,38). Because of space restriction, only a limited selection of original articles can be included here. We refer to recent review articles and to the original papers for details. Of the various parts of the CNS, the hypothalamus, especially the median eminence, often contains neurohormones in the highest concentrations. For a detailed description of the distribution of neurohormones in the hypothalamus, see Chapter 7.

The exact knowledge of the topography of the "endocrine" brain requires localization of perikarya, pathways, and nerve terminals containing certain neurohormones. In general, neurohormones are present in high concentrations in nerve terminals and much less in axons or in perikarya. Immunocytochemical demonstration of extensive networks of neurohormone-containing fibers and nerve terminals provides direct evidence of their topographical localization. The pathways and neurohormone-producing perikarya, however, in many cases may be visualized only with difficulty.

These considerations prompted us to deal with the topography of the "endocrine" brain by concentrating on two basic aspects: (a) the topography of neurohormone-producing cells and (b) the transport of neurohormones.

TOPOGRAPHY OF NEUROHORMONE-PRODUCING CELLS

In addition to original research reports, reviews were published summarizing recent immunocytochemical advances (17,22,23). Information is available concerning the localization of the following neurohormone-producing cells: luteinizing hormone releasing hormone (LHRH), thyrotropin releasing hormone (TRH), somatostatin, vasopressin, oxytocin, substance P, enkephalins, angiotensin II, vasoactive intestinal peptide (VIP), gastrin, prolactin, α-MSH (12), β-lipotropin (61,66), and growth hormone (56). Except for the latter three, the localizations of these structures in nerve terminals and perikarya were tabulated by Hökfelt et al. (23). In general, the immunocytochemical observations are in good agreement with the related radioimmunoassays. Most of the above neurohormones are present in measurable concentrations in many brain regions (see ref. 38 for references). Other neurohormones, which have not yet been visualized immunocytochemically, are also present in the CNS. The topographical distribution of neurotensin (27,58), β-endorphin (30,43), and ACTH (28–30,43) in the CNS has already been mapped by radioimmunoassay. For further description of the topography of active neuronal peptides, see also Chapter 8.

Although substantial fractions of neurohormones are found in various extrahypothalamic sites, biochemical, physiological, and endocrine studies unequivocally indicate that the most important part of the "endocrine" brain is the hypothalamus, especially if regarded in combination with the preoptic area. Immunocytochemical (17,22,23) and radioimmune studies (9,37–39) give support to the statement that all hypothalamic nuclei contain almost all known neurohormones; neurohormone-producing cell bodies are found less frequently in the CNS.

According to current knowledge, several nuclei of the hypothalamus and the preoptic region contain cells that synthesize one or more neurohormones. These are summarized in Table 1 without critical remarks and are meant only for general orientation of the reader. Some of the data leave room for a degree of skepticism about the experimental techniques used.

In addition to the preoptic and hypothalamic nuclei, other brain regions also contain neurohormone-producing perikarya (see refs. 17,22,23 for references). In some cortical areas the neurons contain somatostatin, gastrin, and VIP. In the hippocampus, somatostatin and gastrin are present in cell bodies. In the amygdala, a number of neuropeptides (e.g., somatostatin, substance P, VIP, enkephalins, and gastrin) have been found in the perikarya; and in the septum LHRH, in the thalamus substance P and β-lipotropin-containing cell bodies have been visualized. Substance P, enkephalins, and sporadically LHRH are present in mesencephalic neurons. Substance P has also been found in a few cells in the globus pallidus and caudate putamen. Enkephalin-containing perikarya have been found in regions of the medulla oblongata (e.g., the nucleus raphe magnus and pallidus) as well as in the nucleus tractus solitarii, which also has substance P-containing cells. With the aid of immunofluorescence, sub-

TABLE 1. *Topography of identified neurohormone-producing neurons in the hypothalamus and preoptic area of the rat*

Area	Hormone and references
Preoptic region	
Medial preoptic nucleus	LHRH (20,51,52); enkephalins (17)
Preoptic periventricular nucleus	Somatostatin (1,13,21); vasopressin (10); enkephalins (17)
Lateral preoptic area	Substance P (17,22)
Bed nucleus of the stria terminalis	LHRH (20); substance P (17,22)
Hypothalamic nuclei	
Periventricular hypothalamic nucleus	TRH (17); somatostatin (1,18,21)
Suprachiasmatic nucleus	Vasopressin (31,60,64)
Supraoptic nucleus	Somatostatin (13); vasopressin (10,16,54,59); oxytocin (59)
Paraventricular nucleus	TRH (17); somatostatin (13); vasopressin (10, 16,54,59); oxytocin (10,59); enkephalins (17,22); angiotensin II (22,23)
Arcuate nucleus	LHRH (20); enkephalins (17,22); β-lipotropin (61); α-MSH (12)
Ventromedial nucleus	Substance P (17,22); enkephalins (17,22)
Dorsomedial nucleus	TRH (17,22,24); substance P (17,22)
Lateral hypothalamic area	TRH (17)
Perifornical area	TRH (17,22); enkephalins (17,22); angiotensin II (22,23)

stance P- and enkephalin-synthesizing neurons have been demonstrated in the spinal cord.

The termination of the axons of these neurons, and hence the site of action of their neurohormones, is obscure. Since the possibility of extracerebral transport of neurohormones from the above territories is rather limited, it seems likely that neurohormones produced outside the hypothalamus exert a local action. Thus they would be mainly of the neurotransmitter type.

TRANSPORT OF NEUROHORMONES

Neurohormones act far from the site of their synthesis. To understand their mechanism of action, knowledge of alternative ways of transport is essential (see Chapter 9). Neurohormones may reach the target organ through axons, blood vessels, or the cerebrospinal fluid (CSF); as a rule, these routes exist in parallel.

Neuroanatomical Evidence for Axonal Transport of Neurohormones

The most straightforward evidence for the axonal transport of neurohormones is their direct visualization inside the axon by a specific technique. Unfortunately, even this direct information is of limited value without the demonstration of the perikarya to which the axons belong. In such cases, indirect approaches (pathway transections, deafferentations, lesions, surgical interventions in combination with chemicals like colchicine, methanol, melatonin, or barbiturates, which are able to affect the synthetic activity of neurohormone-synthesizing cell bodies) may be of help in determining the direction of transport. Within deafferented neurons, neurohormones disappear after some time from the distal segments of transected axons, whereas they accumulate in the segments proximal to the cut. Temporal relationships must also be taken into account: A minimum period of 4 to 7 days is required for the complete disappearance of the substance. It is notable that after transection, as a result of "flowing back," neurohormones may also accumulate in the distal segment (45). The "flowing back" material is resorbed within 7 to 10 days; after this period accumulated neurohormones are found only in the proximal segment.

Other means are available for the visualization of axonal transport. Horseradish peroxidase, cobalt chloride, and procion yellow are suitable tracers for demonstrating delicate long axons. These methods, however, owing to their nature yield no information about the chemical character of the axon.

The final destination of transport of neurohormones is the blood circulation or the CSF unless they have no neurotransmitter or neuromodulatory functions. However, blood–brain and liquor–brain barriers are bidirectionally impermeable to peptides.

Therefore the CNS areas that allow free passage of neurohormones are restricted to the median eminence and circumventricular organs.

Extra and Intrahypothalamic Neuronal Components of the Median Eminence

The special structure of the median eminence ensures a free transport of neurotransmitters. The pericapillary space surrounding the fenestrated capillaries of the primary portal plexus is practically open toward the vessels, the external and internal liquor spaces on one side, and toward the nerve terminals on the other. Depending on actual gradients, neurohormones may readily reach the pituitary, the liquor space, and the mediobasal hypothalamus.

All the known neurohormones can be demonstrated in the median eminence (38,39). Several extra and intrahypothalamic pathways converge onto this region. The most important are (see ref. 47 for details): (a) Supraopticohypophysial tract from the magnocellular neurosecretory nuclei (supraoptic and paraventricular). The bulk of its fibers pass through the internal layer of the median eminence to terminate in the neurohypophysis. Some of the axons or axon collaterals end around the capillaries of the external zone of the median eminence (49,53, 65,67). (b) Axons from the "parvicellular neurosecretory" nuclei (55). Most of these arise from the arcuate, anterior periventricular, ventromedial, posterior hypothalamic, and premammillary nuclei (47,63), as well as from the suprachiasmatic nucleus (67). Fibers from the latter cell group contain vasopressin; the chemical nature of fibers from the other parvicellular nuclei has not been identified yet. A percentage of these, from the arcuate and anterior periventricular cells are dopaminergic, and the others might be peptidergic. In fact, a number of various neuropeptide-synthesizing cell bodies have been demonstrated immunocytochemically in the parvicellular nuclei (Table 1). (c) The periventricular system (see ref. 47 for references). Along the third ventricle are several rostrocaudally directed fibers. These emerge mainly from the preoptic area and from the hypothalamus, but fibers from other forebrain areas are also included, many of which end in the median eminence (63). It seems likely that some LHRH fibers from the preoptic area (51,52) run in the periventricular system, as do some of the TRH and somatostatin fibers that have their perikarya in the periventricular region. (d) Intra- and extrahypothalamic fibers are conveyed by the medial forebrain bundle to the median eminence. Most of them turn from the lateral hypothalamus to the medial through the lateral retrochiasmatic area, then take a caudal turn and enter the median eminence from the anterior end (11,36,45). Among these fibers are some limbic ones, but presumably numerous preoptic fibers (maybe some of the LHRH-containing axons) and ascending noradrenergic pathways also project by this route to the mediobasal hypothalamus and median eminence (42). (e) There are a number of other neurotransmitter-containing fibers of brainstem origin whose topography is not completely known. Their termination in the median eminence was demonstrated with electron microscopy (Fig. 2) after electrolytic or chemical lesions of various brainstem areas (44).

Efforts to demonstrate synaptic contacts of axons ending in the median eminence have proved to be unsuccessful. There is little doubt that many of the thousands of axons entering the median eminence terminate there since only a small number of axons can be followed to the pituitary stalk. However, nerve terminals in the pericapillary spaces of the median eminence lack the synaptic specialization characteristic of CNS synapses. This is to some extent understandable as release of neurohormones takes place in the median eminence rather than neurotransmission. On the other hand, it would be a gross oversimplification to suppose that neurohormones leak passively from the terminals to the pericapillary space. The high concentrations in the median eminence of several neurotransmitters (see refs. 9,39 for references) are indicative of a regulatory mechanism for the storage and release of neurohormones. This might be realized at the level of the perikarya by stimulating or inhibiting neurohormone synthesis or at the level of the terminals in the median eminence by inducing or blocking the release of neurohormones. However, these two actions cannot be regarded as separate effects. Golgi preparations show that fibers entering the hypothalamus give off several collaterals, forming an abundant network (Fig. 3). This system of collaterals may establish connections not only within a single nucleus but

FIG. 2. Degenerated nerve elements *(arrows)* in the median eminence after electrolytic lesions in various brain areas. **A:** Pontine (locus ceruleus) lesion. **B:** Lesion in the arcuate nucleus. **C:** Surgical transection between the medial and lateral hypothalamus.

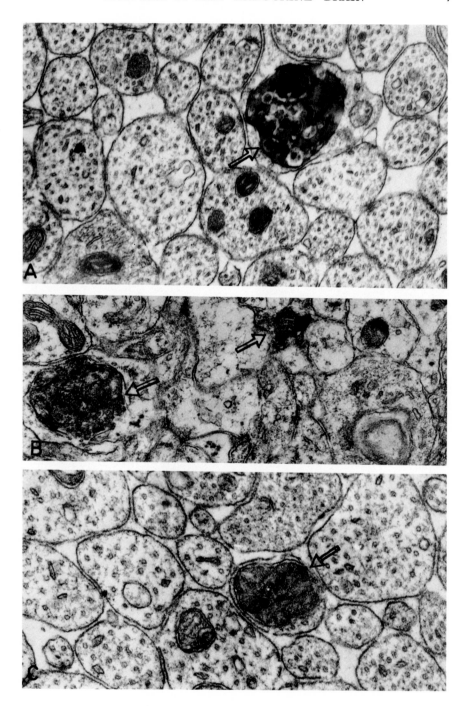

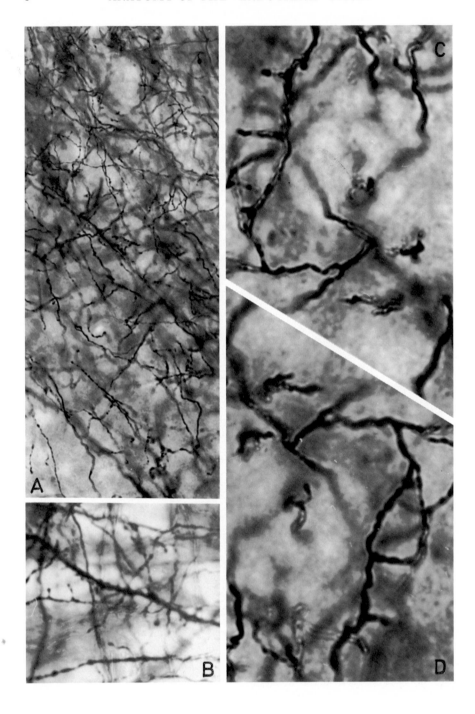

with practically the entire hypothalamus, including the median eminence. Hence neural inputs to the hypothalamus are never confined to individual neurons, or even to a population that produces one type of neurohormone, but affect the production of all hypothalamic neurohormones. As was shown by silver impregnation methods, an axon entering the hypothalamus may terminate in one or more hypothalamic nuclei and may have collaterals ending in the median eminence. This implies that the single neural input may exert perikaryal and terminal effects simultaneously. Thus the production and release of neurohormones is a much more integrated process than was once thought.

Neurohormones and Nerve Terminals in Circumventricular Organs

Although the central site of neuroendocrine regulation is the median eminence, there are some other places in the CNS where neural, vascular, and liquor transport of neurohormones is possible. Among such are the circumventricular organs. In mammals, probably four of these—the organum vasculosum laminae terminalis (OVLT), the subfornical organ (SFO), the subcommissural organ (SCO), and the area postrema—participate in the transport of neurohormones.

Circumventricular organs are characteristically located in prominent sites of the ventricular system, e.g., at transitions between ventricular portions (Fig. 4). Being situated between the external and internal liquor spaces, they have close topographical connections with both. They possess an abundant network of special fenestrated capillaries. No liquor–brain and blood–brain barriers exist within their boundaries. These are the features that enable neurohormones to be transported through the circumventricular organs. Consistent with morphological predisposition, biochemical studies (8,26,41) verified the presence of high concentrations of neurohormones.

With the aid of immunocytochemistry, it was possible to demonstrate that neurohormones present in the circumventricular organs are not produced by local perikarya but are obviously transported from elsewhere as they are confined to nerve terminals (23,48,62). Although the data on the origin of axons terminating in the circumventricular organs are sporadic and those few available concentrate on the OVLT, it is not unrealistic to regard the OVLT, SFO, SCO, and area postrema as "free harbors" for the products of the preoptic area, septal region, epithalamus, and solitary tract nucleus (obex area), respectively. Axons terminating in the above circumventricular organs may discharge their neurohormones either into the external or internal liquor spaces, or into capillaries.

FIG. 3. Neuronal network in the mediobasal hypothalamus of the rat. Golgi impregnation. **A:** Axon and axon collaterals in the arcuate nucleus. Horizontal section. ×16. **B:** Impregnated axons and dendrites in the ventromedial nucleus. ×140. **C** and **D:** Axonal branches with a number of collaterals in the arcuate nucleus. ×900. (Courtesy of Dr. H. V. Cuc, 1st Department of Anatomy, Budapest.)

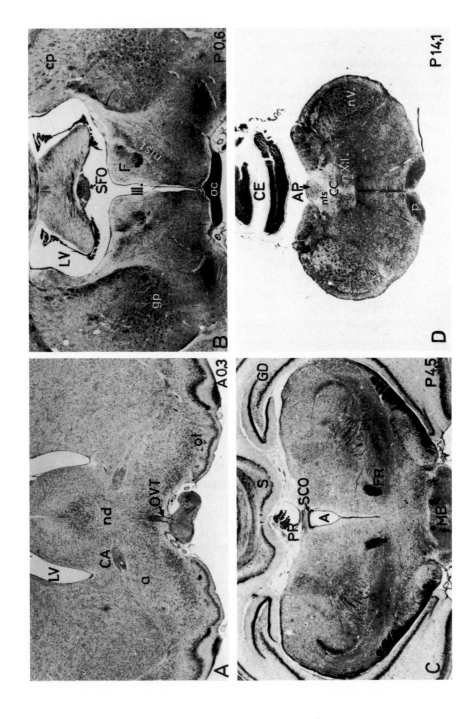

Possible Transport of Neurohormones by CSF

Sophisticated biochemical methods enabled neurohormones to be determined in the CSF (5,25,35,50). Theoretically they may be derived from all axons ending in the ependyma or under the pia mater. Although direct evidence is not available, it seems likely that neurohormones of the external and internal liquor spaces are transported through the circumventricular organs.

Neurohormones may be transported in three directions from the CSF: (a) to another CNS area; (b) to the systemic circulation; or (c) to the pituitary gland through the portal vessels. (For the functional role of the CSF in neuroendocrine integration, see Chapter 10.)

The first two routes are hypothetical at the present state of our knowledge. Therefore, only the third one, for which there is experimental support, is dealt with.

Role of Tanycytes in the Transport of Neurohormones

It has long been supposed that substances from the third ventricle may enter the median eminence. Tanycytes were thought to be instrumental in this process. Tanycytes are modified ependymal cells situated in the lower half of the ventricle, starting from the retrochiasmatic area and extending caudally to the posterior wall of the inframammillary recess. Long processes emerge from their cell bodies, starting at the ventricular wall and traversing the mediobasal hypothalamus with an arciform course (Fig. 5). They may end either on the other surface of the median eminence, in the pericapillary spaces of the median eminence, or on the capillary walls in the mediobasal hypothalamus (arcuate and ventromedial nuclei).

In the first case connection is established between the external and internal liquor spaces. The external liquor space at the base of the hypothalamus is that which communicates mainly rostrally with other external liquor spaces of the cerebral surface (Fig. 5A,B). In the second case, tanycytes are connected with the liquor space surrounding fenestrated capillaries of the median eminence. There are several nerve terminals here. Potentially this seems to be the most obvious way of transport. The significance of the third possible way of transport

---

FIG. 4. Circumventricular organs in the rat brain. Coronal sections at various distances rostral (A) and caudal (P) to the bregma level (in mm). **A:** Organum vasculosum laminae terminalis (OVLT). **B:** Subfornical organ (SFO). **C:** Subcommissural organ (SCO). **D:** Area postrema (AP). (a) accumbens nucleus. (A) cerebral aqueduct. (CA) anterior commissure. (CC) central canal. (CE) cerebellum. (cp) caudatus-putamen. (F) fornix. (FR) fasciculus retroflexus. (GD) dentate gyrus. (gp) globus pallidus. (LV) lateral ventricle. (MB) mammillary body. (nd) nucleus of the diagonal band. (nist) bed nucleus of the stria terminalis. (nts) nucleus tractus solitarii. (nV) nucleus tractus spinalis of the fifth nerve. (nXII) motor nucleus of the hypoglossal nerve. (oc) optic chiasm. (ot) olfactory tubercle. (P) pyramidal tract. (PR) pineal recess. (S) subiculum. (III) third ventricle.

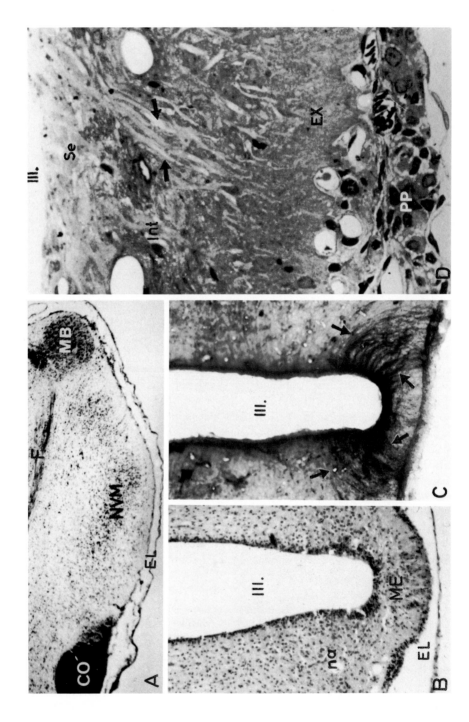

cannot be judged at present owing to insufficient knowledge. At any rate, since capillaries of the arcuate and ventromedial nuclei drain into the basal and not into the portal veins (40), neurohormone transport, if any, must be directed to the systemic circulation.

The topographical situation of tanycytes is, at the moment, no more than an anatomical possibility for neurohormone transport; nor has the direction of the supposed tanycyte transport been unequivocally decided. Generally, substances are thought to be transported from the ventricle to the median eminence. However, it cannot be ruled out that tanycytes are able to take up neurohormones in the median eminence and to transport them into the third ventricle (33).

Vascular Transport of Neurohormones

There is little doubt that the most important route of neurohormonal transport is vascular. This role is dual in the "endocrine" brain: (a) transport of neurohormones; (b) feedback to neurohormone-producing neurons. Since the blood–brain barrier is impermeable to neurohormones, these substances may enter the circulation or may be resorbed from the blood at CNS areas possessing fenestrated capillaries—the median eminence and the circumventricular organs. They are characterized not only by the lack of a blood–brain barrier but also by an abundant vascular network (15) surrounded by a wealth of axons, tanycytes, and other specialized glial structures.

Possibilities of Vascular Transport in the Circumventricular Organs

The vascular link of the organum vasculosum laminae terminalis (OVLT) with the medial preoptic nucleus was recently discovered (2,46). Arterioles supplying this organ form an abundant plexus in the OVLT. Some of them run as slender metarterioles to the medial preoptic nucleus to join its capillary network. From there veins drain either directly to the basal veins or to the venous system of the OVLT. In the OVLT several neuropeptide-containing nerve fibers are in close contact with fenestrated capillaries. Moreover, the preoptic region rich in neuropeptide-synthesizing cells (Table 1) is also connected with this microcirculatory unit (46). This may serve as a morphological basis for a feedback mechanism.

FIG. 5. Hypothalamic external (subarachnoidal) and internal (third ventricle) liquor spaces in the rat. Tanycytes *(arrows)* between the external (EL) and internal (III) liquor spaces. **A:** Parasagittal section (1 mm lateral to the midline) of the hypothalamus with the external liquor space lateral to the median eminence. **B:** Coronal section of the hypothalamus at the rostral level of the median eminence (ME). **C:** Coronal section of the hypothalamus at the same level of **B** with tanycyte processes visualized by nonspecific acetylcholinesterase staining. **D:** Semithin section of the median eminence. Internal (Int) and external (Ex) layers of the median eminence. (se) subependymal layer. (pp) primary plexus. (Courtesy of Dr. L. Záborszky, 1st Department of Anatomy, Budapest.)

The subfornical organ also has a rich vascular plexus. The pericapillary space is directly connected with the liquor lacunae penetrating into the organ. Arteries to the organ are also supplying the neighboring choroid plexuses. The neurohormone content is lower than that of the OVLT (8,21,46).

As compared to other circumventricular organs, the subcommissural organ has a relatively sparse vascular plexus which communicates with the choroid vessels of the habenula, pineal body, and pineal recess. The cells of this organ (transitional forms between tanycytes and ependymal cells) connect the ventricular system (third ventricle and cerebral aqueduct) with the above vessels and the external liquor space.

The area postrema is also abundantly vascularized. Its vessels anastomose with those supplying the choroid plexus of the fourth ventricle. This abundant network of fenestrated vessels has a direct link with the underlying nucleus of the solitary tract that contains several neurotransmitter- and neurohormone-producing neurons (2,4).

Vascular Transport of Neurohormones in the Median Eminence

In the median eminence the most important route of transport is the classical neurohumoral one of Harris (19). At the basal surface of the median eminence–pituitary stalk, hypophysial arteries form a rich vascular network, the "primary plexus." The portal veins originate from here and from the "capillary loops" of deeper layers of the median eminence. Neurohormones are transported via axons or perhaps tanycytes to the pericapillary space of fenestrated capillaries, from where they may enter the portal circulation. The site of neurohumoral transport is mainly the external layer of the median eminence, but "capillary loops" penetrate along the midline high into the internal layer (4,14) up to the subependymal layer of the third ventricle. (For a detailed description of the pituitary portal system see refs. 3,13).

For almost 50 years, since the discovery of the portal circulation, the direction of circulation in the median eminence has been a matter of debate (see ref. 3 for references). Although it is proved that in the median eminence and in the hypophysial stalk the blood flows toward the pituitary gland, this is not the only direction. Data are accumulating that support the existence of significant backflow. The anatomical possibility for this has been demonstrated (4,6,57). In addition to the primary plexus–portal vein system, a subependymal plexus is also present, formed secondarily from the "capillary loops." This is, like the "capillary loops," a metarteriolar plexus (4) communicating at the dorsal surface of the stalk with the branches of the posterior hypophysial artery. These supply the neurohypophysis and the posterior part of the median eminence. A strong plexus is formed in the caudal part of the hypophysial stalk (4,6), enabling the blood to flow in either direction depending on the actual pressure gradients. The experiments of Török (57) provided evidence that this backflow is a reality. From the pituitary gland the blood flows through the median eminence to the hypothalamus. The route for this is the subependymal plexus whose branches terminate in the capillary network of the arcuate nucleus (4). The existence of retrograde transport is supported by the observations that pituitary hormones are present in high concentrations in the blood of the median eminence (34) and that labeled ACTH fragments microinjected into the pituitary appear within minutes in the CNS (32). Backflow from the pituitary gland to the median eminence is certainly vascular. For further transport, three possibilities can be taken into consideration (32): (a) further vascular transport to the hypothalamus; (b) transport to the external and/or internal liquor space(s); (c) axonal transport, suggested by the verified ability of neurons to take up substances from the blood (7).

Newly gained information confirms repeatedly that the median eminence is by far the most important region with regard to neurohormone transport. All potential ways of transport have their anatomical substrates in this area. Hormones, irrespective of their cerebral, hypophysial, or peripheral origin, enter the pericapillary spaces of the median eminence and from here may reach all regions of the CNS and the pituitary gland. Therefore it is not unreasonable to consider the pericapillary spaces of the median eminence to be the key structures in the operation of the "endocrine" brain.

CONCLUDING REMARKS

The "endocrine" brain is a relatively novel term for a recently discovered control system. Its individual constituents have long been known, but their present grouping is the result of a new concept of their function.

Rapid expansion of neuroendocrinological knowledge adds continuously to the understanding of this function. There are about 20 chemically identified substances known to act as neurohormones. Most can be localized and measured quantitatively. Other CNS substances are putative neurohormones by having a bioactivity. However, their chemical identification, a prerequisite for topographic localization, has not yet been successful. Of course, the "endocrine" brain may have additional neurohormones whose functional and chemical properties are still hidden.

The "endocrine" brain is a topographically diffuse system. In the present context, "diffuse" does not mean, as it usually does, the lack of exact knowledge. Owing to the chain of control mechanisms involved and to the high number of interrelationships, it is not surprising that almost all CNS regions participate more or less in the endocrine control system. Although much of the "endocrine" brain is concentrated in the hypothalamus, neurohormone production occurs at other sites as well. Hence the hypothalamo-hypophysial system is by no means equivalent to the "endocrine" brain; it is a part of it.

The topography of the "endocrine" brain cannot be approached by conventional means of descriptive anatomy. The main reason for this is that the distribution of neurohormone-producing cells cannot be defined in terms of CNS nuclei, areas, layers, etc. In addition, it often happens that a topographically circumscribed cell group contains cells synthetising different neurohormones. Thus it would be highly unrealistic to regard an anatomical unit as the center of production of a single type of neurohormone. The same applies to pathways with respect to the transport of a neurohormone.

Introduction of the concept of the "endocrine" brain will certainly modify orthodox neuroanatomical and neuroendocrinological views without devaluating classical findings. These were necessary steps to the development of present ideas about the "endocrine" brain. There seems to be little doubt that further advances from research in this field will add substantially to our knowledge and, at the same time, refine the present interpretation of the "endocrine" brain.

REFERENCES

1. Alpert, L. C., Brawer, J. R., Patel, Y. C., and Reichlin, S. (1976): Somatostatinergic neurons in anterior hypothalamus: Immunohistochemical localization. *Endocrinology,* 98:255–258.
2. Ambach, G., Kivovics, P., and Palkovits, M. (1978): The arterial and venous blood supply of the preoptic region in the rat. *Acta Morphol. Acad. Sci. Hung.,* 26:21–41.
3. Ambach, G., and Palkovits, M. (1979): The blood supply of the hypothalamus in the rat. In: *Handbook of the Hypothalamus,* edited by P. J. Morgane and J. Panksepp. Dekker, New York *(in press).*
4. Ambach, G., Palkovits, M., and Szentágothai, J. (1976): Blood supply of the rat hypothalamus. IV. Retrochiasmatic area, median eminence, arcuate nucleus. *Acta Morphol. Acad. Sci. Hung.,* 24:93–118.
5. Ben-Jonathan, N., Mical, R. S., and Porter, J. C. (1974): Transport of LRF from CSF to hypophysial portal and systemic blood and the release of LH. *Endocrinology,* 95:18–25.
6. Bergland, R. M., and Page, R. B. (1978): Can the pituitary secrete directly to the brain? (Affirmative anatomical evidence.) *Endocrinology,* 102:1325–1338.
7. Broadwell, R. D., and Brightman, M. W. (1976): Entry of peroxidase into neurons of the central and peripheral nervous system from extracerebral and cerebral blood. *J. Comp. Neurol.,* 166:257–283.
8. Brownstein, M., Palkovits, M., and Kizer, J. S. (1975): On the origin of luteinizing hormone-releasing hormone (LH-RH) in the supraoptic crest. *Life Sci.,* 17:679–682.
9. Brownstein, M. J., Palkovits, M., Saavedra, J. M., and Kizer, J. S. (1976): Distribution of hypothalamic hormones and neurotransmitters within the diencephalon. In: *Frontiers in Neuroendocrinology,* Vol. 4, edited by L. Martini and W. F. Ganong, pp. 1–23. Raven Press, New York.
10. Buijs, R. M., Swaab, D. F., Dogterom, J., and van Leeuwen, F. W. (1978): Intra- and extrahypothalamic vasopressin and oxytocin pathways in the rat. *Cell Tissue Res.,* 186:423–433.
11. Cuc, H. van, Léránth, Cs., and Palkovits, M. (1980): Light and electron microscopic studies on the medial forebrain bundle in rat. III. Degenerated nerve elements in the medial hypothalamic nuclei following surgical transections of the medial forebrain bundle. *Brain Res. Bull. (in press).*
12. Dubé, D., and Pelletier, G. (1977): Immunohistochemical localization of alpha-melanocyte stimulating hormone (α-MSH) in the rat brain. In: *Program 59th Meet. Endocrine Soc.,* p. 216.
13. Dubois, M. P., and Kolodziejczyk, E. (1975): Centres hypothalamiques du rat sécrétant la somatostatine: Répartition des péricaryons en 2 systèmes magno et parvocellulaires (étude immunocytologique). *C R Acad. Sci. (Paris),* 281:1737–1740.
14. Duvernoy, H. (1972): The vascular architecture of the median eminence. In: *Brain-Endocrine Interaction. Median Eminence: Structure and Function,* edited by K. M. Knigge, D. E. Scott, and A. Weindl, pp. 79–108. Karger, Basel.
15. Duvernoy, H., and Koritké, J. G. (1964): Contribution à l'étude de l'angioarchitectonie des organes circumventriculaires. *Arch. Biol. (Liege),* 75:693–748.

16. Elde, R. P. (1973): Methods for the localization of vasopressin-containing neurons in the hypothalamus and pars nervosa by immunoenzyme histochemistry. *Anat. Rec.,* 175:255–258.

17. Elde, R., and Hökfelt, T. (1978): Distribution of hypothalamic hormones and other peptides in the brain. In: *Frontiers in Neuroendocrinology,* Vol. 5, edited by W. F. Ganong and L. Martini, pp. 1–33. Raven Press, New York.

18. Elde, R. P., and Parsons, J. A. (1975): Immunocytochemical localization of somatostatin in cell bodies of the rat hypothalamus. *Am. J. Anat.,* 144:541–548.

19. Harris, G. H. (1955): *Neural Control of the Pituitary Gland.* Edward Arnold, London.

20. Hoffman, G. E., Joseph, S. A., and Knigge, K. M. (1977): Evidence for two different fields of gonadotropin releasing factor (GnRF) neurons in mouse and rat brain. In: *Program 59th Meet. Endocrine Soc.,* p. 65.

21. Hökfelt, T., Efendić, S., Hellerström, C., Johansson, O., Luft, R., and Arimura, A. (1976): Cellular localization of somatostatin in endocrine-like cells and neurons of the rat with special references to the A1 cells of the pancreatic islets and to the hypothalamus. *Acta Endocrinol. [Suppl] (Kbh),* 200:1–41.

22. Hökfelt, T., Elde, R., Fuxe, K., Johansson, O., Ljungdahl, Å., Goldstein, M., Luft, R., Efendić, S., Nilsson, G., Terenius, L., Ganten, D., Jeffcoate, S. L., Rehfeld, J., Said, S., Perez de la Mora, M., Possani, L., Tapia, R., Teran, L., and Palacios, R. (1978): Aminergic and peptidergic pathways in the nervous system with special reference to the hypothalamus. In: *The Hypothalamus,* edited by S. Reichlin, R. J. Baldessarini, and J. B. Martin, pp. 69–135. Raven Press, New York.

23. Hökfelt, T., Elde, R., Johansson, O., Ljungdahl, Å., Schultzberg, M., Fuxe, K., Goldstein, M., Nilsson, G., Pernow, B., Terenius, L., Ganten, D., Jeffcoate, S. L., Rehfeld, J., and Said, S. (1978): Distribution of peptide-containing neurons. In: *Psychopharmacology: A Generation of Progress,* edited by M. A. Lipton, A. DiMascio, and K. F. Killam, pp. 39–66. Raven Press, New York.

24. Hökfelt, T., Fuxe, K., Johansson, O., Jeffcoate, S., and White, N. (1975): Distribution of thyrotropin-releasing hormone (TRH) in the central nervous system as revealed with immunocytochemistry. *Eur. J. Pharmacol.,* 34:389–392.

25. Joseph, S. A., Sorrentino, S., and Sundberg, D. K. (1975): Releasing hormones: LRF and TRF in the cerebrospinal fluid of the third ventricle. In: *Brain-Endocrine Interaction. II. The Ventricular System in Neuroendocrine Mechanisms,* edited by K. M. Knigge and D. E. Scott, pp. 306–312. Karger, Basel.

26. Kizer, J. S., Palkovits, M., and Brownstein, M. J. (1976): Releasing factors in the circumventricular organs of the rat brain. *Endocrinology,* 98:311–317.

27. Kobayashi, R. M., Brown, M., and Vale, W. (1977): Regional distribution of neurotensin and somatostatin in rat brain. *Brain Res.,* 126:584–588.

28. Krieger, D. T., Liotta, A., and Brownstein, M. J. (1977): Presence of corticotropin in limbic system of normal and hypophysectomized rats. *Brain Res.,* 128:575–579.

29. Krieger, D. T., Liotta, A., and Brownstein, M. J. (1977): Presence of corticotropin in brain of normal and hypophysectomized rats. *Proc. Natl. Acad. Sci. USA,* 74:648–652.

30. Krieger, D. T., Liotta, A., Suda, T., Palkovits, M., and Brownstein, M. J. (1977): Presence of immunoassayable β-lipotropin in bovine brain and spinal cord: Lack of concordance with ACTH concentrations. *Biochem. Biophys. Res. Commun.,* 16:930–936.

31. Krisch, B. (1978): Light- and electron microscopic localization of vasopressin or a vasopressin-like substance in the neurons of the rat suprachiasmatic nucleus. *Cell Tissue Res.,* 194:361–365.

32. Mezey, E., Palkovits, M., De Kloet, E. R., Verhoef, J., and De Wied, D. (1978): Evidence for pituitary-brain transport of a behaviorally potent ACTH analog. *Life Sci.,* 22:831–838.

33. Nakai, Y., and Naito, N. (1975): Uptake and bidirectional transport of peroxidase injected into the blood and cerebrospinal fluid by ependymal cells of the median eminence. In: *Brain-Endocrine Interaction. II. The Ventricular System,* edited by K. M. Knigge, D. E. Scott, H. Kobayashi, and S. Ishii, pp. 94–108. Karger, Basel.

34. Oliver, D., Mical, R. S., and Porter, J. C. (1977): Hypothalamic-pituitary vasculature: Evidence of retrograde blood flow in the pituitary stalk. *Endocrinology,* 101:598–604.

35. Ondo, J. G., Eskay, R. L., Mical, R. S., and Porter, J. C. (1973): Release of LH by LRF into the CSF: A transport role for the median eminence. *Endocrinology,* 93:231–237.

36. Palkovits, M. (1977): Neural pathways involved in ACTH regulation. *Ann. NY Acad. Sci.,* 297:455–476.
37. Palkovits, M. (1978): Neurochemical anatomy of the neuroendocrine hypothalamus. *Bull. Schweiz. Akad. Med. Wiss.,* 34:113–130.
38. Palkovits, M. (1978): Topography of chemically identified neurons in the central nervous system: A review. *Acta Morphol. Acad. Sci. Hung.,* 26:211–290.
39. Palkovits, M. (1979): Microchemistry of the microdissected hypothalamic nuclear areas. *Int. Rev. Cytol.,* 56:315–339.
40. Palkovits, M. (1979): Regional distribution of neurohormones in the central nervous system. In: *Cell Biology of Hypothalamic Neurosecretion,* edited by J. D. Vincent and C. Kordon, pp. 339–356. CNRS, Paris.
41. Palkovits, M., Brownstein, M., Arimura, A., Sato, H., Schally, A. V., and Kizer, J. S. (1976): Somatostatin content of the hypothalamic ventromedial and arcuate nuclei in the circumventricular organs in the rat. *Brain Res.,* 10:430–434.
42. Palkovits, M., Fekete, M., Makara, G. B., and Herman, J. P. (1977): Total and partial hypothalamic deafferentation for topographical identification of catecholaminergic innervations of certain preoptic and hypothalamic nuclei. *Brain Res.,* 127:127–136.
43. Palkovits, M., Gráf, L., Hermann, I., Borvendég, J., and Láng, T. (1978): Regional distribution of enkephalins, endorphins and ACTH in the central nervous system of rats determined by radioimmunoassay. In: *Endorphins '78,* edited by L. Gráf, M. Palkovits, and A. Z. Rónai, pp. 187–195. Akadémiai Kiadó, Budapest.
44. Palkovits, M., Léránth, Cs., Záborszky, L., and Brownstein, M. J. (1977): Electron microscopic evidence of direct neuronal connections from the lower brain stem to the median eminence. *Brain Res.,* 136:339–344.
45. Palkovits, M., Makara, G. B., and Stark, E. (1976): Hypothalamic region and pathways responsible for adrenocortical response to surgical stress in rats. *Neuroendocrinology,* 21:280–288.
46. Palkovits, M., Mezey, É., Ambach, G., and Kivovics, P. (1978): Neural and vascular connections between the organum vasculosum laminae terminalis and preoptic nuclei. In: *Brain-Endocrine Interaction. III. Neural Hormones and Reproduction,* edited by D. E. Scott, G. P. Kozlowski, and A. Weindl, pp. 302–313. Karger, Basel.
47. Palkovits, M., and Záborszky, L. (1979): Neural connections of the hypothalamus. In: *Handbook of the Hypothalamus,* edited by P. J. Morgane and J. Panksepp. Dekker, New York *(in press).*
48. Pelletier, G., Leclerc, R., and Dubé, D. (1976): Immunohistochemical localization of hypothalamic hormones. *J. Histochem. Cytochem.,* 24:864–871.
49. Pittman, Q. J., Blume, H. W., and Renaud, L. P. (1978): Electrophysiological indications that individual hypothalamic neurons innervate both median eminence and neurohypophysis. *Brain Res.,* 157:364–368.
50. Schaub, C., Bluet-Pajot, M. T., Szikea, G., Lornet, C., and Talairach, J. (1977): Distribution of growth hormone and thyroid-stimulating hormone in cerebrospinal fluid and pathologic compartments of the central nervous system. *J. Neurol. Sci.,* 31:123–131.
51. Sétáló, G., Vigh, S., Schally, A. V., Arimura, A., and Flerkó, B. (1975): Immunohistological investigations on the LH-RH-synthesizing neuron system of the rat. In: *Cellular and Molecular Bases of Neuroendocrine Processes,* edited by E. Endrőczy, pp. 77–88. Akadémiai Kiadó, Budapest.
52. Sétáló, G., Vigh, S., Schally, A. V., Arimura, A., and Flerkó, B. (1976): Immunohistological study of the origin of LH-RH containing nerve fibres of the rat hypothalamus. *Brain Res.,* 103:597–602.
53. Silverman, A. J. (1976): Ultrastructural studies on the localization of neurohypophysial hormones and their carrier proteins. *J. Histochem. Cytochem.,* 24:816–827.
54. Swaab, D. F., Pool, C. W., and Nijveldt, F. (1975): Immunofluorescence of vasopressin and oxytocin in the rat hypothalamo-neurohypophyseal system. *J. Neural. Transm.,* 36:195–215.
55. Szentágothai, J. (1964): The parvicellular neurosecretory system. *Prog. Brain Res.,* 5:135–146.
56. Tan Pacold, S., Hojuat, S., Kirsteins, L., Yarragary, L., Kisla, J., and Lawrence, A. M. (1977): Brain growth hormone: Evidence for the presence and production of biologically active GH-like immunoreactivity from the amygdaloid nucleus. *Clin. Res.,* 25:299A.
57. Török, B. (1964): Structure of the vascular connections of the hypothalamo-hypophysial region. *Acta Anat. (Basel),* 59:84–99.

58. Uhl, G. R., and Snyder, S. H. (1976): Regional and subcellular distributions of brain neurotensin. *Life Sci.*, 19:1827–1832.

59. Vandesande, F., and Diericky, K. (1975): Identification of the vasopressin producing and of the oxytocin producing neurons in the hypothalamic magnocellular neurosecretory system of the rat. *Cell Tissue Res.*, 164:153–162.

60. Vandesande, F., Dierickx, K., and DeMey, J. (1975): Identification of vasopressin-neurophysin neurons of the rat suprachiasmatic nuclei. *Cell Tissue Res.*, 156:377–380.

61. Watson, S. J., Barchas, J. D., and Li, C. H. (1977): β-Lipotropin: Localization of cells and axons in rat brain by immunocytochemistry. *Proc. Natl. Acad. Sci. USA*, 74:5155–5158.

62. Weindl, A., and Sofroniew, M. W. (1978): Neurohormones and circumventricular organs: an immunohistochemical investigation. In: *Brain-Endocrine Interaction. III. Neural Hormones and Reproduction*, edited by D. E. Scott, G. P. Kozlowski, and A. Weindl, pp. 117–137. Karger, Basel.

63. Záborszky, L., and Makara, G. B. (1979): Intrahypothalamic connections: An electron microscopic study in the rat. *Exp. Brain Res.*, 34:201–215.

64. Zimmerman, E. A. (1976): Localization of hypothalamic hormones by immunocytochemical techniques. In: *Frontiers in Neuroendocrinology*, Vol. 4, edited by L. Martini and W. F. Ganong, pp. 25–62. Raven Press, New York.

65. Zimmerman, E. A., Carmel, P., and Husain, M. K. (1973): Vasopressin and neurophysin: High concentrations in monkey hypophyseal portal blood. *Science*, 182:925–927.

66. Zimmerman, E. A., Liotta, A., and Krieger, D. T. (1978): β-Lipotropin in brain: Localization in hypothalamic neurons by immunoperoxidase technique. *Cell Tissue Res.*, 186:393–398.

67. Zimmerman, E. A., Stillman, M. A., Recht, L. D., Antunes, J. L., and Carmel, P. W. (1977): Vasopressin and corticotropin-releasing factor: An axonal pathway to portal capillaries in the zona extrema of the median eminence containing vasopressin and its interaction with adrenal corticoids. *Ann. NY Acad. Sci.*, 297:405–419.

The Endocrine Functions of the Brain,
edited by Marcella Motta.
Raven Press, New York © 1980

2

The "Endocrine" Brain: Electrophysiological Aspects

James N. Hayward and Troy A. Reaves Jr.

Departments of Neurology and Medicine, Neurobiology Program, University of North Carolina, Chapel Hill, North Carolina 27514

The "endocrine" brain contains two major classes of neurosecretory "endocrine" hypothalamic neurons, the magnocellular neuroendocrine cell and the parvocellular neuroendocrine cell. We define vertebrate magnocellular neuroendocrine cells (MgC) physiologically as those neurosecretory hypothalamic neurons which are antidromically identified by reason of pituitary stimulation. This class of MgC have large, peptide-positive somata lying in the preoptic nucleus, pars magnocellularis, of fishes and amphibia and in the supraoptic, paraventricular, and accessory nuclei (49) of reptiles, birds, and mammals. Their axons end at the neurohemal junction in the pituitary gland for control of the neurohypophysis. Some of these MgC send fibers to the median eminence, septum, amygdala, brainstem, and spinal cord (26,37; see also Chapter 7). The inclusive term "magnocellular neuroendocrine cell" not only specifies one kind of neurosecretory hypothalamic endocrine neuron, it also allows for analysis of data across species and across hypothalamic anatomical boundaries (24,25,37,56,70).

The other class of neurosecretory endocrine hypothalamic neuron, the parvocellular neuroendocrine cell (PvC), we define physiologically as the neurosecretory neuron which is antidromically identified by reason of median eminence stimulation. The small, peptide-positive somata of these PvC lie scattered in the mediobasal and periventricular hypothalamus of mammals. These peptidergic neurons synthesize and release hypophysiotropic peptide hormones into the primary portal plexus of the median eminence and control adenohypophysial secretion (25,26,56,72).

For two decades an established method for determining how the single hypothalamic endocrine neuron responds to discrete physical, chemical, or behavioral stimuli has been electrophysiological mapping of the input–output connections and the neurophysiological response patterns of neuronal populations (25). Since Cross and Green's (11) initial study, subsequent workers expanded hypothalamic single-cell recording methods to include current techniques of antidromic identification, microiontophoresis, intracellular recording, and dye-marking (25). Experimental models for electrophysiology range from the awake–behaving mammal to the isolated brain slice and hypothalamic cells cultured *in vitro* (25). Despite these refinements, investigators have labored long to produce incomplete results, lacking as they do the ability to identify hypothalamic endocrine cells chemically and to study the same chemical cell type from one animal to another. Today, however, sophisticated progress in peptide biochemistry and immunocytochemistry enables researchers to visualize and analyze a complex network of peptidergic cells, fibers, and terminals in the hypothalamus (26). This well developed technology is most amenable to the electrophysiology of chemically identified MgC.

This review comments briefly on those electrophysiological studies of hypothalamic endocrine neurons published since our last major review of this subject (25) and describes the authors' initial experiments on chemically defined MgC (50,52).

MAGNOCELLULAR NEUROENDOCRINE CELLS

In 1975 the immunohistochemists Vandesande and Dierickx (65) discovered a mixture of vasopressin (VP) and oxytocin (OT) neurons in the supraoptic (NSO) and paraventricular (NPV) nuclei in the mammalian hypothalamus. In 1979 Reaves and Hayward (49) found VP and OT neurons mixed in the accessory nuclei (NAC) of mammals. In 1977 Goossens et al. (19) found a mixture of vasotocin and isotocin neurons in the preoptic nucleus of teleost fish. The recent discovery of a third peptidergic cell type, the enkephalinergic (ENK), in MgC of mammals (26,57) and the preoptic nuclei (NPO) of fish (51) and the possible presence of at least four other peptidergic MgC cell types—β-endorphin, somatostatin, gastrin-cholecystokinin, angiotensin (20,26,62; see also Chapters 7 and 9) further complicate the problem of MgC electrophysiological identification.

Under the influence of osmometric, volumetric, and neural regulation, MgC synthesize the mammalian neurohypophysial hormones vasopressin and oxytocin. Enclosed in membrane-bound vesicles, these peptides flow axoplasmically to the neural lobe, where under the influence of the action potential they are released by exocytosis for the regulation of water balance and milk ejection (see Chapters 9 and 17). The older bioassay data, suggestive of selective release of VP and OT from the neurohypophysis, have been proved incorrect by the newer radioimmunoassay data, which indicate VP and OT release simultaneously to osmotic, volumetric, and neural stimuli (12,68). The MgC roles of ENK in mammals, as well as ENK, vasotocin, and isotocin in fishes, and their patterns of secretion remain to be determined (26,51,57,62).

Electrophysiological Strategies

When Cross and Green (11) recorded single neurons electrophysiologically from the nonidentified NSO and NPV of urethane-anesthetized rabbits, they interpreted their data according to the "nuclear" hypothesis of the day. They assumed that VP neurons lay in the NSO and OT neurons lay in the NPV (see ref. 25 for references). Subsequently, Kandel (28) in the goldfish and Yagi et al. (69) in the rat stimulated the pituitary gland in order to drive antidromic potentials in the hypothalamus, thus identifying MgC physiologically. However, not until the publication of Vandesande and Dierickx's 1975 data (65) did researchers realize that VP and OT neurons were mixed throughout NSO and NPV. They could no longer rely on antidromic identification alone, and on assumed nuclear location for the study of VP and OT neurons (see ref. 25 for references). The work of Dyball and co-workers (5,6,25,47,67), using the lactating, suckling, milk-ejecting rat preparation to identify VP and OT neurons physiologically, has been superseded by the finding of three to seven peptidergic cell types in MgC (20,25,26,57,62; see also Chapter 7) and by the simultaneous release of VP and OT to physiological stimuli (12,68).

The techniques of intracellular recording with measurement of the resting membrane, postsynaptic, and axosomatic spike potentials were first applied to the hypothalamus of the goldfish by Kandel (28), with antidromic identification of MgC in the NPO. Other workers subsequently applied these techniques of intracellular recording of MgC to the mammalian hypothalamus (34) and *in vitro* MgC (1,18,25). Hayward (24), extending this approach, stained goldfish MgC intracellularly with procion yellow, a fluorescent dye, identifying three morphological cell types. More recently Reaves and Hayward (50,52), in their search for an electrophysiological approach to the study of single, chemically identified peptidergic MgC, found that intracellularly dye-marked goldfish preoptic neurons could be immunocytochemically stained for isotocin, vasotocin, or enkephalin. This promises to be another major step for the study of single, antidromically identified, physiologically characterized peptidergic neurons of a specific chemical type in vertebrate and invertebrate species (50,52).

Spontaneous Activity

The majority of studies performed on antidromically identified NSO and NPV neurons, whether in the acutely prepared, anesthetized mammal (5,6,13, 25,47,67) or in the chronically prepared, unanesthetized mammal (25,27), revealed three types of spontaneous firing patterns: silent (3 to 10%), continuously active (65 to 77%), and phasic or burster (20 to 25%).

The burster, a discharge pattern unique to the MgC, may represent an intrinsic pacemaker (13) such as that found in invertebrates (25). Alternatively, the burster may be the end result of local or distant facilitatory or inhibitory influences (25). In organ cultures of the newborn rat's rostral–basal hypothalamus (NSO region), Gahwiler et al. (18) found that unidentified neurons containing neurosecretory granules showed spontaneous phasic firing (42% of cells) and synchronous activity between cells in 59% of neurons. Intracellular recording demonstrated action potentials and postsynaptic potentials. Electrical field stimulation in the cultures resulted in a short-latency excitation followed by inhibition. In acutely prepared 200 to 400 μm coronal slices of the rat hypothalamus, Haller et al. (22) and Hatton et al. (23) found the extracellularly recorded, unidentified MgC in NSO silent. Hatton et al. (23) found spontaneous phasic firing of NPV and NAC. Haller et al. (22) found phasic firing of 33% NSO following exposure to high concentrations (5.0 mM) of the excitatory putative neurotransmitter L-glutamic acid. Bioulac et al. (1) found that a clone of mouse hypothalamic VP producing MgC (HT9-C7) was silent electrically. All of these data suggest that the pacemaker neuron for burster (phasic) activity is either exogenous but near MgC nuclei or is endogenous in MgC.

Whether spontaneous burster (phasic) MgC represent VP neurons and milk-ejection bursters represent OT cells (5,6,13,25,47,67) awaits the chemical identification of these peptidergic cells by the intracellular dye-marking, immunocyto-chemical method of Reaves and Hayward (50,52). In our quantitative field analysis of peptidergic neurons in goldfish NPO, we found ENK neurons to be dominant (50,52). These ENK MgC were larger than isotocin and vasotocin (31 μm versus 25 μm) and outnumbered vasotocin and isotocin together by 2:1. Micro field mapping indicated that these ENK neurons were involved in most (78%) of the somasomatic membrane contacts between peptidergic cells (50,52). We suggest that ENK neurons may engage isotocin and vasotocin neurons in field synchrony by synaptic and ephaptic communication (50,52). Perhaps these burster (phasic) spontaneous firing patterns occur in ENK or other peptidergic MgC cell types involved in neurohypophysial activity (20,25,26,51,57,62).

Osmotic Input

Verney's osmometric hypothesis states that the "osmoreceptors," neural elements in the hypothalamus, detect the osmotic pressure of carotid arterial blood and initiate release of vasopressin from the neurohypophysis during hyperosmolal states (25,66; see also Chapter 17). The majority of the antidromically identified NSO and NPV cells, whether in the acutely prepared anesthetized mammal (5,6,13,25,47,67) or the chronically prepared, unanesthetized mammal (25,27), responded to elevation of plasma osmolality with acceleration of cell firing. As in the "chronic" monkey (25), infusion of hypertonic sodium chloride in the "chronic" sheep resulted in accelerated firing patterns of all types (silent, continuously active, burster), with a shift from silent to continuously active, continuously active to burster, burster to hyperburster during hyperosmolal states (27). Whether the burster (phasic) response patterns to osmotic stimulus in the anesthetized, lactating rat preparation indicates putative VP neurons, as claimed by some workers (5,6,13,25,47,67), awaits definitive chemical identification (50,52). What role ENK and other peptidergic neurons play in osmotic response of VP and OT MgC remains to be determined (26,57).

One peptidergic cell type, angiotensin II (AII), known to lie among MgC (26,62), may be involved in osmoreceptor activation of MgC (61). In the rat's organ-cultured hypothalamo-neurohypophysial system, Sladek and Joynt (61) found that saralasin, an AII antagonist, blocks the VP release to AII and osmotic stimulation. These data indicate that AII modulates osmotic control of VP release. The maneuver of adding hexamethonium but not adding atropine blocks VP release in response to acetylcholine (ACh) and osmotic stimulation. Thus a nicotinic cholinergic synapse appears to mediate osmotic stimulation of VP release (61). Hexamethonium was an ineffective blocker of VP release by AII, whereas saralasin was an ineffective inhibitor of VP release by either ACh or nicotine. These data suggest that independent AII and cholinergic mechanisms control VP release (61). The effectiveness of saralasin and hexamethonium, however, in blocking an osmotically stimulated VP release indicates some interaction between these VP regulators. The two hypothetical models of the osmoreceptor suggested by these data are: (a) *Cell 1* is a cholinergic osmoreceptor neuron which impinges on *cell 2*, which is an angiotensin II neuron that impinges on *cell 3*, a VP or OT MgC neuron which also receives other synaptic input. (b) *Cell 1* is a cholinergic osmoreceptor neuron which also receives AII axosomatic and axoaxonal synaptic input and impinges on *cell 2*, a VP or OT MgC neuron that receives other synaptic input as well (61). These recent ideas of the osmoreceptor as a separate neural element confirm the earlier studies of several workers (see ref. 25 for references). The conclusive description of the osmoreceptor of Verney (66) awaits definitive chemical identification (50,52).

Volumetric Input

Hemorrhage and blood volume depletion are recognized as stimuli for the release of VP from the neurohypophysis by means of the baroreceptor action of the 9th and 10th cranial nerves (25,37,66; see also Chapter 17). Recent data indicate, however, that hemorrhage in conscious dogs releases VP and OT (68), thereby complicating the interpretation of single-unit responses in the MgC nuclei during hypovolemic states (25).

In the acutely prepared, anesthetized animal (25,47), acute hemorrhage produces a gradual acceleration without phasic firing of putative OT neurons and a rapid acceleration with phasic firing of putative VP neurons (47). In an analysis of the type of baroreceptor input to NSO, experiments with carotid occlusion (25,29,35,73) caused antidromically identified NSO single units to accelerate. On further analysis of these data, Yamashita (73) concluded that the carotid sinus nerve carried inhibitory input from carotid baroreceptors. When researchers removed such inhibitory input during the carotid occlusion or hemorrhage, "endogenous" acceleration of NSO resulted (73). In addition, when the carotid sinus nerve carried excitatory input from carotid chemoreceptors, which are in turn excited by local hypoxia, acceleration of NSO single units resulted (73). Koizumi and Yamashita (35) found that vagal-mediated left atrial stretch receptors exerted a moderate inhibitory influence on antidromically identified NSO and NPV single units in dogs (98% of cells) and cats (70% of cells). This inhibitory left atrial stretch effect was too weak to inhibit acceleration of NSO and NPV by carotid occlusion or chemoreceptor activity (35). In further studies in the "acute" cat, Menninger (36) found that whereas balloon stretch of the left atrium caused a change in firing of 15% of antidromically identified NSO single cells, 60% of these accelerated, perhaps responding to the associated drop in arterial blood pressure (36). When associated hemodynamic changes were avoided by direct stretch of the left atrium with an atrial suture, he found 72% of the NSO cells responsive, and all were inhibited (36). All neurons inhibited by atrial stretch were excited by hypertonic saline (36). These data are consistent with the high concentration of VP neurons in the NSO of the cat (49). In similar studies in the anesthetized rat, Kannan and Yagi (29) found three types of antidromically identified NSO cells: (a) MgC with input from osmoreceptors alone; (b) MgC with input from carotid baroreceptors alone; and (c) MgC with inputs from osmoreceptors and carotid baroreceptors. The inhibition of NSO unit acceleration to intracarotid osmotic stimulation by simultaneous pressure stimulation of the carotid sinus was of particular interest (29). Further exploration of the interaction of volumetric and osmometric input to MgC awaits cell chemical identification studies (50,52).

Reproductive Activity

Behavioral states related to reproduction and the milk-ejection reflex release oxytocin and perhaps vasopressin (12,68) from the magnocellular neuroendocrine neurons (4,25). As discussed under *Electrophysiological Strategies* (above), the use of the lactating, suckling, milk-ejecting rat preparation to identify OT and VP neurons physiologically is based on the assumption that the burst discharge which occurs prior to suckling-induced milk ejection represents activity of OT neurons (5,6,13,25,47,67). Whether this assumption is valid awaits studies of OT and VP with radioimmunoassay and chemical identification of these MgC (50,52).

In an attempt to study the various cell types in the paraventricular nucleus, Freund-Mercier and Richard (17) recognized three categories: type I cells, antidromically driven; type II cells, orthodromically driven; and type III cells, unresponsive to pituitary stimulation. Only the type I neurosecretory cells showed changes in spontaneous firing rates related to the endocrine state: The fastest rates (3.6 spikes/sec) were during lactation and the lowest rates (1.2 spikes/sec) during metestrus; the highest incidence of phasic units was during proestrus (17). Although a small percentage of the type I cells were activated by vaginal distention, this activity was not influenced by the state of estrous cycle or lactation (17). Only the evoked activity (vaginal distention) of type III cells was affected by the endocrine state: 52% responsive (32% excited, 20% inhibited) during estrus, in contrast to 12% responsive (4% excited, 8% inhibited) during proestrus (17).

In a study of antidromically identified paraventricular units recorded during labor and the estrous cycle in the rat, Boer and Nolten (4) found the highest firing rates (3.2 spikes/sec) during labor before expulsion and the lowest firing rates (1.6 spikes/sec) during metestrus–diestrus. The increased firing during labor resulted from: (a) a marked reduction (>25%) in the percentage of totally silent cells; and (b) an increase in the magnitude of the mean firing rate of the phasically firing units (1.6 to 3.4 spikes/sec) (4). These workers found no bursts of activity during labor as have been described to precede suckling-induced milk ejections (5,6,13,25,47,67). On the basis of these data obtained during labor in the rat, Boer and Nolten (4) raise some serious questions about the ability of researchers to establish the chemical cell type based solely on electrophysiological criteria. Definitive chemical identification of MgC during reproductive activity awaits more precise methods (50,52).

Synaptic Input and Putative Chemical Neurotransmitters

Chemical identification of MgC (50,52) during microiontophoresis of putative neurotransmitters on the membranes of VP and OT neurons would improve the confusing literature in this field (25,56,70). In studies in the anesthetized rat, Bioulac et al. (2) divided antidromically identified NSO units into putative OT cells ("continuously active") and putative VP units ("phasic"). "OT" cells were inhibited by iontophoretic application of acetylcholine (ACh) and γ-amino-butyric acid (GABA) and accelerated by glutamate (GLU). The "phasic" "VP" cells were excited by ACh and GLU and inhibited by GABA. Some variable effects depended on the phase of the periodic discharge cycle. That microionto-phoresis of several putative neurotransmitters on three to seven potentially different peptidergic MgC neurons in the hypothalamus (25,26,62) would yield inconclusive results is no surprise (25). Chemical identification of MgC and appropriate neurotransmitter application is the apparent next step (50,52).

Summary

To effect the regulation of water balance, blood volume, labor, and milk ejection, the MgC in the NSO, NPV, and NAC synthesize, transport, and release the neurohypophysial hormones VP and OT. The rate of neurohypophysial hormone release depends on the intensity of action-potential firing in the MgC. At least three MgC of the neuronal types VP, OT, and ENK coexist in the NSO, NPV, and NAC, having been characterized as silent, continuously active, and burster by their spontaneous activity patterns. Whether these functional states of activity relate to the chemical cell type is unclear. The cell membrane of the MgC has excitatory receptors for nicotinic cholinergic and angiotensin II putative transmitters. Driven by osmotic, volumetric, and neural stimuli, MgC provide important support for self-preservation of the organism and for propagation of the species.

PARVOCELLULAR NEUROENDOCRINE CELLS

Three hypophysiotropic (releasing and inhibiting) peptidergic hormones have been chemically identified, synthesized, and localized in the parvocellular neuroendocrine cells in the hypothalamus: thyrotropin releasing hormone (TRH), luteinizing hormone releasing hormone (LHRH), and somatostatin (20,26). Synthesized in 1969, the simple cyclic tripeptide TRH induces the release of adenohypophysial thyroid stimulating hormone (TSH). TRH is localized immunohistochemically in the dorsomedial nucleus and perifornical area PvC, in fibers in the median eminence, and elsewhere in the brain (20,26; see also Chapter 7). Synthesized in 1972, the simple linear decapeptide LHRH induces the release of adenohypophysial follicle stimulating hormone (FSH) and luteinizing hormone (LH). LHRH is localized immunohistochemically in the periventricular–basal hypothalamic and preoptic area PvC and in fibers in the median eminence and elsewhere in the brain (20,26; see also Chapter 7). Synthesized in 1973, the simple cyclic tetradecapeptide somatostatin inhibits the release of basal and stimulated adenohypophysial growth hormone (GH) and inhibits the secretion of TRH-induced TSH as well as insulin and glucagon by pancreatic islet cells. Somatostatin is localized immunohistochemically in the periventricular hypothalamus PvC and in fibers in the median eminence and elsewhere in the brain (20,26; see also Chapter 7). Other recently discovered hypothalamic peptidergic neurons which may project to the median eminence neurohemal junction onto the primary portal plexus for action on adenohypophysis include vasopressin (VP), oxytocin (OT), lipotropin-endorphin-ACTH, substance P, enkephalin (ENK), angiotensin II (AII), vasoactive intestinal peptide (VIP), gastrin-(G17)-cholecystokinin, and neurotensin (20,26,62; see also Chapters 7 and 9). Most of these putative hypophysiotropic release-inhibiting factors are also candidates for possible peptide neurotransmitter–neuromodulators at synaptic junctions in hypothalamus and extrahypothalamic areas (20,26,62; see also Chapter 1).

Under the influence of releasing peptides and pituitary hormones and adrenal and gonadal steroids, physical influences such as temperature, blood gases, light, chemicals (e.g., glucose, free fatty acids, and amino acids), and neurobehavioral effects, PvC synthesize the mammalian hypophysiotropic hormones. While enclosed in membrane-bound vesicles, the hormones TRH, LHRH, somatostatin, and others flow axoplasmically down the unmyelinated axons to the external zone of the median eminence (see also Chapter 9). There, under the influence of the action potentials, they are released by exocytosis into the primary plexus of the portal vessels for action on adenohypophysial glandular cells. These cells release TSH, FSH, and LH, and inhibit the release of GH and TSH (see also Chapter 11). The roles of these other peptides in the hypothalamus and on the adenohypophysis remain to be determined (20,26,62).

Electrophysiological Strategies

Workers studying PvC face considerable technical problems because of the wide dispersion of small cells in the hypothalamus (20,26; see also Chapters 1 and 7) and the lack of a discrete, isolated tract available for electrical stimulation and antidromic identification such as the MgC have (25). In spite of these difficulties, however, several experimental designs have developed (25,56,72). The most desired approach for single-cell recording is electrical stimulation of the median eminence, which attempts to effect antidromic identification of PvC with terminals at the portal vessel–neurohemal junction in the median eminence (25,56,72). The major problem here is the inability to insulate stimulating electrodes from current spread to adjacent hypothalamic cells and fibers. A second difficulty is the uncertainty of the peptidergic cell type being stimulated and its adenohypophysial-target gland system (25).

Other experimental designs for studying hypothalamic unit activity (e.g., multiunit recording) present greater technical problems (10,25). The use of microwires of various sizes, the filtering of the signal, the presence of muscle contraction artifact, and the indeterminate nature of the biological signal which may be cell somata, axons, muscle activity, or cable-amplifier noise further complicate data interpretation (10,25). For example, if a microwire is placed into the supraoptic or paraventricular magnocellular nuclei, there may be three to seven peptidergic neurons intermixed there (20,26,57,62). It is unlikely that summated electrical activity from these adjacent, closely packed, dissimilar peptidergic neurons would be significant electrophysiologically (25). Intracellular dye-marking and immunocytochemical identification together may be the only way to elucidate meaningful data from such heterogeneous peptidergic neuronal fields (50,52).

Tuberoinfundibular Hypophysiotropic Neurons

Parvocellular tuberoinfundibular hypophysiotropic neurons (TH-PvC) are small, slow-firing hypothalamic cells found in the acutely prepared, urethane-anesthetized mammals. Since single-unit recording without antidromic identification would be biased toward larger, faster firing nonendocrine neurons, the strategy for studying these smaller TH-PvC electrophysiologically involves stimulation of the median eminence stalk junction electrically in urethane-anesthetized rats (25,56,72). The difficulties encountered in these studies relate to possible current spread beyond the median eminence to axons *en passant,* the presence of other axon terminals in the area, and the difficulty of identifying the various hypophysiotropic neuron types, e.g., LHRH, TRH, and somatostatin. Resolution of the TH-PvC chemical identification requires intracellular dye-marking and immunocytochemical staining (50,52).

Anatomical Distribution

Antidromically identified TH-PvC have been located electrophysiologically in the suprachiasmatic nucleus (15%) (72), ventromedial nucleus (6%), and mediobasal hypothalamus–arcuate nucleus (13 to 36%) (25,56,72). Blume et al. (3) found that electrical stimulation of the median eminence yielded 8% short-latency (6 msec) cells in mediobasal hypothalamus (MBH) and 23% longer-latency (12 msec) cells in the vicinity of the paraventricular nucleus (NPV). These results contrasted with neurohypophysial stalk stimulation, where 11% short-latency cells (11 msec) were located in the MBH and 21% longer-latency cells (14 msec) in the vicinity of NPV. These workers (43) demonstrated that a single MgC could send one process to the median eminence and another to the neural lobe. The injection of horseradish peroxidase into the arcuate–median eminence region by Poulain (44) demonstrated horseradish peroxidase-positive cells in the NPV as well as in the suprachiasmatic, preoptic, and septal nuclei, confirming the physiological findings of Blume et al. (3,43). In the *in vitro* slice preparation, Kelly et al. (30) found two morphologically distinct procion-yellow-filled TH-PvC neuron types in preoptic–anterior hypothalamus and arcuate–ventromedial hypothalamus: (a) a large, multipolar with polygonal perikaryon; and (b) a small, fusiform cell. These initial data suggest the possibility for chemical identification in the TH-PvC system (50,52).

Afferent Neural Connections

Electrophysiological study of single neurons in the ventromedial nucleus demonstrated orthodromic and antidromic responses from electrical stimulation of sites in the amygdala and stria terminalis (55). Horseradish peroxidase injected into the amygdala moved by retrograde axoplasmic transport to many ipsilateral ventromedial hypothalamic neurons and to a few cells in the ipsilateral arcuate nucleus, periventricular region, and contralateral ventromedial nucleus (55). These data confirm the presence of reciprocal connections between the amygdala and the hypothalamic ventromedial nucleus in the rat (55). TH-PvC located in the ventromedial nucleus (46%), arcuate nucleus (39%), and periventricular region (15%) in the rat were found to respond to electrical stimulation of the medial preoptic and anterior hypothalamic areas and the amygdala with orthodromic responses (54). These and other data (25,56,72) indicate that several hypothalamic and extrahypothalamic areas, including the medial preoptic–anterior hypothalamic area and the amygdala, may send fibers to the TH-PvC for adaptive neuroendocrine reflexes.

Recurrent Facilitation and Inhibition

In the adult female rat antidromic activation of TH-PvC axons by stimulation of the median eminence produces inhibition and excitation in identified TH-PvC (59,72). The recurrent inhibition in TH-PvC neurons probably involves peptidergic TH-PvC axon collateral excitation of GABA-releasing inhibitory interneurons located in the MBH (59). The recurrent *excitation* in TH-PvC probably involves peptidergic TH-PvC axon collateral inhibition of catecholaminergic releasing inhibitory interneurons. The latter are located in the medial preoptic area where excitatory neurons project back to the MBH (25,59,72). The wide distribution of recurrent inhibition in TH-PvC suggests that inhibitory mechanisms are basic to all peptidergic TH-PvC types (72). The restricted distribution of recurrent excitation suggests that when disinhibition occurs the recurrent excitatory neural circuit becomes a reverberating neural circuit, resulting in an abrupt increase in the secretion rate of a particular releasing peptide (25, 56,59,72). Determination of the particular peptidergic TH-PvC neuron collaterals involved in recurrent inhibition and recurrent excitation awaits the dye-marking specificity and immunocytochemical identification (50,52).

Putative Neurotransmitters: Chemosensitivity

In the adult female rat Moss et al. (40) microiontophoretically applied various biogenic amines to antidromically identified TH-PvC in the median preoptic area (MPO) and arcuate–ventromedia nucleus (ARC-VM) to test chemosensitivity. Although the majority (59 to 82%) of MPO neurons failed to respond to iontophoretic application of norepinephrine (NE), dopamine (DA), 5-hydroxytryptamine (5-HT), and acetylcholine (ACh), approximately one-fourth (25%) showed inhibition following microiontophoresed NE and DA. In the ARC-VM, NE accelerated 72% of TH-PvC, with 55% of these cells unresponsive to ACh. These data support the suggestion that catecholamines (NE and DA) and ACh play a role in the regulation of neurons projecting toward the median eminence. With chemical identification of these TH-PvC, a more precise definition of specific neurotransmitters may become possible (50,52).

Gonadotropin-Related Regulatory Interneurons

Preoptic–Anterior Hypothalamic Neurons

The preoptic–anterior hypothalamic area (PO-AH) is important for cyclic gonadotropin release. In these areas neurons connect orthodromically and antidromically to the amygdala, hippocampus, and mediobasal hypothalamus (MBH) (9,25,56). In order to document structuring and orderliness in these hypothalamic connections, Dyer et al. (15) examined the responses of two groups of PO-AH neurons: those groups clustered within 100 μm and those scattered greater than 1,000 μm apart. The widely separated PO-AH ($>$1,000 μm) cells showed a random distribution of connections with corticomedial amygdala and MBH. The clustered PO-AH cells ($<$100 μm) showed a significant correlation between orthodromic responses from the amygdala and PO-AH cells. Those cells antidromically activated and orthodromically excited by stimulation of the MBH were frequently adjacent to one another. Clustered cells in the ventral half of the PO-AH received significantly more inhibitory inputs from the MBH and the corticomedial amygdala than those situated more dorsally (15). These data indicate the availability of PO-AH neuronal fields with structured, shared amygdala and MBH connections (15) for further analysis of chemical cell types and connections (50,52).

By recording single units in the MPO and stimulating median eminence electrically, Yagi and Sawaki (71) demonstrated that axon collaterals of the tuberoinfundibular neurosecretory cells mediated inhibition and excitation of certain MPO neurons. They also showed that stimulation of the median eminence precedes the catecholaminergic excitatory response. These data support the hypothesis that some MPO PvC are involved in neural pathways mediating recurrent inhibition and recurrent facilitation of TH-PvC (71).

Perkins and Whitehead (42) stimulated the medial forebrain bundle (MFB) electrically while recording single cells in PO-AH, revealing orthodromic excitation (45%), orthodromic inhibition (42%), and antidromic activation (13%). These data suggest the MFB neural circuits' importance for extrahypothalamic modulation of gonadotropin secretion. Carrer and Sawyer (8) found that electrochemical stimulation of the midbrain raphe nucleus increased multiunit spike activity in the MPO, whereas stimulation of the dorsal tegmentum decreased multiunit spike activity in the MPO.

Estrogen

Neurons of the hypothalamus concentrate estrogen (25,56; see also Chapter 3). Studies in various hypothalamic neuronal populations have shown that estrogen excites or inhibits cell firing patterns depending on the anatomical or behavioral substrate (25,56). In the unanesthetized rabbit, hypothalamic neurons projecting to the median eminence–arcuate region responded to intravenous estradiol benzoate dually: (a) spontaneous activity decreased, and (b) a transient increase preceded the decrease (14). Confirming the data of earlier workers in anesthetized mammals (25,56), these results suggest that increased electrical activity following injection of estrogen may indicate that estrogen facilitates LH secretion. The decreased firing rate may indicate the negative feedback effects of estradiol (25,56). In order to determine the specific effects of estrogen on hypothalamic neurons, Kelly et al. (33) applied an active (17β-estradiol hemisuccinate) and inactive isomer (17α-estradiol hemisuccinate) form of this ovarian steroid microiontophoretically to single MPO PvC. They found that the active steroid inhibited 33% of MPO cells tested whereas the inactive form failed to affect any cell. These and other control studies lead to the conclusion that the changes in MPO neuronal responses to estrogen relate to a specific membrane receptor mechanism (33). They also found that the nonantidromically identified neurons were most responsive to local estrogen, showing excitation on late diestrus 1 and inhibitory responses on late diestrus 2, proestrus, and estrus (31). In addition, these workers demonstrated the loss of responsiveness of MPO nonantidromically identified neurons to local application of estrogen 3 to 4 months after ovariectomy (32). Ovarian steroids, estrogen, and/or progesterone seem to be necessary for maintaining this electrical sensitivity, confirming neuronal estrogen receptor mechanisms in the MPO region of female rats (32).

Electrochemical Stimuli

In order to determine the neuronal mechanisms involved in LH release and ovulation induced by electrochemical stimulation of the preoptic area of the brain of the proestrous rat, van der Schoot et al. (60) recorded single neurons in the anterior hypothalamus. Earlier workers had suggested an increased and a decreased anterior hypothalamic unit activity to explain electrochemically induced LH release and ovulation (25,56). Using a variety of experimental approaches that included single-unit recording and plasma LH levels, van der Schoot et al. (60) showed that the plasma LH and the anterior hypothalamic unit firing increased in parallel 15 to 120 min after ipsilateral preoptic electrochemical stimulation. These data support earlier studies which suggested that electrolytic deposition of iron in the preoptic area enhanced preoptic–anterior hypothalamic neuronal activity, resulting in LH release and ovulation (25,56).

LHRH

LHRH, a gonadotropic neuropeptide, may function as a hypothalamic hormone and as a synaptic neurotransmitter (neuromodulator) in the regulation of gonadal activity in the rat (25), as microiontophoresis of LHRH onto hypothalamic and extrahypothalamic neurons suggests. Although some workers found PO-AH, ventromedial, and TH-PvC hypothalamic and cortical neurons responsive (excitation and inhibition), other laboratories could not duplicate all of these results (see ref. 25 for references). Recently Moss et al. (39) found that LHRH appears to have a "specific" excitatory action on nonantidromically driven (AD−) ARC-VM neurons (46%) in comparison to antidromically driven (AD+) ARC-VM neurons (30%), AD+ MPO neurons (32%), and AD− MPO cells (27%) in urethane-anesthetized, ovariectomized, adult female rats. These workers found 41% MPO neurons (AD+ = 48% responsive; AD− = 33% responsive) and 49% of ARC-VM neurons (AD+ = 40% responsive; AD− = 58% responsive) to microiontophoretic application of LHRH (39). Some of the differences among groups of workers probably indicate the presence of important uncontrolled factors, e.g., sex and hormonal state of the animals under study (25,56). Poulain and Carette (46) examined the responses of septal-diagonal band (SP-DBB) neurons driven antidromically or orthodromically from arcuate–median eminence stimulation. They found 20% of SP-DBB cells responded to LHRH: 13% excited, 7% inhibited. Many of the inhibited neurons were AD+ SP-DBB neurons (46).

In an attempt to evaluate contradictory results and to examine the importance of the hormonal state, Moss and Dudley (38) studied the responses of MPO neurons to LHRH microiontophoresis using LHRH agonistic analog and LHRH inactive analog in untreated and estrogen–progesterone-primed, ovariectomized female rats. In the estrogen–progesterone-primed rat, LHRH and its analogs influenced slightly more (54% versus 46%) MPO neurons than in the untreated animals. Hormone treatment apparently increased the percentage of excitatory (from 33% to 51%) and decreased the inhibitory (from 13% to 3%) effects of LHRH and its analogs on MPO neurons (38). Paradoxically, the inactive LHRH analog (des-Pro[9]-Gly[10]-LHRH) was as effective in inducing changes in MPO neurons as LHRH and its agonistic analog (38). These data indicate the seeming randomness with which microiontophoresed LHRH or its analogs affect the spontaneous firing of a rat MPO neuron. Considering the heterogeneous neuronal population studied, the nonspecific effects of urethane and microiontophoresis, and the uncontrolled nature of the "spontaneous" firing patterns, it seems unlikely that microiontophoresis here can produce meaningful data. The basic requirements are that cell firing must be controlled, and the cell types studied need to be better defined physiologically, morphologically, and chemically (50,52).

Adrenocorticotropin-Related Regulatory Interneurons

The secretion of corticotropin releasing factor (CRF), adrenocorticotropin (ACTH), and adrenal cortical steroids is a complex phenomenon involving a number of control factors that include stress, circadian rhythms, feedback mechanisms, and input pathways to the MBH (25,26; see also Chapters 3 and 4). Feldman et al. (16) studied single mediobasal hypothalamic units in response to electrical stimulation of sciatic nerve (Sc), ventrolateral pontine reticular formation (PRF), mammillary peduncle (MP), medial forebrain bundle (MFB), and suprachiasmatic nucleus (SCN). Approximately half of the units recorded responded significantly to one of these input pathways by a change in firing rate. The MP produced inhibition primarily, and the SCN produced facilitation with changes in poststimulus histograms. Different input pathways showed convergence on a single MBH unit. Stimulation of the MBH activated units synaptically (orthodromically) in the PRF, MP, and MFB. These data demonstrate electrophysiological connections between extrahypothalamic sites participating in adrenocortical regulation and the hypophysiotropic area of the hypothalamus. Other earlier studies demonstrated the feedback effects of systemically administered and microiontophoretically applied adrenocortical steroids on single hypothalamic neuronal activity (25,56). Future studies of adrenocorticotropin-related regulatory interneurons should involve chemical, morphological, and physiological definition (50,52).

Suprachiasmatic Parvocellular Vasopressin Neurons

The suprachiasmatic nucleus (SCN) is heterogeneously populated with PvC, some producing vasopressin and neurophysin (25,63), and some receiving input from visual pathways (21). Evidence suggests that this direct visual input is essential for synchronizing circadian rhythms with environmental day–night cycles (25). In the adult female rat, lesions of the SCN cause spontaneous ovulation to fail, behavioral estrus to persist, and the circadian rhythms of corticosterone, pineal serotonin N-acetyl transferase, and motor, feeding, and drinking behavior to be disturbed (48). Whether vasopressin pathways which emanate from SCN are involved in the regulation of these circadian rhythms remains enigmatic (25,63). The fine-caliber vasopressin–neurophysin fibers from SCN run to lateral septum, medial dorsal thalamus, lateral habenula, nucleus of diagonal tract, posterior hypothalamus, interpeduncular nucleus, and nucleus of solitary tract, ending as axosomatic contacts with neurons in these widely scattered projection areas (63).

Confirming earlier studies (25), Sawaki (58) found 38% of SCN units responsive to ipsilateral or contralateral visual input, i.e., photic or electrical stimulation of optic nerve. Twenty-five percent of these units were excitatory, 13% inhibited. Sawaki (58) found for the first time that 15% of SCN cells driven by visual input were antidromically identified as TH-PvC. In order to determine the possible central neurotransmitters involved in SCN neurons, Nishino and Koizumi (41) found that microiontophoresis of ACh and GLU excited most cells (70 to 80%). The monoamines 5-HT, NE, and DA, in the majority (60 to 100%) of cells excited by visual input, depressed the response of SCN neurons. Where visual input inhibited a few SCN neurons, 5-HT and NE depressed 50%, DA inhibited none, NE excited 40%, and ACh and GLU excited 65% (41). These data suggest the involvement of suprachiasmatic neurons in those light-mediated hypothalamic circadian rhythms which are of importance to endocrine and nonendocrine neurons. Whether visual input to the hypothalamus relies on vasopressinergic or the nonvasopressinergic neurons of the SCN to relay information is still unknown. A combination of cell recording, cell marking, and immunohistochemical techniques (50,52) may clarify suprachiasmatic nucleus function.

Thyrotropin-Related Regulatory Interneurons

The thyrotropin releasing hormone (TRH)-positive cell bodies in the hypothalamus lie in the dorsomedial nucleus and the perifornical area (26). The external layer of the median eminence, dorsomedial nucleus, perifornical region, parvocellular and magnocellular part of the paraventricular nucleus, ventromedial nucleus, suprachiasmatic nucleus, and median forebrain bundle contain TRH nerve fibers and terminals (26). In support of a possible synaptic action and in confirmation of earlier studies (25,56), Moss et al. (39) applied TRH microiontophoretically onto nonantidromically identified hypothalamic and extrahypothalamic neurons. Thirty-four percent of the cells responded: 14% excited primarily in the mediobasal hypothalamus, 20% inhibited throughout the brain (39). In an attempt to control the endocrine state of the animal, Moss and Dudley (38) compared the responses of nonidentified medial preoptic neurons to microiontophoretically applied TRH in untreated and estrogen–progesterone-primed ovariectomized female rats. TRH produced more excitation in untreated animals (28%) than in hormone-primed female rats (5%), whereas TRH had no effect on untreated (65%) and hormone-primed (85%) animals (38). In a study of the interaction of TRH and ACh, Yarborough (74) found that microiontophoresis of ACh accelerated cortical neurons. Simultaneous application of TRH iontophoretically enhanced the action of ACh, thus suggesting that TRH be a modulator of certain chemical transmitters (74). In the future, identifying the cells where TRH originates by physiological, morphological, and immunohistochemical methods (50,52) will aid our study of the functional role of this brain peptide.

Other Pituitary Hormones, Monoamines, and Opioid Peptides

Prolactin

Examining the effects of systemic and locally administered prolactin on single hypothalamic neurons, several workers found a complex effect which indicates several possible prolactin feedback sites in the diencephalon (see ref. 25 for references). In a recent study in the female guinea pig Poulain and Carette (45) found two types of response of septal–preoptic neurons to iontophoretic application of prolactin: (a) inhibition (17%) or excitation (8%), rapid in onset and recovery; (b) excitation (75%), slow in onset and long-lasting. The cells which were unresponsive to prolactin or had rapid onset–offset were anatomically distributed diffusely throughout the septal–preoptic area. The long-lasting excitatory effects of prolactin were primarily from cells in the preoptic area (45). There was no particular difference in response to prolactin between cells with or without projections to the median eminence area (45). These data indicate that more than half the units in the septal–preoptic area in the guinea pig change spontaneous firing rates in response to iontophoretically administered prolactin, suggesting the direct feedback effects of this pituitary hormone on hypothalamic neurons.

Monoamines

The hypophysiotropic system is influenced by the dopaminergic (DA), noradrenergic (NE), adrenergic (E), serotonergic (5-HT), and histaminergic (HA) pathways that impinge on the mediobasal hypothalamus (26). Studying the effects of microiontophoretic application of HA on identified ventromedial nucleus (VMN) neurons, Renaud (53) found that 71% were inhibited, 20% excited, and 9% nonresponsive. In those VMN cells tested with other putative transmitters, most were also inhibited by iontophoretic application of GABA, ACh, somatostatin, LHRH, and TRH. In contrast to the earlier studies where HA enhanced activity of the majority (50 to 85%) (25) of unidentified hypothalamic neurons, these inhibitory effects on VMN cells (53) suggest regional differences in histamine sensitivity, perhaps related to regional differences in histamine levels in hypothalamic nuclei (26).

Opioid Peptides

The opioid pentapeptides methionine-enkephalin (met-ENK) and leucine-enkephalin (leu-ENK), are found in cell bodies throughout the hypothalamus with nerve fibers ending in the external layer of the median eminence and in the adenohypophysis (20,26,62,64; see also Chapter 7). It has been suggested that these ENK peptides are synaptic neurotransmitters (neuromodulators) in the brain and hypophysiotropic factors in adenohypophysial regulation (20, 26,62,64). In a study of iontophoretically applied met-ENK and leu-ENK on single tuberal hypothalamic neurons (perifornical area, arcuate, ventromedial and dorsomedial nuclei and adjacent periventricular areas), Carette and Poulain (7) found three patterns of inhibition of cell activity: those inhibited by (a) met-ENK alone; (b) leu-ENK alone; and (c) both enkephalins. This inhibition of tuberal hypothalamic neurons by enkephalins suggests that these opioid penta-peptides may be involved in the regulation of nerve cells involved in adenohypo-physial secretory activity. We expect that future studies of chemically identified ENK neurons may further delineate the specific connections of these peptidergic cells on TH-PvC.

Summary

Parvocellular neuroendocrine cells in the hypothalamus synthesize, transport, and release the hypophysiotropic hormones LHRH, TRH, somatostatin, and others into the primary plexus of the median eminence portal vessels for regulating the secretion of anterior pituitary tropic hormones. The exact anatomical locations of most of these parvocellular neuroendocrine cells are well defined by immunohistochemistry. Dopamine, a potential hypophysiotropic hormone, has been found in the cell bodies of the arcuate nucleus. Vasopressin, another potential hypophysiotropic hormone, has been found in unmyelinated fibers projecting to the external zone of the median eminence from the paraventricular nucleus. Vasopressin located in the parvocellular neurons of the suprachiasmatic nuclei and in the fine fiber network from the suprachiasmatic throughout the hypothalamus may serve a transmitter role in the visually triggered circadian endocrine rhythms. Located in the arcuate and ventromedial nucleus and elsewhere in the mediobasal hypothalamus, as well as in the anterior periventricular and dorsal premammillary nuclei, those parvocellular neuroendocrine cells that have been antidromically identified are sensitive to putative transmitters; to hypophysiotropic, pituitary, tropic, and target gland hormones; and to a wide range of sensory inputs. The nonantidromically identified regulatory neurons are similarly sensitive. It has not been possible to study chemically identified parvocellular neurons. Accordingly, these parvocellular neuroendocrine and regulatory neuronal data are inconclusive at the present time.

CLASSIFICATION OF HYPOTHALAMIC NEURONS

At present our newly developed method for chemical identification of hypothalamic neurons provides an excellent approach for classification and study of central nervous system neurons (50,52). This approach makes available three types of data—physiological, morphological, and chemical—from which one can determine the characteristics of the cell under study. The physiological data allow determination of membrane characteristics and of input pathways from various sensory organs and from orthodromic and antidromic pathways. The morphological data allow three-dimensional reconstruction of the soma, axons, and dendrites from the dye-injected cell, providing an anatomical "fingerprint" of the cell. The chemical identification of the cell by immunohistochemical methods characterizes the peptidergic type of hypothalamic neuron and the nature of the peptide released at nerve terminals. Using this approach, investigators will be able to characterize hypothalamic cells precisely, with the ability to study the same functional–morphological–chemical cell type from one animal to another. Highly reproducible experiments on a cell type will provide the most discriminating method for establishing the functional role of a hypothalamic neuroendocrine cell (50,52).

ACKNOWLEDGMENTS

The authors thank Ms. S. Curtis for editorial assistance. The authors' research quoted in this review was supported in part by research grants NS-13411 and NS-05696 from the U.S. Public Health Service and a grant from the North Carolina Heart Association (1977–78–A–3).

REFERENCES

1. Bioulac, B., Dufy, B., De Vitry, F., Fleury, H., Tixier-Vidal, A., and Vincent, J. D. (1977): Intracellular recording from hypothalamic neurosecretory cells in tissue culture (clone HT9-C7). *Neurosci. Lett.,* 4:257–262.
2. Bioulac, B., Gaffori, O., Harris, M., and Vincent, J. D. (1978): Effects of acetylcholine, sodium glutamate and GABA on the discharge of supraoptic neurons in the rat. *Brain Res.,* 154:159–162.
3. Blume, H. W., Pittman, Q. J., and Renaud, L. P. (1978): Electrophysiological indications of a 'vasopressinergic' innervation of the median eminence. *Brain Res.,* 155:153–158.
4. Boer, K., and Nolten, J. W. L. (1978): Hypothalamic paraventricular unit activity during labour in the rat. *J. Endocrinol.,* 76:155–163.
5. Brimble, M. J., and Dyball, R. E. J. (1977): Characterization of the responses of oxytocin- and vasopressin-secreting neurones in the supraoptic nucleus to osmotic stimulation. *J. Physiol. (Lond),* 271:253–271.
6. Brimble, M. J., Dyball, R. E. J., and Forsling, M. L. (1978): Oxytocin release following osmotic activation of oxytocin neurones in the paraventricular and supraoptic nuclei. *J. Physiol. (Lond),* 278:69–78.
7. Carette, B., and Poulain, P. (1978): Inhibitory action of iontophoretically applied methionine-enkephalin and leucine-enkephalin on tuberal hypothalamic neurons. *Neurosci. Lett.,* 7:137–140.
8. Carrer, H. F., and Sawyer, C. H. (1976): Changes in multiunit spike activity in the rat preoptic area induced by stimulating the midbrain. *Exp. Neurol.,* 52:525–534.
9. Carrer, H. F., Whitmoyer, D. ·I., and Sawyer, C. H. (1978): Effects of hippocampal and amygdaloid stimulation on the firing of preoptic neurons in the proestrous female rat. *Brain Res.,* 142:363–367.

10. Clifton, D. K., Rabii, J., Whitmoyer, D. I., and Sawyer, C. H. (1978): Noise detection and reduction by cross-correlation in multiple unit recording systems. *Brain Res.,* 143:186–190.
11. Cross, B. A., and Green, J. D. (1959): Activity of single neurones in the hypothalamus: Effect of osmotic and other stimuli. *J. Physiol. (Lond),* 148:554–569.
12. Dogterom, J., Wimersma-Greidanus, Tj. B. Van, and Swaab, D. F. (1977): Evidence for the release of vasopressin and oxytocin into cerebrospinal fluid: Measurements in plasma and CSF in intact and hypophysectomized rats. *Neuroendocrinology,* 24:108–118.
13. Dreifuss, J. J., Tribollet, E., Baertschi, A. J., and Lincoln, D. W. (1976): Mammalian endocrine neurones: Control of phasic activity by antidromic action potentials. *Neurosci. Lett.,* 3:281–286.
14. Dufy, B., Partouche, C., Poulain, D., Dufy-Barbe, L., and Vincent, J. D. (1976): Effects of estrogen on the electrical activity of identified and unidentified hypothalamic units. *Neuroendocrinology,* 22:38–47.
15. Dyer, R. G., Ellendorff, F., and MacLeod, N. K. (1976): Non-random distribution of cell types in the preoptic and anterior hypothalamic areas. *J. Physiol. (Lond),* 261:495–504.
16. Feldman, S. Kreisel, B., and Conforti, N. (1976): Electrophysiological connections of the rat mediobasal hypothalamus with brain areas mediating adrenocortical responses. *Brain Res. Bull.,* 1:523–528.
17. Freund-Mercier, M. J., and Richard, P. (1977): Spontaneous and reflex activity of paraventricular nucleus units in cycling and lactating rats. *Brain Res.,* 130:505–520.
18. Gahwiler, B. H., Sandoz, P., and Dreifuss, J. J. (1978): Neurones with synchronous bursting discharges in organ cultures of the hypothalamic supraoptic nucleus area. *Brain Res.,* 151:245–253.
19. Goossens, N., Dierickx, K., and Vandesande, F. (1977): Immunocytochemical localization of vasotocin and isotocin in the preopticohypophysial neurosecretory system of teleosts. *Gen. Comp. Endocrinol.,* 32:371–375.
20. Guillemin, R. (1978): Biochemical and physiological correlates of hypothalamic peptides: the new endocrinology of the neuron. In: *The Hypothalamus,* edited by S. Reichlin, R. J. Baldessarini, and J. B. Martin, pp. 155–194. Raven Press, New York.
21. Guldner, F. H. (1978): Synapses of optic nerve afferents in the rat suprachiasmatic nucleus. I. Identification, qualitative description, development and distribution. *Cell Tissue Res.,* 194:17–35.
22. Haller, E. W., Brimble, M. J., and Wakerley, J. B. (1978): Phasic discharge in supraoptic neurones recorded from hypothalamic slices. *Exp. Brain Res.,* 33:131–134.
23. Hatton, G. I., Armstrong, W. E., and Gregory, W. A. (1978): Spontaneous and osmotically-stimulated activity in slices of rat hypothalamus. *Brain Res. Bull.,* 3:497–508.
24. Hayward, J. N. (1974): Physiological and morphological identification of hypothalamic magnocellular neuroendocrine cells in goldfish preoptic nucleus. *J. Physiol. (Lond),* 239:103–124.
25. Hayward, J. N. (1977): Functional and morphological aspects of hypothalamic neurons. *Physiol. Rev.,* 57:574–658.
26. Hökfelt, T., Elde, R., Fuxe, K., Johansson, O., Ljungdahl, A., Goldstein, M., Luft, R., Efendic, S., Nilsson, G., Terenius, L., Ganten, D., Jeffcoate, S. L., Rehfeld, J., Said, S., Perez de la Mora, M., Possani, L., Tapia, R., Teran, L., and Palacios, R. (1978): Aminergic and peptidergic pathways in the nervous system with special reference to the hypothalamus. In: *The Hypothalamus,* edited by S. Reichlin, R. J. Baldessarini, and J. B. Martin, pp. 69–135. Raven Press, New York.
27. Jennings, D. P., Haskins, J. T., and Rogers, J. M. (1978): Comparison of firing patterns and sensory responsiveness between supraoptic and other hypothalamic neurons in the unanesthetized sheep. *Brain Res.,* 149:347–364.
28. Kandel, E. R. (1964): Electrical properties of hypothalamic neuroendocrine cells. *J. Gen. Physiol.,* 47:691–717.
29. Kannan, H., and Yagi, K. (1978): Supraoptic neurosecretory neurons: Evidence for the existence of converging inputs both from carotid baroreceptors and osmoreceptors. *Brain Res.,* 145:385–390.
30. Kelly, M. J., Kuhnt, U., and Wuttke, W. (1979): Morphological features of physiologically identified hypothalamic neurons as revealed by intracellular marking. *Exp. Brain Res.,* 34:107–116.

31. Kelly, M. J., Moss, R. L., and Dudley, C. A. (1977): The effects of microelectrophoretically applied estrogen, cortisol and acetylcholine on medial preoptic-septal unit activity throughout the estrous cycle of the female rat. *Exp. Brain Res.*, 30:53–64.

32. Kelly, M. J., Moss, R. L., and Dudley, C. A. (1978): The effects of ovariectomy on the responsiveness of preoptic-septal neurons to microelectrophoresed estrogen. *Neuroendocrinology*, 25:204–211.

33. Kelly, M. J., Moss, R. L., Dudley, C. A., and Fawcett, C. P. (1977): The specificity of the response of preoptic-septal area neurons to estrogen: 17α-Estradiol versus 17β-estradiol and the response of extrahypothalamic neurons. *Exp. Brain Res.*, 30:43–52.

34. Koizumi, K., and Yamashita, H. (1972): Studies of antidromically identified neurosecretory cells of the hypothalamus by intracellular and extracellular recordings. *J. Physiol. (Lond),* 221:683–705.

35. Koizumi, K., and Yamashita, H. (1978): Influence of atrial stretch receptors on hypothalamic neurosecretory neurones. *J. Physiol. (Lond),* 285:341–358.

36. Menninger, R. P. (1979): Response of supraoptic neurosecretory cells to changes in left atrial distension. *Am. J. Physiol.*, 236:261–267.

37. Moses, A. M., and Share, L. (eds.) (1977): *Neurohypophysis.* Karger, Basel.

38. Moss, R. L., and Dudley, C. A. (1978): Changes in responsiveness of medial preoptic neurons to the microelectrophoresis of releasing hormones as a function of ovarian hormones. *Brain Res.*, 149:511–515.

39. Moss, R. L., Dudley, C. A., and Kelly, M. J. (1978): Hypothalamic polypeptide releasing hormones: Modifiers of neuronal activity. *Neuropharmacology*, 17:87–93.

40. Moss, R. L., Kelly, M. J., and Dudley, C. A. (1978): Chemosensitivity of hypophysiotropic neurones to the microelectrophoresis of biogenic amines. *Brain Res.*, 139:141–152.

41. Nishino, H., and Koizumi, K. (1977): Responses of neurons in the suprachiasmatic nuclei of the hypothalamus to putative transmitters. *Brain Res.*, 120:167–172.

42. Perkins, M. N., and Whitehead, S. A. (1978): Responses and pharmacological properties of preoptic/anterior hypothalamic neurones following medial forebrain bundle stimulation. *J. Physiol. (Lond),* 279:347–360.

43. Pittman, Q. J., Blume, H. W., and Renaud, L. P. (1978): Electrophysiological indications that individual hypothalamic neurons innervate both median eminence and neurohypophysis. *Brain Res.*, 157:364–368.

44. Poulain, P. (1977): Septal afferents to the arcuate-median eminence region in the guinea pig: Correlative electrophysiological and horseradish peroxidase study. *Brain Res.*, 137:150–153.

45. Poulain, P., and Carette, B. (1976): Actions of iontophoretically applied prolactin on septal and preoptic neurons in the guinea pig. *Brain Res.*, 116:172–176..

46. Poulain, P., and Carette, B. (1977): Septal afferents to the arcuate-median eminence region in the guinea pig: Microiontophoretically-applied LRF effects. *Brain Res.*, 137:154–157.

47. Poulain, D. A., Wakerley, J. B., and Dyball, R. E. J. (1977): Electrophysiological differentiation of oxytocin- and vasopressin-secreting neurones. *Proc. R. Soc. Lond. [Biol]*, 196:367–384.

48. Raisman, G., and Brown-Grant, K. (1977): The 'suprachiasmatic syndrome': Endocrine and behavioural abnormalities following lesions of the suprachiasmatic nuclei in the female rat. *Proc. R. Soc. Lond. [Biol]*, 198:297–314.

49. Reaves, T. A., Jr., and Hayward, J. N. (1979): Immunocytochemical identification of vasopressinergic and oxytocinergic neurons in the hypothalamus of the cat. *Cell Tissue Res.*, 196:117–122.

50. Reaves, T. A., Jr., and Hayward, J. N. (1979): Isotocinergic neurons in the goldfish hypothalamus: physiological and morphological studies on chemically identified cells. *Cell Tissue Res.*, 202:17–35.

51. Reaves, T. A., Jr., and Hayward, J. N. (1979): Immunocytochemical identification of enkephalinergic neurons in the hypothalamic magnocellular preoptic nucleus of the goldfish, Carassius auratus. *Cell Tissue Res.*, 200:147–151.

52. Reaves, T. A., Jr., and Hayward, J. N. (1979): Intracellular dye-marked enkephalin neurons in the magnocellular preoptic nucleus of the goldfish hypothalamus. *Proc. Natl. Acad. Sci. USA*, 76:6009–6011.

53. Renaud, L. P. (1976): Histamine microiontophoresis on identified hypothalamic neurons: 3 Patterns of response in the ventromedial nucleus of the rat. *Brain Res.*, 115:339–344.

54. Renaud, L. P. (1977): Influence of median preoptic-anterior hypothalamic area stimulation

on the excitability of mediobasal hypothalamic neurones in the rat. *J. Physiol. (Lond),* 264:541–564.

55. Renaud, L. P., and Hopkins, D. A. (1977): Amygdala afferents from the mediobasal hypothalamus: An electrophysiological and neuroanatomical study in the rat. *Brain Res.,* 121:201–213.

56. Richard, P., Freund-Mercier, M. J., and Moos, F. (1978): Les neurones hypothalamiques ayant une fonction endocrine. *J. Physiol. (Paris),* 74:61–112.

57. Rossier, J., Battenberg, E., Pittman, Q., Bayon, A., Koda, L., Miller, R., Guillemin, R., and Bloom, F. (1979): Hypothalamic enkephalin neurones may regulate the neurohypophysis. *Nature,* 277:653–655.

58. Sawaki, Y. (1977): Retinohypothalamic projection: Electrophysiological evidence for the existence in female rats. *Brain Res.,* 120:336–341.

59. Sawaki, Y., and Yagi, K. (1976): Inhibition and facilitation of antidromically identified tuberoinfundibular neurones following stimulation of the median eminence in the rat. *J. Physiol. (Lond),* 260:447–460.

60. Schoot van der, P., Lincoln, D. W., and Clark, J. S. (1978): Activation of hypothalamic neuronal activity by the electrolytic deposition of iron into the preoptic area. *J. Endocrinol.,* 79:107–120.

61. Sladek, C. D., and Joynt, R. J. (1978): Role of acetylcholine and angiotensin in the osmotic control of vasopressin release by the organ cultured rat hypothalamo-neurohypophyseal system. In: *Program 4th Meet. Neuroscience Soc.,* p. 356.

62. Snyder, S. H. (1978): Peptide neurotransmitter candidates in the brain: focus on enkephalin, angiotensin II and neurotensin. In: *The Hypothalamus,* edited by S. Reichlin, R. J. Baldessarini, and J. B. Martin, pp. 233–242. Raven Press, New York.

63. Sofroniew, M. V., and Weindl, A. (1978): Projections from the parvocellular vasopressin- and neurophysin-containing neurons of the suprachiasmatic nucleus. *Am. J. Anat.,* 153:391–430.

64. Tramu, G., and Leonardelli, J. (1979): Immunohistochemical localization of enkephalins in median eminence and adenohypophysis. *Brain Res.,* 168:457–471.

65. Vandesande, F., and Dierickx, K. (1975): Identification of the vasopressin producing and of the oxytocin producing neurons in the hypothalamic magnocellular neurosecretory system of the rat. *Cell Tissue Res.,* 164:153–162.

66. Verney, E. B. (1947): The antidiuretic hormone and the factors which affect its release. *Proc. R. Soc. Lond. [Biol],* 135:25–106.

67. Wakerley, J. B., Poulain, D. A., and Brown, D. (1978): Comparison of firing patterns in oxytocin- and vasopressin-releasing neurones during progressive dehydration. *Brain Res.,* 148:425–440.

68. Weitzman, R. E., Glatz, T. H., and Fisher, D. A. (1978): The effect of hemorrhage and hypertonic saline upon plasma oxytocin and arginine vasopressin in conscious dogs. *Endocrinology,* 103:2154–2160.

69. Yagi, K., Azuma, T., and Matsuda, K. (1966): Neurosecretory cell: Capable of conducting impulse in rats. *Science,* 142:778–779.

70. Yagi, K., and Iwasaki, S. (1977): Electrophysiology of the neurosecretory cell. *Int. Rev. Cytol.,* 48:141–186.

71. Yagi, K., and Sawaki, Y. (1977): Medial preoptic nucleus neurons: Inhibition and facilitation of spontaneous activity following stimulation of the median eminence in female rats. *Brain Res.,* 120:342–346.

72. Yagi, K., and Sawaki, Y. (1978): Electrophysiological characteristics of identified tuberoinfundibular neurons. *Neuroendocrinology,* 26:50–64.

73. Yamashita, H. (1977): Effect of baro- and chemoreceptor activation on supraoptic nuclei neurons in the hypothalamus. *Brain Res.,* 126:551–556.

74. Yarbrough, G. G. (1976): TRH potentiates excitatory actions of acetylcholine on cerebral cortical neurones. *Nature,* 263:523–524.

The Endocrine Functions of the Brain,
edited by Marcella Motta.
Raven Press, New York © 1980

3

Anatomical Distribution of Steroid Hormone Target Neurons and Circuitry in the Brain

Walter E. Stumpf

Departments of Anatomy and Pharmacology, University of North Carolina, Chapel Hill, North Carolina 27514

ESTROGEN

Through the use of tritium-labeled estradiol and autoradiographic techniques developed in our laboratories, a demonstration of the subcellular localization of the hormone as well as the first mapping of the distribution of estrogen target cells in the diencephalon was accomplished (23). From the results of these early studies[1] three conclusions were derived: (a) the anatomical and functional concept of the "hypophysiotropic area" as the site of steroid feedback and regulation of gonadotropin secretion could not be supported; rather (b) estrogen target cells were found to be arranged in a fashion that follows the distribution of certain neural pathways such as the stria terminalis in the diencephalon; and (c) the nuclear concentration of the hormone was conceived to argue for a stimulatory action, rather than a direct or primary negative feedback, on the grounds of data available for the uterus and other target tissues. These data and concepts have since received increasing support through additional evidence: as predicted, sites of origin of the stria terminalis in the amygdala proved to be target sites for estradiol, and the amygdala was recognized to be complexly organized, similar to the hypothalamus, with regard to functional sites of steroid hormone action. The tendency, often noticed in studies published in the literature, of lumping the amygdala in a single structure or dividing it into a basomedial and dorsolateral unit could not be supported in view of the differential neuronal labeling that includes the nucleus (n.) lateralis anterior, n. basalis medialis, n. medialis, and n. corticalis (24,25). Other estrogen target areas interconnected by the stria terminalis and lying outside of the hypothalamus

---

[1] It is noteworthy that our results were in contrast to those of other investigators. The development of an autoradiographic technique between 1963 and 1968 for the study of noncovalently bound small molecular weight substances was prerequisite (22).

were described, these included the subfornical organ, n. triangularis septi, n. septi lateralis, n. tractus diagonalis, n. olfactorius anterior, n. habenulae lateralis, n. parataenialis, n. periventricularis thalami, hippocampus inferior with subiculum, griseum centrale of the mesencephalon and pons, and the n. tractus solitarii. Thus, by 1970 it was apparent that there is an extensive distribution of estrogen target neurons in the rat brain (25). Three years later this work was confirmed in essence by Pfaff and Keiner (10) who at this time used a technique similar to our thaw-mount autoradiographic technique that eliminated artifacts characteristic of Pfaff's double fixation technique. In our studies in addition to the stria terminalis, the corticomedial hypothalamic tract, the periventricular bundle of Schütz, and other pathways were invoked to constitute portions of the "estrogen-neuron" circuitry. Since the simplistic concept of pituitary regulation through the "hypophysiotropic area" dominated, and still does, only very few investigators in neuroendocrinology advanced into studying extrahypothalamic sites. The importance of extrahypothalamic sites became further apparent as maps of the midbrain, hindbrain, and spinal cord were completed (29,6). Most importantly, anatomical links between estrogen target sites and catecholamine neurons and also peptidergic neurons were repeatedly suggested (23,27,30) and established in our laboratory through the development of combination techniques.

The simultaneous localization within the same section of catecholamines by formaldehyde-induced fluorescence and [³H]estradiol by autoradiography (2,4) showed that catecholaminergic cells are genomic target cells for estradiol. That includes such regions as in the medulla oblongata, the n. reticularis lateralis (A1), and the n. tractus solitarii (A2); in the pons near the n. olivaris superior (A5), the locus coeruleus (A6), and the vicinity of the lemniscus lateralis (A7). While these are mainly norepinephrine-containing cell bodies, dopamine neurons have also been found to be labeled by [³H]estradiol in the basal hypothalamus in the dorsal n. arcuatus and n. periventricularis (A12) (3). Similar to [³H]estradiol, [³H]dihydrotestosterone nuclear labeling is found in select catecholamine neurons in a cell group at the lateral corner of the fourth ventricle (A4), adjacent to the n. olivaris superior (A5), in the locus coeruleus (A6), and in the region of the lemniscus lateralis (A7) (5).

The results of these studies clearly implicate the ventral and dorsal adrenergic bundles as estrogen and, in part, androgen-addressed neuronal systems. Connections between lower brain stem regions such as the n. tractus solitarii and the n. preopticus, the bed nucleus of the stria terminalis as well as the n. paraventricularis (12,21) are also recognized estrogen target neurons, being located at both ends.

The simultaneous localization within the same section of peptide antibodies by immunohistochemistry and [³H]estradiol by autoradiography (17) showed that neurophysin I containing cells are genomic target cells for [³H]estradiol, that estrogen target cells in the pituitary are gonadotrophes, somatotrophes, lactotrophes, and thyrotrophes as well (7), and dihydrotestosterone target cells in the pars distalis of the pituitary are gonadotrophes and thyrotrophes (18). A comparison of the topography of estrogen target neuron distribution in the preoptic-septal hypothalamus agrees with the sites where neuronal perikarya are located that stain with antigonadotropin-releasing hormone. It is, therefore, likely that gonadotropin-releasing hormone producing cells are target cells for estradiol (30). Similar anatomical relationships seem to exist between sites of estrogen action and production of other neurohormones or transmitters.

The available data confirm earlier concepts from this laboratory that estradiol and other steroid hormones are neuronal activators and regulators. The fact that estrogen target cells are found in the brain of all vertebrate species studied to date (8,32), including cyclostomes and primates, indicates the importance of the ovarian steroid hormone-brain interaction for vertebrates. Furthermore, estrogen target sites have been demonstrated in neonates in contradiction to negative biochemical evidence (19,20), and also in the 10-day and 17-day chicken embryo (9) and in 16-day fetal mice (33). Thus, actions of steroid hormones during development at extrahypothalamic as well as hypothalamic sites are indicated.

ANDROGEN

The presence in the brain of androgen receptors has repeatedly been questioned by other investigators, although a specific pattern of distribution of neurons with nuclear labeling after [3H]testosterone or [3H]dihydrotestosterone injection has been demonstrated in autoradiograms (13,15). While there is some overlap with sites of accumulation of estrogen target cells, androgen-specific sites exist in many regions including the dorsolateral septum, the ventromedial nucleus of the hypothalamus, most of the pyramidal cell areas of the hippocampus, and, especially, motor neurons of the brain stem and spinal cord. It is apparent that somatomotor and psychomotor neuronal systems are a domain for androgen steroid action, while, in comparison with estrogen, regions known to modulate sensory perception show stronger representation of estrogen target neurons (31). The behavioral consequences of this dichotomy of emphasis of "male" versus "female" sex steroid hormone sites of action can be recognized, for instance, in the prevalence of motor activation in male sexual approaches to the female, and in male territorial defense.

PROGESTAGEN

The presence in the brain of progestagen receptors has repeatedly been questioned by other investigators, although a specific pattern of distribution of neurons with nuclear labeling has been shown in the guinea pig after injection of [3H]progesterone (14) and in the rat after injection of the synthetic progestin [3H]R5020 (16). To date studies with progestagens are incomplete and barely cover the whole forebrain. Progestagen concentrating neurons have been seen only in areas where estrogen target neurons are found, although less extensive than the latter, including in the hypothalamus the n. preopticus, the n. periventricularis, the n. arcuatus, and the n. ventromedialis. Although estrogen pretreatment increases nuclear uptake of progestagen, nuclear labeling can be demonstrated without such pretreatment (14).

GLUCOCORTICOSTEROIDS AND MINERALCORTICOSTEROIDS

The first anatomical demonstration of brain target cells for glucocorticosteroid hormone was published in 1971 (26). At this time the major sites of glucocorticosteroid action in the rat forebrain were recognized as being extrahypothalamic and include the hippocampus, dorsal septum, indusium griseum, as well as areas of the amygdala and the cortex. These results were later confirmed by others, especially Warembourg (36). A more complete mapping of the rat brain reveals an extensive distribution of target cells for [3H]corticosterone (34) as well as [3H]aldosterone (35). Both glucocorticosteroid and mineralcorticosteroid target cells occupy similar sites throughout the central nervous system, although, under the conditions of the experiments, [3H]aldosterone shows a stronger uptake and wider distribution. In contrast to other steroid hormones, in the hypothalamus nuclear concentration of radioactivity in neurons is nonconspicuous in studies with [3H]corticosterone and only scattered with [3H]aldosterone. The strongest nuclear labeling is seen in certain neurons of the precommissural, supracommissural, and infracommissural hippocampus and in structures closely associated with the hippocampal complex such as the dorsolateral septum, certain regions of the amygdala, and the endorhinal cortex. Cortical cell layers show a remarkably extensive neuronal labeling with [3H]corticosterone and [3H]aldosterone. Cortical layers 2, 3, and 5 show strongest nuclear neuronal labeling when compared with neurons in other layers. With both the gluco- and mineral-corticosteroid in the midbrain, the pons, the medulla, the cerebellum, and the spinal cord, neurons that are associated with sensory or motor systems show distinct nuclear labeling with strongest uptake in the large motor neurons of the spinal cord and cranial nerves (1,34). Also neurons in the reticular formation show varying degrees of nuclear labeling.

Studies with [3H]dexamethasone, a synthetic glucocorticosteroid, show a pattern of distribution in the brain different from the patterns obtained with [3H]corticosterone or [3H]aldosterone. While the natural adrenal steroids enter the brain apparently readily, after [3H]dexamethasone injection there is a delayed entry. In autoradiographic studies (11) with mature adrenalectomized rats, 30 min after a single intravenous injection of 0.5 µg/100 g b.w., radioactivity is concentrated in the ventricular system and in its immediate vicinity, while it is largely absent from the neuropil in areas remote from the ventricles. After 3 hr, radioactivity appears equilibrated throughout the brain, without the differential neuronal uptake, for instance, in the hippocampus, as seen so characteristically with the natural adrenal steroid hormones. Further studies need to clarify the reasons for the demonstrated differences between the different adrenal steroids.

CONCLUSIONS

The results obtained through the use of our thaw-mount and dry-mount autoradiographic techniques as well as their combination techniques for the simultaneous localization of catecholamines or antibodies to peptide hormones demonstrate a characteristic and extensive distribution pattern of steroid hormone target neurons in the brain and close relationships to neurotransmitter and peptide messenger systems. The topographical distribution or hormone architecture that is specific for each individual hormone led to the early questioning of concepts engrained in contemporary neuroendocrinology that attribute to neurons of the basal hypothalamus or the "hypophysiotropic area" a dominant role in the neural regulation of endocrine gland functions (23,27,28). The advent of additional information since 1975 through the use of immunohistochemistry supports concepts advanced earlier by us about the importance of circuitry in the periventricular brain and the possible dominance of extrahypothalamic sites in neuroendocrine regulations. For instance, the demonstrated anatomical links between steroid hormone uptake sites and production sites of catecholamines indicate that for many of the neuroendocrine events the stimuli are originated outside of the hypothalamus, probably not only for "modulation" but for the essential events such as the cyclic release of gonadotropins. The fact that lesions in the preoptic-septal area abolish cyclicity does not contradict this if one considers the catecholaminergic innervation of hypothalamic regions. It is likely that steroid hormone action in the brain, as in other tissues, is genomically stimulatory and that what is perceived as "negative feedback" is mediated through the steroidal activation of inhibitory systems or an inhibition through secondary products (23). The differential nuclear uptake in different neurons or neuronal groups of a given steroid hormone argues for a differential activation of target neurons that depends on steroid hormone blood levels and probably can be modulated through actions of other steroid and peptide messengers.

ACKNOWLEDGMENT

This work was supported by Public Health Service grant nos. NS09914 and AE01104.

REFERENCES

1. Birmingham, M. K., Stumpf, W. E., and Sar, M. (1979): Nuclear localization of aldosterone in rat brain cells, assessed by autoradiography. *Experientia,* 35:1240–1241.
2. Grant, L. D., and Stumpf, W. E. (1973): Localization of ³H-estradiol and catecholamines in identical neurons in the hypothalamus. *J. Histochem. Cytochem.,* 21:404.
3. Grant, L. D., and Stumpf, W. E. (1975): Hormone uptake sites in relation to CNS biogenic

amine systems. In: *Anatomical Neuroendocrinology,* edited by W. E. Stumpf and L. D. Grant, pp. 445–464. Karger, Basel.

4. Heritage, A. S., Grant, L. D., and Stumpf, W. E. (1977): ^{3}H-estradiol in catecholamine neurons of rat brain stem: Combined localization by autoradiography and formaldehyde-induced fluorescence. *J. Comp. Neurol.,* 176:607–630.

5. Heritage, A. S., Stumpf, W. E., Sar, M., and Grant, L. D. (1979): ^{3}H-dihydrotestosterone in catecholamine neurons of rat brain: Combined localization by autoradiography and formaldehyde-induced fluorescence. *J. Comp. Neurol. (in press).*

6. Keefer, D. A., Stumpf, W. E., and Sar, M. (1973): Topographical localization of estrogen-concentrating cells in the rat spinal cord following ^{3}H-estradiol administration. *Proc. Soc. Exp. Biol. Med.,* 143:414–417.

7. Keefer, D. A., Stumpf, W. E., and Petrusz, P. (1976): Quantitative autoradiographic assessment of ^{3}H-estradiol uptake in immunocytochemically characterized pituitary cells. *Cell Tiss. Res.,* 166:25–35.

8. Kim, Y. S., Stumpf, W. E., Sar, M., and Martinez-Vargas, M. C. (1978): Estrogen and androgen target cells in the brain of fishes, reptiles, and birds: Phylogeny and ontogeny. *Am. Zool.,* 18:425–433.

9. Martinez-Vargas, M. C., Gibson, D. B., Sar, M., and Stumpf, W. E. (1975): Estrogen target sites in brain of the chick embryo. *Science,* 190:1307–1308.

10. Pfaff, D. W., and Keiner, M. (1973): Atlas of estradiol-concentrating cells in the central nervous system of the female rat. *J. Comp. Neurol.,* 151:121–158.

11. Rees, H. D., Stumpf, W. E., and Sar, M. (1975): Autoradiographic studies with ^{3}H-dexamethasone in the rat brain and pituitary. In: *Anatomical Neuroendocrinology,* edited by W. E. Stumpf and L. D. Grant, pp. 262–269. Karger, Basel.

12. Sakumoto, T., Tohyama, M., Sato, K., Kimoto, Y., Kinugasa, T., Tanizawa, Ò., Kurachi, K., and Shimizu, N. (1978): Afferent fibre connections from lower brain stem to hypothalamus studied by the horseradish peroxidase method with special reference to noradrenaline innervation. *Exp. Brain Res.,* 31:81–94.

13. Sar, M., and Stumpf, W. E. (1971): Androgen localization in the brain and pituitary, *Fed. Proc.,* 30:363.

14. Sar, M., and Stumpf, W. E. (1973): Neurons of the hypothalamus concentrate ^{3}H-progesterone or metabolites of it. *Science,* 182:1266–1268.

15. Sar, M., and Stumpf, W. E. (1977): Distribution of androgen target cells in rat forebrain and pituitary after ^{3}H-dihydrotestosterone administration. *J. Steroid Biochem.,* 8:1131–1135.

16. Sar, M., and Stumpf, W. E. (1978): Progestin-target cells in rat brain and pituitary. *J. Steroid Biochem.,* 9:877.

17. Sar, M., and Stumpf, W. E. (1978): Simultaneous localization of neurophysin I and ^{3}H-estradiol in hypothalamic neurons using a combined autoradiographic and immunohistochemical technique. *J. Histochem. Cytochem.,* 26:227.

18. Sar, M., and Stumpf, W. E. (1979): A combined thaw-mount autoradiography and immunohistochemistry technique for simultaneous localization of steroid and peptide hormones: Localization of androgen in gonadotropes, thyrotropes and pituicytes of rat pituitary. *Cell Tiss. Res. (in press).*

19. Sheridan, P. J., Sar, M., and Stumpf, W. E. (1973): Localization of ^{3}H-estradiol or its metabolites in the CNS of neonatal female rat. *Program 55th Meet. Endocrine Soc.,* p. 67.

20. Sheridan, P. J., Sar, M., and Stumpf, W. E. (1974): Autoradiographic localization of ^{3}H-estradiol or its metabolites in the central nervous systems of the developing rat. *Endocrinology,* 94:1386–1390.

21. Silver, M. A., Jacobovitz, D., Crowley, W., and O'Donohue, T. (1978): Retrograde transport of dopamine-β-hydroxylase antibody (ADβH) by CNS noradrenergic neurons: Hypothalamic noradrenergic innervations. *Anat. Rec.,* 190:541.

22. Stumpf, W. E., and Roth, L. J. (1966): High resolution autoradiography with dry-mounted, freeze-dried, frozen sections. Comparative study of six methods using two diffusible compounds, ^{3}H-estradiol and ^{3}H-mesobilirubinogen. *J. Histochem. Cytochem.,* 14:274–287.

23. Stumpf, W. E. (1968): Estradiol concentrating neurons: Topography in the hypothalamus by dry-mount autoradiography. *Science,* 162:1001–1003.

24. Stumpf, W. E., and Sar, M. (1969): Distribution of radioactivity in hippocampus and amygdala after injection of ^{3}H-estradiol by dry-mount autoradiography. *Physiologist,* 12:368.

25. Stumpf, W. E. (1970): Estrogen-neurons and estrogen-neuron systems in the periventricular brain. *Am. J. Anat.,* 129:207–218.
26. Stumpf, W. E. (1971): Autoradiographic techniques and the localization of estrogen, androgen and glucocorticoid in pituitary and brain. *Am. Zool.,* 11:725–739.
27. Stumpf, W. E., and Sar, M. (1973): Hormonal inputs to releasing factor cells, feedback sites. *Progr. Brain Res.,* 39:53–71.
28. Stumpf, W. E. (1975): The brain: An encodrine gland and hormone target, an introduction. In: *Anatomical Neuroendocrinology,* edited by W. E. Stumpf and L. D. Grant, pp. 2–8. Karger, Basel.
29. Stumpf, W. E., Sar, M., and Keefer, D. A. (1975): Atlas of estrogen target cells in rat brain. In: *Anatomical Neuroendocrinology,* edited by W. E. Stumpf and L. D. Grant, pp. 104–119. Karger, Basel.
30. Stumpf, W. E., and Sar, M. (1977): Steroid hormone target cells in the periventricular brain: Relationship to peptide hormone-producing cells. *Fed. Proc.,* 36:1973–1977.
31. Stumpf, W. E., and Sar, M. (1977): Localization of steroid receptors in relation to function. In: *Endocrinology, Vol. 1,* edited by V. H. T. James, pp. 18–22. Excerpta Medica, Amsterdam.
32. Stumpf, W. E., and Sar, M. (1978): Anatomical distribution of estrogen, androgen, progestin, corticosteroid and thyroid hormone target sites in the brain of mammals: Phylogeny and ontogeny. *Am. Zool.,* 18:435–445.
33. Stumpf, W. E., and Sar, M. (1978): Estrogen target cells in fetal brain. In: *Hormones and Brain Development,* edited by G. Dörner and M. Kawakami, pp. 27–33. Elsevier, Amsterdam.
34. Stumpf, W. E., and Sar, M. (1979): Glucocorticosteroid and mineral corticosteroid hormone target sites in the brain: Autoradiographic studies with corticosterone, aldosterone and dexamethasone. In: *Interactions within the Brain-Pituitary Adrenocortical System,* edited by M. Jones and M. F. Dallman. Academic Press, New York *(in press).*
35. Stumpf, W. E., and Sar, M. (1979): Steroid hormone target cells in the extrahypothalamic brain stem and cervical spinal cord: Neuroendocrine significance. *J. Steroid Biochem. (in press).*
36. Warembourg, M. (1973): Etude radioautographique des retroactions centrales des corticosteroids ^{3}H chez le rat et le cobaye. In: *Neuroendocrinologie de l'Axe Corticotrope, Vol. 22,* pp. 41–66. INSERM, Paris.

The Endocrine Functions of the Brain,
edited by Marcella Motta.
Raven Press, New York © 1980

4

Role of Receptors in the Mechanism of Steroid Hormone Action in the Brain

Thomas G. Muldoon

Department of Endocrinology, Medical College of Georgia, Augusta, Georgia 30912

Exposition of the molecular occurrences which immediately ensue from introducing a steroid hormone into a cell of a responsive tissue is unfolding rapidly through the efforts of an extensive army of investigators. For the most part, the groundwork has been laid through the utilization of organ systems which respond acutely and predictably with a readily measurable endpoint. Thus the uterus of the rat served as a prime model for the study of estrogen action, the chick oviduct for progesterone action, and the rat ventral prostate for androgen action. Given the enormous complexity and interplay of systems within the brain, the task of sorting out individual responses to specific hormones is an overwhelmingly formidable one. Nevertheless, significant progress has been made along these lines through an interdisciplinary attack combining the efforts of biochemists, endocrinologists, physiologists, anatomists, molecular biologists, psychobiologists, and pharmacologists.

Inevitably, this type of approach created a great deal of confusion and apparent contradiction when attempts were made to interrelate the various findings. Profound differences in such critical parameters as tissue source and preparation, the nature and temporal facets of the chosen hormonal action, and experimental methodology and interpretation compounded an already complex situation. Moreover, the invalidity of many crude studies in the light of subsequent, more sophisticated analyses, had to be perceived and dealt with. Because of these difficulties, no comprehensive picture of hormone action in the brain has yet evolved. The aim of this chapter is to present a current analysis of a single aspect of this problem, i.e., the mechanisms which exist within discrete portions of the brain and pituitary gland for specific uptake and retention of steroid hormones. Wherever possible, attempts are made to cut across disciplinary lines and correlate the findings with existing data on the multifarious effects of hormonal steroids in these tissues.

CURRENT CONCEPTS OF THE ROLE OF RECEPTORS IN STEROID HORMONE ACTION

As an immediate result of the remarkable progress of steroid chemistry during the 1930s, clinical assessment of the actions of steroid hormones throughout the body became a flourishing field of investigation, and endocrinology began to develop and mature into a discrete science. Data accumulated at a rapid pace and, without any unified concept or mechanism on which to base the findings, most ideas about steroid hormone action were derived from empirical clinical observations. It was recognized quite early during this period that various interrelationships existed among the actions of steroid hormones and protein hormones, especially as related to ovulation and reproductive function in general. Moreover, the brain was clearly implicated as a primary endocrine control center through which a wide variety of hormonal signals were funneled and were sorted out by unknown means. It was conceded that, in order to modulate functions in remote endocrine glands, the brain needed some mechanisms for the detection of their secretory products.

In 1960 Jensen and Jacobson (65) published a set of experimental data that was to have a profound effect on the development of knowledge concerning the biochemistry of steroid hormone action. Their basic observation was that, following administration to rats *in vivo,* estrogens were specifically retained only within tissues that were known to be responsive to these hormones. Subsequent studies from a number of laboratories rapidly established that the retention mechanism was related to the presence within target tissue cells of proteins which were capable of binding steroid hormones with very high affinity and steroidal specificity, and which were referred to as receptors. The demonstration that sucrose density gradient ultracentrifugational analysis could be utilized to measure and study the properties of these receptors (161) was another early landmark in solving the mystery of the basis for hormonal responsiveness. A multitude of papers has been published to date on the characteristics of receptors for all classes of steroid hormones in many tissues and species, and it is noteworthy that a common mechanistic thread runs through all these diverse systems.

A simple representation of the primary mechanism of action of estrogens is shown in Fig. 1; for details, the reader is directed to several excellent reviews (9,19,64). The estradiol molecule (E) encounters little or no resistance as it traverses the plasma membrane of the cell. Within the cytoplasmic compartment, a limited number of receptor molecules (R) are available for binding the steroid to form an estrogen–receptor complex, thereby effectively eliminating the possibility of these steroid molecules diffusing back out of the cell. In *in vitro* experiments performed at low temperatures, the sequence of events terminates here, and the complex can be shown to sediment in sucrose gradients as either an 8S (in low-salt-containing buffer) or a 4S (in high-salt buffer) moiety. *In vivo* or *in vitro* studies performed at elevated temperatures permit detection of subsequent events, the first of which is rapid transformation of the complex

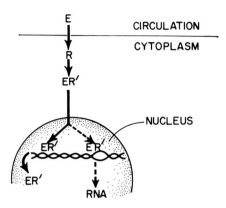

FIG. 1. Initial events in the cellular action of estradiol. (E) estrogen. (R) cytoplasmic receptor. (ER') transformed complex. The solid and dotted lines within the nucleus represent alternate routes for the estrogen–receptor complex following translocation into the nucleus.

to a new form (ER'), which sediments at 5S. The latter complex, in contrast to the untransformed species, accumulates within a short period of time in the cell nucleus; indeed, a highly plausible conceptualization of the intracellular mechanism of steroid hormone action holds that the sole function of the steroid molecule resides in its ability to modify the cytoplasmic receptor to a form capable of transformation into the nucleus. The intricacies of this problem were considered at some length by Gorski and Gannon (53). Having gained access to the nucleus, the estrogen–receptor complex is strongly attracted to the genomic apparatus, where it affects genetic expression by alteration of the nature and extent of transcription. Differential synthesis of RNA species engenders different patterns of protein synthesis, and a logical extrapolation, although still without a great deal of unequivocal substantiation, is that these translational products direct the ultimate display of hormonal activity. As indicated in Fig. 1, the amount of ER' which enters the nucleus can be far in excess of that amount which binds to specific "acceptor" sites in the chromatin structure. The possible functional significance of the surplus nuclear complexes has been virtually ignored, although recent developments are lending support to the existence of extragenomic actions of steroid hormones.

The simplistic nature of the depiction of the intracellular pathway of estrogen biodynamics in Fig. 1 becomes readily apparent when one begins to examine the fate of radiolabeled estradiol within target tissue cells as a function of time following introduction of the hormone. Data from our laboratory were interpreted in the light of existing information from a number of other groups to yield a composite description of intracellular receptor dynamics (26). Our model for this system is presented in Fig. 2. Regulation of the level of cytoplasmic receptor (R_C) is most powerfully effected by estradiol itself (22), and the mechanisms of this control are threefold. Cells of estrogen-responsive tissues have the constitutive property of synthesizing estrogen receptors, a process enhanced

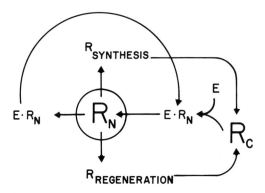

FIG. 2. Dynamics of estrogen–receptor turnover within a responsive cell. The major pools of intracellular receptor are the cytoplasmic (R_C) and the nuclear (R_N) forms. These species are continually fluctuating relative to each other by closely interlocking mechanisms, including: translocation of the activated estrogen–receptor complex ($E \cdot R_N$) into the nucleus and subsequent reappearance of the complex in the cytoplasm for reutilization; *de novo* synthesis of receptor and appearance in the cytoplasm in a form capable of interacting with estradiol; and regeneration of cytosol receptor by a microsome-mediated dissociation of nuclear complexes.

by estradiol and which follows the genetic expression route outlined in Fig. 1. As the circulating levels of estradiol increase, a portion of the nuclear estrogen–receptor complex ($E \cdot R_N$) may be seen to leave the nucleus and become associated with the microsomes for a period of time, after which the intact complex is liberated into the cytoplasm and can immediately re-enter the nucleus, thus describing a reutilization phenomenon. This second nuclear uptake phase was recently confirmed in the mouse uterus (84). When the endogenous titer of estradiol is high, nuclear receptor complexes are dissociated, allowing regeneration of receptor into the cytoplasm, where it is capable of being reactivated by another molecule of estradiol.

Any definitive delineation of the mechanism of estrogen action must take into account the three methods of synthesis, reutilization, and recycling by which receptor levels are regulated by the hormone itself. The implied capability of the steroid hormone to act in ways other than alteration of genetic transcription is reflected in several examples of estrogen action which do not involve nuclear sites of primary action (89,122,130).

This brief description of the role of receptors in steroid hormone action has been limited to the estrogen–receptor system. For the most part, the basic considerations are similar for all steroid hormones, but some very significant differences do exist which are fundamental to our understanding of receptor biodynamics. Irrespective of quantitative variances, which are manifold, the following qualitative differences in receptor systems are essential considerations:

1. Some steroid hormones are metabolized within the cell to more active intermediates or to products with different hormonal properties. Testosterone

is reduced to 5α-dihydrotestosterone (DHT), which has a higher affinity for the androgen receptor than does testosterone. Testosterone can also be aromatized to estradiol, which can utilize the estrogen receptor in the same cell. Estradiol, on the other hand, undergoes minimal metabolic conversion within target cells. Recent evidence favors intracellular reduction of progesterone in a manner totally analogous to that of testosterone.

2. To further complicate the situation, considerable cross reactivity is exhibited with respect to the steroidal specificity of binding. Androgens and estrogens are capable of binding to each other's receptor with varying degrees of affinity; under certain circumstances it can even be demonstrated that androgens can effect nuclear translocation of the estrogen receptor. Progesterone and glucocorticoids can also share common receptors. Although antagonism is often observed between the actions of progesterone and testosterone, it is probably the result of competition for 5α-reductase rather than binding to commonly recognizable receptor binding sites.

3. Progesterone receptors are uniquely dependent on the presence of estrogen through an estrogen–receptor-mediated induction process. In the brain, recent evidence (which is discussed later in the chapter) indicates that this may not be a ubiquitous requirement.

4. Receptor lability is a decisive factor for quantifying and relating various steroid hormone–tissue interactions. All receptors are thermolabile, but to varying degrees. The estrogen receptor is inherently more stable than either the androgen or the progesterone receptor. Glucocorticoid–receptor complexes are relatively unstable because the affinity of binding is several orders of magnitude lower than that of the estrogen–receptor complex. In general, the binding of a ligand enhances the thermostability of a receptor, and the more firmly bound the ligand, the greater the amount of protection. For this reason it is sometimes necessary to use synthetic steroids with very high avidity for given receptors in order to satisfactorily measure receptor levels [e.g., the synthetic progestin, promegestone (R-5020), allows measurement of progesterone receptors in samples where levels are too low to be quantified using the less strongly bound natural progesterone].

5. Steroid hormones bind with high affinity to proteins other than receptors. These proteins may be intracellular or of plasma origin; they are different for different steroids; and they often vary in amount as a function of the stage of development of the organism. The presence of these binding proteins limits accessibility of the hormone to its receptor and imposes severe methodological restrictions on accurate analysis of receptor levels and properties. A related problem is the *in vivo* difference in rate of penetration of steroid hormones from the blood into discrete areas such as the brain. It is important to realize that these and many other of the factors mentioned herein dictate the need for great caution when attempting to correlate data obtained from *in vivo* and *in vitro* studies.

RECEPTORS FOR ESTROGENS, ANDROGENS, PROGESTERONE, AND CORTICOSTEROIDS THROUGHOUT THE BRAIN AND PITUITARY

Two recent reviews on steroid hormone receptors in the brain (71,108) provide a scholarly and elegant exposition of various aspects of this field. This chapter therefore is geared toward an overview of the subject, with particular emphasis on the most recent developments available to the author.

To the uninitiated, a survey of the literature on hormone receptors in the brain can be confusing because no uniformity exists among investigators with respect to method of dissection and the terminology used to describe discrete portions of the brain. Except where specifically noted otherwise, this chapter is limited to studies performed using the rat and, for clarification and consistency, areas of the brain are designated in accordance with their localization as shown in Fig. 3. The telencephalic structures are those with the lower numbers, and the diencephalic region is roughly numbers 7 through 11, with the midbrain area encompassing the mesencephalic reticular formation structure and interpe-

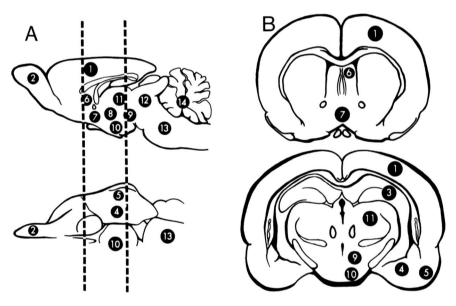

FIG. 3. Loci of steroid hormone receptors in the central nervous system. **A:** The rat brain is shown in: midsagittal view *(top)* and external view of the right hemisphere from the ventral surface *(bottom)*. **B:** Frontal cross section through the left vertical dotted line in **A** *(top)*, and frontal cross section through the right vertical dotted line in **A** *(bottom)*. The numbered regions are: (1) cerebral cortex; (2) olfactory bulb; (3) hippocampus; (4) amygdala; (5) pyriform cortex; (6) septum; (7) anterior hypothalamic-preoptic area; (8) middle hypothalamus; (9) posterior hypothalamus; (10) basal hypothalamus and median eminence; (11) thalamus; (12) midbrain (lower portion containing mesencephalic reticular formation structure and interpeduncular region); (13) pons; and (14) cerebellum.

duncular region. The pituitary gland is not included as part of the brain but is considered in the ensuing discussion because of its vital connections and correlations with the brain receptor systems. Autoradiographic studies are not dealt with herein, as they are expertly handled in Chapter 3 and in a recent review (159).

Tissue Localization and Subcellular Distribution

In an extensive analysis of estrogen binding in the rat brain, McEwen and Pfaff (111) established that specific saturable retention of radiolabeled estradiol 2 hr after intraperitoneal injection was highest in the pituitary, hypothalamus, preoptic region, and septum. Significantly lower retention was observed in amygdala, hippocampus, cerebellum, and brainstem. Maurer and Woolley (104) subsequently showed that anterior hypothalamic-preoptic area and basal hypothalamic-median eminence regions concentrate estradiol 10 and 8 times, respectively, more extensively than cortical tissue; the tissue/cortex ratio was 1.0:2.3 for other brain areas. To demonstrate estrogenic specificity, these authors used competition studies with diethylstilbestrol (DES), which is known to bind with very high affinity to estrogen receptors. Competition was very effective in anterior hypothalamic-preoptic and basal hypothalamic-median eminence areas, less effective in septum and dorsal hypothalamus, and totally absent in cortex, hippocampus, brainstem, and plasma.

McEwen and Pfaff (111) found very little difference in the uptake patterns among male, female, neonatally castrated male, and neonatally androgenized female rats, with the female hypothalamus showing a greater amount of uptake than the hypothalamus of any other group. Interestingly, Barley et al. (7) reported that cytosol binding in the female hypothalamus is most prevalent in the anterior portion of the gland, whereas the male favors the middle hypothalamus; moreover, in castrate males the pattern shifts to that of the female. The question of sex differences in estrogen retention in the brain has been raised many times and has still not been laid to rest. Conflicting reports appear which must be the result of dissimilarities in experimental conditions, particularly that of the time periods used in the studies. Although some investigators (94,105) confirm the absence of a sex distinction in brain uptake, others (166) find diminished uptake into nuclei of pituitary and hypothalamus of androgenized females. Circulating testosterone levels may be an important factor, since nuclear estradiol binding in the anterior hypothalamic-preoptic, basal hypothalamic-median eminence, amygdaloid, and septal regions (but not in the anterior pituitary) is lower in intact males and testosterone-treated castrate males than in untreated castrate males (131). Significantly, Whalen and Olsen (179) recently reported that isolated hypothalamic chromatin from castrate male rats specifically binds estradiol less extensively than do analogous female samples at short intervals after injection; this is more a measure of kinetics than extent of binding and seems to be a true sex-related difference. There appears to be little variance in tissue distribution of specific binding of estradiol in the cytoplasmic or nuclear compartment of the cell 1 hr after steroid administration (103), but long-term changes in cytosol/nuclear distribution are different in the anterior pituitary from those in the hypothalamus (116).

The rat posterior pituitary contains specific estradiol binding sites, as demonstrated *in vivo* and *in vitro* in cytosol and nuclear fractions (133). Oddly, however, estradiol–receptor complexes cannot be demonstrated by sucrose gradient analysis in this tissue (71). Since oxytocin levels rise following estradiol administration, a possible function of neurohypophyseal receptors is predesignated. The pineal gland, known to be involved in reproductive function (140), contains estrogen (16) and androgen (17) receptors. This system is particularly intriguing because these receptors, at least in part, are regulated through a β-adrenergic receptor by noradrenergic neurons originating in the superior cervical ganglia.

Metabolism of estradiol has not been extensively examined in relation to brain receptors, since it is not an intracellular event of any considerable magnitude. However, mindfulness of peripheral conversion to estrone prompted two studies of interest. Luttge (95) found that, following injection of tritiated estradiol, the estradiol accumulates in a specific saturable manner in the anterior portion of the diencephalon, whereas estrone becomes localized nonspecifically in the posterior diencephalon–anterior mesencephalon area. In sheep, receptors are present in the pituitary which bind estradiol and estrone with equivalent high affinity, but no specific binding of estrone can be detected in the hypothalamus (183). Clearly, more investigation is warranted in this area.

Specific androgen binding in the brain occurs at a markedly reduced level compared to that of estradiol, but the pattern of tissue distribution is similar. In fact, early studies hinted that the same receptor system might function for both classes of steroid, but subsequent competition studies dispelled this notion. Testosterone binding sites sensitive to competition by unlabeled testosterone are located in highest concentration in the pituitary, septum, hypothalamus, and preoptic area, with somewhat lower levels in the amygdala and olfactory bulb (112). In addition, testosterone-specific binding has been discerned in the cerebellum (50), cerebral cortex, and pineal of mature and immature rats (58), although the presence in immature cortex is controversial (60).

Testosterone and DHT manifest similar distribution patterns, with the possible exception of cortex binding (151), although the authors suggest that the low specific activity of their radiolabeled DHT might not have allowed detection of the cortical binding. There is no evidence for the existence of separate brain receptors for testosterone and DHT. Following injection of [³H]testosterone, large amounts of testosterone and DHT are found in nuclei of brain and pituitary. Moreover, testosterone 5α-reductase is present in brain primarily in the diencephalic regions where binding activity is most pronounced (106). The nuclear binding of DHT is saturable and can be inhibited by the presence of cyproterone acetate but not by progesterone, corticosterone, or 5β-DHT (90). Cytoplasmic uptake and nuclear retention are enhanced following attenuation of circulating androgen levels by castration or adrenalectomy; this accounts for the fact that early studies on intact animals failed to uncover the existence of androgen receptors in neural tissue.

The steroidal specificity of androgen binding in brain tissues has been problematic enough to indicate that heterogeneous groups of binding sites are being studied by various workers. Naess (125) reports the following decreasing order of affinity, similar in hypothalamus, preoptic area, and cortex: DHT > testosterone > cyproterone acetate > progesterone > androstenedione > estradiol. Attardi et al. (4) find that estradiol binds quite well to the DHT-specific receptors (10% of the affinity of DHT), but DHT does not interact at all with the estradiol-specific binding proteins. Other investigators report that testosterone, DHT, 3β-androstanediol, and estradiol compete with greater than 85% efficacy for hypothalamic androgen receptors, and that 3α-androstanediol and progesterone compete to better than 50% (60). It is difficult to correlate these findings with the lack of estradiol binding reported by several other groups. There may be some indication that androgen receptor specificity changes with age, but even such an unusual happenstance as this would not resolve all the conflicting reports. Fox (48) presented interesting data concerning the existence of two classes of high-affinity binding sites in mouse hypothalamic-preoptic area. One set of sites binds estradiol; the other binds estradiol, testosterone, and DHT. In normal animals the latter sites exhibit partial blocking of estradiol binding by testosterone. The same group of investigators found that hypothalamic-preoptic receptors for estradiol and testosterone can be separated by differential elution from DNA-cellulose columns (182), a promising approach for future separation and analysis of receptor systems in the central nervous system. It is perhaps of significance at this point to present a cautionary note emphasized by studies in our laboratory (172), as well as in others (126). In anterior pituitary cytosol, testosterone and DHT appear to bind with equal affinity, whereas DHT binds twice as well as testosterone in hypothalamic cytosol. In actuality, 50% of the DHT in the pituitary cytosol is being converted to 3α-androstanediol during the competition experiment, but minimal conversion occurs in hypothalamic cytosol. Correction for the interference by metabolism yields the same relative affinities of the hormones for the receptor of either tissue.

Using an electron capture technique, Robel et al. (142) determined that intracellular pituitary testosterone is concentrated 25 times over plasma levels, whereas intracellular pituitary DHT concentration is equal to that of plasma. In the hypothalamus the intracellular level of either hormone is five times that of plasma. This is a good indication that testosterone is an important androgen in neural tissue. It would be remiss at this point not to mention that estradiol accumulates in limbic and hypothalamic cell nuclei following [3H]testosterone administration to neonatal animals; this is discussed in a later section on developmental function of steroid receptors.

Localization of specific progesterone binding sites in the brain was investigated during the early 1970s with puzzling results (177). Retention of progesterone appeared highest in mesencephalic areas (interpeduncular region and reticular formation structures) with somewhat lower levels in the anterior and posterior hypothalamus, and pretreatment with estrogen had no effect on progesterone retention in any portion of the brain (177). Additionally, pretreatment with unlabeled progesterone did not influence subsequent accumulation of radiolabeled progesterone in the brain (97,176). One hour after injection of progesterone, less than 5% of the compound localized in the median eminence was confined to the nuclear fraction (153). Thus the highest binding was observed in areas lacking estrogen receptor activity; it was not inducible by estrogen; it was not saturable; and it did not appear to result in translocation to the nucleus. There remained little reason to suspect that the species being monitored truly represented progesterone receptors.

Only recently has the enigma of progesterone receptors in the brain been resolved, thanks to the utilization of promegestone (R-5020). This synthetic progestin binds specifically to progesterone receptors (without interference binding to corticosteroid-binding globulin) with higher affinity than progesterone itself. Use of this compound allowed discovery of saturable, estrogen-dependent, steroid-specific cytoplasmic (45,75) and nuclear (12,119) receptors for progesterone in the brain and pituitary. The order of greatest nuclear accumulation was: pituitary > hypothalamus > preoptic area = cortex > midbrain (12). It was satisfying to find a distribution similar to that of estrogen receptors, since it was difficult to imagine how diencephalic estrogen action could produce mesencephalic progesterone receptors (assuming universality of the phenomenon of estrogen inducibility of these receptors). The binding specificity of the receptors followed the order: R-5020 > norgestrel $\simeq$ norprogesterone > progesterone >> estradiol, with no detectable affinity for testosterone, dexamethasone, or aldosterone (119).

In clear contradistinction to the receptors discussed thus far, corticosterone is preferentially accumulated by nuclei of the rat hippocampus, with lower levels in the amygdala and septum, and very little binding in pituitary, hypothalamus, preoptic area, or cortex (107). This distribution confirms earlier autoradiographic analysis (141,170). Nuclear retention of dexamethasone is high in the pituitary and that of corticosterone low (109). In pituitary cytosol *in vitro,* unlabeled dexamethasone does not compete for [³H]corticosterone binding, but either unlabeled dexamethasone or unlabeled corticosterone competes equally for [³H]dexamethasone binding. Furthermore, cortisol, desoxycorticosterone, and progesterone, but not estradiol, bind to the sites for which corticosterone is able to compete (107). These data are consistent with high levels of corticosteroid-binding globulin (or similar proteins) in the pituitary cytosol (which binds corticosterone but not dexamethasone) and significant receptor concentration (which has an appreciable attraction for dexamethasone). In *in vivo* studies, [³H]dexamethasone accumulation in cell nuclei is distributed quite uniformly throughout the brain; *in vitro,* however, its ability to compete for specific nuclear [³H]corticosterone binding sites in the hippocampus is much greater than would be predicted from the *in vivo* results. This may be partially attributable to an impeded rate of penetration from the blood into the brain, or *in vivo* to metabolic events. The heterogeneity of the nature and intracellular localization of glucocorticoid receptors in the brain (100) also cannot be overlooked as a factor contributing to the differential patterns of retention of these steroids.

Mineralocorticoid interactions with brain receptors have not been accorded much attention. In a study by Anderson and Fanestil (2), the antagonist SC-9420, known to compete for renal aldosterone receptors, blocked whole brain cytosol binding of either [^{3}H]aldosterone or [^{3}H]dexamethasone, when used in large molar excess. Equimolar concentrations of SC-9420, however, competed for [^{3}H]aldosterone binding but not for that of [^{3}H]dexamethasone, indicating some degree of selectivity for presumably different sites. A recent autoradiographic analysis of aldosterone retention (44) favors preferential binding in hippocampal nuclei, with lesser amounts in anterior pituitary glandular cells, septum, amygdala, and pyriform cortex. Further analysis is required before the latter studies can be accepted as evidence for mineralocorticoid-specific receptors, since competition by unlabeled steroids was not investigated. The function of putative aldosterone receptors in the brain remains obscure.

Ontogeny

In the neonatal rat, estrogen receptors are detectable in the anterior hypothalamus, preoptic area, amygdala, and cerebral cortex (98,175). The cortical receptors sediment as 8S complexes, with transformation to a 5S nuclear form and evidence for translocation (98), just as do the receptors from the limbic tissues. The fate of the cortical receptors as the animal grows toward adulthood is highly contentious. It has been reported variously that these receptors are (58,125) or are not (60,98) present in immature and adult rats. The investigators are apparently measuring different binding species, since they publish widely divergent data on the steroidal specificity of the "receptors" they are describing.

The estrogen receptor levels in the hypothalamus increase gradually from day 5 to 7, then more rapidly at 2 to 3 weeks of age, to a full adult complement at about 28 days of age (6,72,73). Testosterone does not bind to neonatal cortex but does bind to the hypothalamus in neonatal animals, although competition experiments indicate that the latter binding utilized the estrogen receptor, rather than suggesting the presence of neonatal androgen receptors (174). This final point, however, is challenged by Kato's observation (69) of steroid-specific testosterone-binding proteins in female rat hypothalamus at 3 or 7 days of age. In support of this finding, diencephalic tissue of the neonatal rat is capable of reducing testosterone to DHT (18). Kato (70) also reported androgen-specific binding sites in neonatal male rat hypothalamus by sucrose gradient measurements, and the ontogenic development of this receptor class closely parallels that of the estrogen receptors.

Apposite to these considerations of receptor ontogeny is the work of Attardi and Ohno (5) in the mouse. In this species, brain estrogen receptor levels appear to be constant during the first 3 weeks of age, an interval during which DHT receptor levels increase threefold. There are no sex differences in this pattern. The concentration of DHT receptors in the hypothalamic-preoptic area is higher than that in the cortex, and the differential remains constant as the receptor levels rise with age. However, the ratio of hypothalamic-preoptic to cortical estrogen receptors increases 12-fold during this period. Thus the deceptive constancy of total estrogen receptor concentration must arise from counterbalancing increases in hypothalamic-preoptic sites and decreases in cortical binding sites.

Progesterone receptor activity has not been reported in the brains of young animals, in keeping with the presumptive requirement for a background of estrogen priming being causal to the appearance of these receptors. Along these lines, however, MacLusky and McEwen (99) recently made the unprecedented observation that R-5020-specific progesterone receptors in the midbrain, amygdala, cortex, and hippocampus of the rat are not sensitive to estrogen induction as are tissue receptors for this hormone in hypothalamic-preoptic area, pituitary, and uterus. Glucocorticoid receptors in the rat brain mature between 10 and 21 days of age (30). This temporal pattern coincides nicely with the maturation of the adult response to stress and the development of circadian periodicity in circulating glucocorticoid levels, implicating these receptors in pituitary-adrenal regulatory mechanisms.

Physicochemical Characteristics

Of all facets of our knowledge of steroid hormone receptors, the information on their physical nature easily ranks highest with respect to uniformity and continuity. With few exceptions, receptors for different types of steroid hormones are similar molecules, and standard receptor methodology is generally applicable to all of them, with some modifications being necessary as a result of the way in which the receptors interact with their ligands. Relatively little is known about the receptors in higher brain centers, but appreciable work has been done on the characterization of hypothalamic and anterior pituitary receptors. Kato (71) reviewed and presented much of his data on these receptors. Work from our laboratory on pituitary estrogen receptors was also covered in some detail recently (123). Therefore no attempt is made herein to present a comprehensive analysis of this subject; rather, the basic principles and results are set forth for the single system of the hypothalamic (or pituitary) estrogen receptors, and selective correlations are made with other steroid hormone receptors.

Gel filtration and centrifugation through a sucrose density gradient are the simplest and most commonly employed methods for demonstrating some basic features of steroid receptors. The patterns of [^{3}H]estradiol-incubated cytosol elution from Sephadex G-200 are shown in Fig. 4 for male and female hypothalami. The results tell us that all the macromolecule-bound estrogen elutes as a single symmetrical peak followed later by a sharp rise in radioactivity represent-

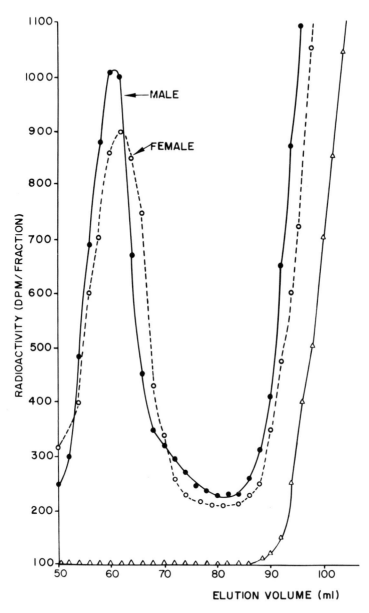

FIG. 4. Sephadex G-200 gel filtration patterns of male and female hypothalamic cytosol following incubation with [³H]estradiol. A cytosol sample incubated with [³H]testosterone is also shown. No macromolecular-bound testosterone species is detectable in these tissues from intact animals. The elution patterns shown are exclusive of the column void volume.

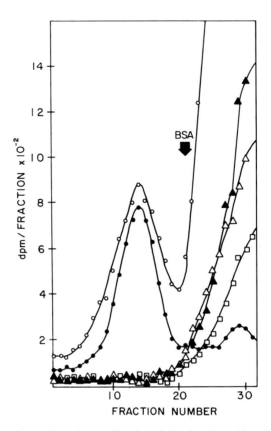

FIG. 5. Sucrose density gradient ultracentrifugal analysis of male and female rat hypothalamic cytosol following addition of [³H]estradiol. Cytosol samples were applied to a 5 to 20% linear sucrose gradient prepared in low-salt buffer and centrifuged for 15.5 hr at 45,000 rpm. The estrogen–receptor complex had a sedimentation constant of 8S and was undetectable in samples which had been incubated in the presence of either pronase or a large molar excess amount of unlabeled estradiol. (BSA) bovine serum albumin.

ing unbound steroid which percolates slowly through the gel. Thus the presence of a single rather heavy species is indicated, and the quantity is not different between the sexes. Sucrose gradient analysis of similar samples in a low-salt gradient (Fig. 5) also shows a single peak sedimenting in the 8S region, totally displaceable by unlabeled estradiol and abolished by addition of a proteolytic enzyme to the cytosol. The absence of male–female disparity is confirmed.

Steroid–receptor interactions are customarily defined in terms of the concentration of receptor binding sites and the affinity of the receptor for the ligand. Data may be obtained by saturation binding analysis, whereby a constant level of receptor is exposed to increasing amounts of steroid, the mixture is allowed to come to a predetermined equilibrium state, and the protein-bound and unbound steroid species are separated by any of a number of methods and quantified. For more details, the reader is referred to the recent review by Clark and Peck (28). The results may then be graphically dissected in several ways. The use of the direct linear plot method (43,184) is exemplified in Fig. 6 for hypothalamic and anterior pituitary cytosol. With this procedure, values can be read directly from the graph. The binding affinity is high for the two samples and identical at $K_A = K_D^{-1} = 4 \times 10^{10}$ M^{-1}. There are 10 times as many receptor binding sites in the anterior pituitary (1.5×10^{-10} M) as in the hypothalamus (2.0×10^{-11} M).

This simple introduction is the basis on which virtually all receptors are initially studied, permitting definition in terms of finite binding capacity, high affinity of interaction, and steroidal specificity. Tissue specificity is an additional

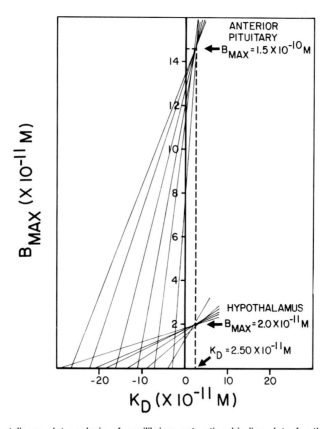

FIG. 6. Direct linear plot analysis of equilibrium saturation binding data for the interaction between estradiol and the cytoplasmic estrogen receptors from rat anterior pituitary and hypothalamus. Cytosol was incubated to equilibrium with varying amounts of [³H]estradiol. Specific binding was assessed, and molar quantities of unbound and bound steroid at each point were plotted in K_D, B_{max} space. Values for the equilibrium dissociation constant and the respective concentrations of receptor binding sites were read directly from the graph, as indicated.

factor to determine within an organism before all physicochemical criteria of designation as "receptors" are satisfied. The other, far more difficult touchstone is functionality, which is considered in some detail in other portions of this chapter. Other methodologies (e.g., electrophoretic analysis, behavior in gradients under different buffer conditions, effects of heat and other denaturing devices, and competitive effects of other compounds) are refinements of the basic characterization procedures. Perhaps the most revealing of any other major types of additional analyses are measurements of kinetic parameters. Association and dissociation rate kinetics have been determined with several receptor systems and afford information on receptor nature, turnover, lability, and metabolism which cannot be obtained from equilibrium studies. This subject has been discussed for the pituitary estrogen receptors (123).

In immature rats the estrogen receptor of the anterior pituitary and hypothalamus is present primarily as a 4S to 5S species, as opposed to the predominant 8S form in the adult (157). Smaller forms of receptor have been recognized for some time (158), but only recently have they received much attention. It seems that in many tissues receptors exist as 4S forms during periods when hormonal levels are relatively low and transform to 8S moieties after stimulation. This has been observed for progesterone receptors in chick oviduct (162) and recently for mouse mammary tissue estrogen receptors (124). Essentially overlooked was the earlier observation by Milgrom et al. (117) that guinea pig progesterone receptors in the uterus oscillate between 4S and 7S forms during the normal estrous cycle.

Nuclear receptors may be extracted with high-salt concentrations from nuclei following incubation with [³H]estradiol-charged cytosol at elevated temperatures. Uterine nuclear receptors sediment in a high-salt sucrose gradient at about 5S (66). Those of the anterior pituitary and hypothalamus have been reported as somewhat larger (74,121), although other researchers (11,49,88) detect a 5S nuclear species for these tissues also.

Receptors with greatest specificity for either testosterone (148,149) or DHT (71,126) have been discovered in anterior pituitary and hypothalamic tissue. There is disagreement among investigators as to the absolute concentration of these binding sites, but there is a consensus that they are present at about 10-fold lower concentration than the estrogen receptors in the respective tissues, and the anterior pituitary is found by all groups to contain five times as many androgen receptors as the hypothalamus. The preoptic area contains roughly the same concentration of androgen receptors (1.3×10^{-15} moles/mg protein) as does the hypothalamus (60,126), and the cortex has only slightly fewer. It is significant in terms of steroid feedback control that androgen receptors in the anterior pituitary are localized primarily within the gonadotropes (150). Androgen receptors are notoriously more labile than estrogen receptors and appear to require the presence of ligand to maintain their functionality. Estrogen receptor levels in most tissues remain high long after ovariectomy, but androgen receptors disappear quite rapidly following castration.

As discussed elsewhere, progesterone receptors in the brain were only recently characterized to any extent. In agreement with progesterone–receptor systems in other tissues, those in the brain are rather sensitive to *in vitro* conditions, and stabilization by addition of glycerol to buffers is a recommended procedure. The progesterone receptors in some areas of the brain require estrogen stimulation for their existence, whereas those in other areas do not (99). In the estrogen-primed immature female rat, the anterior pituitary level of progesterone receptors has been reported as 9.6 fmoles/mg protein in one study (75) and 140 fmoles/ mg protein in another (119). In an analysis of the anterior pituitary receptors in estrogen-treated ovariectomized-adrenalectomized animals, the level was 273 fmoles/mg protein (99). Hypothalamic levels were generally lower but also varied widely depending on the researcher. It is possible that the dose responsiveness of the progesterone receptor induction by estradiol has not yet been sufficiently defined to allow comparison between one experimental protocol and another. Cerebral cortex progesterone receptors, not inducible by estradiol, are present at levels similar to those in the hypothalamus (99). In the few instances tested to date, cytosol progesterone receptors in the brain were characterized as 6S to 7S binding proteins, and a 5S nuclear form was detected in the anterior pituitary (45,75). There is no statistically significant basis for assuming differences among progesterone–receptor, androgen–receptor, and estrogen–receptor interactions with respect to binding affinity.

Glucocorticoid receptors differ from those of other steroid hormones, principally in the lower affinity with which they bind naturally occurring ligands. In the brain, corticosterone–receptor interactions are half-maximally saturated at concentrations two to three orders of magnitude lower than those required for other receptor systems. The equilibrium binding affinity is slightly higher for the nuclear complex ($K_A = 5 \times 10^8$ M^{-1}) than for the cytoplasmic complex ($K_A = 1$ to 2×10^8 M^{-1}) (113). Dexamethasone and triamcinolone acetonide are synthetic glucocorticoids known to bind to glucocorticoid receptors with high affinity but have little propensity for corticosterone-binding plasma proteins. The use of these steroids seemed logical, therefore, for examination of brain corticoid receptors. It was found, however, that these compounds interact with binding proteins in the brain and anterior pituitary in a manner different from that of corticosterone. Either triamcinolone (135,171) or dexamethasone (35) interacts with a very labile receptor species in the pituitary, thereby conferring on this receptor a great deal of stability. Corticosterone binds to a much greater extent in the pituitary cytosol and to more stable proteinaceous moieties, but does not impart appreciable additional stability to the binder. In pituitary cell nuclei, the situation is reversed quantitatively, with the synthetic steroids having the higher capacity (35). *In vivo,* nuclear retention of corticosterone is of a higher magnitude than that of dexamethasone in the hippocampus (109). Possible explanations for this unusual behavior among these ligands include the presence of several cell types within a specified tissue sample having different patterns of uptake for the steroids, different classes of glucocorticoid-binding sites with varying specificities of binding, or dissimilarities in the intracellular nuclear uptake and processing machinery for different compounds.

Role in Development

When testosterone is administered to a neonatal female rat, she develops into a sterile adult with permanent acyclicity of gonadotropin secretion. This imprinting of a male pattern on a female organism in this manner is referred to as neonatal androgenization. Since it is now known that estrogen and androgen receptors are present in the neonatal rat brain, it is of considerable interest to determine the role of these receptors in sexual differentiation of the brain.

A great deal of information has been amassed on the induction of neonatal androgenization, much of which tends to support the concept that testosterone is active by virtue of aromatization to estradiol, which then acts through its own receptors. There are, however, some recent findings which strongly suggest involvement of androgens and androgen receptors. The basic arguments supporting both views on the subject are summarized in Table 1. It should be noted that "androgenization" denotes anovulatory sterility, and "defeminization" refers to the sex behavioral response of lordosis. There can be little doubt from the data that aromatization is an important feature of the overall response, since the nonaromatizable DHT is ineffective in inducing androgenization and

TABLE 1. *Evidence for receptor mediation of sexual differentiation of the brain*

Estrogen Receptors

1. Estradiol is at least equally as effective as testosterone in inducing androgenization (39,40).
2. Estradiol receptors are present in the neonatal rat brain (98,175).
3. DHT is ineffective as an androgenizing agent.
4. Following administration of radiolabeled testosterone, high levels of radiolabeled estradiol are found in nuclei of hypothalamus and limbic tissues (91,173).
5. Accumulation of [^{3}H]estradiol following administration of [^{3}H]testosterone is reduced by the presence of an inhibitor of aromatization (92).
6. The ability of testosterone to abolish development of gonadotropin cyclicity in female rats can be negated by an inhibitor of aromatization (167).
7. The antiestrogen MER-25 administered simultaneously to neonatal animals with either estrogen or androgen prevents defeminization (41,42). (See also item 6 below.)

Androgen Receptors

1. Androgen receptors are found in neonatal rat brain (69).
2. Estradiol is ineffective as an inducer of androgenization in testicular-feminized animals, which have very low androgen receptor levels but normal estrogen receptor concentration (4,127).
3. Serum transcortin and several hepatic steroid-interconverting enzymes have distinct brain-modulated patterns in the male which are imprinted by testosterone on the female rat but not by estradiol (36).
4. Progesterone protects against neonatal androgenization of the female (78).
5. The antiestrogen CI-628 prevents testosterone-induced androgenization but not defeminization (110).
6. MER-25 does not block steroid induction of defeminization (15,61).

since nuclear radiolabeled estradiol can account for as much as half of the recovered radioactivity following injection of radiolabeled testosterone.

It is also becoming clear that androgen receptors are involved in androgenization. The protective effect of progesterone is most readily interpretable on the basis of its interaction with androgen receptors (for which it is known to have an appreciable attraction), since it does not interact with estrogen receptors and since progesterone receptors do not appear to be present at this stage of development. The most convincing argument for androgen receptor involvement is the information obtained from studies on testicular-feminized mice and rats (4,127). These animals are acutely deficient in brain androgen receptors but have normal complements of estrogen receptors; in spite of this fact, neonatal administration of estradiol does not result in masculinization, as would be expected if only estrogen receptors were mediating the response. The likeliest explanation for the mechanism of neonatal androgenization incorporates participation by androgens and estrogens (probably with overlapping steroidal specificities). Testosterone is effective because it binds to the androgen receptor and is converted to estradiol, which utilizes the estrogen receptor. Estradiol works by virtue of its recognition of both androgen–receptor and estrogen–receptor binding sites. A satisfying corollary to this proposal is the observation that estradiol synergizes with DHT to elicit male sexual behavior in castrate male rats (87). The possible role of androgens in suppressing development of female characteristics in normal perinatal rats (51) is supported by the observation (167) that normal male rat copulatory behavior is seen in adult male rats treated neonatally with an inhibitor of aromatization.

A number of investigators (25,104,105,111) report that uptake of estradiol into the brain and pituitary of adult neonatally androgenized female rats is not different from that seen in normal adult rats, although the uterine uptake is decreased by about half. On the surface, then, it appears that estrogen receptors are not involved in stimulation of ovulation. Vertes and King (166) claimed diminished nuclear estradiol uptake in the pituitary and hypothalamus of androgenized animals, and suggested (165) that the defect in these rats resides in abnormal acceptor binding within the nucleus, resulting in an inability to properly synthesize new receptor and a concomitant loss of estrogen responsiveness. An alternate proposal (115), similar in concept, is that lack of periodic estrogen stimulation in androgenized animals leads to degeneration of the existing receptors and loss of responsivity. These working hypotheses have been refuted on the basis of analysis of receptor dynamics, which is discussed in the section Dynamics of Turnover, below.

An interesting concept has arisen for an alternate mechanism as the foundation of sexual differentiation. Toran-Allerand (163) described the actions of testosterone and estradiol on enhancement of neurite outgrowth of mouse hypothalamic explant cultures. This suggests that differential axonal growth may be important in brain development and is certainly an area to be watched with intense interest.

There is little evidence to indicate that there are critical changes in receptor levels or activity announcing the onset of puberty. More likely, the receptor systems are fully primed at this time, awaiting their signal from a steroidal messenger. Indeed, it has been amply demonstrated that injection of estradiol can promote precocious puberty in the female rat (138,155). A single notable exception to this idea is the study by Monbon et al. (120) to the effect that, although the actual amount of testosterone binding in male hypothalamus and pituitary does not change with sexual maturation, the pituitary has a higher affinity for testosterone in the mature, in contrast to the immature, animal. No analogous change in affinity was seen in hypothalamic samples over the same age increment.

Regulation of Receptor Activity

Estrogens are capable of inducing synthesis of their own receptors and, as such, represent the most active regulators of these proteins. The details of this process are discussed in the following section of this chapter, dealing specifically with receptor dynamics. For now, considerations are limited to the modulatory effects of thyroid hormones, androgens, and progesterone on estrogen receptor activity.

Thyroxine has a specific stimulatory effect on estrogen receptors in the anterior pituitary but not in the hypothalamus or uterus (23,123). Recent evidence (124) indicates that this effect is also seen in mouse mammary tissue. The anterior pituitary and hypothalamic responses are compared in Table 2. Thyroidectomy leads to decreased anterior pituitary receptor levels, and this effect can be totally reversed by administration of thyroxine to an approximate euthyroid state. Further augmentation of thyroid hormone levels to a distinctly hyperthyroid state dramatically increases receptor concentration in the ovariectomized, but not

TABLE 2. *Thyroid hormone effects on anterior pituitary and hypothalamic estrogen receptors*

Treatment	Estrogen receptor concentration (% of vehicle control)	
	Castrated	Intact
Anterior pituitary		
Thyroidectomy	62	58
Thyroidectomy + thyroxine	106	112
Intact + thyroxine	177	116
Hypothalamus		
Thyroidectomy	97	92
Thyroidectomy + thyroxine	93	98
Intact + thyroxine	108	92

Thyroidectomy and/or ovariectomy were performed 3 or 2 weeks prior to sacrifice, respectively. Thyroxine treatment in these experiments consisted of 300 μg L-thyroxine per day for 5 days.

in the intact, animal, suggesting an additional undefined control point. To study the effect under more clearly definable conditions, castrate estrogen-primed rats were used to maintain relatively constant levels of circulating estrogen. As may be seen in Fig. 7, thyroxine once again enhanced receptor activity in the anterior pituitary, but not in the uterus or hypothalamus of the control castrate animals. Estrogen treatment led to diminished receptor levels in all tissues because the animals were killed 5 hr after the final injection of estradiol, a period when cytosol receptors are still appreciably depleted. A combination of thyroxine and estradiol pretreatment effectively reversed the action of estradiol in the anterior pituitary but not in the other tissues. Thus the effect of thyroxine was not simply the result of the removal of endogenous estradiol from the circulation. Manipulation of thyroid hormone levels had no effect on hypothalamic estrogen receptor levels under any of the conditions used. The results observed in the pituitary were unrelated to the ability of the receptor system to respond to estradiol or to competition for estrogen–receptor binding sites.

Androgens are capable of causing estrogen–receptor translocation into the nucleus (144,147). This important observation has now been explained in molecular terms (85,172) as the result of low-affinity interactions of androgens with the receptors, which can be measured accurately only in kinetic, rather than equilibrium, experiments. The initial velocity of the formation of an estradiol–receptor complex is inhibited selectively by androgens in a competitive, dose-

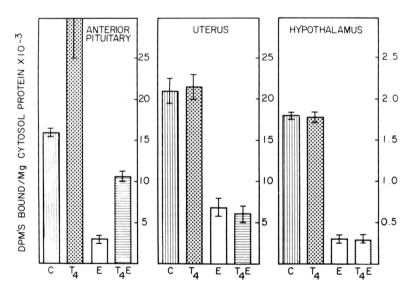

FIG. 7. Influence of thyroxine and estradiol alone and in combination on cytosol estrogen receptor binding in the anterior pituitary, hypothalamus, and uterus of ovariectomized rats. Animals were injected with vehicle (C), 300 μg thyroxine (T_4), or 0.2 μg estradiol (E) or thyroxine plus estradiol (T_4E) for 5 days. They were then sacrificed 5 hr after the final injection, and specific receptor binding in the target tissue cytosols was measured.

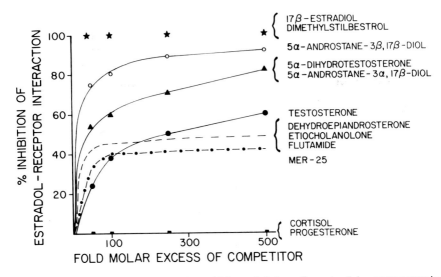

FIG. 8. Effectiveness of various types of steroidal agents in impeding estradiol–receptor complex formation in anterior pituitary cytosol. The putative competitors listed at the right were added to cytosol at levels in excess of [³H]estradiol, as specified on the abscissa. Association rate experiments were then performed, and the initial velocity of the [³H]estradiol–receptor interaction in the presence of the inhibitor was compared to that in its absence.

related process which does not involve any variation in concentration of the receptors. The efficacy of various types of hormonal agents in impeding estradiol–receptor interaction is presented in Fig. 8. Strong androgens are effective as: 5α-androstane-3β,17β-diol > DHT = 5α-androstane-3α,17β-diol > testosterone. Weak androgens and antiandrogens (represented by flutamide) and weak antiestrogens (MER-25) inhibited in a fashion independent of their concentration. The strong antiestrogen dimethylstilbestrol was as potent as estradiol in blocking complex formation, and the complete failure of cortisol or progesterone to inhibit the reaction was testament to the specificity of the effect.

A direct influence of progesterone on estrogen receptors was indicated by the autoradiographic results of Anderson and Greenwald (1), which illustrated that, whereas preinjection of unlabeled estradiol resulted in decreased subsequent [³H]estradiol labeling in the brain and anterior pituitary, preinjection of progesterone diminished labeling only in the brain. Cortisone acetate under the same conditions had no effect on uptake into either tissue. The state of the animals apparently dictates the nature of the progesterone effect. In estrogen-primed animals, progesterone injection leads to a decrease in the estradiol retention capability of the uterus, pituitary, and hypothalamus (21). Long-term administration of progesterone to ovariectomized rats, however, causes increased retention of estradiol in the median eminence, anterior hypothalamic-preoptic area, amygdala, and cerebral cortex (93). These antipodal actions of progesterone are reflected in its biological actions on estrogen-dependent processes.

Hypophysectomy leads to decreased estradiol uptake in all brain structures (111). An interesting putative explanation is that gonadotropins, through the "short-loop" feedback mechanism, maintain estrogen receptors at a level which effectively allows estrogen inhibition of gonadotropin secretion.

Control of estrogen receptors in the pineal differs somewhat with age in an extraordinary manner (16). In adult rats, superior cervical ganglionectomy depresses nuclear estrogen–receptor complex accumulation, and this can only partially be reversed by estradiol treatment. Isoproterenol permits return of receptor levels to basal control values. Thus the receptors in these mature animals are regulated by estradiol and by noradrenergic neuron stimulation. In the 6-day-old rat, however, nuclear receptors can be demonstrated and respond to estrogen stimulation. Since this is a period during which most pinealocytes lack innervation, the ontogenesis of the receptors appears to be similar to that in other tissues (i.e., under the influence of estrogen), whereas the neuronal influence is superimposed at a later stage of life.

The most obvious regulator of androgen receptor activity is the nature of the hormone which serves as ligand, since the direction and extent of metabolism and interconversion of androgens provide a series of compounds of widely divergent affinities for the receptor. This general phenomenon does not require extensive elaboration; a few interesting examples from the literature should suffice to exemplify its role in androgen action. Whalen et al. (178) demonstrated that cyproterone acetate had no effect on testosterone binding in pituitary, brain, or muscle, whereas it reduced similar binding in seminal vesicles. This was consonant with an inability of cyproterone acetate to inhibit androgen-mediated sexual behavior in male rats and an ability to cause regression of seminal vesicles of mature animals. It was considered possible that the antiandrogen interfered with a metabolite formed in the seminal vesicles but not in the other tissues examined. Androstenedione seemed a likely candidate, but subsequent work from the same group (180) showed that this metabolite is formed in the brain as well as in the seminal vesicles. It is still conceivable that another metabolite is involved in this differential competitive effect. Pertinent to these considerations is the provocative suggestion that pituitary hormones can alter the metabolism of testosterone in some androgen-responsive tissues and not in others (36).

It might be reasonably assumed that since DHT has a greater affinity for brain receptors than does testosterone the former steroid represents the preferred ligand and testosterone utilizes the receptor only when DHT levels are low. However, this is a dangerous assumption because there are instances in which testosterone is not capable of assuming the role of the missing DHT. Walsh et al. (168) convincingly showed that patients lacking 5α-reductase manifest normal development of testosterone-responsive, but not DHT-responsive, male reproductive organs.

An important related issue with respect to control of androgen receptor activity is the increased stability of the receptors elicited by ligand binding. This has played a crucial role in detection and characterization of brain androgen receptors. In intact adult or chronically orchidectomized male rats, brain androgen receptor levels are undetectable, explaining why early studies using these animal models suggested that such receptors did not exist. It appears that endogenous androgen levels in intact animals are sufficiently high to obviate measurement of unoccupied binding sites. At 1-day postcastration, these levels abated to the point where receptors could be readily quantified and analyzed. At longer intervals after castration, the labile ligand-free receptors have been metabolically degraded to such a degree that the levels again fall below the detectable range.

The question of alteration of binding affinity with animal age has been addressed apropos of the androgen receptor. The saturation binding level of male pituitary and hypothalamus is not different between immature and mature rats, but the pituitary of the mature animal has a higher affinity for testosterone than that of the immature animal; this age-dependent change in binding activity is not observed in the hypothalamus (120). Preliminary results (52) also indicate that a decrease in affinity for DHT occurs with cytosol receptors of cortex, amygdala, hypothalamus, and anterior pituitary as male animals increase in age from young adult to 18-month-old animals. Interestingly, in this study, the opposite effect was observed in female rats, i.e., the affinity for DHT increased with age.

The extensive overlap in tissue distribution of estrogen and androgen receptors in the brain permits the inference that the two steroid hormones at least partially share the same binding sites; if true, this would represent a very important control mechanism of receptor activity. McEwen et al. (112) showed that uptake of [³H]estradiol into the pituitary, hypothalamus, and preoptic area is suppressed by unlabeled estradiol more effectively than by unlabeled testosterone, whereas uptake of [³H]testosterone within the same structures is diminished to an equal extent by either unlabeled hormone (except in the pituitary, where testosterone is the preferential competitor). This can be interpreted as a demonstration of two sets of binding sites, one having greater affinity for estradiol than testosterone, and the other having equal affinity for either steroid or a greater affinity for testosterone. It then appears that the brain receptor mechanisms for these two hormones operate more as a function of the relative concentrations of estrogen and androgen than by independent detection of the absolute concentration of each.

Thyroxine increases the concentration of glucocorticoid receptors in the anterior pituitary (83), reminiscent of its action on estrogen receptors in the same tissue (23). In addition, thyroxine treatment also results in elevated levels of the transcortin-like anterior pituitary corticosterone binder. Estradiol also increases the concentration of the latter protein but has no effect on glucocorticoid receptors in either the anterior pituitary or hippocampus (34). It seems likely that the transcortin-like protein competes with the receptor for corticosterone, thereby effectively interfering with steroid translocation into the nucleus and ensuing biological activity. This protein is largely localized in association with the anterior pituitary cell plasma membranes and is not simply a plasma contaminant (82). The situation here is analogous to that of androgen-binding protein, which is found only in the testis and seems to serve as a storage depot for maintenance of high tissue levels of the steroid.

Dynamics of Turnover

If one accepts the central role of receptor interactions in the mechanism of steroid hormone action, it follows that the single most critical feature of the system is the level and activity of the cytoplasmic receptor, since this is the sole determinant of the initial uptake capacity of the cell and therefore controls all subsequent intracellular events leading to the hormone's action. In this section, a number of the biochemical features of receptor dynamics in the cell are explored as they function to regulate tissue responsiveness. In the succeeding section, various physiological aspects of this phenomenon are presented.

The regulation of estrogen receptor activity by estradiol itself has been characterized as a triphasic phenomenon dependent on circulating estrogen levels (Fig. 2). For considerations at this point, the entire process representing reappearance of receptor following depletion of cytosol (by nuclear translocation) is referred to as replenishment. The basic features of the depletion–replenishment response are presented in Fig. 9 for the anterior pituitary and hypothalamus of different rat models, as summarized from work in this laboratory (22,25,26). Patterns

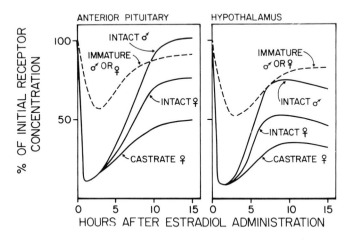

FIG. 9. Depletion–replenishment process of estrogen receptor turnover in the anterior pituitary and hypothalamic cytosol of various rat models. The patterns shown are schematic representations derived from numerous experimental determinations. Animals were injected with estradiol at time zero and killed in groups at various times thereafter. Specific binding capacity of the cytosols for estradiol was assessed at each interval and expressed as the percentage of the zero-time concentration determined in nonestrogen-treated animals at the time of the injections into the respective experimental groups.

are similar in both tissues. Following injection of estradiol, it is possible to effect virtually complete translocation of receptor into the nucleus. Reappearance is always observed at a faster rate and to a greater extent in mature male rats than in mature females, but the sex differences in replenishment are not manifest in immature animals. This might indicate that androgens play a role in the replenishment process, although this idea has not been tested. It is of some interest that depletion is much more difficult to achieve in immature animals than in adults. In a recent preliminary report, Chouknyiska and Vassileva-Popova (20) state that testosterone receptor dynamics in male rat anterior pituitary, hypothalamus, cortex, and testes change with age, the variation between the 10-day-old and the mature animal being of particular significance. They claim differential rates of formation of cytosol testosterone–receptor complexes with age, a unique observation to date.

Intact adult animals of either sex invariably replenish receptors to a higher level than do castrate animals, exemplifying the regulatory control by endogenous estrogen concentration. As measured by autoradiography, the cellular turnover of estrogen is appreciably faster than that of the receptors, being maximal at 2 hr and decreasing by a third every subsequent 2 hr, so that there are no labeled cells remaining after 8 hr (1). In this vein, it is pertinent to mention the unusual finding that it is not possible to significantly deplete hippocampal cytosol of glucocorticoid receptors with steroid, even under conditions where nuclear translocation is known to transpire (164); this suggests an uncommonly rapid mechanism for receptor replenishment. There may, however, be some other factors involved here since, following adrenalectomy, a rapid phase of increased corticosterone binding is seen concomitant with the fall in endogenous corticosterone. The second phase, however, probably representing receptor synthesis, occurs only between 12 hr and 5 days after adrenalectomy (114).

Progesterone and DHT have some effects on estrogen receptor depletion and replenishment. Hsueh et al. (63) discerned that administration of progesterone during the phase of estrogen-induced replenishment caused a rapid and dramatic fall in the replenishment rate in the rat uterus. With respect to depletion and 15-hr replenishment levels, the modulatory influences of progesterone and DHT are illustrated in Fig. 10. In the anterior pituitary, hypothalamus, and uterus, pretreatment with either progesterone or DHT diminished the extent of depletion caused by an estradiol injection, progesterone being slightly more effective than the androgen. When interpreting the effect on replenishment shown in Fig. 10, it must be kept in mind that these values are the sum of the actual amount replenished plus the amount not originally depleted. With this in mind, DHT had no appreciable effect on replenishment in any of the three tissues. Progesterone was effective only in the anterior pituitary, where it caused a marked decrease in the replenishment level.

Studies of the dynamics of estrogen receptor turnover have provided some valuable information concerning the mechanism of actions of antiestrogens. These compounds generally compete well for receptor binding sites, the order

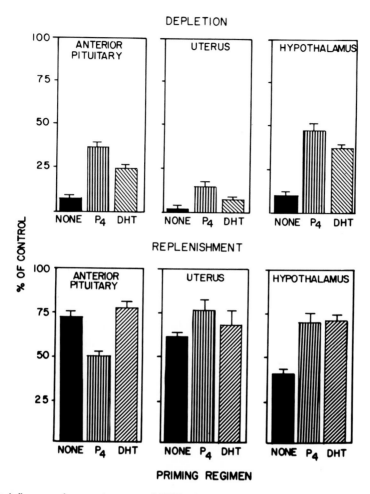

FIG. 10. Influence of progesterone and DHT priming on estrogen receptor depletion and replenishment in estrogen-sensitive tissues. Ovariectomized animals received progesterone (8 mg/kg body weight) or DHT (4 mg/kg body weight) each day for 5 days. On day 6 these animals, plus a group of vehicle-injected control animals, were administered a single injection of estradiol. At 1 hr (depletion) or 15 hr (replenishment) thereafter the animals were sacrificed, and the cytosol receptor content was determined in anterior pituitary, uterus, and hypothalamus. Values are expressed as a percentage of zero-time receptor concentration for each group.

of effectiveness for several of them in the anterior pituitary and hypothalamus being: dimethylstilbestrol = estradiol > CI-628 > MER-25 (24). Antiestrogens are intrinsically estrogenic (160), probably by virtue of their ability to bind and translocate estrogen receptors when estrogen levels are low (143,146). In the presence of estradiol, some antiestrogens inhibit translocation of the estradiol–receptor complex, whereas others appear to be ineffective in this respect (76,146). Kurl and Morris (86) recently measured depletion 24 hr after injection of different antiestrogens and found that their order of effectiveness was: clomiphene > tamoxifen > MER-25 for depleting receptors in the pituitary and uterus, but that it was exactly the reverse order when assessed in amygdala and anterior and middle hypothalamus. It is quite possible that this puzzling result is occasioned by differential capabilities for penetration into the brain, as appears to be the case for CI-628 (24).

Long-term nuclear retention of antiestrogen–receptor complexes, with accompanying suppression of the replenishment process, is a tenable explanation for the mechanism of action of some antiestrogens (29), stressing the importance of intact depletion–replenishment machinery for normal hormonal responsiveness. This is not, however, the only mechanism of action of antiestrogens. Large differences in rates, amounts, tissue specificity, and sex specificity of various facets of depletion and replenishment resulting from administration of different antiestrogens (24) clearly accentuate the need for careful individual examination of the subcellular events induced or altered by each compound.

In a previous section of this chapter, the curious failure to discern differences in receptor levels of animals after neonatal androgenization was described, as were several hypothetical explanations involving defective receptor dynamics in this animal model. An analysis of this system (25) revealed that the processes of depletion and replenishment are quite dramatically altered in the anterior pituitary of the neonatally androgenized female rat. In the anterior pituitary, hypothalamus, and uterus, the 1-hr depletion level is similar for untreated and

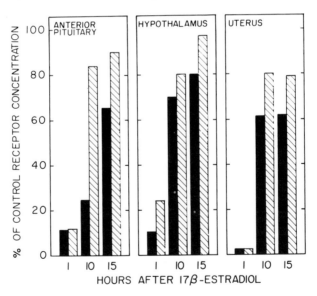

FIG. 11. Influence of estradiol administration on cytosol receptor concentration in target tissues from normal *(solid bars)* and neonatally androgenized *(hatched bars)* female rats. Receptor depletion (1 hr after estradiol), rate of replenishment (10-hr level), and extent of replenishment (15-hr level) were measured at intervals after injection of estradiol. (From ref. 25.)

androgenized animals (Fig. 11). The 10- and 15-hr replenishment levels in the uterus and hypothalamus are slightly elevated in the androgenized animals, but no gross differences in the patterns are observed (Fig. 11). Worth mentioning in this regard is the observation by Lobl (94) that neonatal androgenization alters the mechanism of nuclear estradiol uptake in the uterus (from an unsaturable to a saturable system) but has no effect on the hypothalamic nuclear receptors, which remain unsaturable. In the anterior pituitary, the rate (10-hr level) and the extent (15-hr level) of replenishment are markedly enhanced in the androgenized animals as compared to the intacts. The replenishment pattern in the androgenized female is not significantly different from that of the intact male; thus the imposition of a male pattern of tonic gonadotropin secretion by neonatal androgenization of the female rat is paralleled by the establishment in these animals of a male pattern of intracellular receptor dynamics. These results may have implications in elucidation of the molecular components underlying the physiological manifestations of androgenization.

Functional Correlates

There are various cogent arguments in favor of a role for estrogen and androgen receptors as mediators in the control of sexual behavior and gonadotropin secretion by these hormones. The localization of these receptors throughout the brain is similar for the two gonadal steroid groups and is quite highly specific. The receptors are confined to discrete topographical areas, centering around neurons in the diencephalic structures known to be instrumental in control of reproductive function (8,54,57,59,152) including gonadotropin secretion and sexual behavior, as well as in specific neurons of various telencephalic nuclear structures. The localization of androgen and estrogen receptors in the anterior pituitary is also consistent with a direct action of estrogens (13,38,55,128) and androgens (68,79,118) on the anterior pituitary gland. Moreover, sexual differentiation of the brain at an early stage of postnatal development in the rat, leading to the superimposition of tonicity on an established pattern of cyclicity, is generally conceded to be mediated through the hypothalamus directly or through higher brain centers feeding impulses into the hypothalamus; in animals at this stage, heavy neuronal labeling of estrogen or androgen is seen in the preoptic area and mediobasal hypothalamus. Other evidence for a link between receptor binding and reproductive function is based on empirical observations of correlations in temporal, dose-dependency, and specificity parameters with physiological responses and is therefore of an unavoidably indirect and inductive nature.

The role of estrogen receptors in the normal ovulatory process has been examined in a number of ways. Measurement of anterior pituitary levels throughout the rat estrous cycle (154) revealed that the receptor concentration decreases by 40% from diestrus-2 to proestrus (while estrogen levels are rising) and replenishes during estrus. White et al. (181) found similar oscillations in hypothalamic estrogen receptor levels during the estrous cycle. In studies from our laboratory,

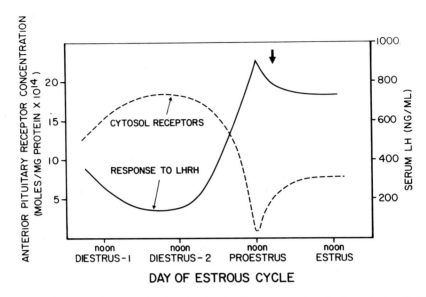

FIG. 12. Correlation between levels of cytosol estrogen receptors in the anterior pituitary and responsiveness of the pituitary to LHRH stimulation. Groups of animals were killed at various times throughout the normal estrous cycle 10 min after administration of LHRH into the carotid artery. Serum LH levels were determined as an indicator of responsiveness of the pituitary, and estrogen receptor content of pituitary cytosol was measured at the same intervals. The composite diagrams are derived from multiple determinations at 10 to 12 intervals during a single cycle. The arrow represents the time of the preovulatory gonadotropin surges.

we attempted to correlate anterior pituitary and hypothalamic receptor levels with anterior pituitary responsiveness to exogenous luteinizing hormone releasing hormone (LHRH) at various times during the estrous cycle (56) and with the events following administration of pregnant mare's serum gonadotropins (PMSG) to 30-day-old immature female rats to induce an initial ovulation in a predictable manner (132).

The patterns of pituitary responsiveness to LHRH and the simultaneous values for cytosol estrogen–receptor levels are shown in Fig. 12 (actual data are found in ref. 56). The sensitivity to LHRH rises dramatically from noon of diestrus-2 to noon of proestrus, an interval during which cytosol estrogen receptors are precipitously depleted by translocation into the nucleus. The preovulatory surges of LH and FSH occurred 6 to 8 hr after maximal depletion. A steady phase of receptor replenishment was seen from late proestrus to mid-diestrus-2, during which time responsiveness to LHRH steadily diminished. Clearly, an inverse relationship exists between efficacy of LHRH in releasing gonadotropin and cytoplasmic estrogen receptor levels in the anterior pituitary; stated in a perhaps more functionally significant way, there is a positive correlation between nuclear receptor content and LHRH responsiveness. Hypothalamic

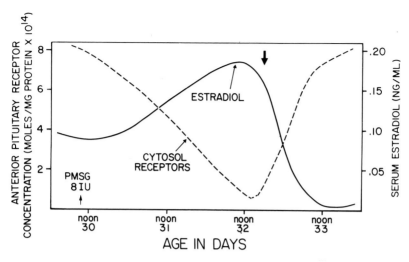

FIG. 13. Serum estradiol and anterior pituitary cytosol estrogen receptor levels during initial ovulation induced by PMSG in immature female rats. On the morning of day 30 of age, animals were administered 8 IU of PMSG and were sacrificed in groups at 10 to 12 intervals spaced throughout the successive 3 days. The preovulatory surges of FSH and LH occurred on the afternoon of day 32, at a time when estradiol levels were falling and receptors were recovering from a full depletion phase.

cytosol receptors were also measured in these studies and were found to vary in a manner similar to that in the anterior pituitary.

When immature animals at 30 days of age were induced to ovulate with PMSG, serum estradiol and anterior pituitary estrogen receptors fluctuated during the 3 successive days following PMSG administration as depicted in Fig. 13 and as described in detail in Parker et al. (132). In this animal model, serum estradiol levels rose and fell in almost exact opposite fashion from those of cytosol estrogen receptors in the anterior pituitary (and hypothalamus, not shown). In addition, the preovulatory gonadotropin surge again occurred shortly after maximal depletion, when nuclear activity of estradiol was presumably at its highest level. In the normal rat estrous cycle, Clark et al. (27) observed parallelism between anterior pituitary nuclear estrogen–receptor complex concentration and secretory rate of estradiol. All these data strongly implicate anterior pituitary and hypothalamic estrogen receptors in the critical sequence of events leading to gonadotropin secretion and ovulation.

Several lines of evidence converge to give a plausible receptor-based explanation for differences between male and female rats in their tonic versus cyclic pattern of gonadotropin secretion. The suppression of cyclicity by androgens appears to be expressed through alterations at the level of the hypothalamic-preoptic region of the brain (54). Flerko et al. (47) reported that estradiol uptake by the hypothalamus of castrate female adults was higher than that in neonatally androgenized castrate female adults (the latter group having chronically elevated androgen levels). In a similar vein, McEwen and Pfaff (111) demonstrated that normal female hypothalamus retains more estradiol than either normal male or neonatally androgenized female hypothalamus. These results suggest that androgen-mediated reduction in the sensing mechanism for estradiol in the hypothalamus might underlie the action of the androgen in abolishing gonadotropin cyclicity. This concept is reinforced by the observation that estradiol binding in the male favors the middle hypothalamus, whereas that in the female prefers the anterior hypothalamus (7). Thus the simple scarcity of anterior hypothalamic-preoptic receptors in the male may create a situation in which threshold stimulation of cyclicity cannot be achieved. Closely related in concept is the fact that hypothalamic chromatin binding of estradiol is lower in males than in females (179). Finally, an intriguing sexual dichotomy in receptor specificity in the brain lends further credence to this idea. McEwen et al. (112) demonstrated that competition by unlabeled estradiol for [^{3}H]testosterone uptake is greater in the male brain than in the female; on the opposite side of the coin, however, competition by unlabeled testosterone for [^{3}H]estradiol uptake is greater in females than in males. These data indicate not only that different classes of androgen and estrogen binding sites exist with differential specificities, but that there is an additional sex-related variation imposed on these differences.

The direct involvement of androgen receptors in the brain in regulation of sexual behavior is perhaps most simply and elegantly authenticated by the fact that testicular feminized mice, deficient in androgen receptors, show virtual absence of male sex behavior (129). This same animal model provides convincing reason to believe that androgen receptors play a role in control of gonadotropin secretion. Very high levels of DHT or testosterone administered to castrate testicular feminized rats suppress gonadotropin levels, apparently by utilization of the very low levels of androgen receptors present in these animals (127). A cautionary note is in order here concerning metabolism, as exemplified by the inability to demonstrate appreciable receptor binding of androstenedione, even though this steroid is as effective as testosterone in maintaining sexual behavior in castrate male animals (134). It is probable that androstenedione is effective by virtue of its metabolic conversion to testosterone.

The recency of the characterization of brain progesterone receptors has not allowed extensive experimentation on correlations between receptor activity and physiological implications. This is also of exceptional difficulty with progesterone because it, more than perhaps any other steroid hormone, is dependent on the hormonal milieu for the very nature of its action on a given tissue. There can be little doubt, however, that neural loci of progesterone action are vital to its role in sexual behavior and reproductive biology.

Sexual receptivity in the female rat is initially facilitated by the action of progesterone on neural tissue previously primed with estrogen (10,136), whereas higher levels of progesterone can inhibit receptivity. The intracerebral site of this action of progesterone is not clear. Some workers (96,145) find progesterone activity following implantation into mesencephalic, but not diencephalic, structures. Others (137,169) report activity only following implantation into the hypothalamic-preoptic or mediobasal hypothalamic area. It may be that experimental manipulations were different enough in these studies to allow arrival at opposing conclusions. It must also be kept in mind that, although R-5020-detectable receptors are localized primarily in the diencephalic brain, appreciable progesterone uptake of a "nonspecific" nature occurs in mesencephalic tissue. It is entirely conceivable that the unsaturable binding sites in the latter regions are also of physiological import through a mechanism differing in some or all respects from the receptor concept.

Progesterone injection to cycling rats can either advance or delay ovulation, depending on the time at which it is administered (46,185). Both of these actions are mediated through neural influences, in the general vicinity of the preoptic-hypothalamic-median eminence region (80,156). It appears that these activities may be related to an ability of progesterone to elevate estradiol retention in this brain area (93). Since estrogen priming is a prerequisite for these progesterone actions, as it is for appearance of progesterone receptors in these regions of the brain, the effects of progesterone on the ovulatory parameters very likely involve receptor mediation.

The hypothalamus is a recognized site of corticosteroid feedback control of ACTH secretion through its secretory product corticotropin releasing factor (CRF) (61,101). It has also been recognized for some time that corticoids can interfere with ACTH by modulation of extrahypothalamic regions in the central nervous system (31,33). Studies using specific electrical stimulation and lesioning have now established that these actions also operate through hypothalamic intervention and CRF regulation (76a). The presence of glucocorticoid receptors in the hippocampus, amygdala, and septum is highly suggestive of their involvement in the feedback control of ACTH, since these brain structures are the areas which have the most pronounced input effects on hypothalamic control of ACTH secretion. Stimulation of the hippocampus results in decreased ACTH secretion, whereas lesions in this area enhance ACTH secretion. Electrical stimulation of the amygdala or septum produces the opposite effect from that seen in the hippocampus (139; see also Chapter 14).

The negative feedback mechanisms of glucocorticoids may be distinguished as a fast response related to an acute reaction to stress and a delayed phase showing dose proportionality (32). The steroidal specificity of these responses is different (67), and it appears that the fast response may be mediated through higher brain centers, whereas the delayed response is effected directly at the hypothalamic level or possibly at the anterior pituitary level where modulation of the pituitary responsiveness to CRF is involved (81). It has been shown that dexamethasone is capable of inhibiting CRF-induced ACTH release from pituitary cells (3). Oddly enough, corticosterone implants into the hippocampus result in potentiation of ACTH release, which would be inconsistent with a negative feedback action. Amygdaloid implants, however, produce attenuated

ACTH levels. The studies of Mason's group (102) on the amygdala–hippocampus interrelationships in the stress response, indicating a role for the amygdala in initiating ACTH secretion and for the hippocampus in terminating its release, suggest that endogenous glucocorticoids may function as buffers of this system, having more of a relative role in determining ACTH levels than an absolute function as positive or negative effectors. In fact, Kawakami et al. (77) presented evidence that, under stress conditions where ACTH is rapidly elevated, the hippocampus is highly effective in decreasing ACTH secretion, whereas hippocampal stimulation has little effect on adrenal corticoid synthesis in the unstressed animal.

There is considerable evidence for an influence of glucocorticoids on the nature and extent of a number of behavioral responses. A promising correlation with receptors evolves from an analysis of the corticosterone-induced forced extinction of a passive avoidance response (14). At high dosages (but not at low levels), progesterone and dexamethasone are capable of diminishing this response; this is in keeping with the ability of large amounts of progesterone or dexamethasone to decrease corticosterone binding to hippocampal cytosol receptors.

Alteration in intracellular protein composition, including induction of specific enzymes, is a common action of steroid hormones. DeVellis et al. (37) looked at glycerol phosphate dehydrogenase inducibility by dexamethasone in a rat glioma cell line and defined a dexamethasone-binding protein whose concentration in the nucleus correlates well with the enzyme induction pattern. This protein has many characteristics of a receptor, including specificity; i.e., corticosterone, cortisol, and dexamethasone are inducers whereas progesterone is antagonistic by virtue of its competition for cytosol binding of glucocorticoids.

CONCLUSIONS

The most striking feature of the brain as a target tissue for steroid hormones is its nearly unfathomable complexity. It is clearly impossible to study this organ in the same way as one can readily investigate interactions in a tissue such as the uterus, where steroid receptors are rather uniformly distributed through discrete areas and hormonal responses are easy to quantify. An enormous amount of work on steroid receptors in the brain from experts in many diversified scientific disciplines has resulted in some confusion about a number of points, some of which were examined in this chapter; it has also produced many interesting and valuable clues to elucidation of the molecular events fundamental to the central role of the brain as the regulator of reproductive function. Sophisticated and meticulous methodology is primarily responsible for these advances. Refinements of procedures involving tissue dissection, radiolabeled compounds of diverse physiological function and extremely high specific activity, stereotactic implantation and autoradiography under conditions where artifactual migration of substances is minimized, and various experimental approaches developed because of the unique properties of the brain have been indispensable in the advancement to our current state of knowledge in this area.

The designer of the steroid hormone receptor systems in the brain was an eminently clever scientist. Considering that the hormonal responses being measured generally involve higher brain structures, hypothalamus, pituitary, and endorgans, with feedback control mechanisms certainly existing at all of these sites and probably at many others, the number of possibilities for malfunction is virtually limitless; nevertheless, things usually work pretty well. This is certainly the result, at least in large part, of the system of checks and balances built into the machinery, and receptors are likely candidates as the molecular bearers of this mediatory action. The data available at the present time indicate that the simple presence of circulating hormones in the serum has little significance if the tissue cells do not contain the mechanisms for selective hormonal retention. As measurable by the physicochemical binding parameters, the ability of the cell to discern among a battery of hormones being presented to it is dictated by the attraction between the hormone and the receptor, and often it appears that one hormone may act by virtue of binding to a receptor for which it has relatively little affinity, in the relative absence of the favored ligand. Such overlapping specificity is probably no more accidental than any other selected genetic mutation; on the contrary, the actions resulting from these anomalous receptor interactions are often different qualitatively and quantitatively from those induced by the higher-affinity binding ligand and may well be of considerable physiological import. In turn, of course, the activity of the receptors depends on the availability of the hormones, and here the vital consideration of steroid metabolism enters the picture. Thus the relative amounts of a given ligand are controlled by the activity of steroid-interconverting enzymes present at that time, and this is further regulated by the nonreceptor-binding proteins in plasma and cells.

It is hard to imagine a more exciting, challenging, and functionally vital area of research than the molecular action of hormones at the brain level. A logical approach to further understanding, from our present vantage point, is investigation of the factors which control receptor synthesis, metabolism, structural characteristics, and physiological activity. This promising area is under intensive investigation and can be counted on to produce many additional stimulating findings relative to our understanding of hormone–receptor interactions and receptor–activity interrelationships.

ACKNOWLEDGMENTS

Work presented herein from the author's laboratory was supported by U.S. Public Health Service grant AM-17650 from NIAMDD, National Institutes of Health.

REFERENCES

1. Anderson, C. H., and Greenwald, G. S. (1969): Autoradiographic analysis of estradiol uptake in the brain and pituitary of the female rat. *Endocrinology,* 85:1160–1165.

2. Anderson, N. S., and Fanestil, D. D. (1976): Corticoid receptors in rat brain: Evidence for an aldosterone receptor. *Endocrinology*, 98:676–684.
3. Arimura, A., Bowers, C. Y., Schally, A. V., Saito, M., and Miller, M. C. (1969): Effect of corticotropin-releasing factor, dexamethasone and actinomycin D on the release of ACTH from rat pituitaries in vivo and in vitro. *Endocrinology*, 85:300–311.
4. Attardi, B., Geller, L. N., and Ohno, S. (1976): Androgen and estrogen receptors in brain cytosol from male, female, and testicular feminized (tfm/y) mice. *Endocrinology*, 98:864-874.
5. Attardi, B., and Ohno, S. (1976): Androgen and estrogen receptors in the developing mouse brain. *Endocrinology*, 99:1279–1290.
6. Barley, J., Ginsburg, M., Greenstein, B. D., MacLusky, N. J., and Thomas, P. J. (1974): A receptor mediating sexual differentiation? *Nature*, 252:259–260.
7. Barley, J., Ginsburg, M., MacLusky, N. J., Morris, I. D., and Thomas, P. J. (1977): Sex differences in the distribution of cytoplasmic oestrogen receptors in rat brain and pituitary: Effects of gonadectomy and neonatal androgen treatment. *Brain Res.*, 129:309–318.
8. Bar-Sela, M. E., and Critchlow, V. (1966): Delayed puberty following electrical stimulation of amygdala in female rats. *Am. J. Physiol.*, 211:1103–1107.
9. Baulieu, E-E., Atger, M., Best-Belpomme, M., Corvol, P., Courvalin, J-C., Mester, J., Milgrom, E., Robel, P., Rochefort, H., and deCatalogne, D. (1975): Steroid hormone receptors. *Vitam. Horm.*, 33:649–736.
10. Beach, F. A. (1942): Importance of progesterone to induction of sexual receptivity in spayed female rats. *Proc. Soc. Exp. Biol. Med.*, 51:369–371.
11. Bieglmayer, C., Pockl, E., Spona, J., Adamiker, D., and Jettmar, W. (1977): Nuclear translocation of the rat pituitary cytosol 17β-estradiol receptor. *FEBS Lett.*, 81:342–346.
12. Blaustein, J. D., and Wade, G. N. (1978): Progestin binding by brain and pituitary cell nuclei and female rat sexual behavior. *Brain Res.*, 140:360–367.
13. Bogdanove, E. M. (1963): Direct gonad-pituitary feedback: An analysis of effects of intracranial estrogenic depots on gonadotrophin secretion. *Endocrinology*, 73:696–712.
14. Bohus, B., and DeKloet, E. R. (1977): Behavioural effects of corticosterone related to putative glucocorticoid receptor properties in the rat brain. *J. Endocrinol.*, 72:64P–65P.
15. Brown-Grant, K. (1974): Failure of ovulation after administration of steroid hormones and hormone antagonists to female rats during the neonatal period. *J. Endocrinol.*, 62:683–684.
16. Cardinali, D. P. (1977): Nuclear receptor estrogen complex in the pineal gland: Modulation by sympathetic nerves. *Neuroendocrinology*, 24:333–346.
17. Cardinali, D. P., Nagle, C. A., and Rosner, J. M. (1975): Control of estrogen receptors in the rat pineal gland by catecholamine transmitter. *Life Sci.*, 16:81–91.
18. Chamberlain, J., and Rogers, A. W. (1972): The appearance of dihydrotestosterone-^{3}H in the diencephalon of neonatal rats after subcutaneous injection of testosterone-[3]H. *J. Steroid Biochem.*, 3:945–947.
19. Chan, L., and O'Malley, B. W. (1976): Mechanism of action of the sex steroid hormones. *N. Engl. J. Med.*, 294:1322–1328.
20. Chouknyiska, R., and Vassileva-Popova, J. G. (1977): Effect of age on the bonding of ^{3}H-testosterone with receptor protein from rat brain and testes. *C. R. Acad. Bulg. Sci.*, 30:133–135.
21. Ciaccio, L. A., and Lisk, R. D. (1972): Effect of hormone priming on retention of ^{3}H-estradiol by males and females. *Nature [New Biol.]*, 236:82–83.
22. Cidlowski, J. A., and Muldoon, T. G. (1974): Estrogenic regulation of cytoplasmic receptor populations in estrogen-responsive tissues of the rat. *Endocrinology*, 95:1621–1629.
23. Cidlowski, J. A., and Muldoon, T. G. (1975): Modulation by thyroid hormones of cytoplasmic estrogen receptor concentrations in reproductive tissues of the rat. *Endocrinology*, 97:59–67.
24. Cidlowski, J. A., and Muldoon, T. G. (1976): Dissimilar effects of antiestrogens upon estrogen receptors in responsive tissues of male and female rats. *Biol. Reprod.*, 15:381–389.
25. Cidlowski, J. A., and Muldoon, T. G. (1976): Sex-related differences in the regulation of cytoplasmic estrogen receptor levels in responsive tissues of the rat. *Endocrinology*, 98:833–841.
26. Cidlowski, J. A., and Muldoon, T. G. (1978): The dynamics of intracellular estrogen receptor regulation as influenced by 17β-estradiol. *Biol. Reprod.* 18:234–246.
27. Clark, J. H., Anderson, J. N., and Peck, E. J. (1973): Nuclear receptor-estrogen complexes of rat uteri: Concentration-time-response parameters. *Adv. Exp. Med. Biol.*, 36:15–59.

28. Clark, J. H., and Peck, E. J. (1977): Steroid hormone receptors: Basic principles and measurements. In: *Receptors and Hormone Action,* Vol. 1, edited by B. W. O'Malley and L. Birnbaumer, pp. 383–410. Academic Press, New York.

29. Clark, J. H., Peck, E. J., and Anderson, J. N. (1974): Oestrogen receptors and antagonism of steroid hormone action. *Nature,* 251:446–448.

30. Clayton, C. J., Grosser, B. I., and Stevens, W. (1977): The ontogeny of corticosterone and dexamethasone receptors in rat brain. *Brain Res.,* 134:445–453.

31. Corbin, A., Mangili, G., Motta, M., and Martini, L. (1965): Effect of hypothalamic and mesencephalic steroid implantations on ACTH feedback mechanisms. *Endocrinology,* 76:811–818.

32. Dallman, M. F., and Yates, F. E. (1969): Dynamic asymmetries in the corticosteroid feedback pathway and distribution, binding and metabolism elements of the adrenocortical system. *Ann. NY Acad. Sci.,* 156:696–721.

33. Davidson, J. M., and Feldman, S. (1967): Effects of extrahypothalamic dexamethasone implants on the pituitary adrenal system. *Acta Endocrinol. (Kbh),* 55:240–246.

34. DeKloet, E. R., Burbach, P., and Mulder, G. H. (1977): Localization and role of transcortin-like molecules in the anterior pituitary. *Mol. Cell. Endocrinol.,* 7:261–273.

35. DeKloet, E. R., Wallach, G., and McEwen, B. S. (1975): Differences in corticosterone and dexamethasone binding to rat brain and pituitary. *Endocrinology,* 96:598–609.

36. DeMoor, P., Verhoeven, G., Heyns, W., and VanBaelen, H. (1976): Diversity in androgenic effect as studied in rat and mouse. In: *The Endocrine Function of the Human Ovary,* edited by V. H. T. James, M. Serio, and G. Giusti, pp. 159–173. Academic Press, London.

37. DeVellis, J., McGinnis, J. F., Breen, G. A. M., Leveille, P., Bennett, K., and McCarthy, K. (1977): Hormonal effects on differentiation in neural cultures. In: *Cell, Tissue and Organ Culture in Neurobiology,* edited by S. Federoff and L. Hertz, pp. 485–511. Academic Press, New York.

38. Docke, F., and Dorner, G. (1974): Oestrogen and the control of gonadotrophin secretion in the immature rat. *J. Endocrinol.,* 63:285–298.

39. Docke, F., and Dorner, G. (1975): Anovulation in adult female rats after neonatal intracerebral implantation of oestrogen. *Endokrinologie,* 65:375–377.

40. Doughty, C., Booth, J. E., McDonald, P. G., and Parrott, R. F. (1975): Effects of oestradiol-17β, oestradiol benzoate and the synthetic oestrogen RU2858 on sexual differentiation in the neonatal female rat. *J. Endocrinol.,* 67:419–424.

41. Doughty, C., Booth, J. E., McDonald, P. G., and Parrott, R. F. (1975): Inhibition, by the anti-oestrogen MER-25, of defeminization induced by the synthetic oestrogen RU2858. *J. Endocrinol.,* 67:459–460.

42. Doughty, C., and McDonald, P. G. (1974): Hormonal control of sexual differentiation of the hypothalamus in the neonatal female rat. *Differentiation,* 2:275–285.

43. Eisenthal, R., and Cornish-Bowden, A. (1974): The direct linear plot: A new graphical procedure for estimating enzyme kinetic parameters. *Biochem. J.,* 139:715–720.

44. Ermish, A., and Ruhle, H. J. (1978): Autoradiographic demonstration of aldosterone-concentrating neuron populations in rat brain. *Brain Res.,* 147:154–158.

45. Evans, R. W., Sholiton, L. J., and Leavitt, W. W. (1978): Progesterone receptor in the rat anterior pituitary: Effect of estrogen priming and adrenalectomy. *Steroids,* 31:69–81.

46. Everett, J. W. (1944): Evidence in normal albino rat that progesterone facilitates ovulation and corpus luteum formation. *Endocrinology,* 34:136–137.

47. Flerko, B., Mess, B., and Illei-Donhoffer, A. (1969): On the mechanism of androgen sterilization. *Neuroendocrinology,* 4:164–169.

48. Fox, T. O. (1975): Androgen- and estrogen-binding macromolecules in developing mouse brain: Biochemical and genetic evidence. *Proc. Natl. Acad. Sci. USA,* 72:4303–4307.

49. Fox, T. O. (1977): Conversion of the hypothalamic estradiol receptor to the "nuclear" form. *Brain Res.,* 120:580–583.

50. Fox, T. O. (1977): Estradiol and testosterone binding in normal and mutant mouse cerebellum: Biochemical and cellular specificity. *Brain Res.,* 128:263–273.

51. Gerall, A. A., Dunlap, J. L., and Wagner, R. A. (1976): Effects of dihydrotestosterone and gonadotrophins on the development of female behavior. *Physiol. Behav.,* 17:121–126.

52. Ginsburg, M., and Greenstein, B. D. (1977): Comparison of the abundances and affinities of androgen receptors in brain, pituitary gland and ventral prostate of 18-month and 12-week old rats. *J. Endocrinol.,* 72:65P.

53. Gorski, J., and Gannon, F. (1976): Current models of steroid hormone action: A critique. *Annu. Rev. Physiol.,* 38:425–450.
54. Gorski, R. A. (1966): Localization and sexual differentiation of the nervous structures which regulate ovulation. *J. Reprod. Fertil. (Suppl),* 1:67–88.
55. Greeley, G. H., Allen, M. B., and Mahesh, V. B. (1975): Potentiation of luteinizing hormone release by estradiol at the level of the pituitary. *Neuroendocrinology,* 18:233–241.
56. Greeley, G. H., Muldoon, T. G., and Mahesh, V. B. (1975): Correlative aspects of luteinizing hormone-releasing hormone sensitivity and cytoplasmic estrogen receptor concentration in the anterior pituitary and hypothalamus of the cycling rat. *Biol. Reprod.,* 13:505–512.
57. Green, J. D., Clemente, C. D., and DeGroot, J. (1957): Rhinencephalic lesions and behavior in cats. *J. Comp. Neurol.,* 108:505–545.
58. Gustafsson, J. A., Pousette, A., and Svensson, E. (1976): Sex specific occurrence of androgen receptors in rat brain. *J. Biol. Chem.,* 251:4047–4054.
59. Halasz, B. (1969): The endocrine effects of isolation of the hypothalamus from the rest of the brain. In: *Frontiers in Neuroendocrinology,* Vol. 1, edited by W. F. Ganong and L. Martini, pp. 307–342. Oxford University Press, London.
60. Hannouche, N., Thieulant, M-L., Samperez, S., and Jouan, P. (1978): Androgens binding proteins in the cytosol from prepubertal male rat hypothalamus, preoptic area and brain cortex. *J. Steroid Biochem.,* 9:147–151.
61. Hayashi, S. (1974): Failure of intrahypothalamic implants of antiestrogen, MER-25, to inhibit androgen sterilization in female rats. *Endocrinol. Jpn.,* 21:453–457.
62. Hedge, G. A., and Smelik, P. G. (1969): The action of dexamethasone and vasopressin on hypothalamic CRF production and release. *Neuroendocrinology,* 4:242–253.
63. Hsueh, A. J. W., Peck, E. J., and Clark, J. H. (1976): Control of uterine estrogen receptor levels by progesterone. *Endocrinology,* 98:438–444.
64. Jensen, E. V., and DeSombre, E. R. (1972): Mechanism of action of the female sex hormones. *Annu. Rev. Biochem.,* 41:203–230.
65. Jensen, E. V., and Jacobson, H. I. (1960): Fate of steroid estrogens in target tissue. In: *Biological Activities of Steroids in Relation to Cancer,* edited by G. Pincus and E. P. Vollmer, pp. 161–178. Academic Press, New York.
66. Jensen, E. V., Suzuki, T., Kawashima, T., Stumpf, W. E., Jungblut, P. W., and DeSombre, E. R. (1968): A two-step mechanism for the interaction of estradiol with rat uterus. *Proc. Natl. Acad. Sci. USA,* 59:632–638.
67. Jones, M. T., Hillhouse, E. W., and Burden, J. L. (1977): Structure-activity relationships of corticosteroid feedback at the hypothalamic level. *J. Endocrinol.,* 74:415–424.
68. Kamberi, I. A., and McCann, S. M. (1972): Effects of implants of testosterone in the median eminence and the pituitary on FSH secretion. *Neuroendocrinology,* 9:20–29.
69. Kato, J. (1976): Nuclear and cytosol receptors for 5α-dihydrotestosterone and testosterone in the hypothalamus and hypophysis and testosterone receptors from neonatal female rat hypothalamus. *J. Steroid Biochem.,* 7:1179–1187.
70. Kato, J. (1976): Ontogeny of 5α-dihydrotestosterone receptors in the hypothalamus of the rat. *Ann. Biol. Anim. Biochim. Biophys.,* 16:467–469.
71. Kato, J. (1977): Steroid hormone receptors in brain, hypothalamus and hypophysis. In: *Receptors and Mechanism of Action of Steroid Hormones,* Part II, edited by J. R. Pasqualini, pp. 603–672. Dekker, New York.
72. Kato, J., Atsumi, Y., and Inaba, M. (1971): Development of estrogen receptors in the rat hypothalamus. *J. Biochem.,* 70:1051–1053.
73. Kato, J., Atsumi, Y., and Inaba, M. (1974): Estradiol receptors in female rat hypothalamus in the developmental stages and during pubescence. *Endocrinology,* 94:309–317.
74. Kato, J., Atsumi, Y., and Muramatsu, M. (1970): Nuclear estradiol receptor in rat anterior hypophysis. *J. Biochem.,* 67:871–872.
75. Kato, J., Onouchi, T., and Okinaga, S. (1978): Hypothalamic and hypophyseal progesterone receptors: Estrogen-priming effect, differential localization, 5α-dihydroprogesterone binding, and nuclear receptors. *J. Steroid Biochem.,* 9:419–427.
76. Katzenellenbogen, B. S., and Ferguson, E. R. (1975): Antiestrogen action in the uterus: Biological ineffectiveness of nuclear bound estradiol after antiestrogen. *Endocrinology,* 97:1–12.
76a. Kawakami, M., Sato, K., Tarasawa, E., Yoshida, K., Miyamoto, T., Sekiguchi, M., and

Hattori, Y. (1968): Influence of electrical stimulation and lesion in limbic structure upon biosynthesis of adrenocorticoid in the rabbit. *Neuroendocrinology,* 3:337–348.

77. Kawakami, M., Sato, K., Yoshida, K., and Miyamoto, T. (1969): Biosynthesis of ovarian steroids in the rabbit: Influence of progesterone or estradiol implantation into the hypothalamus and limbic structures. *Neuroendocrinology,* 5:303–321.

78. Kincl, F. A., and Maqueo, M. (1965): Prevention by progesterone of steroid-induced sterility in neonatal male and female rats. *Endocrinology,* 77:859–862.

79. Kingsley, T. R., and Bogdanove, E. M. (1973): Direct feedback of androgens: Localized effects of intrapituitary implants of androgens on gonadotrophic cells and hormone stores. *Endocrinology,* 93:1398–1409.

80. Kobayashi, F., Hara, K., and Miyoke, T. (1970): Facilitation of luteinizing hormone release by progesterone in proestrous rats. *Endocrinol. Jpn.,* 17:149–155.

81. Koch, B., Lutz, B., Briaud, B., and Mialhe, C. (1975): Glucocorticoid binding to adenohypophysis receptors and its physiological role. *Neuroendocrinology,* 18:299–310.

82. Koch, B., Lutz-Bucher, B., Briaud, B., and Mialhe, C. (1977): Glucocorticoid binding to plasma membranes of the adenohypophysis. *J. Endocrinol.,* 73:399–400.

83. Koch, B., Lutz-Bucher, B., Briaud, B., and Mialhe, C. (1978): Inverse effects of corticosterone and thyroxine on glucocorticoid binding sites in the anterior pituitary gland. *Acta Endocrinol. (Kbh),* 88:29–37.

84. Korach, K. S., and Ford, E. B. (1978): Estrogen action in the mouse uterus: An additional nuclear event. *Biochem. Biophys. Res. Commun.,* 83:327–333.

85. Korach, K. S., and Muldoon, T. G. (1975): Inhibition of anterior pituitary estrogen-receptor complex formation by low-affinity interaction with 5α-dihydrotestosterone. *Endocrinology,* 97:231–236.

86. Kurl, R. N., and Morris, I. D. (1978): Differential depletion of cytoplasmic high affinity oestrogen receptors after the in vivo administration of the antioestrogens, clomiphene, MER-25 and tamoxifen. *Br. J. Pharmacol.,* 62:487–493.

87. Larsson, K., and Sodersten, P. (1973): Sexual behavior in male rats treated with estrogen in combination with dihydrotestosterone. *Horm. Behav.,* 4:289–299.

88. LeGuellec, C., Thieulant, M-L., Samperez, S., and Jouan, P. (1978): A specific estradiol-17β receptor in cell nuclei from anterior hypophysis of immature male rats. *J. Steroid Biochem.,* 9:393–398.

89. Liang, T., and Liao, S. (1975): A very rapid effect of androgen on initiation of protein synthesis in prostate. *Proc. Natl. Acad. Sci. USA,* 72:706–709.

90. Lieberburg, I., MacLusky, N. J., and McEwen, B. S. (1977): 5α-Dihydrotestosterone receptors in rat brain and pituitary cell nuclei. *Endocrinology,* 100:598–607.

91. Lieberburg, I., and McEwen, B. S. (1975): Estradiol-17β: A metabolite of testosterone recovered in cell nuclei from limbic areas of neonatal rat brains. *Brain Res.,* 85:165–170.

92. Lieberburg, I., Wallach, G., and McEwen, B. S. (1977): The effects of an inhibitor of aromatization (1,4,6-androstatriene-3,17-dione) and an antiestrogen (CI-628) on in vivo formed testosterone metabolites recovered from neonatal rat brain tissues and purified cell nuclei: Implications for sexual differentiation of the rat brain. *Brain Res.,* 128:176–181.

93. Lisk, R. D., and Reuter, L. A. (1977): In vivo progesterone treatment enhances [³H]estradiol retention by neural tissue of the female rat. *Endocrinology,* 100:1652–1658.

94. Lobl, R. T. (1975): Alterations in the mechanism of intracellular transport. *Psychoneuroendocrinology,* 1:131–140.

95. Luttge, W. G. (1972): The estrous cycle of the rat: Effects on the accumulation of estrogen metabolites in brain and peripheral tissues. *Brain Res.,* 38:315–325.

96. Luttge, W. G., and Hughes, J. R. (1976): Intracerebral implantation of progesterone: Reexamination of the brain sites responsible for facilitation of sexual receptivity in estrogen-primed ovariectomized rats. *Physiol. Behav.,* 17:771–775.

97. Luttge, W. G., Wallis, C. J., and Hall, N. R. (1974): Effects of pre- and posttreatment with unlabeled steroids on the in vivo uptake of [³H]progestins in selected brain areas, uterus and plasma of the female mouse. *Brain Res.,* 71:105–115.

98. MacLusky, N. J., Chaptal, C., Lieberburg, I., and McEwen, B. S. (1976): Properties and subcellular inter-relationships of presumptive estrogen receptor macromolecules in the brains of neonatal and prepubertal female rats. *Brain Res.,* 114:158–165.

99. MacLusky, N. J., and McEwen, B. S. (1978): Oestrogen modulates progestin receptor concentrations in some rat brain areas but not in others. *Nature,* 274:276–278.

100. MacLusky, N. J., Turner, B. B., and McEwen, B. S. (1977): Corticosteroid binding in rat brain and pituitary cytosols: Resolution of multiple binding components by polyacrylamide gel based isoelectric focusing. *Brain Res.,* 130:564–571.

101. Mangili, G., Motta, M., and Martini, L. (1966): Control of adrenocorticotropic hormone secretion. In: *Neuroendocrinology,* Vol. 1, edited by L. Martini and W. F. Ganong, pp. 298–370. Academic Press, New York.

102. Mason, J. W. (1958): The central nervous system regulation of ACTH secretion. In: *Reticular Formation of the Brain,* edited by H. H. Jasper, L. D. Proctor, R. S. Knighton, W. C. Noshay, and R. T. Costello, pp. 645–662. Little Brown, Boston.

103. Maurer, R. A., and Woolley, D. E. (1974): Demonstration of nuclear ^{3}H-estradiol binding in hypothalamus and amygdala of female, androgenized-female, and male rats. *Neuroendocrinology,* 16:137–147.

104. Maurer, R. A., and Woolley, D. E. (1974): ^{3}H-Estradiol distribution in normal and androgenized female rats using an improved hypothalamic dissection procedure. *Neuroendocrinology,* 14:87–94.

105. Maurer, R. A., and Woolley, D. E. (1975): ^{3}H-Estradiol distribution in female, androgenized female, and male rats at 100 and 200 days of age. *Endocrinology,* 96:755–765.

106. McEwen, B. S. (1975): Hormones, receptors and brain function. *Adv. Pathobiol.,* 1:56–69.

107. McEwen, B. S. (1977): Glucocorticoid receptors in neuroendocrine tissues. In: *Endocrinology,* Vol. 1, edited by V. H. T. James, pp. 23–28. Excerpta Medica, Amsterdam.

108. McEwen, B. S. (1978): Gonadal steroid receptors in neuroendocrine tissues. In: *Receptors and Hormone Action,* Vol. 2, edited by B. W. O'Malley and L. Birnbaumer, pp. 353–400. Academic Press, New York.

109. McEwen, B. S., DeKloet, R., and Wallach, G. (1976): Interactions in vivo and in vitro of corticoids and progesterone with cell nuclei and soluble macromolecules from rat brain regions and pituitary. *Brain Res.,* 105:129–136.

110. McEwen, B. S., Lieberburg, I., MacLusky, N., and Plapinger, L. (1977): Do estrogen receptors play a role in the sexual differentiation of the rat brain? *J. Steroid Biochem.,* 8:593–598.

111. McEwen, B. S., and Pfaff, D. W. (1970): Factors influencing sex hormone uptake by rat brain regions. I. Effects of neonatal treatment, hypophysectomy, and competing steroid on estradiol uptake. *Brain Res.,* 21:1–16.

112. McEwen, B. S., Pfaff, D. W., and Zigmond, R. E. (1970): Factors influencing sex hormone uptake by rat brain regions. III. Effects of competing steroids on testosterone uptake. *Brain Res.,* 21:29–38.

113. McEwen, B. S., and Wallach, G. (1973): Corticosterone binding to hippocampus: Nuclear and cytosol binding in vitro. *Brain Res.,* 57:373–386.

114. McEwen, B. S., Wallach, G., and Magnus, C. (1974): Corticosterone binding to hippocampus: Immediate and delayed influences of the absence of adrenal secretion. *Brain Res.,* 70:321–334.

115. McGuire, J. L., and Lisk, R. D. (1968): Estrogen receptors in the intact rat. *Proc. Natl. Acad. Sci. USA,* 61:497–503.

116. Menon, K. M. J., and Gunaga, K. P. (1976): Cytoplasmic and nuclear receptor-estradiol complex in the hypothalamus and pituitary: Relationship with pituitary sensitivity to gonadotropin releasing hormone and gonadotropin secretion in the rat. *Neuroendocrinology,* 22:8–17.

117. Milgrom, E., Atger, M., Perrot, M., and Baulieu, E-E. (1972): Progesterone in uterus and plasma. VI. Uterine progesterone receptors during the estrous cycle and implantation in the guinea pig. *Endocrinology,* 90:1071–1078.

118. Mittler, J. C., and Meites, J. (1966): Effects of hypothalamic extract and androgen on pituitary FSH release in vitro. *Endocrinology,* 78:500–504.

119. Moguilewsky, M., and Raynaud, J-P. (1977): Progestin binding sites in the rat hypothalamus, pituitary and uterus. *Steroids,* 30:99–109.

120. Monbon, M., Loras, B., Reboud, J. P., and Bertrand, J. (1974): Binding and metabolism of testosterone in the rat brain during sexual maturation. I. Macromolecular binding of androgens. *J. Steroid Biochem.,* 5:417–423.

121. Mowles, T. F., Ashkanazy, B., Mix, E., and Sheppard, J. H. (1971): Hypothalamic and hypophyseal estradiol-binding complexes. *Endocrinology,* 89:484–491.

122. Muldoon, T. G. (1971): Characterization of steroid-binding sites by affinity labeling: Further

studies of the interaction between 4-mercuri-17β-estradiol and specific estrogen-binding proteins in the rat uterus. *Biochemistry,* 10:3780–3784.

123. Muldoon, T. G. (1977): Pituitary estrogen receptors. In: *The Pituitary, A Current Review,* edited by M. B. Allen and V. B. Mahesh, pp. 295–329. Academic Press, New York.

124. Muldoon, T. G. (1978): Characterization of mouse mammary tissue estrogen receptors under conditions of differing hormonal backgrounds. *J. Steroid Biochem.,* 9:485–494.

125. Naess, O. (1976): Characterization of the androgen receptor in the hypothalamus, preoptic area and brain cortex of the rat. *Steroids,* 27:167–185.

126. Naess, O., Attramadal, A., and Hansson, V. (1977): Receptors for testosterone and 5α-dihydrotestosterone in the anterior pituitary and various areas of the brain. In: *The Testis in Normal and Infertile Men,* edited by P. Troen and H. R. Nankin, pp. 227–241. Raven Press, New York.

127. Naess, O., Haug, E., Attramadal, A., Aakvaag, A., Hansson, V., and French, F. (1976): Androgen receptors in the anterior pituitary and central nervous system of the androgen "insensitive" (Tfm) rat. *Endocrinology,* 99:1295–1303.

128. Nicoll, C. S., and Meites, J. (1962): Estrogen stimulation of prolactin production by rat adenohypophysis in vitro. *Endocrinology,* 70:272–277.

129. Ohno, S., Geller, L. N., and Younglai, E. V. (1974): Tfm mutation in masculinization versus the feminization of the mouse central nervous system. *Cell,* 3:235–242.

130. Ohno, S., and Lyon, M. F. (1970): X-linked testicular feminization in the mouse as a non-inducible regulatory mutation of the Jacob-Monod type. *Clin. Genet.,* 1:121–127.

131. Ogren, L., Vertes, M., and Woolley, D. E. (1976): In vivo nuclear ^{3}H-estradiol binding in brain areas of the rat: Reduction by endogenous and exogenous androgens. *Neuroendocrinology,* 21:350–365.

132. Parker, C. R., Costoff, A., Muldoon, T. G., and Mahesh, V. B. (1975): Correlative aspects of luteinizing hormone-releasing hormone sensitivity and cytoplasmic estrogen receptor concentration in the anterior pituitary and hypothalamus of the cycling rat. *Biol. Reprod.,* 13:505–512.

133. Pedroza, E., and Rosner, J. M. (1975): Some characteristics of in vitro ^{3}H-estradiol binding by the rat posterior pituitary. *Neuroendocrinology,* 19:193–200.

134. Perez, A. E., Ortiz, A., Cabezza, M., Beyer, C., and Perez-Palacios, G. (1975): In vitro metabolism of ^{3}H-androstenedione by the male rat pituitary, hypothalamus, and hippocampus. *Steroids,* 25:53–62.

135. Portonova, R., and Sayers, G. (1974): Corticosterone suppression of ACTH secretion: Actinomycin D sensitive and insensitive components of the response. *Biochem. Biophys. Res. Commun.,* 56:928–933.

136. Powers, J. B. (1970): Hormonal control of sexual receptivity during the estrous cycle of the rat. *Physiol. Behav.,* 5:831–835.

137. Powers, J. B. (1972): Facilitation of lordosis in ovariectomized rats by intracerebral progesterone implants. *Brain Res.,* 48:311–325.

138. Ramirez, V. D., and Sawyer, C. H. (1965): Advancement of puberty in the female rat by estrogen. *Endocrinology,* 76:1158–1168.

139. Redgate, E. S., and Fahringer, E. E. (1973): A comparison of the pituitary-adrenal activity elicited by electrical stimulation of preoptic, amygdaloid and hypothalamic sites in the rat brain. *Neuroendocrinology,* 12:334–343.

140. Reiter, R. J. (1973): Comparative physiology: Pineal gland. *Annu. Rev. Physiol.,* 35:305–328.

141. Rhees, R., Grosser, B., and Stevens, W. (1975): The autoradiographic localization of [^{3}H]dexamethasone in the brain and pituitary of the rat. *Brain Res.,* 100:151–156.

142. Robel, P., Corpechot, C., and Baulieu, E-E. (1973): Testosterone and androstanolone in rat plasma and tissues. *FEBS Lett.,* 33:218–220.

143. Rochefort, H., Lignon, F., and Capony, F. (1972): Formation of estrogen nuclear receptor in the uterus: Effect of androgens, estrone and nafoxidine. *Biochem. Biophys. Res. Commun.,* 47:662–670.

144. Rochefort, H., and Garcia, M. (1976): Androgens on the estrogen receptor. I. Binding and in vivo nuclear translocation. *Steroids,* 28:549–560.

145. Ross, J., Claybough, C., Clemens, L. G., and Gorski, R. A. (1971): Short latency induction of estrous behavior with intracerebral gonadal hormones in ovariectomized rats. *Endocrinology,* 89:32–38.

146. Ruh, T. S., and Ruh, M. F. (1974): The effect of antiestrogens on the nuclear binding of the estrogen receptor. *Steroids,* 25:257–273.
147. Ruh, T. S., Wassilak, S. G., and Ruh, M. F. (1974): Androgen-induced nuclear accumulation of the estrogen receptor. *Steroids,* 24:209–224.
148. Samperez, S., Thieulant, M-L., and Jouan, P. (1969): Mise en evidence d'une association macromoleculaire de la testosterone 1-2-³H dans l'hypophyse anterieure et l'hypothalamus du rat normal et castre. *C. R. Acad. Sci. (Paris),* 268:2965–2967.
149. Samperez, S., Thieulant, M. L., Mercier, L., and Jouan, P. (1974): A specific testosterone receptor in the cytosol of rat anterior hypophysis. *J. Steroid Biochem.,* 5:911–915.
150. Sar, M., and Stumpf, W. E. (1973): Cellular and subcellular localization of radioactivity in the rat pituitary following injection of 1,2-³H-testosterone using dry-autoradiography. *Endocrinology,* 92:631–635.
151. Sar, M., and Stumpf, W. E. (1977): Distribution of androgen target cells in rat forebrain and pituitary after [³H]-dihydrotestosterone administration. *J. Steroid Biochem.,* 8:1131–1135.
152. Sawyer, C. H. (1960): Reproductive behavior. In: *Handbook of Physiology: Neurophysiology,* Vol. II, edited by J. Field, pp. 1225–1240. American Physiological Society, Washington, D.C.
153. Seiki, K., and Hattori, M. (1973): In vivo uptake of progesterone by the hypothalamus and pituitary of the female ovariectomized rat and its relationship to cytoplasmic progesterone-binding protein. *Endocrinol. Jpn.,* 20:111–119.
154. Sen, K. K., and Menon, K. M. J. (1978): Oestradiol receptors in the rat anterior pituitary gland during the oestrous cycle: Quantitation of receptor activity in relation to gonadotrophin releasing hormone-mediated luteinizing hormone release. *J. Endocrinol.,* 76:211–218.
155. Smith, E. R., and Davidson, J. M. (1968): Role of estrogen in the cerebral control of puberty in female rats. *Endocrinology,* 82:100–108.
156. Smith, E. R., Weick, R. F., and Davidson, J. M. (1969): Influence of intracerebral progesterone on the reproductive system of female rats. *Endocrinology,* 85:1129–1136.
157. Spona, J., Bieglmayer, C., Adamiker, D., and Jettmar, W. (1977): Ontogeny of 17β-estradiol-binding protein in female rat hypothalamus and anterior pituitary. *FEBS Lett.,* 76:306–310.
158. Steggles, A. W., and King, R. J. B. (1970): The use of protamine to study [6,7-³H]-oestradiol-17β binding in rat uterus. *Biochem. J.,* 118:695–701.
159. Stumpf, W. E., and Sar, M. (1977): Autoradiographic localization of estrogen, androgen, progestin, and glucocorticosteroid in "target tissues" and "nontarget tissues." In: *Receptors and Mechanism of Action of Steroid Hormones,* Part 1, edited by J. R. Pasquali, pp. 41–84. Dekker, New York.
160. Terenius, L. (1970): Two modes of interaction between oestrogen and antiestrogen. *Acta Endocrinol. (Kbh),* 64:47–58.
161. Toft, D. O., and Gorski, J. (1966): A receptor molecule for estrogens: Isolation from the rat uterus and preliminary characterization. *Proc. Natl. Acad. Sci. USA,* 55:1574–1581.
162. Toft, D. O., and O'Malley, B. W. (1972): Target tissue receptors for progesterone: The influence of estrogen treatment. *Endocrinology,* 90:1041–1045.
163. Toran-Allerand, C. D. (1976): Sex steroid and the development of the newborn mouse hypothalamus and preoptic area in vitro: Implications for sexual differentiation. *Brain Res.,* 106:407–412.
164. Turner, B. B., and McEwen, B. S. (1976): Hippocampal cytosol binding capacity of corticosterone: no depletion with nuclear receptor loading. In: *Program 58th Meet. Endocrine Soc.,* p. 93.
165. Vertes, M., Barnea, A., Lindner, H. R., and King, R. B. J. (1973): Studies on androgen and estrogen uptake by rat hypothalamus. *Adv. Exp. Med. Biol.,* 36:137–173.
166. Vertes, M., and King, R. J. B. (1971): The mechanism of oestradiol binding in rat hypothalamus: Effect of androgenization. *J. Endocrinol.,* 51:271–282.
167. Vreeburg, J. T. M., van der Vaart, P. D. M., and van der Schoot, P. (1977): Prevention of central defeminization but not masculinization in male rats by inhibition neonatally of oestrogen biosynthesis. *J. Endocrinol.,* 74:375–382.
168. Walsh, P. C., Madden, J. D., Harrod, M. J., Goldstein, J. L., McDonald, P. C., and Wilson, J. D. (1974): Familial incomplete male pseudohermaphroditism, type 2. *N. Engl. J. Med.,* 291:944–949.
169. Ward, I. L., Crowley, W. R., and Zemlan, F. P. (1975): Monoaminergic mediation of female sexual behavior. *J. Comp. Physiol. Psychol.,* 88:53–61.

170. Warembourg, M. (1975): Radioautographic study of the rat brain and pituitary after injection of ³H-dexamethasone. *Cell Tissue Res.,* 161:183–191.

171. Watanabe, H., Orth, D. N., and Toft, D. O. (1973): Glucocorticoid receptors in pituitary tumor cells. I. Cytosol receptors. *J. Biol. Chem.,* 248:7625–7630.

172. Watson, G. H., Korach, K. S., and Muldoon, T. G. (1977): Obstruction of estrogen-receptor complex formation: Further analysis of the nature and steroidal specificity of the effect. *Endocrinology,* 101:1733–1743.

173. Weisz, J., and Gibbs, C. (1974): Metabolites in the brain of the newborn female rat after an injection of tritiated testosterone. *Neuroendocrinology,* 14:72–86.

174. Westley, B. R., and Salaman, D. F. (1977): Nuclear binding of the oestrogen receptor of neonatal rat brain after injection of oestrogens and androgens: Localization and sex differences. *Brain Res.,* 119:375–388.

175. Westley, B. R., Thomas, P. J., Salaman, D. F., Knight, A., and Barley, J. (1976): Properties and partial purification of an oestrogen receptor from neonatal rat brain. *Brain Res.,* 113:441–447.

176. Whalen, R. E., and Gorzalka, B. B. (1974): Estrogen-progesterone interactions in uterus and brain of intact and adrenalectomized immature and adult rats. *Endocrinology,* 94:214–223.

177. Whalen, R. E., and Luttge, W. G. (1971): Differential localization of progesterone uptake in brain: Role of sex, estrogen pretreatment and adrenalectomy. *Brain Res.,* 33:147–155.

178. Whalen, R. E., Luttge, W. G., and Green, R. (1969): Effects of the anti-androgen cyproterone acetate on the uptake of 1,2-³H-testosterone in neural and peripheral tissues of the castrate male rat. *Endocrinology,* 84:217–222.

179. Whalen, R. E., and Olsen, K. L. (1978): Chromatin binding of estradiol in the hypothalamus and cortex of male and female rats. *Brain Res.,* 152:121–131.

180. Whalen, R. E., and Rezek, D. L. (1972): Localization of androgenic metabolites in the brain of rats administered testosterone or dihydrotestosterone. *Steroids,* 20:717–724.

181. White, J. O., Lim, L., and Thomas, S. (1977): Hypothalamic and peripheral relations during the oestrous cycle of the female rat: The oestrogen receptor in the hypothalamus. *Biochem. Soc. Transact.,* 5:1072–1073.

182. Wieland, S. J., Fox, T. O., and Savakis, C. (1978): DNA-binding of androgen and estrogen receptors from mouse brain: Behavior of residual androgen receptor from tfm mutant. *Brain Res.,* 140:159–164.

183. Wise, P. M., and Payne, A. H. (1975): Estrone and estradiol binding by a cytoplasmic receptor in the sheep pituitary and hypothalamus. In: *Program 57th Meet. Endocrine Soc.,* p. 361.

184. Woosley, J. T., and Muldoon, T. G. (1976): Use of the direct linear plot to estimate binding constants for protein-ligand interactions. *Biochem. Biophys. Res. Commun.,* 71:155–160.

185. Zeilmaker, G. H. (1966): The biphasic effect of progesterone on ovulation in the rat. *Acta Endocrinol. (Kbh),* 51:461–468.

The Endocrine Functions of the Brain,
edited by Marcella Motta.
Raven Press, New York © 1980

5

Metabolism of Steroid Hormones in the Brain

Pierre Jouan and Suzanne Samperez

Laboratoire de Neurobiologie Moléculaire, Centre Régional de Recherche en Endocrinologie, Rennes Cedex, France

In males, the main androgen found in blood is testosterone. However, it is now well established that in target organs, testosterone is chiefly metabolized into 5α-reduced steroids, and it may be considered to be a prehormone. For that reason, the intracellular metabolism of testosterone in the pituitary gland as well as in some brain areas appears to be the essential step in the control exerted by androgens over several events, such as sexual differentiation, sexual behavior, reproductive function, and regulation of gonadotropin secretion.

Consequently, the study of testosterone metabolism was a prerequisite for further investigation of the mechanisms of androgen action at the central level, especially for their possible binding to specific receptors. In this and other laboratories, thorough studies were devoted to this topic, and the results are summarized in this chapter.

ANDROGEN METABOLISM IN THE ANTERIOR PITUITARY GLAND OF THE MALE

In the anterior pituitary gland of the male, testosterone is metabolized through several pathways.

Oxidative Pathway

The oxidative pathway leads to the formation of androstenedione through the action of 17β-hydroxysteroid dehydrogenase (Fig. 1). The conversion of testosterone into androstenedione has been observed in the pituitaries of a number of animal species (intact and castrated animals) (4,13,18,24,32,36,40,41,50, 51,53).

This pathway appears to be of little importance, since androstenedione per se is a weak androgen, and is not, at the pituitary level, convertible into estrone. Moreover, androstenedione is easily transformed into 5α-androstanedione by

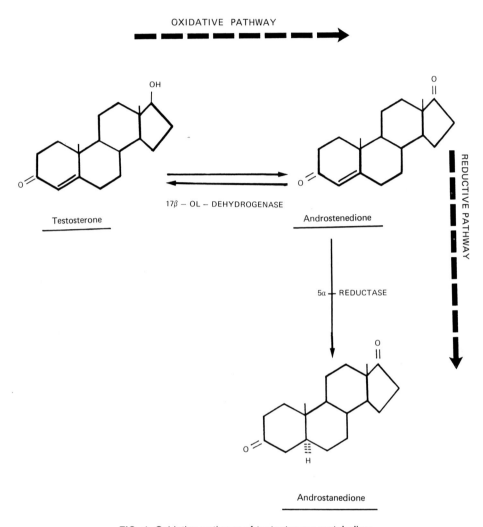

FIG. 1. Oxidative pathway of testosterone metabolism.

means of a 5α-reductase (35,36) (Fig. 1). 5α-Androstanedione is a weak androgen devoided of action on gonadotropin secretion. Furthermore, androstenedione is likely to be reconverted into testosterone (35,36,41). Nevertheless, androstanedione is the metabolite formed in the largest quantity.

Reductive Pathway

In all respects this is the most important pathway in testosterone metabolism. The conversion of testosterone into 5α-dihydrotestosterone (5α-DHT) was first observed in the rat and in the human fetal pituitary (18). It was then demonstrated in the pituitary from several animal species, both *in vivo* and *in vitro* (4,19,24,25,32,36,41,51,53).

The successive steps in the reduction of testosterone are summarized in Fig. 2. The first step, as mentioned, leads to the formation of 5α-DHT and the enzyme responsible for this transformation (5α-reductase) should be considered as the key enzyme of testosterone metabolism. The synthesis of 5α-DHT is important because: (a) the conversion of testosterone into 5α-DHT is a nonreversible process; (b) 5α-DHT is the main metabolite of testosterone and the main androgen bound in the nuclei of pituitary cells; (c) 5α-DHT is not aromatizable to estrogens; (d) 5α-DHT is more effective in the regulation of gonadotropin secretion than testosterone itself; (e) 5α-DHT is the precursor of 5α-androstane-3α,17β-diol (3α-adiol) and of 5α-androstane-3β,17β-diol (3β-adiol).

When the metabolism of testosterone in the pituitary is compared with the metabolism of testosterone in the prostate a great difference can be observed. The synthesis of 5α-DHT in the prostate is much greater than in the pituitary, probably because in the pituitary testosterone is exclusively metabolized in the gonadotrophs. Two sets of experiments supported this statement: first, Sar and Stumpf (45,46,48), using dry-autoradiography, studied the cellular and subcellular localization of tritiated testosterone and of 5α-DHT. Their results clearly demonstrated that androgens were selectively concentrated in gonadotrophs, whereas thyrotrophs, acidophils, and chromophobes did not retain radioactivity.

Second, velocity sedimentation at unit gravity of isolated pituitary cells was used as a suitable method to obtain enriched populations of various cell types (17). It was demonstrated that the conversion of testosterone into 5α-DHT was several times higher in fractions containing enriched populations of gonadotrophs than in fractions containing somatotrophs or chromophobes (3,23). When monodispersed cells from male rat pituitary were incubated with tritiated testosterone for 1 hr and then divided into six fractions of enriched populations of cells, the following results were reported (23): the greatest uptake of radioactivity was found in the enriched population of gonadotrophs; it was 1.8 to 2.6 times greater than that found in other fractions. The amount of 5α-reduced metabolites of testosterone in the enriched fraction of gonadotrophs was three times greater than in the enriched population of somatotrophs or chromophobs (23). Testosterone was the main androgen identified in all fractions except in the enriched fraction of gonadotrophs, where 5α-DHT represented 12%, 3α-adiol 4.5%, and androstenedione 2.3% of the total radioactivity (23).

From these results it might be concluded that the uptake and metabolism of testosterone were greater in the enriched population of gonadotrophs than in other fractions.

In our laboratory, the localization of the 5α-reductase activity in a number of enriched populations of different cells was studied. It was clearly demonstrated that the 5α-reductase activity was mainly located in the enriched population of gonadotrophs. Furthermore, there was a good correlation between the presence of 5α-reductase activity and that of LH and FSH.

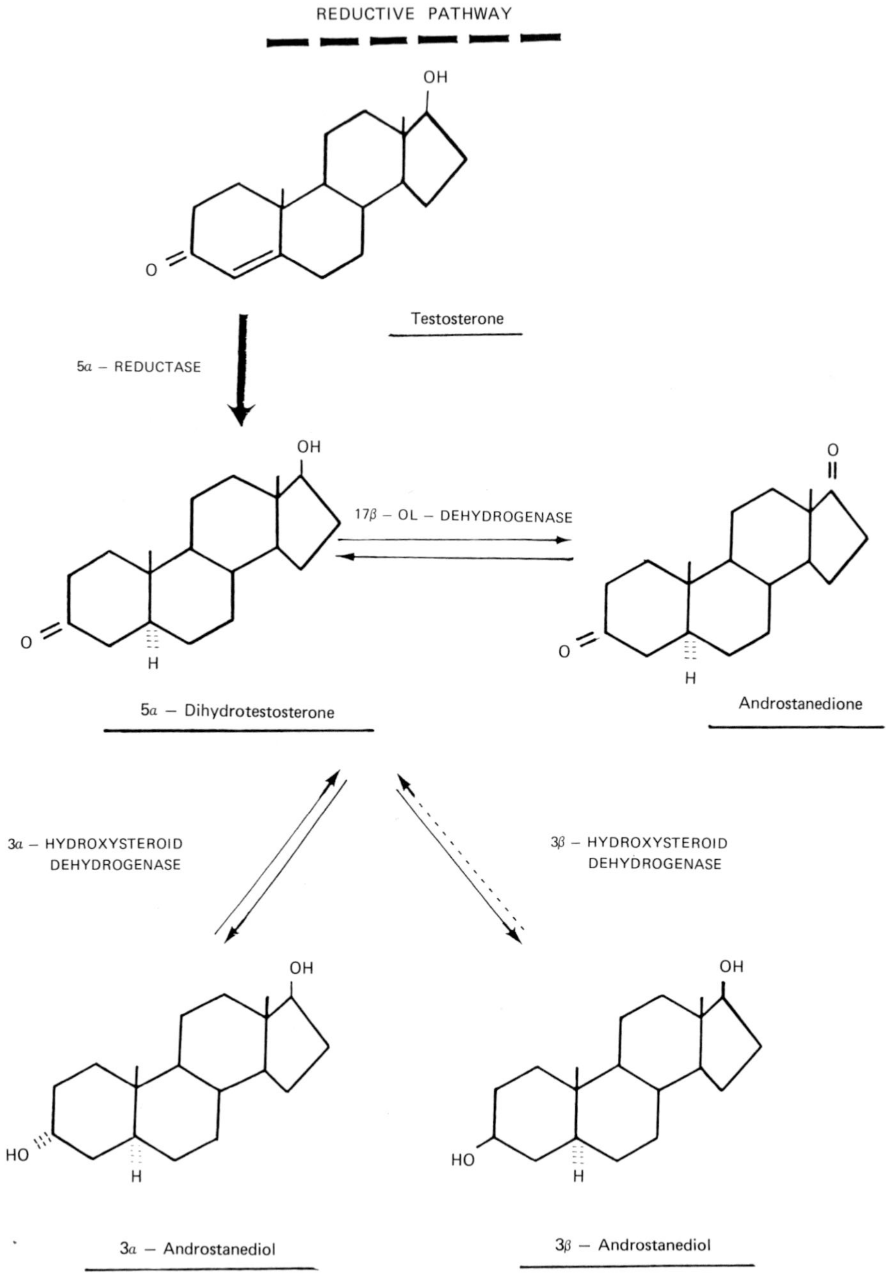

FIG. 2. Reductive pathway of testosterone metabolism.

The second step in the reductive pathway of testosterone is the partial conversion of 5α-DHT into 3α-adiol and 3β-adiol. Two enzymes are involved in this process, the 3α- and 3β-hydroxysteroid dehydrogenases (Fig. 2). The formation of 3α-adiol and 3β-adiol in the pituitary has been demonstrated in several laboratories (4,13,18,24,33,41,51)

The conversion of 5α-DHT into 3α-adiol is a reversible process that might be involved in the regulation of the intracellular level of 5α-DHT. Indeed, when pituitaries were incubated with tritiated 3α-adiol or when tritiated 3α-adiol was injected into male rats, a rapid and intensive conversion of 3α-adiol into 5α-DHT occurred (37). Seventy-three percent of the radioactivity was recovered as 5α-DHT within 30 min. It was mainly found in the 105,000 × g supernatant and in the cellular nuclei. In these two subcellular compartments, 5α-DHT was almost equally recovered in bound and unbound fractions. Moreover, when the hypothalamus or the brain were studied under the same conditions, it appeared that the conversion of 3α-adiol into 5α-DHT was less extensive than in the pituitary; 5α-DHT represented only 28% and 29% of the total radioactivity recovered from the hypothalamus and the brain, respectively. The rapid and extensive conversion of 3α-adiol into 5α-DHT is an important process because: (a) in pituitary cytosol there is no receptor for 3α-adiol; (b) the level of 3α-adiol found in the pituitary is never high is spite of the large amount of 3α-hydroxysteroid dehydrogenase; and (c) it seems to be one of the mechanisms involved in the regulation of the intracellular level of 5α-DHT. The extensive conversion of 3α-adiol into 5α-DHT was confirmed by Kao et al. (57).

From these data the conclusion is that 3α-adiol per se has no physiological action and that it exerts its biological effects via 5α-DHT. At the same time the physiological role of 5α-DHT is confirmed to be prevalent.

As shown in Fig. 2, 5α-DHT is also metabolized into 3β-adiol through the action of the 3β-hydroxysteroid dehydrogenase. Unlike 3α-adiol, 3β-adiol is not reconverted to a significant extent into 5α-DHT, and the major products of the 3β-adiol metabolism are highly polar steroids (15,27). The production of the 3β-adiol surely stands for an important aspect of the 5α-DHT metabolism insofar as it offers some interesting biological possibilities. It could be involved in the processes of sexual maturation, since, when it is injected into immature female rats, it induces precocious puberty (2,8,9).

Moreover, no receptor specific to 3β-adiol was found in the pituitary cytosol, and it is not bound to the androgen receptor. However, preliminary studies showed that it was specifically bound to cytosol proteins (55). The sedimentation coefficient of the hormone-protein complex was 3 S, and androgens did not compete for its binding sites, whereas estrogens did compete to a larger extent than 3β-adiol itself. More recent investigations have demonstrated that in the male rat pituitary cytosol, 3β-adiol was bound with high affinity and specificity to the estradiol receptor (55). Thus, it appears that 3β-adiol is an androgen that may have antagonistic or synergistic properties with regard to estradiol. Its biological action could be henceforth investigated with respect to these findings.

Hydroxylative Pathway

In the male pituitary, 3β-adiol is, to a large extent, converted into polar steroids (27) (Fig. 3). These are trihydroxysteroids, identified as 5α-androstane-3β, 6α, 17β-triol (6α-triol) and 5α-androstane-3β, 7α, 17β-triol (7α-triol) (15,27). They account, respectively, for 53% and 28% of the total 3β-adiol metabolites. The remaining percentage is 6β and 7β-triols.

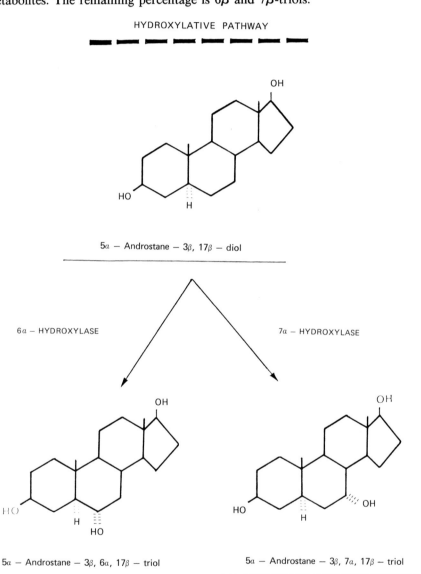

FIG. 3. Conversion of 5α-androstane-3β,17β-diol to 5α-androstane-3β,6α,17β-triol and 5α-androstane-3β,7α,17β-triol.

Triols were found during incubations of whole pituitaries in the presence of tritiated 3β-adiol. When whole pituitaries were incubated with tritiated 3β-adiol for 1 hr, triols accounted for 51% of the total radioactivity recovered in tissues, and for 56% of the total radioactivity found in the incubation medium.

The conversion of 3β-adiol into triols is a rapid process leading to the recovery of 370 fmoles per one pituitary within 5 min. The major part of the triols was released in the incubation medium in direct ratio to time. The release was estimated to be 30 fmoles/1 min/1 pituitary (Fig. 4). At the present time, the biological properties of 6α- and 7α-triols are unknown, but the synthesis of the triols could be an interesting mechanism for the regulation of the intracellular level of 3β-adiol. In any case, attention must be drawn to the binding of 3β-adiol to the estrogen receptor as well as to the synthesis of triols.

Properties and Subcellular Localization of the Main Enzymes Involved in the Metabolism of Androgens

5α-Reductase (3-oxo-5α-Steroid-Δ₄-Reductase)

5α-Reductase, as previously mentioned, is the key enzyme of testosterone metabolism because the synthesis of 5α-DHT is the first event in the metabolic sequence and is a nonreversible process.

The properties and the subcellular localization of 5α-reductase were studied in the pituitary as well as in different brain areas. In any case, the highest activity was found in microsomes (32,41). In the male rat pituitary, the specific activity of 5α-reductase, expressed as fmoles of 5α-DHT formed per 100 μg proteins and per 30 min, was 30 in the 600 × g pellet, 58 in the 10,000 × g pellet, 97 in the 105,000 × g pellet, and 36 in the 105,000 × g supernatant (32). The apparent K_m of the microsomal 5α-reductase was 1.8 μM and the enzyme activity was dependent on NADPH⁺ (32). Some 5α-reductase activity was found in cellular nuclei; it was less than in the microsomes, but was significant (32,41,53,54,56). However, the presence in the nuclear fraction of outer nuclear membranes raised the question of the biological significance of this enzyme activity. In purified nuclei it was demonstrated that 5α-reductase activity exhibited a behavior different from DNA. The 5α-reductase activity relative to DNA decreased during purification (41). That could have been due to decreased microsomal contamination or to disappearance of outer nuclear membranes. When these membranes were separated from the nucleoplasm, the 5α-reductase activity was exclusively found in the membrane fraction (6). Consequently, the 5α-reductase activity observed in cellular nuclei must be related to the presence of outer nuclear membranes.

3α-Hydroxysteroid Dehydrogenase (3α-Hydroxysteroid Oxidoreductase)

The enzyme responsible for the conversion of 5α-DHT into 3α-adiol was found in the pituitary gland as well as in several brain regions. The greatest activity was observed in the 105,000 × g supernatant (cytosol) (33,41). In the

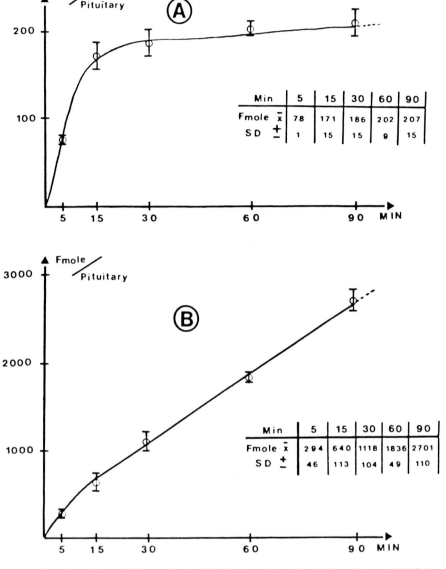

FIG. 4. Kinetic studies of triols synthesis. **(A)** Triols synthesis in pituitary tissue at 37°C for various times. Results are expressed as fmoles of triols produced per pituitary. **(B)** Triols release in the incubation medium. Results are expressed as fmoles of triols released per pituitary. (From Jovan et al., *unpublished data.*)

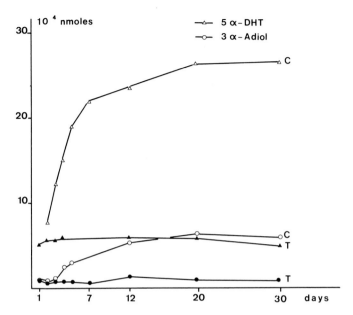

FIG. 5. Time course of the increase in pituitary 5α-reductase activity after castration. **C** = Castrated rats; **T** = sham-operated rats. (From Thien et al., ref. 32, with permission.)

male rat pituitary, the apparent K_m was 2 μM, the optimum pH 6.5 to 7.0, and the optimal temperature 37 to 40°C (33). The thermolability of the enzyme was particularly noticed: raising the temperature of pituitary incubations to 45°C for 30 min resulted in a considerable decrease (47%) in the enzyme activity (33).

The pituitary 3α-hydroxysteroid dehydrogenase activity is dependent on NADPH⁺ concentration. It has been shown that high concentrations of NADPH⁺ favor the synthesis of 3α-adiol, whereas low concentrations favor the formation of 5α-DHT (33).

In the pituitary gland, the 3α-hydroxysteroid dehydrogenase activity is 300 times greater than that of the 5α-reductase; therefore, 3α-adiol should be the major reduced metabolite of testosterone found in the tissue. That is not the case because the conversion of 5α-DHT into 3α-adiol is a reversible process, and because the reverse reaction is favored by a low tissue level of NADPH⁺ (37). Therefore, in the pituitary the formation of either 3α-adiol or 5α-DHT is selectively directed by the tissue concentration of NADPH⁺ (33).

As will be demonstrated elsewhere, the 3α-hydroxysteroid dehydrogenase activity is not modified, whereas the 5α-reductase activity is markedly increased by gonadectomy (33).

3β-Hydroxysteroid Dehydrogenase (3β-Hydroxysteroid Oxidoreductase)

3β-Hydroxysteroid dehydrogenase is responsible for the conversion of 5α-DHT into 3β-adiol. Obviously, this enzyme has not been thoroughly studied,

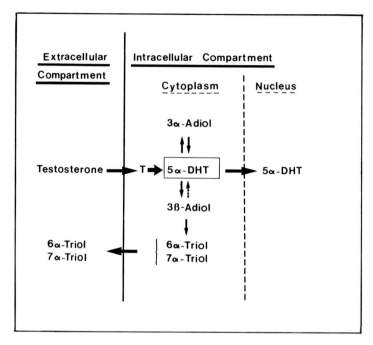

FIG. 6. Central position of 5α-DHT in testosterone metabolism in the male rat pituitary.

in spite of the very special properties of 3β-adiol. Studies are still in progress in this laboratory. From preliminary work, it appears that in the immature male rat pituitary, two enzymes are involved in the 3β-reduction of 5α-DHT: the first of these is located in the microsomes and is $NADPH^+$-dependent; the second is found in cytosol and is $NADH^+$-dependent.

3β-Hydroxysteroid-6α-Hydroxylase (6α-hydroxylase) and 3β-Hydroxysteroid-7α-Hydroxylase (7α-Hydroxylase)

These enzymes are responsible for the metabolism of 3β-adiol to 6α- and 7α-triols. They were studied in the male rat pituitary, and the highest activity was found in microsomes (15). The hydroxylase activity found in nuclei was probably due to the presence in nuclear preparations of outer nuclear membranes: The two hydroxylases were strictly dependent on $NADPH^+$ and were completely inactive in the absence of coenzyme.

It is possible to conclude that the 5α-reductase can be considered as the key enzyme of testosterone metabolism, at least in the anterior pituitary (Fig. 6).

Hormonal Regulation of the 5α-Reductase Activity

Effect of Gonadectomy

The pituitary 5α-reductase activity is dramatically increased by gonadectomy (Fig. 5). This has been demonstrated either *in vivo,* after injection of tritiated testosterone into castrated animals (51), or *in vitro,* after incubations of whole pituitaries (5,19,20,25) or of pituitary microsomes with tritiated testosterone (32). It was demonstrated that: (a) the increase in 5α-DHT production became evident by 2 days after gonadectomy and was very significant 2 days later (4, 25,32) (Fig. 5); (b) the increase continued for at least 2 weeks, then a plateau was reached. At that time, the enzyme activity was five times greater than the control value (4,32) (Fig. 5); (c) the synthesis of 3α-adiol paralleled that of 5α-DHT (4,25,32), due to the large amount of 3α-hydroxysteroid dehydrogenase in the pituitary tissue (33), although the 3α-hydroxysteroid dehydrogenase activity per se was not modified by castration (33); (d) the 17β-hydroxysteroid oxidoreductase activity was not affected by gonadectomy, and the production of androstenedione was unchanged; (e) the increase in 5α-reductase activity was observed both in the male and in the female rat (4); (f) the increase in 5α-DHT production was observed in the pituitary exclusively; In the hypothalamus or in other brain areas, the 5α-reductase activity was not modified by castration (4,5,25,32); and (g) the increase in 5α-reductase activity was related to gonadectomy exclusively. Neither adrenalectomy nor thyroidectomy were able to significantly modify the synthesis of 5α-DHT in the rat pituitary (4).

At the present time there is no available explanation for the postcastration rise in the pituitary 5α-reductase activity. The disappearance of endogenous testosterone might be involved. It would prevent the dilution of the tritiated hormone in the tissue. Thus, the increase in 5α-reductase activity would be more apparent than real. However, this is not the case, since the increase was observed whatever the concentration of labeled substrate used (up to 10^{-5}M) (32). One could also postulate that some inhibitor of 5α-reductase was present in microsomes from intact rats and disappeared after castration. This assumption was discarded when the incubation of a mixture of microsomes from intact and castrated rats did not result in a decrease in 5α-reductase activity (7).

It seems likely that the increase in 5α-reductase activity could be due to the synthesis of new molecules of enzyme. Administration of some antibiotics to castrated animals afforded more complete explanations. Cycloheximide, which is known to inhibit protein biosynthesis, was administered to castrated animals for 3 days, starting on the day of gonadectomy. It was shown that the rise in 5α-reductase activity was completely suppressed (32). Moreover, there was no modification of the enzyme activity in control animals receiving cycloheximide. On the other hand, actinomycin D was without effect on the 5α-reductase activity (32). Taking into account the inefficiency of actinomycin D and the specific action of cycloheximide, it was postulated that 5α-reductase biosynthesis is regulated at the posttranscriptional level, and that castration induces a gradual increase in the intracellular amount of the enzyme.

It is now well established that castration leads to the proliferation and enlargement of gonadotrophs as well as to an increase in LH and FSH secretion. Therefore, a parallel seems to be drawn between gonadotroph cell change, gonadotropin secretion and 5α-reductase activity. This statement emphasizes the biological importance of 5α-DHT in the pituitary gland.

Effect of Hormonal Treatment

It is possible to inhibit the postcastration rise in 5α-DHT by hormonal treatment. Daily administration of testosterone propionate (40 μg/100 g body weight/day), starting on the day of castration, prevented the increase in 5α-reductase activity (5). The same dose of 5α-DHT propionate was less effective (5). Estradiol benzoate (0.05 μg/100 g body weight/day) was slightly effective, whereas 3β-adiol (100 μg/100 g body weight/day) was completely ineffective (5). It was also demonstrated that the *in vitro* conversion of testosterone into 5α-DHT in pituitaries from castrated rats previously injected with testosterone was inhibited, whereas it was not modified in pituitaries from castrated animals given progesterone or corticosterone (2 mg/100 g body weight/day) (20).

The 5α-reductase activity in microsomes from pituitaries of castrated rats treated with androgens or estrogens was also studied (7,32). It appeared that the postcastration rise in microsomal 5α-reductase activity was prevented by the administration of testosterone, 5α-DHT, and 3α-adiol to castrated animals (7,32). Their relative efficacy was: 5α-DHT > 3α-adiol > testosterone (7). The action of 3α-adiol was attributed to its intracellular conversion into 5α-DHT (37). Administration of estradiol or of 3β-adiol did not modify the microsomal 5α-reductase activity (7). Thus, 5α-DHT appeared to be the most effective hormone for the regulation of the microsomal 5α-reductase activity. The mechanism by which 5α-DHT regulates the enzyme activity and its own secretion is still unknown.

The effect of the hypothalamus on the pituitary 5α-reductase activity was studied, and it was demonstrated that there was a direct effect of hypothalamic factors on the enzyme activity (16). Coincubation of pituitary and hypothalamus of intact male rats resulted in an increase in 5α-DHT production. On the contrary, when the pituitary from a castrated rat was incubated with the hypothalamus from an intact rat, there was an inhibition of the pituitary 5α-reductase activity (16). Coincubation of the pituitary and the hypothalamus from castrated rats, or coincubation of the pituitary from intact rats with the hypothalamus from castrated rats, did not modify the 5α-reductase activity (16). Moreover, the luteinizing hormone releasing hormone (LHRH) added to the incubation medium with pituitaries was able to promote the formation of 5α-DHT in intact rats, and to inhibit its formation in castrated rats (16). The mechanism of action of LHRH or of other hypothalamic factors is still obscure. Further investigation is necessary to ascertain the role of LHRH, and to explain its possible action.

Changes in Testosterone Metabolism During Sexual Maturation

Some experiments have been performed to study the metabolism of testosterone in pituitaries from rats of various ages and to correlate any changes found with sexual development and maturation.

The metabolism of testosterone was studied at 5-day intervals from birth to puberty (5). In all cases, 5α-DHT, and to a lesser extent 3α-adiol, were the main metabolites recovered. In males and in females, the production of 5α-DHT was greater at birth than in the adult age (5). In females the synthesis of 5α-DHT reached a high level between days 10 and 15 (5). Then it gradually fell from day 15 to day 30. In males, following a slight increase up to day 10, there was a decrease and a second and significant rise between days 30 and 34 (5). Parallel changes in the pituitary gonadotropic activity were observed.

The *in vitro* study of testosterone metabolism during sexual maturation allowed us to identify separately the metabolites released into the incubation medium and those which were bound to cytosol or nuclear proteins (13,24). In the incubation medium, there was no obvious modification of the metabolites with respect to age (24). On the contrary, there was less testosterone and more 5α-DHT bound to cytosol proteins at puberty than before or after puberty (24). Furthermore, there was more 5α-DHT bound to nuclear proteins in prepubertal and pubertal male rats than in younger or adult animals (24). Modifications of gonadotropin secretion and sexual maturation might result from these changes.

The synthesis of polar steroids and of androstanediols in the male rat pituitary was also studied during sexual maturation (13). In 6-week-old rats the amounts of polar steroids and androstanediols found in the incubation medium were greater than in 3-week or 9-week-old rats (13).

The *in vitro* study of testosterone metabolism during postnatal development and puberty provides some data concerning the enzymes involved in the metabolism of androgens. However, it should be remembered that in females the 5α-reductase function is devoted to the metabolism of progesterone and of hormones with a double bond in the position 4–5.

To really understand the role of androgens in sexual maturation and gonadotropin modulation, it would be necessary to estimate the intrapituitary levels of various hormones from birth to adult age, and to correlate these with the amount of cytosol and nuclear receptors for androgens and with the pituitary and blood levels of LH and FSH.

ANDROGEN METABOLISM IN THE HYPOTHALAMUS OF THE MALE

Testosterone Metabolism

Uptake and distribution of tritiated testosterone into brain regions were studied in intact and castrated animals by several methods, such as injections of tritiated hormone, constant infusions or incubation of slices. It was demonstrated that the relative uptakes of testosterone were as follows: anterior pituitary>hypothalamus>midbrain>cerebral cortex (40,42).

In cerebral tissue, testosterone is metabolized along the same pathways as in the pituitary gland. The hormone is converted into 5α-DHT, 3α-adiol, 3β-adiol, androstenedione, and androstanedione (4,13,18,19,24,25,34–36,41,50,

51,56,57,59). 5α-DHT is the main metabolite produced, but in the hypothalamus, testosterone is converted into 5α-DHT to a lesser extent than in the anterior pituitary.

In the hypothalamus, the subcellular distribution of the enzymes involved in testosterone metabolism is the same as in the pituitary gland. 5α-Reductase was predominantly found in microsomes (34,41). It was also found in nuclei, but that was due to the presence in the nuclear pellet of outer nuclear membranes.

The ratios of the specific activities of 5α-reductase in some brain areas relative to that in total brain were: hypothalamus 1.0, cerebellum 1.6, cortex 0.3 (51). 3α-Hydroxysteroid dehydrogenase and 17β-hydroxysteroid dehydrogenase were found in the 105,000 × g supernatant (41). The activity was equally distributed throughout the different brain areas (41).

As in the pituitary gland, the 5α-reduction of testosterone is a nonreversible process. When homogenates of whole hypothalami were incubated in the presence of tritiated 5α-DHT, no testosterone was recovered; the main metabolite was 3α-adiol (34,57). 3α-Adiol was to some extent reconverted into 5α-DHT (34,57). Incubations of hypothalami in the presence of 3α-adiol led to the recovery of a large amount of polar metabolites (57). They were not identified, but it is likely that, as in the pituitary, they are trihydroxysteroids (15,27).

No differences related to the sex of the animals could be detected (4,10,56). Moreover, the metabolism of testosterone was the same in newborn rats (4 to 12 days old) as in prepubertal animals (32 days old) (10). There was no correlation between the production of 5α-reduced steroids and age (13,24), and the hypothalamic 5α-reductase activity was not modified by castration (4,25,32,34).

In brief, when the metabolism of testosterone in the brain of male and female animals was studied, some similarities to and some differences from the pituitary gland could be established. In the brain, as in the pituitary gland, testosterone is mainly metabolized into 5α-reduced steroids. The differences are summarized as follows: (a) in the hypothalamus, the metabolism of testosterone is less extensive than in the pituitary gland; (b) there is no change in testosterone metabolism related to sex or age; and (c) the metabolism of testosterone is not modified by castration. Whether the lack of change in the androgen metabolism is real or due to the difficulties encountered in isolating small and defined brain areas has not been accurately ascertained. One must remember that androgens, as well as estrogens, are located in some discrete areas of the brain, as was shown clearly by dry-autoradiography (44,47,48).

Aromatization of Androgens

It was first demonstrated in 1971 that androstenedione could be converted into estrone and estradiol (29,30). Incubations of diencephalon, including the hypothalamus and the median eminence, from human fetuses at 10 and 22 weeks with [14C]-androstenedione led to the recovery of estrone and estradiol

(29). Since that time, several works have been devoted to studying estrogen synthesis in the brain (1,11,12,14,21,22,28–31,38,39,43,49,58).

Distribution of Aromatase Through Brain Areas

The ability to convert testosterone and adrostenedione into estrogens is not a general property of the central nervous system, but is found only in some specific brain areas. No aromatase activity was found in the pituitary gland or in the frontal cortex (12,14,22,30,38,39,58). It was generally demonstrated that aromatization is greater in the hypothalamus and limbic structures than in other brain areas.

Limbic Structures

Limbic structures from human male fetuses at 17 weeks were able to aromatize androstenedione to estrone and estradiol (30). Estrone was identified with conversion factors of 0.11% in one experiment and 0.05% in another experiment, and estradiol with a conversion factor of 0.019% (30). Conversion of androstenedione to estrone in the limbic system of both male and female adult rabbits, intact or castrated, was also observed (38).

Aromatase activity was present in the rat limbic system during the critical period of sexual differentiation (39). Incubations of limbic structures from rat fetuses at 21 days with androstenedione resulted in the formation of estrone (39). Synthesis of estrone was also observed in the limbic areas from 1, 5, or 10-day-old rats and from adult rats (39). The aromatase activity observed in fetuses or in newborn rats equaled or exceeded that observed in adults. Moreover, it was demonstrated that the estrogens produced were concentrated in the cell nuclei (21,22). Two hr after injection of tritiated testosterone into newborn rats of both sexes, approximately 50% of the radioactivity recovered in limbic cell nuclei occurred as estradiol. The nuclear amount represented a five-fold concentration of estrogens over the level in whole homogenate (21). In limbic areas from adult male rats the same results were obtained (22). In every case, estradiol accounted for 4 to 7% of the total radioactivity and for 36 to 52% of the nuclear radioactivity (22). In three successive experiments, the amounts of estradiol in whole limbic homogenate were 0.8, 0.4, and 1.1 fmoles/mg proteins, whereas they were 16.3, 6.7, and 5.8 fmoles/mg proteins in cell nuclei (22). These results clearly indicated that the estradiol synthesized in the limbic area was to a large extent transferred into the cell nuclei.

Hypothalamus

The hypothalamus was the first brain area identified as the site of androgen aromatization. The conversion of androstenedione into estrone was observed in the hypothalamus from several animal species, such as rat, rabbit, monkey, and human fetus (43). The conversion of androstenedione into estrone and of testosterone into estradiol was demonstrated in the hypothalamus from the rhesus monkey (11). The conversion factors were, respectively, 0.01% and 0.0036%. When expressed as pmoles of estrogens synthesized per g of tissue and per hour, the values were 5.26 for estrone and 1.83 for estradiol (11). Thus, the rate of androstenedione aromatization was three times greater than that of testosterone. Moreover, the aromatizing system was more active in the hypothalamus than in the limbic area; the amounts of estrone and estradiol produced in the hypothalamus were, respectively, 11 and 21 times greater than that produced in the limbic system (11). Perfusions of isolated brains from immature male rhesus monkeys with labeled androstenedione led to the same results. The conversion of androstenedione into estrone was 0.01% of the starting substrate (12). The conversion into estrogens of either androstenedione or testosterone has been observed in hypothalami from fetal, neonatal, immature, and adult male or female rats (14,39,58).

Most of the studies related to the aromatization of androgens in the brain were carried out by incubating either homogenates or slices of tissue. A new approach to the problem consisted of primary monolayer cultures of hypothalamic cells from rat fetuses (1). Eight-day-old cultures were tested for their ability to convert androgens into estrogens. After they had been incubated with either androstenedione or 19-hydroxyandrostenedione for 4 days, estrone was identified in the medium. The formation of estrone was in direct ratio to incubation time and 19-hydroxyandrostenedione appeared to be a more efficient precursor of estrone than androstenedione (1). It produced three times more estrone than did androstenedione. This result correlates with the fact that 19-hydroxyandrostenedione is an intermediate in the aromatization of testosterone. Moreover, the treatment of monolayer cell cultures with cytosine arabinoside, which is known to inhibit the proliferation of non-neuronal cells and to promote the growth of neuronal cells, enhanced the synthesis of estrone. On a per mg protein basis, the production of estrone in treated cultures was six times greater than in untreated cultures (1). These findings suggested that the aromatizing activity was located in the neurons.

The aromatization of androgens was studied in different hypothalamic regions separately. In human fetuses, as well as in rat or in rabbit, it was demonstrated that the conversion of androstenedione into estrone was greater, or was exclusively present, in the anterior part of the hypothalamus (31). No aromatization was found in the posterior part of the hypothalamus from male or female rats (31) or rabbits (38). In 7-day-old and in 120-day-old female rats, the amount of testosterone metabolized to estradiol was greater in the hypothalamus and the amygdala than in the septal or the preoptic areas (58). Within the hypothalamus, some specific regions appeared to be more efficient than others in converting androgens into estrogens (49). The medial preoptic nucleus-anterior hypothalamic nucleus exhibited the highest aromatase activity in male and in female rats. (The highest level of estrone synthesized was 30 pmoles/100 mg proteins/hr in males and 12 pmoles/100 mg proteins/hr in females) (49). The mediobasal hypothalamus exhibited the second highest level of aromatase activity (5 pmoles/100 mg proteins/hr and 3.6 pmoles/100 mg proteins/hr, respectively, in males and females). The conversion of androgens to estrogens was very small in the lateral preoptic nucleus, the lateral hypothalamic nucleus, and the amygdaloid complex (49).

Physiological Modifications of Aromatase Activity

Different physiological states are able to modify the aromatase activity in the brain.

Age

In general, aromatization is greater in the hypothalamus from a fetal or new-born animal than in the hypothalamus from an adult animal (39,58). The aromatizing activity appeared to decrease on and after the 10th day of life. Variations in aromatase activity were thoroughly studied in the developing brain of the rabbit (14). It was demonstrated that in the teleencephalon, the rate of conversion of androgens was very low on day 13. Then it increased to 0.3 pmole/100 mg proteins/hr on day 16 and fell thereafter (14). In the diencephalon, the aromatase activity increased 10-fold from day 16 to day 19, then remained at a high level up to day 25 and fell at the time of delivery to the same level as that observed on day 16 (14).

Sex

Aromatization was greater in males than in females, whether it was studied in the hypothalamus or the limbic area from fetal, neonatal, prepubertal, or adult animals (31,39,43). However, no significant differences appeared in forebrain tissue from male and female embryos (14).

Castration

The aromatase activity was increased by castration (43). It was studied in rabbits castrated 1 month before sacrifice. It appeared that in castrated males the aromatase activity was two to three times greater than in intact males. In castrated females a five-fold increase was observed (28,38) (Fig. 7). It was especially noticed that gonadectomy tended to abolish sex differences.

Hormone Administration

Administration of estradiol to castrated male or female rabbits resulted in a significant increase in aromatase activity in the hypothalamus and the limbic

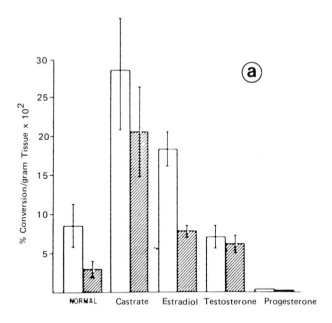

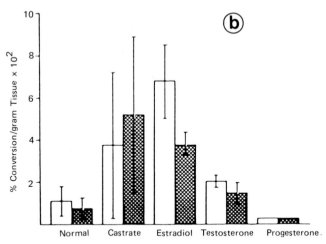

FIG. 7. The effects of castration and hormonal pretreatment on the aromatization of [³H]androstenedione by rabbit hypothalamus **(a)** and limbic tissues **(b).** □, male; ▨, female. (From Naftolin et al., ref. 28, with permission.)

area (28,38) (Fig. 7). Testosterone administration abolished the sex differences in the hypothalamus by increasing activity in females without changing that in males. The limbic system of both sexes exhibited a significant increase in activity, which also decreased the sex differences. Administration of progesterone resulted in a decrease in the aromatase activity in male and female hypothalami, so that sex differences were abolished (28,38) (Fig. 7). Incubation of hypothalami from adult rabbits with cyproterone or cyproterone acetate resulted in a dramatic decrease in hypothalamic aromatase activity (28).

In conclusion, the aromatization of androgens in some definite areas of the central nervous system has been accurately demonstrated. This could be involved in several biologial events, such as brain differentiation, puberty timing, sexual behavior, or gonadotropin regulation. Although the role of additional formation of estrogens can be explained in males, it is not so clear in females, where estrogens from ovarian origin should be enough to ensure such biological regulation.

REFERENCES

1. Canik, J. A., Vaccaro, D. E., Ryan, K. J., and Leeman, S. E. (1977): The aromatization of androgens by primary monolayer cultures of foetal rat hypothalamus. *Endocrinology,* 100:250–253.
2. David, R., and Eckstein, B. (1976): Androstanediol sulphates in peripheral blood of immature rats and some of their biological effects. *J. Endocrinol.,* 71:299–304.
3. Denef, C. (1976): Partial purification of different pituitary cell types in the rat: A study in developmental changes in cell type distribution and correlation with in situ conversion of testosterone to 5α-dihydrotestosterone. *Ann. Biol. Anim. Biochim. Biophys.,* 16:409–412.
4. Denef, C., Magnus,C., and McEwen, B. S. (1973): Sex differences and hormonal control of testosterone metabolism in rat pituitary and brain. *J. Endocrinol.,* 59:605–621.
5. Denef, C., Magnus, C., and McEwen, B. S. (1974): Sex-dependent changes in pituitary 5α-dihydrotestosterone and 3α-androstanediol formation during postnatal development and puberty in the rat. *Endocrinology,* 94:1265–1274.
6. Ducouret, B., Samperez, S., and Jouan, P. (1977): Localization d'une activité 5α-réductase dans les membranes nucléaires de l'hypophyse antérieure du rat mâle adulte, normal et castré. *C.R. Soc. Biol. (Paris),* 171:639–643.
7. Ducouret, B., Samperez, S., and Jouan, P.: Régulation hormonale de l'activité de la 5α-réductase des microsomes de l'hypophyse antérieure du rat mâle. *C.R. Soc. Biol. (Paris) (in press).*
8. Eckstein, B. (1975): Studies on the onset of puberty in the female rat. *J. Steroid Biochem.,* 6:873–878.
9. Eckstein, B., and Springer, C. (1971): Induction of an ovarian epimerase system catalyzing the transformation of 5α-androstane-3α, 17β-diol to 5α-androstane-3β, 17β-diol after treatment of immature rat with gonadotrophins exhibiting FSH-like activity. *Endocrinology,* 89:347–352.
10. Farquhar, M. N., Namik, H., and Gurbman, A. (1976): Cytoplasmatic and nuclear metabolism of testosterone in the brains of neonatal and prepubertal rats. *Neuroendocrinology,* 20:358–372.
11. Flores, F., Naftolin, F., and Ryan, K. J. (1973): Aromatization of androstanedione and testosterone by rhesus monkey hypothalamus and limbic system. *Neuroendocrinology,* 11:177–182.
12. Flores, F., Naftolin, F., Ryan, K. J., and White, R. J. (1973): Estrogen formation by the isolated perfused rhesus monkey brain. *Science,* 180:1074–1075.
13. Genot, A., Loras, B., Monbon, M., and Bertrand, J. (1975): *In vitro* metabolism of testosterone in the rat brain during sexual maturation. III. Studies of the formation of main androstanediols and androstene-diols. *J. Steroid Biochem.,* 6:1247–1252.
14. George, F. W., Tobleman, W. T., Milewich, L., and Wilson, J. D. (1978): Aromatase activity in the developing rabbit brain. *Endocrinology,* 102:86–91.
15. Guiraud, J. M., Morfin, R., Ducouret, B., Samperez, S., and Jouan, P. (1979): Pituitary metabolism of 5α-androstane-3β, 17β-diol: Intense and rapid conversion into 5α-androstane-3β, 6α, 17β-triol and 5α-androstane-3β, 7α, 17β-triol. *Steroids,* 241–248.
16. Has, B., Kniewald, S., and Milkovic, S. (1975): Effects of coincubation of the pituitary and hypothalamus of intact and castrated male rats and the influence of LH-RH on pituitary 5α-reductase activity. *Neuroendocrinology,* 19:36–43.

17. Hymer, W. C., Evans, W. H., Kraicer, J., Mastro, A., Davis, J., and Grisworld, E. (1973): Enrichment of cell types from rat adenohypophysis by sedimentation. *Endocrinology,* 92:275–287.

18. Jaffe, R. B. (1969): Testosterone metabolism in target tissues: Hypothalamic and pituitary tissues of the adult rat and human fetus and the immature rat epiphysis. *Steroids,* 14:483–498.

19. Kniewald, Z., Massa, R., Motta, M., and Martini, L. (1971): Feedback mechanisms and the control of the hypothalamo-hypophysial complex. In: *Steroid Hormone and Brain Function,* edited by C. H. Sawyer and R. A. Gorski, pp. 289–299. University of California Press, Los Angeles.

20. Kniewald, Z., and Milkovic, S. (1973); Testosterone: A regulator of 5α-reductase activity in the pituitary of male and female rats. *Endocrinology,* 92:1772–1775.

21. Lieberburg, I., and McEwen, B. S. (1975): Estradiol-17β: A metabolite of testosterone recovered in cell nuclei from limbic areas of neonatal rat brains. *Brain Res.,* 85:165–170.

22. Lieberburg, I., and McEwen, B. S. (1975): Estradiol-17β: A metabolite of testosterone recovered in cell nuclei from limbic areas of adult male rat brains. *Brain Res.,* 91:171–174.

23. Lloyd, R. V., and Karavolas, H. J. (1975): Uptake and conversion of progesterone and testosterone to 5α-reduced product by enriched gonadotropic and chromophobic rat anterior pituitary cell fractions. *Endocrinology,* 97:517–526.

24. Loras, B., Genot, A., Monbon, M., Buecher, F., Reboud, J. P., and Bertrand, J. (1974): Binding and metabolism of testosterone in the rat during sexual maturation. II. Testosterone metabolism. *J. Steroid Biochem.,* 5:425–431.

25. Massa, R., Stupnicka, E., Kniewald, Z., and Martini, L. (1972): The transformation of testosterone into dihydrotestosterone by the brain and the anterior pituitary. *J. Steroid Biochem.,* 3:385–399.

26. Mercier, L., Leguellec, C., Thieulant, M. L., Samperez, S., and Jouan, P. (1976): Androgen and estrogen receptors in the cytosol from male rat anterior hypophysis; further characteristics and differentiation between androgen and estrogen receptors. *J. Steroid Biochem.,* 7:779–785.

27. Morfin, R., Guiraud, J. M., Ducouret, B., Samperez, S., and Jouan, P. (1979): Mise en évidence du 5α-androstane-3β, 6α, 17β-triol et du 5α-androstane-3β, 7α, 17β-triol dans l'hypophyse antérieure du rat mâle prépubère. *C.R. Acad. Sci. (Paris),* 288:437–440.

28. Naftolin, F., Ryan, K. J., Davies, I. J., Reddy, V. V., Flores, F., Petro, Z., Kuhn, M., White, R. J., Takoaka, Y., and Wolin, L. (1975): The formation of estrogens by central neuroendocrine tissues. *Recent Prog. Horm. Res.,* 31:295–315.

29. Naftolin, F., Ryan, K. J., and Petro, Z. (1971): Aromatization of androstenedione by the diencephalon. *J. Clin. Endocrinol. Metab.,* 33:368–370.

30. Naftolin, F., Ryan, K. J., and Petro, Z. (1971): Aromatization of androstenedione by limbic system tissue from human fetuses. *J. Endocrinol.,* 51:795–796.

31. Naftolin, F., Ryan, K. J., and Petro, Z. (1972): Aromatization of androstenedione by anterior hypothalamus of adult male and female rats. *Endocrinology,* 90:295–298.

32. Nguyen Cong Thien, Duval, J., Samperez, S., and Jouan, P. (1974): Testosterone 5α-reductase of microsomes from rat anterior hypophysis: properties, increase by castration and hormonal control. *Biochimie,* 56:899–906.

33. Nguyen Cong Thien, Samperez, S., and Jouan, P. (1975): Properties of 3α-hydroxysteroid dehydrogenase in the male rat pituitary gland. *J. Steroid Biochem.,* 6:1165–1169.

34. Noma, K., Sato, B., Yano, S., and Yamamura, Y. (1975): Metabolism of testosterone in hypothalamus of male rats. *J. Steroid Biochem.,* 6:1261–1266.

35. Perez, A. E., Ortiz, A., Carbeza, M., Beyer, C., and Perez-Palacios, G. (1975): *In vitro* metabolism of ³H-androstenedione by the male rat pituitary, hypothalamus and hippocampus. *Steroids,* 26:5.–62.

36. Perez-Palacios, G., Castaneda, E., Gomez-Perez, F., Perez, A. E., and Gual, C. (1970): *In vitro* metabolism of androgens in dog hypothalamus, pituitary and limbic system. *Biol. Reprod.,* 3:205–213.

37. Pilven, A., Thieulant, M. L., Ducouret, B., Samperez, S., and Jouan, P. (1976): Rapid and intensive conversion of 5α-androstane-3α, 17β-diol into 5α-dihydrotestosterone in the male rat anterior pituitary: *In vivo* and *in vitro* studies. *Steroids,* 28:349–358.

38. Reddy, V. V. R., Naftolin, F., and Ryan, K. J. (1973): Aromatization in the central nervous system of rabbits: Effects of castration and hormone treatment. *Endocrinology,* 92:589–594.

39. Reddy, V. V. R., Naftolin, F., and Ryan, K. J. (1974): Conversion of androstenedione to estrone by neural tissues from fetal and neonatal rats. *Endocrinology,* 94:117–121.

40. Resko, J. A., Goy, R. W., and Phoenix, C. H. (1967): Uptake and distribution of exogenous testosterone-1,2-^{3}H in neural and genital tissues of the castrated guinea pig. *Endocrinology,* 80:490–498.

41. Rommerts, F. F. G., and Van der Molen, H. J. (1971): Occurrence and localization of 5α-steroid reductase, 3α and 17β-hydroxysteroid dehydrogenases in hypothalamus and other brain tissues of the male rat. *Biochim. Biophys. Acta,* 248:489–502.

42. Roy, S. K., and Laumas, K. R. (1969): 1,2-^{3}H-Testosterone: Distribution and uptake in neural and genital tissues of intact male, castrated male and female rats. *Acta Endocrinol. (Kbh),* 61:629–640.

43. Ryan, K. J., Naftolin, F., Reddy, V., Flores, F., and Petro, Z. (1972): Estrogen formation in the brain. *Am. J. Obstet. Gynecol.,* 114:454–460.

44. Sar, M., and Stumpf, W. E. (1972): Cellular localization of androgen in the brain and pituitary after injection of tritiated testosterone. *Experientia,* 28:1364–1366.

45. Sar, M., and Stumpf, W. E. (1973): Pituitary gonadotrophs: Nuclear concentration of radioactivity after injection of (^{3}H)-testosterone. *Science,* 179:389–391.

46. Sar, M., and Stumpf, W. E. (1973): Cellular and subcellular localization of radioactivity in the rat pituitary after injection of 1,2-^{3}H-testosterone using dry-autoradiography. *Endocrinology,* 92:631–635.

47. Sar, M., and Stumpf, W. E. (1973): Autoradiographic localization of radioactivity in the rat brain after the injection of 1,2-^{3}H-testosterone. *Endocrinology,* 92:251–256.

48. Sar, M., and Stumpf, W. E. (1977): Distribution of androgen target cells in rat forebrain and pituitary after (^{3}H)-dihydrotestosterone administration. *J. Steroid Biochem.,* 8:1131–1135.

49. Selmanoff, M. K., Brodkin, L. D., Weiner, R. I., and Siiteri, P. K. (1977): Aromatization and 5α-reduction of androgens in discrete hypothalamic and limbic regions of the male and female rats. *Endocrinology,* 101:841–848.

50. Sholiton, L. J., and Werk, E. E. (1969): The less-polar metabolites produced by incubation of testosterone-^{14}C with rat and bovine brain. *Acta Endocrinol. (Kbh),* 61:641–648.

51. Stern, J. M., and Eisenfeld, A. J. (1971): Distribution and metabolism of ^{3}H-testosterone in castrated male rat: Effect of cyproterone, progesterone and unlabeled testosterone. *Endocrinology,* 88:1117–1125.

52. Thieulant, M. L., Pelle, G., Samperez, S., and Jouan, P. (1974): Augmentation de la 5α-stéroide réductase des noyaux cellulaires purifiés d'hypophyses de rats mâles castrés. *C.R. Acad. Sci. (Paris),* 278:1281–1284.

53. Thieulant, M. L., Samperez, S., and Jouan, P. (1973): Binding and metabolism of (^{3}H)-testosterone in the nuclei of rat pituitary *in vivo. J. Steroid Biochem.,* 4:677–685.

54. Thieulant, M. L., Samperez, S., and Jouan, P. (1973): Etude du métabolisme de la testosterone-^{3}H dans des noyaux purifiés d'hypophyses antérieures de rats mâles normaux et castrés. *C.R. Soc. Biol. (Paris),* 167:1445–1450.

55. Thieulant, M. L., Samperez, S., and Jouan, P.: 5α-Androstane-3β,17β-diol: An androgen which binds to the estradiol receptor with high affinity, in the male rat hypophysis. *J. Steroid Biochem. (in press).*

56. Verhoeven, G., Lamberigts, G., and De Moor, P. (1974): Nucleus-associated steroid 5α-reductase activity and androgen responsiveness. A study in various organs and brain regions of rats. *J. Steroid Biochem.,* 5:93–100.

57. Wei liu Kao, Perez, L., Perez, A., Loret, L., and Weisz, J. (1977): Metabolism *in vitro* of dihydrotestosterone, 5α-androstane-3α,17β-diol and its 3β-epimer, three metabolites of testosterone, by three of its target tissues, the anterior pituitary, the medial basal hypothalamus and the seminiferous tubules. *J. Steroid Biochem.,* 8:1109–1115.

58. Weisz, J., and Gibbs, C. (1974): Conversion of testosterone and androstenedione to estrogens *in vitro* by the brain of female rats. *Endocrinology,* 94:616–620.

59. Whalen, R. E., and Rezek, D. L. (1972): Localization of androgenic metabolites in the brain of rats administered testosterone or dihydrotestosterone. *Steroids,* 20:717–725.

The Endocrine Functions of the Brain,
edited by Marcella Motta.
Raven Press, New York © 1980

6

Role of Hormones in Perinatal Brain Differentiation

Bernard T. Donovan

Department of Physiology, Institute of Psychiatry, De Crespigny Park, London SE5 8AF, England

The effects of hormones on the brain, and hence the influences hormones exert on behavior, can be reviewed in a variety of ways. Even so, it is always important to distinguish between the organizational effects of hormones, which is the burden of this chapter, and the hormonal state prevailing at the time a behavioral pattern is elicited. The hormonal background influences such parameters as the general metabolic state, the sensitivity of receptors to stimulation, the response of certain receptors, and the psychic outlook, so that generalizations must be made with caution. Nevertheless, the actions of hormones during development set the stage for subsequent behavioral responses.

CRITICAL PERIODS

When considering the effects of hormones on brain development, it is as well to recall that the brain is composed of many parts, each with its own maturational pattern. For example, myelination begins in the phylogenetically older parts of the brain (e.g., the brainstem), so that the vulnerability of specific areas to a factor affecting myelination changes. Similarly, in the newborn rat, neuronal multiplication in the cerebellum is more vulnerable to experimental insults than that of spinal cord neurons, which have developed further (32). Moreover, the brain nuclei essential for the survival of the young develop first. Thus the neurons controlling suckling mature ahead of other cells in the facial nucleus (3).

Although the sequence of developmental changes in the brain is probably common to all mammals, the timing can be very different, a point that must never be neglected when comparing experimental observations. Growth of the human brain is most rapid between the middle of gestation until around 2 years after birth, whereas that of the rat is maximal around 10 days after birth, and most of the development of the guinea pig brain occurs *in utero*. Expressed in another way, the newborn rat or rabbit may be regarded as equivalent, in brain development terms, to that of a 5-month human fetus, and a newborn guinea pig to a 2- to 3-year-old human child (35).

The brain is not uniformly susceptible to the organizational effects of hormones. Alongside the differential sensitivity of various parts of the brain, the sensitivity of a particular structure varies with time and may be permanently affected only when a hormone is given at a particular phase of development, or critical period. Sex hormones are most effective in influencing the pattern of sexual differentiation of the brain of the rat when given during the first few days after birth.

The concept of the critical period has a long history and wide applicability through the behavioral sciences (131,132), although it must be emphasized that many critical periods exist which may overlap or be widely separated in time, depending on the function or process studied. Naturally, the basis of a critical period can vary from one situation to another but may simply represent the phase at which the process under study is proceeding at maximum velocity (130). The growth spurt of the brain has been studied particularly closely, for at this time it is likely to be especially susceptible to disturbance (35).

THYROID HORMONES

The influence of thyroid hormones on brain development and function was well surveyed by Sokoloff and Kennedy (137). They point out that in the mature individual the effects of thyroid dysfunction in most tissues are prominently manifested by changes in energy exchange, but that the brain does not react in this way. On the other hand, in the young mammal the effects of thyroid hormones on growth, development, and maturation predominate, and the brain is most dramatically affected. Consequently, cretinism produces a morphologically and functionally undeveloped brain and mental deficiency. Thyroid hormones promote, and are essential for, the postnatal maturation of the brain, but once mature the brain appears to become insensitive to their actions. This development change in response is reflected in a variety of biochemical indices. Oxygen consumption by the cerebral cortex of the rat is normally low at birth and remains so for about the first 10 days of life; it then rises sigmoidally, reaching the adult level at about 45 days of age. Thyroxine administration accelerates the rise in oxygen consumption, but once the adult level is reached thyroxine treatment is no longer effective. Sokoloff (136) found the relationship between mitochondrial activity and the response to thyroid hormone particularly intriguing ever since the finding that replacement of the mitochondria in preparations of euthyroid liver tissue with those from hyperthyroid animals produced hyperthyroid rates of protein synthesis, whereas hyperthyroid preparations in which the mitochondria were replaced by euthyroid mitochondria showed euthyroid rates of protein synthesis. Somewhat similar results emerged from experiments with adult and immature brain, where the source of the mitochondria determined the presence or absence of stimulation by thyroxine. Protein synthesis was stimulated by mitochondria from immature brain but not by those from adult brain, regardless of the source of the microsomes or cell sap. On this basis, the mitochondria of immature brain appear to be directly responsive to thyroid hormone and seem to lose their sensitivity on maturation.

Morphological Effects

The morphological effects of thyroid hormones on the developing brain have been most closely studied in the rat, although it is well known that the brain weight of human cretins may be 40% below normal, that the cerebral gyri are narrow, and that the thickness of the cerebral cortex is reduced. However, Adams and Rosman (1) emphasized the considerable doubt that any reliable brain lesions have been demonstrated microscopically in hypothyroidism, even when cretinism is accompanied by lifelong idiocy. Experimentally, hypothyroidism in the neonatal rat reduces the size of the perikarya in the cerebral cortex, reduces the growth of axons and dendrites, discourages the ingrowth of axonal processes from the thalamus and elsewhere, and produces a variety of subtle changes in the neuropil, thereby leading to a cerebral cortex in which the cells are closely packed (46,79).

Thyroid hormones, at least in rats and mice, influence the rate of cell proliferation in the postnatal brain. In hypothyroid infant rats, cell acquisition is normal in the forebrain and reversibly retarded in the cerebellum, whereas cell numbers are permanently depressed in the olfactory bulbs. The ultimate restoration of cell numbers in the cerebellum to normal results from the persistence of the germinal zone, as shown histologically and by measuring the rate of DNA synthesis (11). As summarized by Adams and Rosman (1), the inward migration of external granular cells, which cross the molecular layer to form the internal granular layer of the rat cerebellum, is retarded, with delay in the disappearance of the external granular layer. Dendritic arborization of the Purkinje cells is severely retarded; there is a marked reduction in the numbers of basket cells in the cerebellar cortex; and synaptogenesis is reduced significantly. Morphological changes in the cerebellar cortex of hypothyroid animals have been reversed by treatment with thyroid hormones. Balázs et al. (11) propose that as a result of the lack of postsynaptic sites for their axons the survival of a proportion of the granule cells becomes prejudiced. Neonatal treatment with thyroid hormone permanently reduces the number of cells in the brain, probably through acceleration and premature ending of the cell proliferation associated with brain maturation (11,42). In these animals innately organized behavior appeared sooner than in controls, but the subsequent performance of thyroid-hormone-treated animals in adaptive behavior tests was impaired. These changes are mirrored, to a large extent, by changes in protein synthesis in the immature brain, which is three to four times greater than that of the adult. Alongside the effects of thyroid hormone on the mitochondria, alluded to earlier, the affinity of rat cerebellar cytosol for triiodothyronine is high during infancy, when cytodifferentiation is most intense, and declines dramatically with age without a fall in the number of binding sites (49). Additionally, it may be that thyroid hormones influence the formation of the microtubules in nerve cells that are required for axon growth and the formation of interneuronal links (47).

Myelination of the brain of the rat is delayed by thyroidectomy soon after birth and lags 3 to 6 days behind that of controls (124,125), whereas the addition of thyroxine to tissue cultures of newborn rat cerebellum held at optimal temperature advanced the time of appearance of myelin by several days (58). When searching for the precise nature of the defect, Freundl and van Wynsberghe (48) applied quantitative electron microscopic methods to the brains of hypothyroid young rats, and of radiothyroidectomized animals given thyroxine or triiodothyroacetic acid. The number of myelinated axons was normal in the 25-day-old hypothyroid rats, but there was a decrease in the area of the axons. Thyroxine treatment produced an increased number of smaller axons, whereas triiodothyroacetic acid produced fewer but larger axons than thyroxine. The thickness of the myelin sheath never changed. Myelin formation was defective in the visual cortex of hypothyroid infant rats, but this could have arisen from the delayed arrival of visual signals in the developing cortex as a result of prolongation of the neonatal period of eye closure (59).

The density of blood capillaries in the cerebrospinal cortex of cretinous animals is much below that of euthyroid controls, which could account for the disruptive changes of cretinism on adult brain function. However, in view of the evidence that the local metabolic rate is a major factor when determining vascular ingrowth, it seems more likely that the lower capillary density of the cretinous brain is secondary to the lower metabolic rate (137).

Behavioral Effects

When assessing the behavioral effects of neonatal hypothyroidism in the rat, it is necessary to distinguish between the effects on innate and adaptive behaviors. So far as innate behavior is concerned, the appearance of automatic responses (e.g., the startle response to auditory stimuli or the placing reflex) is retarded by thyroidectomy and slightly advanced by the administration of thyroid hormone. However, these forms of innately organized behavior eventually appear in the absence of thyroid hormones so that the thyroid gland appears to influence the rate of development of a neural mechanism rather than directing any patterning (41). On the other hand, more sophisticated tests of learning in a T-maze showed that cretinoid rats take longer to learn and make more errors in learning than euthyroid littermate controls. This situation can be corrected by giving thyroxine and would imply that hypothyroidism during infancy is not necessarily permanent in effect were it not for the results of other experiments using the Hebb Williams closed field test, which provides a critical functional index. As described by Eayrs (41), the test consists of a series of 12 maze-like problems which are explored by the thirst-motivated rat in search of water. Each animal is given eight successive attempts at each problem and its performance measured in terms of the number of errors, not in the amount of time taken, which could be expected to be longer in the less-active thyroidectomized rat. Under these circumstances, the behavior of rats thyroidectomized during infancy is grossly impaired, with the degree of impairment being correlated with the age at which thyroidectomy was carried out and with the age at which replacement therapy was begun.

Clinical Studies

It is fortunate that human brain function need not be irreversibly affected by hypothyroidism *in utero* or during infancy. Brain growth was not affected in monkeys subjected to intrauterine hypothyroidism (64), but protein and RNA synthesis and ganglioside deposition were depressed, although DNA synthesis was not altered. The content of carbonic anhydrase, an enzyme restricted to the glia, was greatly reduced. These changes did not seem to result from maternal malnutrition. Even in cases where the thyroid gland fails to differentiate, the cretin may appear normal. Alongside somatic changes (e.g., slowed growth) inertia and indifference to the environment develop during early childhood, and speech development is delayed. Disturbances in motor function may also emerge. The electroencephalogram is usually marked by the occurrence of slow waves, often of low amplitude. Overall, mental development is slowed and ultimately defective (137).

More marked cretinous changes are apparent in cases of endemic cretinism arising from a dietary deficiency of iodine. In one study in New Guinea (23), it seemed that defective development of upper motor neurons in the pyramidal system produced severe weakness and hypotonia in the arms and legs, so that walking was achieved late during childhood. Severely defective young children could not stand or walk unsupported, and some could not even sit. The face lacked expression, and most afflicted children were also mute and deaf (23). When tests for general intelligence, motor skills, concentration, and perceptual capacity especially adapted to the Indonesian situation were applied to villagers subject to endemic goiter, and were compared with the findings from a control village, significant differences emerged (114).

Although in untreated cretinism intelligence is unquestionably impaired, with adequate and early replacement therapy the prognosis can be extremely good. According to Money (98), there is a general tendency for the intelligence quotient (IQ) to increase as development proceeds, and in a few spectacular cases the IQ may jump by 30 to 40 points. The variability in response to treatment may result from familial circumstances and educational opportunity, the time of onset of thyroid deficiency, the degree and duration of thyroid hormone lack prior to treatment, and the adequacy of replacement therapy. Nevertheless, it is important that treatment begins before 3 to 4 months of age, and some argue that it is necessary to commence therapy almost immediately after birth (13). Indeed efforts have been made to make a test for hypothyroidism mandatory in children treated in the nurseries of federally related health care services in the United States (56).

Neonatal hyperthyroidism transiently advances neuromuscular development and, if sustained, results in a growth spurt and perhaps precocious puberty in children. The seizures and upper motor neuron syndromes of the thyrotoxic adult are rare in children, but tremor is common at all ages. Hyperkinesis, irritability, and abbreviated attention span occur (98,137). Long-lasting changes (hyperactivity as well as intellectual and perceptual–motor difficulties) have been reported in children with neonatal Graves disease rendered euthyroid (63). Sometimes children suffering from sporadic cretinism fail to achieve satisfactory intellectual development despite early and seemingly adequate treatment with thyroid hormone. This lack of response has been attributed to the inadvertent induction of hyperthyroidism in the course of therapy (1). In the rat, overdosage with thyroid hormones during the first 2 weeks of life permanently impairs growth and resets the activity of the hypothalamo-hypophysial-thyroid axis to a low level (7,9).

GROWTH HORMONE

The effects of growth hormone on brain development are controversial, and the findings in clinical and animal experimental work appear to conflict. There seems little doubt that treatment of pregnant rats with growth hormone affects brain growth in the fetuses. Among the responses may be noted an increase in the number and length of dendrites (25); increased brain weight, DNA content, and cortical cell density; and an increase in the ratio of neurons to glia (157) and in the number of cortical neurons; learning ability is also enhanced (126). However, the increase in fetal cerebral DNA after maternal treatment with growth hormone was not reproducible in the later work of Zamenhof et al. (158), although an increase in cerebral weight was again observed. The possibility that growth hormone was exerting its action through changes in maternal metabolic activity and not directly on the fetus seemed plausible on the basis that exogenous growth hormone was unlikely to cross the placental barrier and because the decreases in fetal brain weight, cerebral DNA, and cerebral protein produced by maternal caloric restriction could be corrected by treating the mother with growth hormone. This explanation did not find favor with Sara et al. (127), who again observed that growth hormone treatment of pregnant rats enhanced brain weight and brain DNA activity in the fetuses, although there was no increase in fetal body weight. Maternal food intake and protein metabolism appeared to be unaltered, but there was an increase in placental growth. As indicated by Sara et al. (127), it is possible that maternal somatomedin, produced in response to growth hormone administration, may cross the placenta to affect the embryo, but the passage of somatomedin and any effect it may have remains to be proved. Baláz et al. (11) were uncertain whether the changes in labeled DNA content following a single injection of tritiated thymidine, as reported by Sara et al. (127), reflected a genuine increase in cell proliferation or resulted from changes in the availability of thymidine to the embryo. The claims that growth hormone promotes cell proliferation in the fetal brain conflicted with the histological work of Clendinnen and Eayrs (25) as well as some biochemical studies, where the weights and the DNA, RNA, and protein contents in the brains of offspring of mothers treated with growth hormone from the 7th to the 19th days of pregnancy did not differ from controls when compared from birth to 35 days of age (11). Croskerry et al. (29) were unable to demonstrate any effect of growth hormone treatment on total brain DNA, total brain protein, or total brain weight at birth, or any differential effects on the cerebellum and cerebrum; later Croskerry and Smith (28) argued that, since growth hormone treatment prolonged pregnancy, studies in which this response was not taken into account would lead to spurious differences in body and brain weight and total brain protein. Additionally, the maternal behavior of growth hormone-treated mothers differed from that of controls over the first 2 weeks postpartum. It is also relevant that growth hormone treatment had no effect on the brains of rats hypophysectomized at 6 days of age, when thyroxine administration was beneficial (34), although Pelton et al. (110) found that brain growth was retarded in rats given growth hormone antiserum on postnatal days 2 to 7 to induce a specific growth hormone deficiency.

In neonatal rats bovine growth hormone acts to ameliorate the consequences of thyroidectomy. Eayrs (40) regarded the effect simply as a growth response, whereas Gómez (51) believed that the reaction was of maturational significance.

Growth hormone deficiency during childhood does not seem to be associated with changes in cognition and memory, although there may be psychological immaturity. The effects on intelligence have been the subject of greater debate, as emerges in the report of Meyer-Bahlburg et al. (93). They point out that: (a) previous diagnostic endocrine procedures are below current standards; (b) medical data regarding diagnostic classification, associated endocrine abnormalities, and the onset of growth hormone deficiency, as well as possible factors of brain damage, are usually not presented; and (c) the socioeconomic status of the patient is rarely taken into account. Taking these points into consideration, their study of 29 patients indicated that those with growth hormone deficiency show a basically normal IQ distribution and are not defective in specific mental abilities (93). Commenting on the discrepancies between the results of animal and clinical studies, they note that most investigators who study animals tested the effects of growth hormone administration on the pregnant mother, so that studies of growth hormone deficiency are few. Meyer-Bahlburg et al. (93) also emphasize that in man social factors overlay the effects of biological factors on behavior to a much larger extent than in laboratory animals, and that since in many growth-hormone-deficient dwarfs the growth retardation does not become apparent before the second year of life the exact onset of growth hormone deficiency is not known. Recently a specific effect of maternal deprivation on growth hormone secretion in neonatal rats was reported (75). Separation of the pups from the mother for 2 hr reduced the concentration of growth hormone in the plasma, as well as the activity of ornithine decarboxylase in the brain, without affecting the plasma concentrations of prolactin, thyrotropin, or corticosterone.

ADRENAL HORMONES

Overall, rather little is known about the effect of adrenal steroids on brain maturation in the human infant, although Weichsel (151) emphasized the potential neurological hazards of glucocorticoid therapy during infancy and childhood. Work on the rat and mouse indicates caution, for overdosage with adrenal corticoids during the first few days of life permanently reduces the total number of cells in the brain, probably by inhibiting cell multiplication (10). In the human cerebellum division and migration of granule cell precursors in the external granule layer occurs throughout the first year of life, although appreciable cell division is not evident in the hippocampus (151).

Spine formation of cortical neurons in newborn rats given cortisol was transiently reduced at 14 days (128), the maturation of evoked cortical potential responses retarded (129), and the development of characteristic adult seizure patterns delayed (155). Other inhibitory effects of adrenal glucocorticoids on brain growth and differentiation are summarized by Weichsel (151). The critical nature of the age at treatment was again underlined by Vernadakis and Woodbury (148), who found that cortisol has a biphasic effect on the nervous system. Maturation was delayed and brain excitability decreased when cortisol was given acutely or chronically between the first and seventh days after birth, but brain maturation was accelerated and excitability increased when cortisol was given after the eighth day, perhaps through an effect on brain myelination.

Although the effects of overdosage with corticosteroids and thyroid hormone appear to be similar, in that the brain cell number is reduced, the behavioral consequences differ. There is a retardation in some forms of innate behavior (e.g., swimming); the animals are emotionally more labile; and their ability to perform fine motor coordination is impaired. Adaptive behavior is not impaired, in contrast to the response to overdosage with thyroid hormones. Balázs (10) notes that the timing of the consequences of overdosage with adrenal or thyroid hormones differs in that corticoids inhibit cell multiplication mainly during the treatment period whereas thyroid hormones affect cell formation mainly after a delay of 1 to 2 weeks from the start of treatment. Since the differentiation of various cell types within the brain occurs at various times during development, it is not surprising that the outcome of different forms of hormone treatment varies. In the cerebellum peak differentiation of the basket cells occurs at 2 to 6 days, that of the stellate cells at 13 days, and half of the granule cells develop during the third week after birth.

Numerous effects of adrenal steroids on the growth of cells in explants of the cerebellum of chick embryos were described by Vernadakis et al. (146) in a continuation of earlier work (145). Cortisol and corticosterone, together with estradiol but not progesterone, prevented the fall in acetylcholinesterase activity and RNA content that occurred in their absence. Glial cells, like neurons, accumulated tritiated corticosterone but with less selectivity. In rats hydrocortisone inhibited cerebral RNA and DNA synthesis, although ACTH treatment enhanced the synthesis of brain nucleic acids, a paradoxical finding attributed in part to the catabolic action of a high dosage of hydrocortisone and to a possible direct action of ACTH on brain metabolism (5). Aldosterone and thyroxine also increased RNA and DNA synthesis in the brain.

The limbic system may also be specifically affected by corticosteroid action during development. Studies with labeled hormones show that corticosteroids are taken up and retained in the limbic system although with marked individual differences (33). Howard and Granoff (65) suggested that the emotional lability of corticosterone-treated mice may be attributable to changes in the development of this system.

Neonatal treatment of rats with a glucocorticoid (e.g., hydrocortisone or dexamethasone) delays the establishment of the circadian rhythm in adrenal activity but not when deferred to days 12 to 14 (73,74). The circadian rhythm became established by 55 days in females but took much longer in males (26,95). It may be relevant that the hypothalamic concentration of norepinephrine and serotonin was raised in rats given 1 mg hydrocortisone acetate at birth and killed 30 days later (143).

Information of the kind outlined above takes on added significance in the light of work on the psychophysiological effects of stimulation early in infancy in rats. Daily removal of the pups from the nest for 3 min produced lasting changes in behavior and endocrine function. The emotional reactivity of the manipulated animals was reduced, and the concentration of plasma corticosterone in the disturbed animals at the end of the tests was below that of controls (82). Further, stresses applied during gestation may subsequently affect the reproductive performance of the offspring of rats, with a noticeable trend toward the feminization and demasculinization of the males (150), which is reflected in a variety of neurochemical and neuroanatomical parameters. Thus exposure of rats to heat, restraint, and bright light for days 14 to 21 of gestation permanently affected the concentration of monoamines in various regions of the brain (101).

GONADAL HORMONES

The changes in brain function brought about by gonadal hormones during fetal and neonatal life are profound and have attracted much attention. They provide not only a physiological explanation for some of the differences in the function of the hypothalamo-pituitary-gonadal axis in adult life but, more significantly, a biological basis for the differences in sexual outlook and behavior of the two sexes, even to the extent of attributing homosexual behavior in the human male to a paucity of male sex hormone during a critical period of brain differentiation during fetal life. Put another way, the testosterone secreted by the testis of the male fetus acts on the brain to impose a masculine imprint on a mechanism that is fundamentally female. This view evolved from much earlier studies on the hormonal control of differentiation of the genital tract during embryonic life and was developed by Phoenix et al. (113) on the basis of the effects of exposure to testosterone during intrauterine life on the subsequent sexual behavior of female guinea pigs. When pregnant guinea pigs were injected with the androgen, the young showed masculinization of the genitalia and, later, an increase in mounting behavior and aggressiveness as well as a reduction in the expression of lordosis after treatment with estrogen and progesterone. These effects never resulted from treatment of adult females with androgen. Subsequently, most studies on the sexual differentiation of the brain employed the rat, for the effect of androgen is exercised in this species during the first 5 to 10 days of postnatal life and experimental intervention is accordingly facilitated. Thus castration of neonatal male rats, or treatment with antiandrogen, particularly during the first few days after birth, facilitated the later expression of lordosis after injection of estrogen and progesterone. Lordosis was much less common in similarly hormonally treated intact males or in treated males castrated when adult. Nevertheless, the neonatally castrated males retained some capacity for mounting behavior, which, although less than that of males castrated when adult, was much greater than comparable gonadectomized females. Such findings tend to negate the conclusion of Harris and Levine (62), for example, that rats of both sexes are born with a sexually undifferentiated nervous system of the female pattern. Indeed it is hard to reconcile the occurrence of a female pattern with sexual undifferentiation, and it is perhaps advisable to use the phraseology of MacKinnon (87) that the testes must be present to prevent certain functions and activities which are typically female. Alternatively, the view championed by Reinisch (119) may be preferred wherein androgens act definitively not to imprint male patterns of behavior but rather to predispose the nervous system to react to stimuli in a masculine fashion. Even these cautious generalizations encounter difficulty when applied to other brain systems affected by androgen during development. Urination behavior in the dog is sexually differentiated: Males raise one leg while standing on the other three, and females squat. Female dogs masculinized *in utero* display male mounting behavior when adult, but only when treated with testosterone before and during the test period, whereas the masculinized females show the male urination pattern as adults in the absence of any prior treatment with male hormone. Beach (14) regards these observations as important in reflecting the function of a behavioral system separate from those concerned with mating behavior but nevertheless sexually dimorphic.

The occurrence of bisexuality among mammals is not a new finding and appears to be more common among females than males. Goy and Goldfoot (55) extended this concept by suggesting that there appears to be an inverse relation between the sexes with regard to bisexuality, so that for a given species the greater the bisexuality of the male the less the bisexuality of the female and *vice versa*. The relationship is exemplified by the rhesus monkey: Rhesus males show a conspicuous bisexuality throughout early development, and to some extent even into adult life, whereas among rhesus females male behavior is rare or infrequent during the first years of life and is not favored by treating the adult female with testosterone. Hamsters react rather like rhesus monkeys, but guinea pigs illustrate the opposite situation; male guinea pigs show little or no bisexuality, and lordosis is difficult to detect during adult life, even after treatment with large amounts of estradiol and progesterone. Female guinea pigs show lordosis and mounting in a variety of endocrine states. In this respect, dogs, rats, and mice are more akin to guinea pigs. Further, the definitions of the terms masculinization and defeminization are gradually becoming refined, with masculinization referring to an enhancement of the capacity to show male-like mounting behavior, and defeminization being concerned with the induction of anovulatory sterility and a reduction of the capacity to show lordosis. Masculinization may begin before birth in the rat, whereas the critical period of defeminization covers the first 4 to 5 postnatal days (90).

Exposure of sheep fetuses to testosterone from days 20, 40, or 60 of gestation inhibited the development of estrous cycles as adults, although laparotomy showed that ovulation occurred occasionally. An intramuscular injection of estradiol, which normally initiated LH release, was ineffective in these animals, as in normal males. These observations suggested to Short (134) that the essential difference between the male and female hypothalamus in sheep lay in the ability to initiate an LH discharge in response to estrogen. Castrated rams given estradiol, with or without prior treatment with the steroid to reduce the resting level of plasma LH, also failed to show the estrogen-induced LH surge demonstrable in the ewe (71); pigs also appear to conform to this pattern (44). In contrast, estrogen caused a surge of LH secretion in male monkeys as well as in females (70,121,139). Prior removal of the testes was necessary for the demonstration of this effect in the male, but in any event it is now established that the primate does not follow the pattern of control of sexual differentiation drawn from work on lower species.

As has been well shown in rats, a graded effect on the brain can be brought about by increasing the dose of androgen (36,121). This variable response has been used to provide some physiological basis for homosexuality, as indicative of a degree of androgen insufficiency during development. Accordingly, Dörner (36) induced LH secretion by an injection of estrogen in homosexual men, as in women, but this treatment was ineffective in heterosexual men. However, an LH surge has been observed in normal men given a course of five daily injections of 17β-estradiol (76); work in this field is bedeviled by difficulties in clearly separating male and female behavior, for a continuum is seen in the shift from one sexual mode to the other. Complete sexual dimorphism in any mammalian species is extremely rare, and in any case there is no sound hormonal basis for the occurrence of homosexuality in man (92).

Morphological masculinization, or pseudohermaphroditism, of female monkeys has been achieved by repeated administration of testosterone propionate *in utero;* but apart from a delay in the onset of menstruation, normal menstrual cycles set in as maturation proceeds. Similarly, regular menstrual cycles develop with treatment in girls unwittingly exposed to the masculinizing action of excess progesterone during fetal life, or in cases of the adrenogenital syndrome; and pregnancy and lactation have occurred (17,97). The critical period for this effect of androgen on the human brain appears to extend between days 60 and 120 of intrauterine life, although the evidence is of necessity indirect (61). Once past puberty, normal heterosexual interests develop. Money and Lewis (100) were struck by the frequent incidence of high IQs in their patients; and since unusually high IQs were later found in a group of progestin-induced pseudohermaphrodites, the effect seemed to result from the operation of hormonal rather than genetic factors. The clinical conclusions of the American workers (100) are supported by observations made in the Soviet Union, for homosexual behavior was lacking in a group of 18 patients suffering from adrenogenital syndrome whose treatment began during adolescence or adult life (83). Again, the general educational level in these patients was exceptionally high, although the IQ was not measured (83). More detailed analysis of the relationship between prenatal exposure to excessive androgen and performance in a variety of intelligence tests confirmed the occurrence of an elevated IQ, although the androgenization itself does not appear to be a causative factor. The IQs of the parents and siblings of patients with the adrenogenital syndrome were similar to those of the patients, so that the operation of a genetic mechanism is postulated (8).

Other behavioral changes in females subjected to increased androgen action have been noted. Female monkeys treated with androgen during intrauterine life (112,121) and girls with the adrenogenital syndrome (43,99) show significantly more rough-and-tumble play, as well as dominance behavior, than their normal peers. Infant male rhesus monkeys show a greater frequency of threat, play initiation, rough and tumble play, and chasing play than females, although these activities are normally enjoyed by females. Hermaphroditic female rhesus monkeys placed and compared with normal females showed a shift in pattern in the male direction (112). Neonatal castration did not inhibit the expression of normal male behavior during infancy.

Before the possible significance of sex steroids in defining the future pattern of sexual behavior was realized, large doses of estrogen and lesser amounts of progesterone were occasionally given to diabetic women to sustain pregnancy. One study subsequently showed that boys exposed prenatally to exogenous female hormones displayed less rough-and-tumble, less aggressive, and less athletic behavior than controls (156), although the difference may have been related to changes in the maternal behavior of the sick mothers. In a more extensive study, the effects of treatment with various preparations of estrogen and progestins on the offspring of mothers treated for threatened pregnancy were assessed and the children compared with siblings born of uncomplicated pregnancies (120). No changes in IQ were detected, but when the subjects were classified on the basis of the estrogen/progesterone ratio [e.g., high estrogen and low progestin—"estrogen" group; intermediate dosages of progestin and low estrogen (with the majority receiving no estrogen)—"progestin" group; and maximal progestin and intermediate amounts of estrogen—"intermediate" group] subtler consequences emerged. The members of the progestin group were more independent, individualistic, self-assured, self-sufficient, and sensitive, whereas those in the estrogen group were more group-oriented and group-dependent and less independent, less sensitive, and less self-assured. There was no masculinization of the genitalia in any of the children studied in this investigation (120). When other studies of the effects of progesterone supplementation during pregnancy on intellectual development were reappraised, it was concluded that there were no beneficial effects (85,86).

Other behavioral patterns in the rat (e.g., wheel-running, emergence, and open-field behavior) have been shown to be affected by neonatal androgen. Female rats are less timid in the emergence and open-field situation, for they emerge more quickly than males, cover more area, and drop fewer fecal boluses. Neonatally testosterone-treated females behave like males, and neonatally castrated males more like females. Similar observations were made in hamsters. Changes in aggressive behavior have also been reported, as reviewed by Goldstein (50) and Reinisch (119).

The consequences of androgen insufficiency during development can be studied clinically in two conditions: Turner's syndrome and the androgen-insensitivity or testicular feminization syndrome. In Turner's syndrome one of the sex chromosomes is missing—the chromosomal complement being XO—and the patients develop phenotypically as females. Gonads are lacking in these individuals, but despite the lack of estrogen they are feminine in appearance and psychosexual outlook. Androgens are present but cannot be utilized in patients with the androgen-insensitivity syndrome, who are genetically male with testes, but phenotypically female. Personality characteristics and gender identification in these individuals are female in orientation with no indication of any masculinization of behavior. Like the adrenogenital syndrome, the condition may be cited in support of the significance of androgens in influencing sexual orientation.

Mechanism of Action

There is surprisingly little understanding of the mechanism of action of androgen on the brain. One attractive view is that early postnatal treatment with androgen in the rat interferes with the normal development of estrogen receptor proteins in the brain and with the accumulation of estrogen by the appropriate neurons. Such estrogen-sensitive neurons might then become desensitized and functionally unresponsive to endogenous fluctuations in blood estrogen concentration (45). In accord with this concept, there are many reports that the responsiveness of peripheral target organs (uterus, vagina) to estradiol is reduced in animals treated with androgen early in life. There are sex differences in the oxygen usage of the hypothalamus, with consumption by the male hypothalamus being greater. Tissue from prepubertal rats, normal males, neonatally androgenized females, and neonatally ovariectomized androgenized females showed a higher rate of oxygen usage than tissue from control females, spayed females, or castrated males. Cyclic changes in oxygen consumption were observed in hypothalamic tissue from females and linked with the estrous cycle (96).

Another view of the process of sexual differentiation of the brain is that it is a consequence not of the action of androgen alone but of the interaction of androgen with progesterone, which is acting in this case as an antiandrogen (121). In the male primate fetus, testosterone levels are high and progesterone levels low, and androgenization occurs; in contrast, in the female not only are blood androgen levels low but the relatively high concentration of progesterone prevents the action of even the small amounts of male hormone in circulation. Progesterone is known to prevent the masculinizing action of testosterone in neonatal rats (22,72), but proof of this supposition in the primate is awaited.

A major part of the action that androgen exerts on the brain is exercised through the hypothalamus. Female rats can be rendered acyclic and anovulatory by the local application of micropellets of testosterone to the hypothalamus, with the most effective region being the ventromedial-arcuate nuclear area (102). There appear to be specific sites where implantation of testosterone or estradiol produces independent masculinization of the gonadotropic hormone secretion pattern, or male or female behavior patterns (24). Implants of gonadal steroid into the dorsal preoptic area perinatally increased the amount of masculine sexual behavior displayed by adults. On the other hand, the ventromedial hypothalamus was the only area where neonatal steroid implants produced gonadotropic hormone acyclicity in adults. Neonatal implants of testosterone or estradiol in the dorsal preoptic area increased adult behavioral responsiveness to estradiol benzoate alone, whereas similar implants in the ventromedial hypothalamus decreased adult behavioral responsiveness to combined treatment with estradiol and progesterone.

An anatomical response to steroid action in the induction of sexually dimorphic variation in the synaptic connections in the preoptic area of the hypothalamus was revealed by Raisman and Field (115). Quantitative electron microscopic study showed that the number of nonamygdaloid synapses on dendritic spines was higher in the preoptic area of normal female rats than in males. Following experiments involving neonatal castration or androgen administration, a high incidence of nonstrial synapses on dendritic spines in the preoptic area of normal females or males castrated within 12 hr of birth was correlated with the ability to initiate a preovulatory surge of gonadotropin and the ability of progesterone to facilitate lordosis. When these capacities were lacking, as in normal males and in neonatally androgenized females, there was a low incidence of spine synapses in the preoptic area. More studies of this kind are needed, particularly as Brown-Grant and Raisman (20) found that destruction of the sexually dimorphic part of the preoptic area did not permanently abolish cyclic reproductive function in female rats. Sex differences in the dendritic field pattern of neurons in the dorsomedial preoptic area of adult golden hamsters were detected by Greenough et al. (57). Males tended to have a central concentration, whereas females showed an irregular dendritic density distribution with concentrations dorsolateral, ventral, and medial to the area of highest dendritic density in the males. The meaning of this difference is unclear, although its reality is underlined by the finding that the volume of the medial preoptic nucleus in the male rat was greater than that of females (53). The volume of this nucleus in adult male rats castrated neonatally was reduced compared with males castrated after weaning, and was increased in females neonatally injected with testosterone.

Sexually dimorphic changes are evident in the brain outside the hypothalamus, for the sizes of the nuclei in the amygdala of squirrel monkeys differ, with the nuclei being larger in males than in females (21). The nuclear diameters in the suprachiasmatic nuclei in males and females were similar. The basis of this difference is again unclear, for it may be attributed to androgenization during fetal life, or it may reflect the variation in circulating hormones in males and females. Nevertheless, Staudt and Dörner (138) observed that the sizes of nuclei in neurons in the medial and central parts of the amygdala were larger in adult male rats castrated soon after birth than in males castrated later in life. Similarly, large nuclei were present in females, whereas the neonatal administration of androgen reduced nuclear size. There is evidence that the neural input from the amygdala to the hypothalamus may be affected by androgen, for the neurons in the mediobasal hypothalamus of males or androgenized females are more likely to be linked synaptically to the amygdala than the same cells in females or in neonatally castrated males (39).

Under organ culture conditions estradiol and hydrocortisone improved the maintenance of chick embryo cerebellar explants (147), and estradiol and testosterone enhanced the proliferation of neuronal processes in fragments of hypothalamic tissue collected from newborn mice (141). This was particularly marked in cultures of the preoptic-anterior hypothalamic area and to a lesser degree of the premammillary region, whereas other parts of the hypothalamus were not steroid-sensitive. Significantly, treatment of cultures with serum containing antibodies to estradiol retarded and reduced the outgrowth of processes. The effect was not related to the sex of the donor of the tissue but could be restricted to the first week of life. Cultures deprived of gonadal steroids also appear to contain fewer neurons reacting to an antibody to luteinizing hormone-releasing factor than controls (142). Corresponding information comes from studies of synapse formation in the arcuate nucleus of rats, where neonatal treatment with estradiol benzoate increased the number of axodendritic synapses and reduced the extracellular space in the neuropil matrix (4). Since the number of axodendritic synapses was similar in control and estrogen-treated animals at 150 days, it appeared that estrogen facilitated the development of synaptic structures. Curry and Timiras (31) earlier suggested that neonatal estrogenization accelerated synapse formation. It is noteworthy that 17β-estradiol, but not testosterone, hydrocortisone, or α-estradiol, increased the production of nerve growth factor by a rat central nervous system glioma cell line (111).

Naftolin et al. (104,105) argued that androgen is converted to estrogen by the hypothalamus of the fetus in the course of defining the future mode of reproductive activiy. Aromatization of androstenedione has been demonstrated in the anterior hypothalamus and limbic system of human fetuses (104,105), as well as in perinatal rats (118,152,153), and tissue from the fetal human hypothalamus or temporal lobe can convert testosterone to estradiol-17β (68,103). Inhibition of aromatization in the neonatal male rat by treatment with androstan-1, 4,6-triene-3,17-dione was associated with the maintenance of cyclic gonadotropic function in the adult (149). Estrogens have been shown to cause anovulatory infertility (37,52), and the action of testosterone can be blocked by pretreatment with an antiestrogen (87), although antiestrogens are not always effective (18,54).

Testosterone is converted to dihydrotestosterone in the course of action on certain peripheral target organs, and the latter hormone is then a highly effective androgen; but dihydrotestosterone does not act like testosterone in causing masculinization of the brain (19,154). According to McDonald and Doughty (89), only aromatizable androgens can induce sterility. Androgens inhibit the establishment of the lordosis response in male rats, and Södersten (135) developed the argument that, paradoxically, the effect is produced by estradiol formed from testosterone. Estradiol benzoate was more effective in this regard than testosterone; dihydrotestosterone benzoate had no inhibitory effect; and treatment with an antiestrogen antagonized the masculinizing effects of the testes or of exogenous estrogen or testosterone. This and allied work illustrate the differential response of the male or female brain to similar hormonal stimulation. Concordantly, Booth (15) showed that the treatment of newborn male rats with an antiestrogen reduced the later incidence of ejaculation as well as the appearance of significantly more lordosis behavior after estrogen and progesterone pretreatment than in controls. An inhibitor of aromatization reduced the effects of testosterone, given simultaneously to neonatal rats, on cyclic gonadotropin secretion and receptive behavior (16).

The aromatase activity of rabbit brain is greater in males than in females. For the hypothalamus the ratio is $2:1$ to $3:1$, and for the limbic system $2:1$. Aromatization of androgen by the limbic system is demonstrable in monkeys, rabbits, and rats, as well as man, and differs strikingly between male and female rat fetuses (103). The activity in the limbic system of 21-day male rat fetuses is in the adult range, climbs after birth, and then falls to adult levels. Conversely, there is no demonstrable activity in the 21-day female rat fetus. Limbic aromatization is evident on postnatal day 1 and thereafter remains around adult levels.

Presumptive receptors for androgens and estrogens have been demonstrated in the brain of the developing mouse and show a high affinity for dihydrotestosterone (6). This finding argues against the aromatization hypothesis, for the failure of dihydrotestosterone to modify sexual differentiation in the female rat may stem from its rapid metabolism to 5α-androstanediols. Dihydrotestosterone prevents the development of female behavior in the hamster, whereas cyproterone acetate, which prevents neonatal masculinization of the brain, inhibits the binding of dihydrotestosterone to the androgen receptor in mouse brain cytosol but interferes only slightly with the estrogen receptor.

High titers of estrogen may be in circulation in the fetus during pregnancy, so it is initially difficult to understand on the basis of the aromatization hypothesis why the brain of the female rat escapes masculinization. Reddy et al. (118) pointed out that in the blood of perinatal rats proteins are present which selectively bind estrogens and may render them unavailable to the brain. Androgens are not similarly bound, so the action of testosterone or androstenedione would not be so impeded. The protein, the so-called α-fetoprotein, comprises some 50% of the plasma proteins of the neonatal rat but gradually disappears over the first 4 weeks of postnatal life. MacKinnon (87) considers that since the estimated concentrations of the biologically active estrogen are low from 0 to 23 days of age, whereas its affinity for α-fetoprotein is very strong, the resultant activity of the hormone is too weak to inhibit FSH levels or to masculinize the brain. An extracellular estrogen-binding protein is present in the brains of neonatal rats (91), as well as a more specifically located cytoplasmic receptor (12). Nevertheless, estrogens are more potent than androgens in modifying sexual development in the female rat. Very little estradiol is present in fetal plasma in the rhesus monkey early in gestation (122), although substantial amounts may be found in human fetal blood as early as 10 weeks of gestation (123). Strong binding of steroids to proteins is not marked in the human fetus: The binding of 17β-estradiol at different ages was of the same order of magnitude as that of adult normal sera of either sex, whereas testosterone binding in the fetus was always lower than in adults but greater than that of estradiol (106).

Alongside their effects on sexual behavior, gonadal hormones influence agonistic behavior. In a number of mammalian species the male is more aggressive than the female, and this may also result from the activity of sex hormones early in development. Thus in mice the treatment of females with androgen postnatally predisposes them to be aggressive after administration of androgen during adult life. Conversely, neonatal castration of males causes them to become less responsive to androgen treatment in terms of the induction of aggressiveness than does castration later in life. There is also an endocrine basis for submissiveness, but this has been less deeply studied (81).

MONOAMINES

In view of the importance of brain monoamines in neuroendocrine function, the prenatal development of the central pathways and the effect of hormones on them is of concern. Most is known about their differentiation in the rat, where the capacity for the synthesis and storage of amines develops very early.

5-Hydroxytryptamine-containing neurons appear at 8 mm, dopamine neurons at 9 mm, and norepinephrine neurons at 11 mm. Several axonal projections capable of synthesizing neurotransmitters have developed by 12 mm (133). Coyle (27) notes that enzymes involved in catecholamine synthesis (e.g., tyrosine hydroxylase, DOPA decarboxylase, and dopamine-β-hydroxylase) as well as dopamine and norepinephrine are detectable in the fetal rat brain as early as 15 days' gestation. During the last week of fetal development, there is a relatively linear and coordinated increase in the levels of the presynaptic markers for the catecholaminergic neurons, reaching about 30% of adult levels by birth. From studies on the incorporation of tritiated thymidine, it seems that division of the noradrenergic neurons in the locus ceruleus ceases by 14 days' gestation and that of the dopaminergic neurons in the substantia nigra by 16 days. There is thus good agreement between the times at which cell division ends and the appearance of neurotransmitters and biosynthetic enzymes. After the first 2 weeks of gestation, differentiation and not multiplication of the catecholaminergic cells predominates in the rat. Monoaminergic fibers are evident in the guinea pig hypothalamus at 30 days and appeared to be fully defined at 43 days (88).

Catecholaminergic and 5-hydroxytryptaminergic neurons were evident in the 7-week human fetal brain (length 2.1 cm), and the basic arrangement of the systems matched that of the rat (108). Marked differentiation and development of these systems emerged between 7 and 23 weeks.

A fluorescence reaction indicative of the presence of catecholamine in nerve fibers first develops in the periventricular region of the human hypothalamus around the 10th week of gestation and reaches the median eminence by the 13th week. Thereafter the intensity of the reaction increases slowly (66). However, Partanen and Hervonen (109) observed a few fibers only near the wall of the third ventricle at 15 weeks, and the number did not increase over the ensuing month.

Hypothyroidism in the developing rat is associated with marked decreases in the concentration of 5-hydroxytryptamine in the cerebellum, midbrain, and striatum, and increases in the concentration of 5-hydroxyindoleacetic acid (117). These changes could be corrected by treatment with L-triiodothyronine. Conversely, the induction of hyperthyroidism in newborn rats by daily administration of triiodothyronine was accompanied by biochemical signs of an increased turnover of dopamine (116). Administration of 1 mg hydrocortisone acetate to rats at birth increased the hypothalamic concentrations of norepinephrine and 5-hydroxytryptamine in the medial hypothalamus at 30 days but not that of dopamine (143).

The presence of monoamines in neurons, although indicative of some maturational change, says little about the functional activity of the nerve cells. However, synaptic connections for the dopaminergic neurons in the substantia nigra are evident in the rat by 18 days' gestation, although the density of the synapses is low until the number begins to markedly increase between 15 and 30 days postpartum. For the locus ceruleus, faint staining of the synaptic profiles of the noradrenergic neurons is first observed at 19 days' gestation and the most rapid phase of synaptogenesis occurs between 5 and 10 days after birth (80).

When drugs interfering with monoaminergic transmission were given to fetal or neonatal rats, long-term changes ensued (2,67,69,78,94,107). On the basis of such findings, and their own observations that reserpine interferes with cell proliferation in the brains of suckling rats, Lewis et al. (84) point out that neurohumoral agents influence the growth and differentiation of glial cells in developing nervous tissue. They elaborate processes, synthesize transmitters, and exhibit characteristic responses to pharmacological agents at a time when most other neuronal types have still to differentiate. It is suggested that neurotransmitters could act as hormones controlling cell replication in the brain, and that drugs which affect neurotransmitter balance could in this way interfere with cell production.

Sex differences in the activity of neurotransmitter enzymes in the brain are well known, although it is less easy to assess the importance of the differential effects of androgens or estrogens in producing them, or their physiological or behavioral significance (30,144). Neonatal androgenization depresses the developmental rise in 5-hydroxytryptamine that is characteristic of the female rat (77), whereas reserpine and chlorpromazine block androgenization of the female rat hypothalamus (60), an effect that may be related to the lasting effect of chlorpromazine given during pregnancy and lactation in raising the concentration of 5-hydroxytryptamine in the brains of the pups (140). Neonatal treatment of rats with a monoamine oxidase inhibitor, a monoamine depletor, or an acetylcholinesterase inhibitor produced changes in the timing of puberty and in subsequent patterns of behavior (38).

REFERENCES

1. Adams, R. D., and Rosman, N. P. (1978): Hypothyroidism: Neuromuscular system. In: *The Thyroid*, edited by S. C. Werner and S. H. Ingbar, 4th ed., pp. 901–910. Harper & Row, New York.
2. Ahlenius, S., Engel, J., and Lundborg, P. (1975): Antagonism by d-amphetamine of learning deficits in rats induced by exposure to antipsychotic drugs during early postnatal life. *Naunyn Schmiedebergs Arch. Pharmacol.,* 288:185–193.
3. Anokhin, P. K. (1964): Systemogenesis as a general regulator of brain development. *Prog. Brain Res.,* 9:54–86.
4. Arai, Y., and Matsumoto, A. (1978): Synapse formation of the hypothalamic arcuate nucleus during post-natal development in the female rat and its modification by neonatal estrogen treatment. *Psychoneuroendocrinology,* 3:31–45.
5. Ardeleanu, A., and Sterescu, N. (1978): RNA and DNA synthesis in developing rat brain: Hormonal influences. *Psychoneuroendocrinology,* 3:93–101.
6. Attardi, B., and Ohno, S. (1976): Androgen and estrogen receptors in the developing mouse brain. *Endocrinology,* 99:1279–1290.
7. Azizi, F., Vagenakis, A. G., Bullinger, J., Reichlin, S., Braverman, L. E., and Ingbar, S. H. (1974): Persistent abnormalities in pituitary function following neonatal thyrotoxicosis in the rat. *Endocrinology,* 94:1681–1688.
8. Baker, S. W., and Ehrhardt, A. A. (1974): Prenatal androgen, intelligence, and cognitive sex differences. In: *Sex Differences in Behavior,* edited by R. C. Friedman, R. M. Richart, and R. L. Vande Wiele, pp. 53–76. Wiley, New York.

9. Bakke, J. L., and Lawrence, N. (1966): Persistent thyrotropin insufficiency following neonatal thyroxine administration. *J. Lab. Clin. Med.,* 67:477–482.
10. Balázs, R. (1972): Hormonal aspects of brain development. In: *The Brain in Unclassified Mental Retardation,* edited by J. B. Cavanagh, pp. 61–72. Churchill Livingstone, London.
11. Balázs, R., Patel, A. J., and Lewis, P. D. (1977): Metabolic influences on cell proliferation in the brain. In: *Biochemical Correlates of Brain Structure and Function,* edited by A. N. Davison, pp. 43–83. Academic Press, London.
12. Barley, J., Ginsburg, M., Greenstein, B. D., MacLusky, N. J., and Thomas, P. J. (1974): A receptor mediating sexual differentiation? *Nature,* 252:259–260.
13. Bass, N. H., Pelton, E. W., and Young, E. (1977): Defective maturation of cerebral cortex: An inevitable consequence of dysthyroid states during early postnatal life. In: *Thyroid Hormones and Brain Development,* edited by G. D. Grave, pp. 199–210. Raven Press, New York.
14. Beach, F. A. (1975): Hormonal modification of sexually dimorphic behavior. *Psychoneuroendocrinology,* 1:3–23.
15. Booth, J. E. (1977): Sexual behaviour of male rats injected with the antioestrogen MER-25 during infancy. *Physiol. Behav.,* 19:35–39.
16. Booth, J. E. (1978): Effects of the aromatization inhibitor androst-4-ene-3,6,17-trione on sexual differentiation induced by testosterone in the neonatally castrated rat. *J. Endocrinol.,* 79:69–76.
17. Brown-Grant, K. (1973): Recent studies on sexual differentiation of the brain. In: *Foetal and Neonatal Physiology,* pp. 527–545. Cambridge University Press, Cambridge, England.
18. Brown-Grant, K. (1974): Failure of ovulation after administration of steroid hormones and hormone antagonists to female rats during the neonatal period. *J. Endocrinol.,* 62:683–684.
19. Brown-Grant, K., Munck, A., Naftolin, F., and Sherwood, M. R. (1971): The effects of the administration of testosterone propionate alone or with phenobarbitone and of testosterone metabolites to neonatal female rats. *Horm. Behav.,* 2:173–182.
20. Brown-Grant, K., and Raisman, G. (1972): Reproductive function in the rat following selective destruction of afferent fibres to the hypothalamus from the limbic system. *Brain Res.,* 46:23–42.
21. Bubenik, G. A., and Brown, G. M. (1973): Morphologic sex differences in primate brain areas involved in regulation of reproductive activity. *Experientia,* 29:619–621.
22. Cagnoni, M., Fantini, F., Morace, G., and Ghetti, A. (1965): Failure of testosterone propionate to induce the 'early androgen' syndrome in rats previously injected with progesterone. *J. Endocrinol.,* 33:527–528.
23. Choufoer, J. C., van Rhijn, M., and Querido, A. (1965): Endemic goiter in Western New Guinea. II. Clinical picture, incidence and pathogenesis of endemic cretinism. *J. Clin. Endocrinol. Metab.,* 25:385–402.
24. Christensen, L. W., and Gorski, R. A. (1978): Independent masculinization of neuroendocrine systems by intracerebral implants of testosterone or estradiol in the neonatal female rat. *Brain Res.,* 146:325–340.
25. Clendinnen, B. G., and Eayrs, J. T. (1961): The anatomical and physiological effects of prenatally administered somatotrophin on cerebral development in rats. *J. Endocrinol.,* 22:183–193.
26. Cost, M. G., and Mann, D. R. (1976): Neonatal corticoid administration: Retardation of adrenal rhythmicity and desynchronization of puberty. *Life Sci.,* 19:1929–1935.
27. Coyle, J. T. (1977): Biochemical aspects of neurotransmission in the developing brain. *Int. Rev. Neurobiol.,* 20:65–103.
28. Croskery, P. G., and Smith, G. K. (1975): Prolongation of gestation by growth hormone: A confounding factor in the assessment of its prenatal action. *Science,* 189:648–650.
29. Croskery, P. G., Smith, G. K., Shepard, B. J., and Freeman, K. B. (1973): Perinatal brain DNA in the normal and growth hormone-treated rat. *Brain Res.,* 52:413–418.
30. Crowley, W. R., O'Donohue, T. L., and Jacobowitz, D. M. (1978): Sex differences in catecholamine content in discrete brain nuclei of the rat: Effects of neonatal castration or testosterone treatment. *Acta Endocrinol. (Kbh),* 89:20–28.
31. Curry, J. J., and Timiras, P. S. (1972): Development of evoked potentials in specific brain systems after neonatal administration of estradiol. *Exp. Neurol.,* 34:129–139.
32. Davison, A. N. (1977): Biochemical, morphological and functional changes in the developing brain. In: *Biochemical Correlates of Brain Structure and Function,* edited by A. N. Davison, pp. 1–13. Academic Press, London.

33. De Kloet, R., Wallach, G., and McEwen, B. S. (1975): Differences in corticosterone and dexamethasone binding to rat brain and pituitary. *Endocrinology,* 96:598–609.
34. Diamond, M. C. (1968): The effects of early hypophysectomy and hormone therapy on brain development. *Brain Res.,* 7:407–418.
35. Dobbing, J. (1974): The later development of the brain and its vulnerability. In: *Scientific Foundations of Paediatrics,* edited by J. A. Davis and J. Dobbing, pp. 565–577. Heinemann, London.
36. Dörner, G. (1974): Environment dependent brain organization and neuroendocrine, neurovegetative and neuronal behavioural functions. *Prog. Brain Res.,* 41:221–236.
37. Dörner, G., Döcke, F., and Hinz, G. (1971): Paradoxical effects of estrogen on brain differentiation. *Neuroendocrinology,* 7:146–155.
38. Dörner, G., Hinz, G., Döcke, F., and Tönjes, R. (1977): Effects of psychotropic drugs on brain differentiation in female rats. *Endokrinologie,* 70:113–123.
39. Dyer, R. G., MacLeod, N. K., and Ellendorff, F. (1976): Electrophysiological evidence for sexual dimorphism and synaptic convergence in the preoptic and anterior hypothalamic areas of the rat. *Proc. R. Soc. Lond. [Biol],* 193:421–440.
40. Eayrs, J. T. (1961): Protein anabolism as a factor ameliorating the effects of early thyroid deficiency. *Growth,* 25:175–189.
41. Eayrs, J. T. (1966): Thyroid and central nervous development. In: *Scientific Basis of Medicine Annual Reviews,* pp. 317–339. Athlone Press, London.
42. Eayrs, J. T. (1968): Developmental relationships between brain and thyroid. In: *Endocrinology and Human Behaviour,* edited by R. P. Michael, pp. 239–255. Oxford University Press, London.
43. Ehrhardt, A. A., and Baker, S. W. (1974): Fetal androgens, human central nervous system differentiation, and behavior sex differences. In: *Sexual Differences in Behavior,* edited by R. C. Friedman, R. M. Richart, and R. L. Vande Wiele, pp. 33–51. Wiley, New York.
44. Elsaesser, F., Parvizi, N., and Ellendorff, F. (1978): Steroid feedback on luteinizing hormone secretion during sexual maturation in the pig. *J. Endocrinol.,* 78:329–342.
45. Flerkó, B. (1974): Hypothalamic mediation of neuroendocrine regulation of hypophysial gonadotrophic functions. In: *Reproductive Physiology,* edited by R. O. Greep, pp. 1–32. Butterworth, London.
46. Ford, D. H., and Cramer, E. B. (1977): Developing nervous system in relation to thyroid hormones. In: *Thyroid Hormones and Brain Development,* edited by G. D. Grave, pp. 1–17. Raven Press, New York.
47. Francon, J., Fellous, A., Lennon, A. M., and Nunez, J. (1977): Is thyroxine a regulatory signal for neurotubule assembly during brain development? *Nature,* 266:188–190.
48. Freundl, K., and van Wynsberghe, D. M. (1978): The effects of thyroid hormones on myelination in the developing rat brain. *Biol. Neonate,* 33:217–223.
49. Geel, S. (1977): Development-related changes of triiodothyronine binding to brain cytosol receptors. *Nature,* 269:428–430.
50. Goldstein, M. (1974): Brain research and violent behavior. *Arch. Neurol.,* 30:1–35.
51. Gómez, C. J. (1971): Hormonal influences of the biochemical differentiation of the rat cerebral cortex. In: *Hormones in Development,* edited by M. Hamburgh and E. J. W. Barrington, pp. 417–435. Appleton-Century-Crofts, New York.
52. Gorski, R. A. (1963): Modification of ovulatory mechanisms by postnatal administration of estrogen to the rat. *Am. J. Physiol.,* 205:842–844.
53. Gorski, R. A., Gordon, J. H., Shryne, J. E., and Southam, A. M. (1978): Evidence for a morphological sex difference within the medial preoptic area of the rat brain. *Brain Res.,* 148:333–346.
54. Gottlieb, H., Gerall, A. A., and Thiel, A. (1974): Receptivity in female hamsters following neonatal testosterone, testosterone propionate, and MER-25. *Physiol. Behav.,* 12:61–68.
55. Goy, R. W., and Goldfoot, D. A. (1975): Neuroendocrinology: Animal models and problems of human sexuality. *Arch. Sex. Behav.,* 4:405–420.
56. Grave, G. D. (1977): Introduction. In: *Thyroid Hormones and Brain Development,* edited by G. D. Grave, pp. xiii–xv. Raven Press, New York.
57. Greenough, W. T., Carter, C. S., Steerman, C., and De Voogd, T. J. (1977): Sex differences in dendritic patterns in hamster preoptic area. *Brain Res.,* 126:63–72.
58. Hamburgh, M. (1966): Evidence for a direct effect of temperature and thyroid hormone on myelinogenesis in vitro. *Dev. Biol.,* 13:15–30.
59. Hamburgh, M., Mendoza, L. A., Bennett, I., Krupa, P., Kim, Y. S., Kahn, R., Hogreff, K.,

and Frankfort, H. (1977): Some unresolved questions of brain-thyroid relationships. In: *Thyroid Hormones and Brain Development,* edited by G. D. Grave, pp. 49–71. Raven Press, New York.

60. Harris, G. W. (1970): Hormonal differentiation of the developing central nervous system with respect to patterns of endocrine function. *Philos. Trans. R. Soc. Lond. [Biol],* 259:165–177.

61. Harris, G. W. (1971): Coordination of the reproductive processes. *J. Biosoc. Sci. (Suppl 3),* 5:5–12.

62. Harris, G. W., and Levine, S. (1965): Sexual differentiation of the brain and its experimental control. *J. Physiol. (Lond),* 181:379–400.

63. Hollingsworth, D. R., and Mabry, C. C. (1976): Congenital Graves disease: Four familial cases with long-term follow-up and perspective. *Am. J. Dis. Child.,* 130:148–155.

64. Holt, A. B., Cheek, D. B., and Kerr, G. R. (1973): Prenatal hypothyroidism and brain composition in a primate. *Nature,* 243:413–415.

65. Howard, E., and Granoff, D. M. (1968): Increased voluntary running and decreased motor coordination in mice after neonatal corticosterone implantation. *Exp. Neurol.,* 22:661–673.

66. Hyyppä, M. T. (1972): Hypothalamic monoamines in human fetuses. *Neuroendocrinology,* 9:257–266.

67. Hyyppä, M. T. (1974): Neuroendocrine control of puberty: Role of perinatal monoamines. In: *Endocrinologie Sexuelle de la Periode Perinatale,* Vol. 32, pp. 395–406. INSERM, Paris.

68. Jenkins, J. S., and Hall, C. J. (1977): Metabolism of [^{14}C]testosterone by human foetal and adult brain tissue. *J. Endocrinol.,* 74:425–429.

69. Joffe, J. M. (1969): *Pre-natal Determinants of Behaviour.* Pergamon Press, Oxford.

70. Karsch, F. J., Dierschke, D. J., and Knobil, E. (1973): Sexual differentiation of pituitary function: Apparent difference between primates and rodents. *Science,* 179:484–486.

71. Karsch, F. J., and Foster, D. L. (1975): Sexual differentiation of the mechanism controlling the preovulatory discharge of luteinizing hormone in sheep. *Endocrinology,* 97:373–379.

72. Kincl, F. A., and Maqueo, M. (1965): Prevention by progesterone of steroid-induced sterility in neonatal male and female rats. *Endocrinology,* 77:859–862.

73. Krieger, D. T. (1972): Circadian corticosteroid periodicity: Critical period for abolition by neonatal injection of corticosteroid. *Science,* 178:1205–1207.

74. Krieger, D. T. (1974): Effect of neonatal hydrocortisone on corticosteroid circadian periodicity, responsiveness to ACTH and stress in prepubertal and adult rats. *Neuroendocrinology,* 16:355–363.

75. Kuhn, C. M., Butler, S. R., and Schanberg, S. M. (1978): Selective depression of serum growth hormone during maternal deprivation in rat pups. *Science,* 201:1034–1036.

76. Kulin, H. E., and Reiter, E. O. (1976): Gonadotropin and testosterone measurements after estrogen administration to adult men, prepubertal and pubertal boys, and men with hypogonadotropism: Evidence for maturation of positive feedback in the male. *Pediatr. Res.,* 10:46–51.

77. Ladosky, W., and Gaziri, L. C. J. (1970): Brain serotonin and sexual differentiation of the nervous system. *Neuroendocrinology,* 6:168–174.

78. Lau, C., Bartolomé, J., Seidler, F. J., and Slotkin, T. A. (1977): Critical periods for effects of prenatal reserpine administration on development of rat brain and adrenal medulla. *Neuropharmacology,* 16:799–809.

79. Lauder, J. M. (1977): Effects of thyroid state on development of rat cerebellar cortex. In: *Thyroid Hormones and Brain Development,* edited by G. D. Grave, pp. 235–252. Raven Press, New York.

80. Lauder, J. M., and Bloom, F. E. (1975): Ontogeny of monoamine neurons in the locus coeruleus, raphe nuclei and substantia nigra of the rat. II. Synaptogenesis. *J. Comp. Neurol.,* 163:251–264.

81. Leshner, A. I. (1975): A model of hormones and agonistic behavior. *Physiol. Behav.,* 15:225–235.

82. Levine, S., Haltmeyer, G. C., Karas, G. G., and Denenberg, V. H. (1967): Physiological and behavioral effects of infantile stimulation. *Physiol. Behav.,* 2:55–59.

83. Lev-Ran, A. (1974): Sexuality and educational levels of women with the late-treated adrenogenital syndrome. *Arch. Sex. Behav.,* 4:27–32.

84. Lewis, P. D., Patel, A. J., Béndek, G., and Balázs, R. (1977): Do drugs acting on the nervous system affect cell proliferation in the developing brain? *Lancet,* 1:399–401.

85. Lynch, A., and Mychalkiw, W. (1978): Prenatal progesterone. II. Its role in the treatment

of pre-eclamptic toxaemia and its effect on the offspring's intelligence: A reappraisal. *Early Hum. Dev.,* 2:323–339.

86. Lynch, A., Mychalkiw, W., and Hutt, S. J. (1978): Prenatal progesterone. I. Its effect on development and on intellectual and academic achievement. *Early Hum. Dev.,* 2:305–322.
87. MacKinnon, P. C. B. (1979): Sexual differentiation of the brain. In: *Human Growth,* Vol. 3, edited by F. Falkner and J. M. Tanner, pp. 183–221. Plenum Press, New York.
88. Maeda, K., and Astic, L. (1972): Développement des neurones monoaminergiques centraux chez le foetus de Cobaye. *C. R. Soc. Biol. (Paris),* 166:1014–1017.
89. McDonald, P. G., and Doughty, C. (1974): Androgen sterilization in the neonatal female rat and its inhibition by an estrogen antagonist. *Neuroendocrinology,* 13:182–188.
90. McEwen, B. S. (1978): Sexual maturation and differentiation: The role of the gonadal steroids. *Prog. Brain Res.,* 48:291–307.
91. McEwen, B. S., Plapinger, L., Chaptal, C., Gerlach, J., and Wallach, G. (1975): Role of fetoneonatal estrogen binding proteins in the associations of estrogen with neonatal brain cell nuclear receptors. *Brain Res.,* 96:400–406.
92. Meyer-Bahlburg, H. F. L. (1977): Sex hormones and male homosexuality in comparative perspective. *Arch. Sex. Behav.,* 6:297–325.
93. Meyer-Bahlburg, H. F. L., Feinman, J. A., MacGillivray, M. H., and Aceto, T. (1978): Growth hormone deficiency, brain development, and intelligence. *Am. J. Dis. Child.,* 132:565–572.
94. Middaugh, L. D., Blackwell, L. A., Santos, C. A., III, and Zemp, J. W. (1974): Effects of d-amphetamine sulfate given to pregnant mice on activity and on catecholamines in the brains of offspring. *Dev. Psychobiol.,* 7:429–438.
95. Miyabo, S., and Hisada, T. (1975): Sex difference in ontogenesis of circadian adrenocortical rhythm in cortisone-primed rats. *Nature,* 256:590–592.
96. Moguilevsky, J. A., Libertun, C., Schiaffini, O., and Scacchi, P. (1969): Metabolic evidence of the sexual differentiation of hypothalamus. *Neuroendocrinology,* 4:264–269.
97. Money, J. (1973): Effects of prenatal androgenization and deandrogenization on behavior in human beings. In: *Frontiers in Neuroendocrinology,* Vol. 3, edited by W. F. Ganong and L. Martini, pp. 249–266. Oxford University Press, New York.
98. Money, J. E. (1975): Intellectual functioning in childhood endocrinopathies and related cytogenetic disorders. In: *Endocrine and Genetic Disorders of Childhood and Adolescence,* edited by L. I. Gardner, 2nd ed., pp. 1207–1218. Saunders, Philadelphia.
99. Money, J., and Ehrhardt, A. A. (1972): *Man and Woman, Boy and Girl.* Johns Hopkins University Press, Baltimore.
100. Money, J., and Lewis, V. (1966): IQ, genetics and accelerated growth: Adrenogenital syndrome. *Bull. Johns Hopkins Hosp.,* 118:365–373.
101. Moyer, J. A., Herrenkohl, L. R., and Jacobowitz, D. M. (1978): Stress during pregnancy: Effect on catecholamines in discrete brain regions of offspring as adults. *Brain Res.,* 144:173–178.
102. Nadler, R. D. (1973): Further evidence on the intrahypothalamic locus for androgenization of female rats. *Neuroendocrinology,* 12:110–119.
103. Naftolin, F., Ryan, K. J., Davies, I. J., Reddy, V. V., Flores, F., Petro, Z., Kuhn, M., White, R. J., Takaoka, Y., and Wolin, L. (1975): The formation of estrogens by central neuroendocrine tissues. *Recent Prog. Horm. Res.,* 31:295–315.
104. Naftolin, F., Ryan, K. J., and Petro, Z. (1971): Aromatization of androstenedione by limbic system tissue from human foetuses. *J. Endocrinol.,* 51:795–796.
105. Naftolin, F., Ryan, K. J., and Petro, Z. (1971): Aromatization of androstenedione by the diencephalon. *J. Clin. Endocrinol. Metab.,* 33:368–370.
106. Nunez, E., Vallette, G., Benassayag, C., and Jayle, M. F. (1974): Comparative study on the binding of estrogens by human and rat serum proteins in development. *Biochem. Biophys. Res. Commun.,* 57:126–133.
107. Nyakas, C., van Delft, A. M. L., Kaplanski, J., and Smelik, P. G. (1973): Exploratory activity and conditioned avoidance acquisition after early postnatal 6-hydroxydopamine administration. *J. Neural. Transm.,* 34:253–266.
108. Olson, L., Boréus, L. O., and Sieger, Å. (1973): Histochemical demonstration and mapping of 5-hydroxytryptamine- and catecholamine-containing neuron systems in the human fetal brain. *Z. Anat. Entwicklungsgesch.,* 139:259–282.
109. Partanen, S., and Hervonen, A. (1973): Monoamine-containing structures in the hypothalamo-hypophyseal system in the human fetus. *Z. Anat. Entwicklungsgesch.,* 140:53–60.

110. Pelton, E. W., Young, E., Bass, N. H., and Grindeland, R. E. (1974): Defective myelinogenesis in developing rat cerebrum induced by selective growth hormone deficiency. *Neurology (Minneap),* 24:377.

111. Perez-Polo, J. R., Hall, K., Livingston, K., and Westlund, K. (1977): Steroid induction of nerve growth factor synthesis in cell culture. *Life Sci.,* 21:1535–1543.

112. Phoenix, C. H. (1974): Prenatal testosterone in the nonhuman primate and its consequences for behavior. In: *Sex Differences in Behavior,* edited by R. C. Friedman, R. M. Richart, and R. L. Vande Wiele, pp. 19–32. Wiley, New York.

113. Phoenix, C. H., Goy, R. W., Gerall, A. A., and Young, W. C. (1959): Organizing action of prenatally administered testosterone propionate on the tissues mediating mating behavior in the female guinea pig. *Endocrinology,* 65:369–382.

114. Querido, A., Bleichrodt, N., and Djokomoeljanto, R. (1978): Thyroid hormones and human mental development. *Prog. Brain Res.,* 48:337–344.

115. Raisman, G., and Field, P. M. (1973): Sexual dimorphism in the neuropil of the preoptic area of the rat and its dependence on neonatal androgen. *Brain Res.,* 54:1–29.

116. Rastogi, R. B., and Singhal, R. L. (1976): Neonatal hypothyroidism: Alterations in behavioural activity and the metabolism of brain norepinephrine and dopamine. *Life Sci.,* 18:851–857.

117. Rastogi, R. B., and Singhal, R. L. (1978): The effect of thyroid hormone on serotonergic neurones: Depletion of serotonin in discrete brain areas of developing hypothyroid rats. *Naunyn Schmiedebergs Arch. Pharmacol.,* 304:9–13.

118. Reddy, V. V. R., Naftolin, F., and Ryan, K. J. (1974): Conversion of androstenedione to estrone by neural tissues from fetal and neonatal rats. *Endocrinology,* 94:117–121.

119. Reinisch, J. M. (1974): Fetal hormones, the brain, and human sex differences: A heuristic, integrative review of recent literature. *Arch. Sex. Behav.,* 3:51–90.

120. Reinisch, J. M., and Karow, W. G. (1977): Prenatal exposure to synthetic progestins and estrogens: Effects on human development. *Arch. Sex. Behav.,* 6:257–288.

121. Resko, J. A. (1975): Fetal hormones and their effect on the differentiation of the central nervous system in primates. *Fed. Proc.,* 34:1650–1655.

122. Resko, J. A., Ploem, J. G., and Stadelman, H. L. (1975): Estrogens in fetal and maternal plasma of the rhesus monkey. *Endocrinology,* 97:425–430.

123. Reyes, F. I., Boroditsky, R. S., Winter, J. S. D., and Faiman, C. (1974): Studies on human sexual development. II. Fetal and maternal serum gonadotropin and sex steroid concentrations. *J. Clin. Endocrinol. Metab.,* 38:612–617.

124. Rosman, N. P., and Malone, M. J. (1977): Brain myelination in experimental hypothyroidism: Morphological and biochemical observations. In: *Thyroid Hormones and Brain Development,* edited by G. D. Grave, pp. 169–194. Raven Press, New York.

125. Rosman, N. P., Malone, M. J., Helfenstein, M., and Kraft, E. (1972): The effect of thyroid deficiency on myelination of brain. *Neurology (Minneap.),* 22:99–106.

126. Sara, V. R., and Lazarus, L. (1974): Prenatal action of growth hormone on brain and behavior. *Nature,* 250:257–258.

127. Sara, V. R., Lazarus, L., Stuart, M. C., and King, T. (1974): Fetal brain growth: Selective action by growth hormone. *Science,* 186:446–447.

128. Schapiro, S. (1968): Some physiological, biochemical and behavioral consequences of neonatal hormone administration: Cortisol and thyroxine. *Gen. Comp. Endocrinol.,* 10:214–228.

129. Schapiro, S., Salas, M., and Vukovich, K. (1970): Hormonal effects on ontogeny of swimming ability in the rat: Assessment of central nervous system development. *Science,* 168:147–151.

130. Scott, J. P. (1962): Critical periods in behavioral development. *Science,* 138:949–958.

131. Scott, J. P. (1970): Foreword. In: *The Post-natal Development of Phenotype,* edited by S. Kazda and V. H. Denenberg, pp. 17–19. Butterworth, London.

132. Scott, J. P., Stewart, J. M., and de Ghett, V. J. (1974): Critical periods in the organization of systems. *Dev. Psychobiol.,* 7:489–513.

133. Seiger, Å., and Olson, L. (1973): Late prenatal ontogeny of central monoamine neurons in the rat: Fluorescence histochemical observations. *Z. Anat. Entwicklungsgesch.,* 140:281–318.

134. Short, R. V. (1975): Sexual differentiation of the brain of the sheep. *J. Endocrinol.,* 66:5P.

135. Södersten, P. (1978): Lordosis behaviour in immature male rats. *J. Endocrinol.,* 76:233–240.

136. Sokoloff, L. (1977): Biochemical mechanisms of the action of thyroid hormones: Relationship to their role in brain. In: *Thyroid Hormones and Brain Development,* edited by G. D. Grave, pp. 73–89. Raven Press, New York.

137. Sokoloff, L., and Kennedy, C. (1973): The action of thyroid hormones and their influence

on brain development and function. In: *Biology of Brain Dysfunction,* Vol. 2, edited by G. E. Gaull, pp. 295–332. Plenum Press, New York.

138. Staudt, J., and Dörner, G. (1976): Structural changes in the medial and central amygdala of the male rat, following neonatal castration and androgen treatment. *Endokrinologie,* 67:296–300.

139. Steiner, R. A., Clifton, D. K., Spies, H. G., and Resko, J. A. (1976): Sexual differentiation and feedback control of luteinizing hormone secretion in the rhesus monkey. *Biol. Reprod.,* 15:206–212.

140. Tonge, S. R. (1973): Permanent alterations in 5-hydroxyindole concentrations in discrete areas of rat brain produced by the pre- and neonatal administration of methylamphetamine and chlorpromazine. *J. Neurochem.,* 20:625–627.

141. Toran-Allerand, C. D. (1976): Sex steroids and the development of the newborn mouse hypothalamus and preoptic area in vitro: Implications for sexual differentiation. *Brain Res.,* 106:407–412.

142. Toran-Allerand, C. D. (1978): The luteinizing hormone-releasing hormone (LH-RH) neuron in cultures of the newborn mouse hypothalamus/preoptic area: Ontogenetic aspects and responses to steroid. *Brain Res.,* 149:257–265.

143. Ulrich, R., Yuwiler, A., and Geller, E. (1975): Effects of hydrocortisone on biogenic amine levels in the hypothalamus. *Neuroendocrinology,* 19:259–268.

144. Vaccari, A., Brotman, S., Cimino, J., and Timiras, P. S. (1977): Sex differentiation of neurotransmitter enzymes in central and peripheral nervous systems. *Brain Res.,* 132:176–185.

145. Vernadakis, A. (1971): Hormonal dependence of embryonic neural tissue in culture. In: *Hormones in Development,* edited by M. Hamburgh and E. J. W. Barrington, pp. 67–74. Appleton-Century-Crofts, New York.

146. Vernadakis, A., Culver, B., and Nidess, R. (1978): Actions of steroid hormones on neural growth in culture: Role of glial cells. *Psychoneuroendocrinology,* 3:47–64.

147. Vernadakis, A., and Timiras, P. S. (1967): Effects of estradiol and cortisol on neural tissue in culture. *Experientia,* 23:467–468.

148. Vernadakis, A., and Woodbury, D. M. (1963): Effect of cortisol on the electroshock seizure thresholds in developing rats. *J. Pharmacol. Exp. Ther.,* 139:110–113.

149. Vreeburg, J. T. M., van der Vaart, P. D. M., and van der Schoot, P. (1977): Prevention of central defeminization but not masculinization in male rats by inhibition neonatally of oestrogen biosynthesis. *J. Endocrinol.,* 74:375–382.

150. Ward, I. L. (1972): Prenatal stress feminizes and demasculinizes the behavior of males. *Science,* 175:82–84.

151. Weichsel, M. E., Jr. (1977): The therapeutic use of glucocorticoid hormones in the perinatal period: Potential neurological hazards. *Ann. Neurol.,* 2:364–366.

152. Weisz, J., and Gibbs, C. (1974): Metabolites of testosterone in the brain of the newborn female rat after an injection of tritiated testosterone. *Neuroendocrinology,* 14:72–86.

153. Weisz, J., and Gibbs, C. (1974): Conversion of testosterone and androstenedione to estrogens in vitro by the brain of female rats. *Endocrinology,* 94:616–620.

154. Whalen, R. E., and Luttge, W. G. (1971): Perinatal administration of dihydrotestosterone to female rats and the development of reproductive function. *Endocrinology,* 89:1320–1322.

155. Woodbury, D. M., and Vernadakis, A. (1967): Influence of hormones on brain activity. In: *Neuroendocrinology,* Vol. 2, edited by L. Martini and W. F. Ganong, pp. 335–375. Academic Press, London.

156. Yalom, I. D., Green, R., and Fisk, N. (1973): Prenatal exposure to female hormones: Effect on psychosexual development in boys. *Arch. Gen. Psychiatry,* 28:554–561.

157. Zamenof, S., Mosley, J., and Schuller, E. (1966): Stimulation of the proliferation of cortical neurons by prenatal treatment with growth hormone. *Science,* 152:1396–1397.

158. Zamenof, S., van Marthens, E., and Grauel, L. (1971): Prenatal cerebral development: Effect of restricted diet, reversal by growth hormone. *Science,* 174:954–955.

The Endocrine Functions of the Brain,
edited by Marcella Motta.
Raven Press, New York © 1980

7

Distribution of Hypothalamic Hormones

Michael J. Brownstein

Laboratory of Clinical Science, National Institute of Mental Health, National Institutes of Health, Bethesda, Maryland 20205

Five peptide hormones are discussed in this review: vasopressin, oxytocin, luteinizing hormone releasing hormone (LHRH), thyrotropin releasing hormone (TRH), and growth hormone release inhibiting hormone (somatostatin). These were isolated from hypothalamic or hypophysial extracts and were assumed to be made by a small, anatomically discrete population of neurons whose processes traveled to or through the median eminence. The isolation of the hypothalamic hormones and the development of sensitive assays for measuring them and immunohistochemical techniques for visualizing them have produced surprising results. It is becoming more and more obvious that the "hypothalamic hormones" are not confined to the hypothalamus and that they must have functions unrelated to the actions that facilitated their discoveries.

VASOPRESSIN, OXYTOCIN, AND THE NEUROPHYSINS

During the late 1940s Bargmann and the Scharrers (8,81) introduced their concept of neurosecretion. They envisioned populations of neurons with certain similarities to endocrine cells. One such population comprises the hypothalamoneurohypophysial system. In this system hormones are made by neurons in the supraoptic (SON) and paraventricular (PVN) nuclei (1,62,93), carried from the hypothalamus to the pituitary in axons, released into a blood capillary network in response to physiological stimuli, and delivered to target organs by the bloodstream. The hormones vasopressin and oxytocin were identified and chemically characterized on the basis of their biological actions (28,29); as a consequence of their purification, the role of the brain and pituitary in regulating the ejection of milk, contraction of the uterus, and conservation of water could be studied in detail.

The magnocellular neurons of the SON and PVN were among the first neurosecretory cells visualized histochemically. In these neurons oxytocin and vasopressin are stored in vesicles along with "binding proteins" called neurophysins.

The neurophysins, oxytocin, and vasopressin are rich in cysteine, and the cysteine is responsible for the staining of "neurosecretory material" observed with Bargmann's modification of Gomori's method.

There are two major neurophysins in the neurohypophysis of most species. One of these is associated with vasopressin and the other with oxytocin (47,48). Antibodies have been raised against the neurophysins from a variety of animals, as well as against vasopressin and oxytocin. The antibodies have been used to develop radioimmunoassays and immunohistochemical techniques, methods employed to study the hormones' distribution, transport, and release (37,38).

Hormone- and neurophysin-containing neurons are concentrated in the SON and PVN. Both nuclei contain oxytocin- and vasopressin-producing cell bodies. The two hormones and their respective neurophysins seem to be made in separate populations of neurons (24,91). In human (101), monkey (100), bovine (104), mouse (103), rat (103), and guinea pig (86) hypothalami, neurophysin is found in the perikarya of magnocellular neurons at all levels along the paraventricular fiber tract between the SON and PVN. In addition, neurophysin-positive cells have been observed extending from the SON and PVN anteriorly as far as the lamina terminalis and the anterior commissure, dorsally as far as the ventral anterior thalamus, laterally beyond the fornix, and caudally to the middle of the median eminence (103). In the rhesus monkey oxytocin, vasopressin, and their respective neurophysins have been visualized in magnocellular perikarya in the preoptic area close to the lamina terminalis (100). These rostrally placed accessory neurons project to the supraoptic crest as the accessory cell groups in other species [e.g., guinea pig (55), cat (15), and rabbit (32)] may also do.

Immunochemical studies in a number of animals have shown that the majority of the axons of neurosecretory cells in the SON and PVN travel via the zona interna of the median eminence to the neural lobe of the pituitary where they terminate on capillaries (101,103). In addition to vasopressin, oxytocin, and the neurophysins, these axons contain two proteins with molecular weights (M.W.) of 20,000 that are the precursors of the two neurophysins (19,34,35). The precursors, which may also give rise to the neurohypophysial hormones, are processed into their respective neurophysins via intermediates (of M.W. 16,000).

Investigators in several laboratories demonstrated that cells of the magnocellular neurosecretory system innervate the zona externa of the median eminence and discharge hormones into the hypophysial portal plexus (24,25,65,75,80, 86,90,92,94,100,102). Unilateral destruction of the PVN results in a loss of vasopressin, oxytocin, and neurophysins from the ipsilateral zona externa (5). Since none of the parvicellular neurons in the PVN appear to contain vasopressin, oxytocin, or neurophysins, the magnocellular neurons in the PVN must provide these substances to the zona externa.

The PVN and SON are not the only nuclei that have neurophysin-containing cells. There are neurons in the dorsal pole of the suprachiasmatic nuclei (SCN) that seem to have neurophysin too (87,90,103). These cells do not appear to have any oxytocin; they make only vasopressin. The SCN have measurable amounts of vasopressin in normal rats but no vasopressin in rats with hereditary diabetes insipidus (Brattleboro rats) (36). The areas of the brain that are innervated by vasopressin-containing cells in the SCN are being sought. Since neurons in the SCN have been shown to serve as circadian clocks, it may be that vasopressin mediates certain rhythmic phenomena in the central nervous system.

Recently Swanson (87) provided evidence that in the rat and the cow there are descending systems of neurophysin-containing pathways that project from the PVN to a variety of extrahypothalamic areas. Among these areas are the medial nucleus of the amygdala, the tract and nucleus of the diagonal band, the mesencephalic central gray, the Edinger–Westphal complex, the marginal nucleus of the brachium conjunctivum, the locus ceruleus, the nucleus of the solitary tract, the nucleus intermedium, the dorsal motor nucleus of the vagus, and the intermediolateral column and central gray and marginal zone of the spinal cord.

LUTEINIZING HORMONE RELEASING HORMONE

During 1960 McCann and his associates (67) showed that the rat hypothalamus contains a substance that releases luteinizing hormone (LH) from the anterior pituitary. Using a bioassay they were able to localize this material more precisely. They assayed extracts of the stalk–median eminence, ventral hypothalamus, dorsal hypothalamus, and suprachiasmatic nucleus. Most of the LH-releasing activity was in the stalk and median eminence; a small amount of activity was detected in the basal hypothalamus. Next, they measured releasing activity in serial sections of the preoptic area and hypothalamus (66). They showed that it was present in a region extending from the preoptic area through the suprachiasmatic area to the median eminence and arcuate nucleus. Subsequently, Wheaton and his co-workers (97) assayed LHRH in brain slices by means of radioimmunoassay and confirmed the earlier bioassay data.

Palkovits and his collaborators (72,73) assayed LHRH in samples of discrete hypothalamic nuclei that were punched out of frozen serial sections of the rat hypothalamus. The amount of LHRH in each tissue homogenate was determined by radioimmunoassay. A very high concentration of LHRH was found in the median eminence; moderate levels were detected in the arcuate nucleus and small amounts in the suprachiasmatic and preoptic regions. In the preoptic area, the bulk of the LHRH seems to reside in the supraoptic crest, a vascular structure that forms part of the rostral tip of the third ventricle (52). The supraoptic crest and the other circumventricular organs are rich in LHRH. The hormone present in these organs may be taken up from the cerebrospinal fluid (CSF) and disposed of, or it may be secreted into the CSF and act on diverse areas of the brain.

LHRH-containing neural structures have been visualized in the human fetus (22), *Saimiri sciurus* (10), *Cebus apella* (10), rhesus monkey (40), sheep (58), cat (11), dog (11), rabbit (91), guinea pig (7,12,13,63), hamster (63), rat (2,7, 40,44,51,57,68,69,76,77,84), duck (23), greenfinch (85), frog (3,39), and toad (26). The neuronal system containing LHRH has been studied most extensively in the guinea pig and the rat. It is unusual in either species to find LHRH-containing perikarya in normal, untreated animals. After treatment with pharmacological agents, LHRH was detected in preoptic and septal neurons in the guinea pig (64). The tuberal region also contains LHRH-positive cells, and LHRH is present in axons and terminals in the median eminence and supraoptic crest. These axons can rarely be traced back to cell bodies in the arcuate region. In fact, the number of LHRH-containing axons in the infundibular region markedly drops after electrolytic lesions are made just caudal to the septum and preoptic areas (13). Therefore the majority of these tuberal axons may originate from cells that are over or rostral to the chiasm.

The results of immunocytochemical studies in the rat are more difficult to understand than those in the guinea pig. A number of workers succeeded in staining preterminal and terminal axons in the rat (14,70,82). These are found in the median eminence, supraoptic crest, septum, preoptic area, perifornical region, and stria terminalis. In spite of this, many investigators (18,95,96) have been unable to visualize LHRH-containing perikarya at all. Weindl and his co-workers (95) reported that there are LHRH-positive cells only in the dorsal preoptic and anterior hypothalamic regions. This is consistent with the finding that total mediobasal hypothalamic deafferentations or frontal deafferentations cause marked decreases in LHRH in the median eminence and arcuate nucleus without affecting LHRH in the supraoptic crest (18,96).

On the other hand, Naik (68,69) and Hoffman (40) visualized LHRH-containing cells in the suprachiasmatic region, arcuate nucleus, and premammillary region. Thus further studies of the location of LHRH-containing neurons and the distribution of their processes in the rat are needed.

According to Sétáló et al. (83), LHRH is especially easy to visualize in neuronal perikarya and processes of the rabbit. LHRH-containing cells were found in the preoptic and tuberal regions, the former region containing the majority of positive cells. LHRH was seen in tuberoinfundibular and preopticoinfundibular tracts, and a dense plexus of LHRH-rich axons was detected in the periventricular area. The latter axons seem to transport LHRH to the median eminence from cells in the preoptic, suprachiasmatic, and septal areas. Small groups of axons or single axons were found in the region of the mammillary body, the medial habenular nuclei, the stria terminalis, the stria medullaris thalami, and the ventral part of the rostral mesencephalon. Scattered neurons and their rostrally projecting processes were described in the diagonal band of Broca as well.

Like the rabbit, the dog and the cat have LHRH-positive perikarya distributed between anterior (preoptic, anterior hypothalamic, septal, and precommissural areas) and posterior (tuberal and premammillary areas) groups (11). In both species there were more cells anteriorly than posteriorly, but in the dog about 40% of the cells stained were located in the posterior group.

In primates most LHRH-containing cell bodies have been found in the mediobasal part of the tuber cinereum, especially in the infundibular and premammillary nuclei (10,40). There are also scattered positive cells in the septal and preoptic area. Although mediobasal hypothalamic deafferentation in rats blocks ovulation, in primates complete surgical isolation of the same region does not interfere with either tonic or cyclic release of gonadotropic hormones (59). Presumably the rostrally located LHRH-containing neurons in primates (those that project to the supraoptic crest, medial habenula, mesencephalon, and telencephalon) have roles in addition to regulating anterior pituitary function (9).

The human fetus has neuronal cell bodies that contain LHRH in the mediobasal hypothalamus (22). These were apparent from the thirteenth week of gestation until birth. LHRH was detected in axons in the median eminence, mediobasal hypothalamus, premammillary area, and epithalamus.

SOMATOSTATIN

Somatostatin is found in the central nervous system (CNS) and the periphery, where it is present in the stomach, duodenum, jejunum, and pancreas (6,79). It has been detected in the brains of several mammals, the pigeon, frog, catfish, and hagfish (88).

Using bioassays and radioimmunoassays, a number of workers (17,54) showed that somatostatin is concentrated in the hypothalamus of the rat where its level is especially high in the median eminence. A number of hypothalamic nuclei contain substantial amounts of somatostatin too: the arcuate, ventromedial, ventral premammillary, periventricular, and medial preoptic nuclei (17,54). Of these, the ventromedial nucleus is unique in being devoid of growth hormone release inhibiting activity (89). It may be that this nucleus is particularly rich in a growth hormone releasing hormone.

The median eminence is not the only circumventricular organ that contains somatostatin. The peptide is present in the supraoptic crest, subfornical organ, subcommissural organ, and area postrema (74).

Outside of the hypothalamus, a number of structures in addition to the circumventricular organs have somatostatin. In fact, only about one-third of the brain's somatostatin is found in the hypothalamus. The septum, preoptic area, and thalamus have moderately high somatostatin concentrations and contribute another 30% to the total (17). The extrahypothalamic somatostatin was recently characterized by Speiss and Vale *(personal communication)*. It appears to have the same amino acid composition as the material that was originally isolated from the hypothalamus.

Because somatostatin was found in the medial hypothalamus and outside of it, the locations of the neurons that provide the median eminence its release inhibiting hormone were not immediately obvious. Complete mediobasal hypothalamic deafferentation and frontal deafferentation caused marked decreases in somatostatin in the median eminence but did not depress somatostatin levels elsewhere (16). Therefore cells in the tuberal area must not supply the remainder of the regions of the central nervous system with their somatostatin. Furthermore, it seems likely that the mediobasal hypothalamus must receive the bulk of its somatostatin from an area rostral to it.

Three groups have succeeded in visualizing somatostatin-containing cell bodies in the rat brain (4,30,46). These cell bodies are located in the anterior periventricular area. When lesions were made in this area in the anterior hypothalamic region or ventromedial preoptic region, somatostatin decreased 90% and 80%, respectively, in the median eminence (31). No changes in the level of the hormone were detected in the ventromedial nucleus; presumably this nucleus has a separate somatostatinergic input from that of the median eminence.

In addition to the dense plexuses of somatostatin-containing fibers observed in the median eminence, arcuate nucleus, and ventromedial nucleus (46,76,78), other fiber systems have been seen. Moderately dense fiber systems have been visualized in the posterior pituitary (42) (which may arise from cells in the magnocellular hypothalamic nuclei), supraoptic crest, subfornical organ, substantia gelatinosa, and dorsal horn of the spinal cord. Neuronal perikarya in the spinal ganglia of the rat have been reported to contain somatostatin (41–43); some somatostatin-containing cells were found in the trigeminal ganglion as well. The somatostatin-positive nerve fibers in the lamina propria of the intestines near the ganglion cells of the myenteric plexus may belong to the spinal ganglion cells mentioned above (42,46). Somatostatin is also present in cells in the thyroid, stomach (42), and the islets of Langerhans (in D cells) (27). In the pancreas somatostatin seems to inhibit insulin and glucagon release (33,56).

THYROTROPIN RELEASING HORMONE

By measuring TSH release from pituitary explants, Krulich and his co-workers (60) showed that TRH is present in the median eminence, dorsomedial hypothalamus, and preoptic area of the rat. Similarly, in discrete hypothalamic nuclei radioimmunoassayed for TRH, the peptide was found to be concentrated in the median eminence (20), and in the cow it was restricted to the middle portion of the zona externa (53). It was present in moderate amounts in the ventromedial, arcuate, dorsomedial, and periventricular nuclei. Modest amounts of TRH were found in the remainder of the hypothalamus, the preoptic area, and the septum pellucidum.

Several investigators reported that immunoassayable TRH is widely distributed in the CNS (49,71,98). The TRH-like material in extracts of extrahypothalamic brain has gel filtration and electrophoretic properties similar to those of TRH, and it seems to be biologically active. In spite of this, the TRH-like substance(s) found outside of the hypothalamus may not all be pyroglutamylhistidyl-prolineamide. Jeffcoate and White (50) found that extracts of sheep, rat, and rabbit cerebral cortex contain an immunoassayable material that differs from synthetic TRH chromatographically. Kubek and his colleagues (61) showed that human brain extracts have less TSH-releasing activity than TRH immunoreactivity. Finally, Youngblood and co-workers (99) stated that molecular structures other than TRH are present in extrahypothalamic brain which are capable of reacting in a "crude" TRH radioimmunoassay. Among the substances that interfere in the radioimmunoassay for TRH are brain lipids that can be removed from samples with ether. Only the hypothalamus, septum, and preoptic area could be shown to contain authentic TRH.

Given the apparent lack of specificity of the antibodies employed to measure TRH, it is not unlikely that this substance has been artifactually localized by means of immunocytochemistry, especially outside the hypothalamus, preoptic area, and septum (45). Within these three regions, TRH has been visualized in the external zone of the median eminence and in dense axonal systems in the dorsomedial nucleus, the paraventricular nucleus, and the perifornical region. Lower numbers of TRH-positive fibers were found in the ventromedial nuclei, periventricular nuclei, and zona incerta; and sparse networks of fibers were found elsewhere in the hypothalamus (43). The supraoptic crest contains a fairly dense collection of TRH-containing processes; the interstitial nucleus of the stria terminalis and the lateral septal nucleus have moderate numbers of positive processes. The above immunocytochemical findings agree reasonably well with radioimmunoassay and bioassay data.

The locations of neurons whose axons supply TRH to the hypothalamus remain to be determined. Complete deafferentation of the mediobasal hypothalamus causes a substantial fall in TRH in this region, as does frontal deafferentation (21). Thus part of the TRH in the tuberal region must come from extratuberal cells. Some of these cells may reside in the periventricular area or the supraoptic area (Hökfelt, *personal communication*).

CONCLUDING REMARKS

The pictures of central distributions of the hypothalamic hormones have been painted to date with rather broad strokes. Studies based on bioassays, radioimmunoassays, and immunocytochemistry are in general agreement but differ from one another in specifics. If anatomical studies are to provide a framework for future biochemical, physiological, and pharmacological work, these differences must be resolved by more careful attention to technical detail.

REFERENCES

1. Adamsons, K., Jr., Engel, S. L., van Dyke, H. B., Schmidt-Nielson, B., and Schmidt-Nielsen, K. (1956): The distribution of oxytocin and vasopressin (antidiuretic hormone) in the neurohypophysis of the camel. *Endocrinology,* 58:272–278.

2. Alpert, L. C., Brawer, J. R., Jackson, J. M. D., and Patel, Y. C. (1975): Somatostatin and LRH: Immunohistochemical evidence for distinct hypothalamic distribution. *Fed. Proc.,* 34:239.

3. Alpert, L. C., Brawer, J. R., Jackson, J. M. D., and Reichlin, S. (1976): Localization of LHRH in neurons in frog brain (Rana pipiens and Rana catesbeiana). *Endocrinology,* 98:910–921.

4. Alpert, L. C., Brawer, J. R., Patel, Y. C., and Reichlin, S. (1976): Somatostatinergic neurons in anterior hypothalamus: Immunohistochemical localization. *Endocrinology,* 98:255–258.

5. Antunes, J. L., Carmel, P. W., and Zimmerman, E. A. (1977): Projections from the paraventricular nucleus to the zona externa of the median eminence of the rhesus monkey: An immunohistochemical study. *Brain Res.,* 137:1–10.

6. Arimura, A., Sato, H., Dupont, A., Nishi, N., and Schally, A. V. (1975): Somatostatin: Abundance of immunoreactive hormone in rat stomach and pancreas. *Science,* 189:1007–1009.

7. Baker, B. L., Dermody, W. C., and Reel, J. R. (1974): Localization of luteinizing hormone-releasing hormone in the mammalian hypothalamus. *Am. J. Anat.,* 139:129–134.

8. Bargmann, W. (1968): Neurohypophysis: Structure and function. In: *Handbook of Experimental Pharmacology, Vol. 23: Neurohypophyseal Hormones and Similar Polypeptides,* edited by B. Berde, pp. 1–39. Springer-Verlag, New York.

9. Barry, J. (1978): Septo-epithalamo-habenular LRF reactive neurons in monkeys. *Brain Res.,* 151:183–187.

10. Barry, J., and Carette, B. (1975): Immunofluorescence study of LRF neurons in primates. *Cell Tissue Res.,* 164:163–178.

11. Barry, J., and Dubois, M. P. (1975): Immunofluorescence study of LRF-producing neurons in the cat and the dog. *Neuroendocrinology,* 18:290–298.

12. Barry, J., Dubois, M. P., and Carette, B. (1974): Immunofluorescence study of the preoptico-infundibular LRF neurosecretory pathway in the normal, castrated, or testosterone-treated male guinea pig. *Endocrinology,* 95:1416–1423.

13. Barry, J., Dubois, M. P., and Poulain, P. (1973): LH-RH producing cells of the mammalian hypothalamus. *Z. Zellforsch. Microsk. Anat.,* 146:351–366.

14. Barry, J., Dubois, M. P., Poulain, P., and Leonardelli, J. (1973): Characterisation et topographie de neurones hypothalamiques immunoreactifs avec des anticorps anti-LRF de synthèse. *C R Acad. Sci. (Paris),* 276:3191–3193.

15. Bisset, G. W., Clark, B. J., and Errington, M. J. (1971): The hypothalamic neurosecretory pathways for the release of oxytocin and vasopressin in the cat. *J. Physiol. (Lond.),* 217:111–131.

16. Brownstein, M. J., Arimura, A., Fernandez-Durango, R., Schally, A. V., Palkovits, M., and Kizer, J. S. (1977): The effect of hypothalamic deafferentation on somatostatin in the rat brain. *Endocrinology,* 100:246–249.

17. Brownstein, M. J., Arimura, A., Sato, H., Schally, A. V., and Kizer, J. S. (1975): The regional distribution of somatostatin in the rat brain. *Endocrinology,* 96:1456–1461.

18. Brownstein, M. J., Arimura, A., Schally, A. V., Palkovits, M., and Kizer, J. S. (1976): The effect of surgical isolation of the hypothalamus on its luteinizing hormone-releasing hormone content. *Endocrinology,* 98:662–665.

19. Brownstein, M., and Gainer, H. (1977): Neurophysin biosynthesis in normal rats and in rats with hereditary diabetes insipidus. *Proc. Natl. Acad. Sci. USA,* 74:4046–4049.

20. Brownstein, M. J., Palkovits, M., Saavedra, J., Bassiri, R., and Utiger, R. D. (1974): Thyrotropin-releasing hormone in specific nuclei of rat brain. *Science,* 185:267–269.

21. Brownstein, M. J., Utiger, R. D., Palkovits, M., and Kizer, J. S. (1975): Effect of hypothalamic deafferentation on thyrotropin releasing hormone levels in rat brain. *Proc. Natl. Acad. Sci. USA,* 72:4177–4179.

22. Bugnon, C., Bloch, B., and Fellmann, D. (1976): Mise en évidence cyto-immunologique de neurones à LH-RH chez le foetus humain. *C R Acad. Sci. (Paris),* 282:1625–1628.

23. Calas, A., Kerdelhue, B., Assenmacher, I., and Jutisz, M. (1974): Les axones à LH-RH de l'éminence médiane: Etude ultrastructurale chez le canard par une technique immunocytochimique. *C R Acad. Sci. (Paris),* 278:2557–2559.

24. De Mey, J., Dierickx, K., and Vandesande, F. (1975): Immunohistochemical demonstration of neurophysin I- and neurophysin II-containing nerve fibers in the external region of the bovine median eminence. *Cell Tissue Res.,* 157:517–519.

25. Dietrickx, K., Vandesande, F., and De Mey, J. (1976): Identification, in the external region

of the rat median eminence, of separate neurophysin-vasopressin and neurophysin-oxytocin containing nerve fibers. *Cell Tissue Res., 168:141–151.*

26. Doerr-Schott, J., and Dubois, M. P. (1975): Localisation et identification d'un centre LH-RF dans l'encephale du crapaud, Bufo vulgaris Laur. *C R Acad. Sci. (Paris),* 280:1285–1287.
27. Dubois, P. M., Paulin, C., Assan, R., and Dubois, M. P. (1975): Evidence for immunoreactive somatostatin in the endocrine cells of human foetal pancreas. *Nature,* 256:731–732.
28. Du Vigneaud, V., Ressler, C., Swan, J. M., Roberts, C. W., Katsoyannis, P. G., and Gordon, S. (1953): Synthesis of an octapeptide amide with the hormonal activity of oxytocin. *J. Am. Chem. Soc.,* 74:4879–4880.
29. Du Vigneaud, V., Lawler, H. C., and Popenoe, A. (1953): Enzymatic cleavage of glycinamide from vasopressin and a proposed structure for the pressor–antidiuretic hormone of the posterior pituitary. *J. Am. Chem. Soc.* 75:4880–4881.
30. Elde, R. P., and Parsons, J. A. (1975): Immunocytochemical localization of somatostatin in cell bodies of the rat hypothalamus. *Am. J. Anat.,* 144:541–548.
31. Epelbaum, J., Willoughby, J. O., Brazeau, P., and Martin, J. B. (1977): Effects of lesions and hypothalamic deafferentation on somatostatin distribution in the brain. *Endocrinology,* 101:1495–1502.
32. Ford, D. H., and Kantounis, S. (1957): The localization of neurosecretory structures and pathways in the male albino rabbit. *J. Comp. Neurol.,* 108:91–107.
33. Fugimoto, W. Y., Ensinck, J. W., and Williams, R. W. (1974): Somatostatin inhibits insulin and glucagon release by monolayer cell cultures of rat endocrine pancreas. *Life Sci.,* 15:1999–2004.
34. Gainer, H., Sarne, Y., and Brownstein, M. (1977): Neurophysin biosynthesis: Conversion of a putative precursor during axonal transport. *Science,* 195:1354–1356.
35. Gainer, H., Sarne, Y., and Brownstein, M. (1977): Biosynthesis and axonal transport of rat neurohypophyseal proteins and peptides. *J. Cell Biol.,* 73:366–381.
36. George, J. M., and Forrest, J. (1976): Vasopressin and oxytocin content of microdissected hypothalamic areas in rats with hereditary diabetes insipidus. *Neuroendocrinology,* 21:275–279.
37. George, J. M., and Jacobowitz, D. M. (1975): Localization of vasopressin in discrete areas of rat hypothalamus. *Brain Res.,* 93:363–366.
38. George, J. M., Staples, S., and Marks, B. (1976): Oxytocin content of microdissected areas of rat hypothalamus. *Endocrinology,* 98:1430–1433.
39. Goos, H. J., Ligtenberg, P. J. M., and Van Oordt, P. G. W. J. (1976): Immunofluorescence studies on gonadotropin releasing hormone (GRH) in the fore-brain and neurohypophysis of the green frog, Rana esculenta L. *Cell Tissue Res.,* 168:325–333.
40. Hoffman, G. E. (1976): Immunocytochemical localization of luteinizing hormone-releasing hormone (LHRH) in murine and primate brain. *Anat. Rec.,* 184:429–430.
41. Hökfelt, T., Efendic, S., Hellerstrom, D., Johansson, O., Luft, R., and Arimura, A. (1975): Cellular localization of somatostatin in endocrine-like cells and neurons of the rat with special references to the A_1-cells of the pancreatic islets and to the hypothalamus. *Acta Endocrinol. [Suppl. 200] (Kbh),* 80:5–41.
42. Hökfelt, T., Elde, R., Johansson, O., Luft, R., Nilsson, G., and Arimura, A. (1976): Immunohistochemical evidence for separate populations of somatostatin-containing and substance P-containing primary afferent neurons in the rat. *Neuroscience,* 1:131–136.
43. Hökfelt, T., Elde, R., Johansson, O., Luft, R., and Arimura, A. (1975): Immunohistochemical evidence for the presence of somatostatin, a powerful inhibitory peptide, in some primary sensory neurons. *Neurosci. Lett.,* 1:231–235.
44. Hökfelt, T., Fuxe, K., Goldstein, M., Johansson, O., Fraser, H., and Jeffcoate, S. L. (1975): Immunofluorescence mapping of central monoamine and releasing hormone (LRH) systems. In: *Anatomical Neuroendocrinology,* edited by W. E. Stumpf and L. D. Grant, pp. 381–392. Karger, Basel.
45. Hökfelt, T., Fuxe, K., Johansson, O., Jeffcoate, S., and White, N. (1975): Thyrotropin releasing hormone (TRH)-containing nerve terminals in certain brain stem nuclei and in the spinal cord. *Neurosci. Lett.,* 1:133–139.
46. Hökfelt, T., Johansson, O., Fuxe, K., Löfström, A., Goldstein, M., Park, D., Ebstein, R., Fraser, H., Jeffcoate, S., Efendic, S., Luft, R., and Arimura, A. (1975): Mapping and relationship of hypothalamic neurotransmitters and hypothalamic hormones. In: *Central Nervous System and Behavioral Pharmacology,* edited by M. Airaksinen, pp. 93–110. Pergamon Press, Oxford.

47. Hollenberg, M. D., and Hope, D. V. (1967): Fractionation of neurophysin by molecular-sieve and ion-exchange chromatography. *Biochem. J.,* 104:122–127.
48. Hope, D. B., Schachter, B. A., and Frankland, B. T. B. (1964): Dissociation of oxytocin, vasopressin and neurophysin by gel filtration. *Biochem. J.,* 93:7P.
49. Jackson, I. M. D., and Reichlin, S. (1974): Thyrotropin-releasing hormone (TRH): Distribution in hypothalamic and extrahypothalamic brain tissues of mammalian and sub-mammalian chordates. *Endocrinology,* 95:854–862.
50. Jeffcoate, S. L., and White, N. (1975): Is there any thyrotropin releasing hormone in mammalian extra-hypothalamic brain tissue? *J. Endocrinol.,* 67:42.
51. King, J. C., Parsons, J. A., Erlandsen, S. L., and Williams, T. H. (1974): Luteinizing hormone-releasing hormone (LH-RH) pathway of the rat hypothalamus revealed by the unlabeled antibody peroxidase-antiperoxidase method. *Cell Tissue Res.,* 153:211–217.
52. Kizer, J. S., Palkovits, M., and Brownstein, M. (1976): Releasing factors in the circumventricular organs of the rat brain. *Endocrinology,* 98:309–315.
53. Kizer, J. S., Palkovits, M., Tappaz, M., Kebabian, J., and Brownstein, M. (1976b): Distribution of releasing factors, biogenic amines, and related enzymes in the bovine median eminence. *Endocrinology,* 98:649–659.
54. Kobayashi, R., Brown, M., and Vale, W. (1977): Regional distribution of neurotensin and somatostatin in rat brain. *Brain Res.,* 126:584–588.
55. Kraggs, G. S., Tindal, J. S., and Turvey, A. (1971): Paraventricular–hypophyseal neurosecretory pathways in the guinea pig. *J. Endocrinol.,* 50:153–162.
56. Koerker, D. J., Ruch, W., Chideckel, E., Palmer, J., Goodner, C. J., Ensinck, J., and Gale, C. C. (1974): Somatostatin: Hypothalamic inhibitor of the endocrine pancreas. *Science,* 184:482–484.
57. Kordon, C., Kerdelhué, B., Pattou, E., and Jutisz, M. (1974): Immunocytochemical localization of LHRH in axons and nerve terminals of the rat median eminence. *Proc. Soc. Exp. Biol. Med.,* 147:122–127.
58. Kozlowski, G. P., and Zimmerman, E. A. (1974): Localization of gonadotropin-releasing hormone (Gn-RH) in sheep and mouse brain. *Anat. Rec.,* 178:396.
59. Krey, L. C., Butler, W. R., and Knobil, E. (1975): Surgical disconnection of the medial basal hypothalamus and pituitary function in the rhesus monkey. I. *Endocrinology,* 96:1073–1087.
60. Krulich, L., Quijada, M., Hefco, E., and Sundberg, D. K. (1974): Localization of thyrotropin-releasing factor (TRF) in the hypothalamus of the rat. *Endocrinology,* 95:9–17.
61. Kubek, M. J., Lorincz, M. A., and Wilber, J. F. (1977): The identification of thyrotropin releasing hormone (TRH) in hypothalamic and extrahypothalamic loci of the human nervous system. *Brain Res.,* 126:196–200.
62. Lederis, M. K. (1961): Vasopressin and oxytocin in the mammalian hypothalamus. *Gen. Comp. Endocrinol.,* 1:80–89.
63. Leonardelli, J., Barry, J., and Dubois, M. P. (1973): Mise en évidence par immunofluorescence d'un constituent immunologiquement apparenté au LH-RF dan l'hypothalamus et l'éminence mediane chez les mammifères. *C R Acad. Sci. (Paris),* 276:2043–2048.
64. Leonardelli, J., and Dubois, M. P. (1974): Commande aminergique et cholinergique de cellules hypothalamiques élaboratrices de LH-RH chez le cobaye. *Ann. Endocrinol. (Paris),* 35:639–645.
65. Livett, B. G., and Parry, H. B. (1971): Accumulation of neurophysin in the median eminence and cerebellum of sheep with natural scrapie. *Br. J. Pharmacol.,* 43:423P–424P.
66. McCann, S. M. (1962): A hypothalamic luteinizing-hormone-releasing-factor. *Am. J. Physiol.,* 202:395–400.
67. McCann, S. M., Taleisnik, S., and Friedman, H. M. (1960): LH-releasing activity in hypothalamic extracts. *Proc. Soc. Exp. Biol. Med.,* 104:432–434.
68. Naik, D. V. (1974): Immunohistochemical and immunofluorescent localization of LH-RF neurons in the hypothalamus of rat. *Anat. Rec.,* 178:424.
69. Naik, D. V. (1975): Immunoreactive LH-RH neurons in the hypothalamus identified by light and fluorescent microscopy. *Cell Tissue Res.,* 157:423–436.
70. Naik, D. V. (1975): Immuno-electron microscopic localization of luteinizing hormone-releasing hormone in the arcuate nuclei and median eminence of the rat. *Cell Tissue Res.,* 157:437–455.

71. Oliver, C., Eskay, R. L., Ben-Jonathan, N., and Porter, J. C. (1974): Distribution and concentration of TRH in the rat brain. *Endocrinology,* 95:540–553.
72. Palkovits, M. (1973): Isolated removal of hypothalamic or other brain nuclei of the rat. *Brain Res.,* 59:449–450.
73. Palkovits, M., Arimura, A., Brownstein, M. J., Schally, A. V., and Saavedra, J. M. (1974): Luteinizing hormone-releasing hormone (LH-RH) content of the hypothalamic nuclei in rat. *Endocrinology,* 96:554–558.
74. Palkovits, M., Brownstein, M., Arimura, A., Sato, H., Schally, A. V., and Kizer, J. S. (1976): Somatostatin content of the hypothalamic ventromedial and arcuate nuclei and the circumventricular organs in the rat. *Brain Res.,* 109:430–434.
75. Parry, H. B., and Livett, B. G. (1973): A new hypothalamic pathway to the median eminence containing neurophysin and its hypertrophy in sheep with natural scrapie. *Nature,* 242:63–65.
76. Pelletier, G., Labrie, F., Arimura, A., and Schally, A. V. (1974): Electron microscopic immunohistochemical localization of growth hormone-release inhibiting hormone (somatostatin) in the rat median eminence. *Am. J. Anat.,* 140:445–450.
77. Pelletier, G., Labrie, F., Puviani, R., Arimura, A., and Schally, A. V. (1974): Electron microscopic localization of luteinizing hormone-releasing hormone in rat median eminence. *Endocrinology,* 95:314–315.
78. Pelletier, G., LeClare, R., Dube, D., Labrie, F., Puviani, R., Arimura, A., and Schally, A. V. (1975): Localization of growth hormone-release inhibiting hormone (somatostatin) in the rat brain. *Am. J. Anat.,* 142:397–400.
79. Reichlin, S., Saperstein, R., Jackson, I. M. D., Boyd, A. E., III, and Patel, Y. (1976): Hypothalamic hormones. *Annu. Rev. Physiol.,* 38:389–429.
80. Robinson, A. G., and Zimmerman, E. A. (1973): Cerebrospinal fluid and ependymal neurophysin. *J. Clin. Invest.,* 52:1260–1267.
81. Scharrer, E., and Scharrer, B. (1954): Hormones produced by neurosecretory cells. *Recent Prog. Horm. Res.,* 10:183–240.
82. Sétáló, G. (1975): LH-RH-containing neural elements in the rat hypothalamus. *Endocrinology,* 96:135–142.
83. Sétáló, G. (1977): Anatomy, using new immunohistological techniques. In: *Endocrinology,* Vol. 1, edited by V. H. T. Janes, pp. 100–104. Excerpta Medica, Amsterdam.
84. Sétáló, G., Vigh, S., Schally, A. V., Arimura, A., and Flerko, B. (1975): LH-RH containing neural elements in the rat hypothalamus. *Endocrinology,* 96:135–142.
85. Sharp, P. J., Haase, E., and Fraser, H. M. (1975): Immunofluorescent localization of sites binding anti-synthetic LHRH serum in the median eminence of the greenfinch (Chloris chloris L). *Cell Tissue Res.,* 162:83–91.
86. Silverman, A. J. (1975): The hypothalamic magnocellular neurosecretory system of the guinea pig. I. Immunohistochemical localization of neurophysin in the adult. *Am. J. Anat.,* 144:433–444.
87. Swanson, L. W. (1977): Immunohistochemical evidence for a neurophysin-containing autonomic pathway arising in the paraventricular nucleus of the hypothalamus. *Brain Res.,* 128:346–353.
88. Vale, W., Ling, N., Rivier, C., Rivier, J., Villarreal, J., and Brown, M. (1976): Anatomic and phylogenetic distribution of somatostatin. *Metabolism,* 25:1491–1494.
89. Vale, W., Rivier, C., Palkovits, M., Saavedra, J. M., and Brownstein, M. J. (1974): Ubiquitous brain distribution of inhibitors of adenohypophyseal secretion. *Endocrinology,* 94:A128.
90. Vandesande, F., DeMey, J., and Dietrickx, K. (1974): Identification of neurophysin producing cells. I. The origin of the neurophysin-like substance-containing nerve fibers of the external region of the median eminence of the rat. *Cell Tissue Res.,* 151:187–200.
91. Vandesande, F., and Dietrickx, K. (1975): Identification of the vasopressin producing and of the oxytocin producing neurons in the hypothalamic magnocellular neurosecretory system of the rat. *Cell Tissue Res.,* 164:153–162.
92. Vandesande, F., Dietrickx, K., and DeMey, J. (1975): Identification of separate vasopressin-neurophysin II and oxytocin-neurophysin I containing nerve fibers in the external region of the bovine median eminence. *Cell Tissue Res.,* 158:509–516.
93. Van Dyke, H. B., Adamson, K., Jr., and Engel, S. L. (1957): The storage and liberation of neurohypophyseal hormones. In: *The Neurohypophysis,* edited by H. Heller, pp. 65–76. Academic Press, New York.

94. Watkins, W. B. (1973): Neurophysin and the neurosecretory fibers of the sheep infundibulum. *Z. Zellforsch. Mikrosk. Anat.,* 145:471–478.
95. Weindl, A., Sofroniev, M. V., and Sehinko, I. (1978): The distribution of vasopressin, oxytocin, neurophysin, somatostatin, and luteinizing hormone releasing hormone producing neurons. In: *Neurosecretion and neuroendocrine activity: evolution, structure, and function,* edited by W. Bargmann, A. Oksche, A. Polenov, and B. Scharrer, pp. 172–190. Springer, Heidelberg.
96. Weiner, R. I., Pattou, E., Kerdelhue, B., and Kordon, C. (1975): Differential effects of hypothalamic deafferentation upon luteinizing hormone-releasing hormone in the median eminence and organum vasculosum of the lamina terminalis. *Endocrinology,* 97:1597–1600.
97. Wheaton, J. E., Krulich, L., and McCann, S. M. (1975): Localization of luteinizing hormone-releasing hormone in the preoptic area and hypothalamus of the rat using radioimmunoassay. *Endocrinology,* 97:30–38.
98. Winokur, A., and Utiger, R. D. (1974): Thyrotropin-releasing hormone: Regional distribution in rat brain. *Science,* 185:265–267.
99. Youngblood, W. W., Lipton, M. A., and Kizer, J. S. (1978): TRH-like immunoreactivity in urine, serum, and extrahypothalamic brain: Non-identity with synthetic pyrogluhist-pro-(NH₂) (TRH). *Brain Res.,* 151:99–116.
100. Zimmerman, E. A., and Antunes, J. L. (1976): Organization of the hypothalamic pituitary system: Current concepts from immunohistochemical studies. *J. Histochem. Cytochem.,* 24:807–815.
101. Zimmerman, E. A., Antunes, J., Carmel, P. W., Defendini, R., and Ferin, M. (1976): Magnocellular neurosecretory pathways in the monkey: Immunohistochemical studies of the normal and lesioned hypothalamus using antibodies to oxytocin, vasopressin, and neurophysins. *Trans. Am. Neurol. Assoc.,* 101:16–19.
102. Zimmerman, E. A., Carmel, P. W., Husain, M. K., Ferin, M., Tannenbaum, M., Frantz, A. G., and Robinson, A. G. (1973): Vasopressin and neurophysin: High concentrations in monkey hypophyseal portal blood. *Science,* 182:925–927.
103. Zimmerman, E. A., Defendini, R., Sokol, H. W., and Robinson, A. G. (1975): The distribution of neurophysin-secreting pathways in the mammalian brain: Light microscopic studies using the immunoperoxidase technique. *Ann. NY Acad. Sci.,* 248:92–111.
104. Zimmerman, E. A., Hsu, K. C., Robinson, A. G., Carmel, P. W., Frantz, A. G., and Tannenbaum, M. (1973): Studies of neurophysin-secreting neurons with immunoperoxidase techniques employing antibody to neurophysin I. *Endocrinology,* 92:931–940.

The Endocrine Functions of the Brain,
edited by Marcella Motta.
Raven Press, New York © 1980

8

Localization of Active Peptides in the Brain

Georges Pelletier

Medical Research Council Group in Molecular Endocrinology, Le Centre Hospitalier de l'Université Laval, Quebec, Quebec G1V 4G2, Canada

It was demonstrated many years ago that some neurons had the characteristics of secretory cells (32). During the late 1940s and the 1950s, with the help of the Gomori staining technique, it was demonstrated that the large neurons of the supraoptic and paraventricular nuclei contained granular elements which were transported down to the posterior pituitary where they were stored (2,33). It was later established that the hypothalamic neurons are involved in the synthesis and release of two hormones, oxytocin and vasopressin. Since some magnocellular neurons of the hypothalamus were known to be able to secrete hormones, and since the influence of the hypothalamus on anterior pituitary secretion was well established, it was suggested that the activity of anterior pituitary function could be influenced by some factors produced by hypothalamic neurons and released into the pituitary portal blood vessels. The recent elucidation of the structures of two hypothalamic releasing hormones, thyrotropin releasing hormone (TRH) and luteinizing hormone releasing hormone (LHRH), and one release inhibiting hormone, somatostatin (1,5,7–9), and the production of specific antibodies against these hormones recently led to extensive studies on the morphology of the parvicellular systems. Using immunoelectron microscopic techniques, it has been shown that LHRH and somatostatin are stored within small secretory granules before being released into the capillaries of the portal vessels (23,25,27,28). This system thus appears to be similar to the magnocellular systems involved in the production of vasopressin and oxytocin.

During the past few years, an increasing number of peptides known to be produced in the pituitary gland—e.g., β-lipotropin (β-LPH), β-endorphin, adrenocorticotropin (ACTH), and α-melanocyte-stimulating hormone (α-MSH)—have been observed in the central nervous system (CNS) (13,16,17,37). Peptides of gastrointestinal origin have also been identified within the CNS (20,23). The physiological action of these peptides in the brain is still almost completely unknown. The immunohistochemical localization of the peptides at the light and electron microscopic levels can help clarify their role by giving information about their site of synthesis and their association with subcellular organelles.

IMMUNOCYTOCHEMICAL METHODS

In all our studies we used the sensitive immunoperoxidase technique developed by Sternberger (34) and involving the use of the peroxidase–antiperoxidase complex. Extensive work performed by Moriarty (21) on the ultrastructural localization of tropic hormones in the pituitary gland provided the methods and principles which are now applied for the localization of peptides in all the tissues, including the CNS. At the light microscope level, the localization studies were performed in consecutive thick (7 μm) paraffin sections. For the immunoelectron microscopic localization studies, positive regions previously identified by light microscopy were carefully dissected and embedded in Araldite. The PAP technique was then applied to the ultrathin sections (postembedding technique). The primary antisera were generally used at a dilution ranging from 1:500 to 1:4,000. All the immunohistochemical reactions were carefully controlled by immunoabsorption of the antiserum with the corresponding and related antigens. Detection of various peptides in consecutive sections was also used as a control of specificity.

LOCALIZATION OF α-MSH

α-MSH, a tridecapeptide known for its pigmentary effect on skin of lower vertebrates, plays a role in a variety of adaptive mechanisms in mammals, including man (10,12,31). Recently, α-MSH was detected by radioimmunoassay in all divisions of the rat brain with a higher concentration in the hypothalamus (22). With the help of immunocytochemistry and a specific antiserum to α-MSH (35), we were able to identify, for the first time, the structures associated with α-MSH in the rat brain (13,24). Nerve fibers containing α-MSH were observed throughout regions of the hypothalamus, thalamus, and midbrain (Fig. 1). Immunoreactive cell bodies were observed only in the arcuate nucleus of the hypothalamus. Essentially the same results were obtained in rats hypophysectomized 2 and 8 weeks previously, thus indicating the extrapituitary origin of brain α-MSH. Since deafferentation of the hypothalamus resulted in complete disappearance of the α-MSH fibers normally found in the extrahypothalamic regions, it was concluded that brain α-MSH is synthesized in neuronal cell bodies located in the arcuate nucleus. Using immunoelectron microscopy, it was possible to determine that immunostaining was restricted to dense-core vesicles (40 to 70 nm in diameter) in the positive nerve fibers or endings (Fig. 2) (24).

In the human hypothalamus, high concentration of nerve fibers staining for α-MSH were observed in the dorsal portion of the periventricular nucleus (11). As observed in the rat, positive neuronal cell bodies could be detected only in

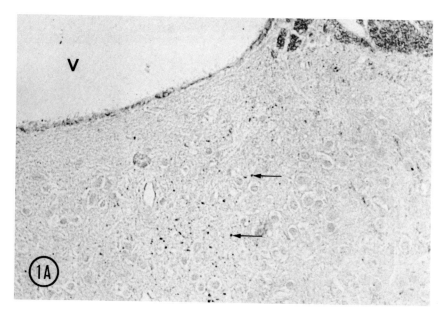

FIG. 1. A: Immunohistochemical detection of α-MSH in a coronal section through the rat thalamus. Immunostained fibers *(arrows)* are present in the paraventricular nucleus. (V) third ventricle. ×200.

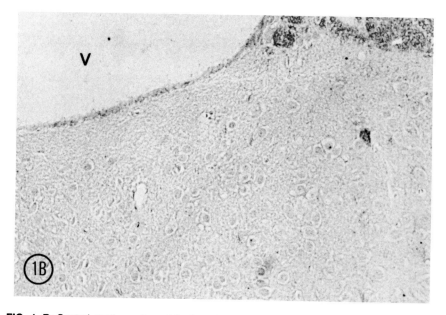

FIG. 1. B: Control section adjacent to that shown in **A.** Immunoabsorption with synthetic α-MSH has completely prevented staining. ×200.

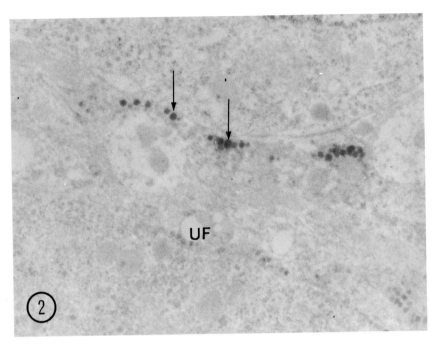

FIG. 2. Ultrastructural localization of α-MSH in the arcuate nucleus. A fiber containing immunoreactive dense-core vesicles *(arrows)* can be observed. Another fiber is unstained (UF). ×25,000.

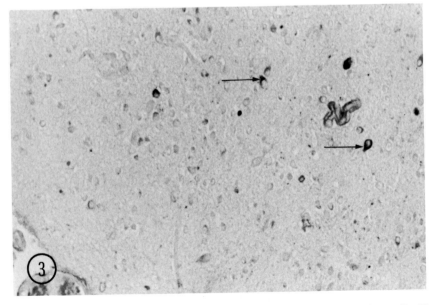

FIG. 3. Localization of α-MSH in a coronal section through the human hypothalamus. Positive cell bodies *(arrows)* are present in the arcuate nucleus. ×200.

the arcuate nucleus (also called the infundibular nucleus in man) (Fig. 3). Since no α-MSH could be detected in the human pituitary gland with the specific antiserum used, it is very likely that α-MSH does not originate from the pituitary but is synthesized in the neurons.

The production of α-MSH by hypothalamic neurons which are sending axons throughout the brain, as well as the presence of this peptide in dense vesicles strongly support the hypothesis that α-MSH could act as a neurotransmitter, the exact function of which remains to be established.

LOCALIZATION OF ACTH

As α-MSH, ACTH is another pituitary hormone which seems to exert some action in the CNS of mammals (12,31,36). Recently immunoreactive and bioreactive ACTH activities were found in the brain of normal and hypophysectomized rats, the highest concentration being in the hypothalamus (16). Using immunofluorescence and an antiserum against the COOH terminus of ACTH, Larsson (19) found ACTH immunoreactive fibers in many regions of the rat brain.

In order to clearly identify the nervous structures containing ACTH, we performed an immunohistochemical study on this peptide using antibodies

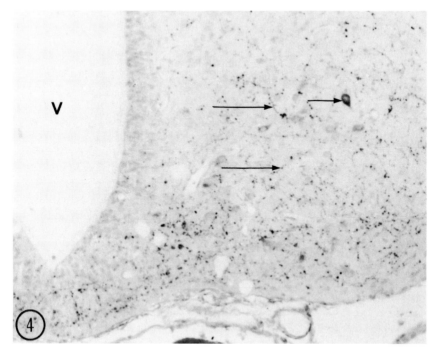

FIG. 4. Localization of ACTH in a coronal section through the rat mediobasal hypothalamus. Immunostained cell bodies *(short arrow)* and fibers *(long arrows)* can be observed in the arcuate nucleus. (V) third ventricle. ×200.

TABLE 1. *ACTH immunoreactivity in different areas of the rat brain*

Area	Immunoreactivity[a]
Telencephalon and diencephalon	
Nucleus lateralis of the septum	++
Nucleus proprius of the stria terminalis	++++
Amygdala	++
Median preoptic area	+++
Anterior hypothalamus	+++
Nucleus periventricularis	++++
Nucleus paraventricularis hypothalamus	++++
Arcuate nucleus and periarcuate area	++++ (cells)
Nucleus ventromedialis	+
Nucleus dorsomedialis	+++
Lateral hypothalamus	+++
Posterior hypothalamus	+++
Nucleus paraventricularis thalamus	++++
Posterior thalamus	++
Mesencephalon	
Periaqueductal grey	++++
Nucleus parabrachialis	++++
Reticular formation	++
Substantia nigra	+
Metencephalon and myelencephalon	
Periventricular grey	++
Nucleus lateralis parabrachialis	++
Nucleus reticularis	+
Spinal nucleus of the trigeminal nerve	+
Spinal cord	+

[a] The intensity of the reaction was graded from + to ++++ according to the concentration of immunostained fibers.

against the NH_2 and COOH termini of this molecule (23,29). Identical localizations were obtained with the two antisera. In the rat brain, immunoreactive nerve fibers were found to be largely distributed throughout regions of the hypothalamus, thalamus, and midbrain (Fig. 4). Semiquantitative evaluation of the concentration of ACTH fibers in various areas of the rat brain is listed in Table 1. Positive fibers are also occasionally observed in the spinal cord. Immunostained neuronal cell bodies could be detected only in the arcuate nucleus and in areas just lateral to that nucleus. As previously demonstrated for α-MSH, hypophysectomy had no effect on the immunostaining for ACTH, indicating that ACTH observed in the brain is not of pituitary origin.

In animals pretreated with colchicine, the intensity in the staining of cell bodies was markedly increased, whereas the concentration of positive fibers throughout the brain was concomitantly decreased. With this treatment, it was not possible to detect ACTH cell bodies outside the hypothalamus. In animals

FIG. 5. Ultrastructural localization of ACTH in the rat arcuate nucleus. Positive dense-core vesicles *(arrows)* are found in a neuronal cell body (N) nucleus. ×28,000.

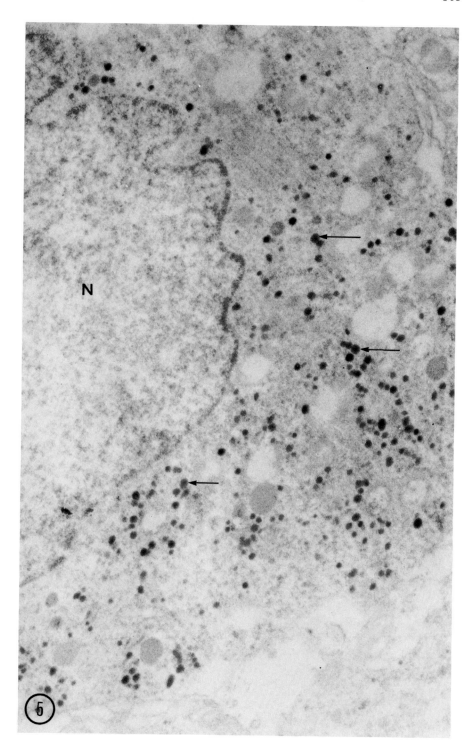

bearing a hypothalamic deafferentation, no ACTH fibers could be detected in the extrahypothalamic areas, whereas normal immunoreactivity was retained in the isolated hypothalamus. In adult rats that had been injected during the neonatal period with monosodium glutamate, immunostaining for ACTH was almost completely abolished in all brain areas. Since this treatment destroys the arcuate nucleus, and since deafferentation produces a disappearance of extrahypothalamic fibers, it must be concluded that ACTH in the regions of the brain is produced by neuronal cell bodies located in the arcuate nucleus.

At the ultrastructural level, the immunostained structures found in the arcuate nucleus were nerve fibers and neuronal cell bodies. In the fibers, specific staining was mostly observed in the dense-core vesicles. The diameter of these ACTH vesicles ranged between 60 and 80 nm. In the immunostained cell bodies, the reaction product was also localized in dense-core vesicles of similar sizes distributed throughout the cytoplasm (Fig. 5). These ultrastructural studies indicate that ACTH is synthesized and stored within dense-core vesicles in the cell body of the ACTH neuron before being transported along the axon. The presence of ACTH in dense-core vesicles support the hypothesis that ACTH could be considered a neurohormone or neuromodulator.

LOCALIZATION OF β-LPH AND ENDORPHINS

β-LPH, which is probably the precursor of endorphins (6), has been detected by radioimmunoassay in bovine CNS (4,17,18). Immunoreactive β-LPH has also been localized by immunofluorescence in axons of many areas of the rat brain (37). Using an antiserum to human β-LPH, we investigated the morphological localization of this peptide in the brain of normal and hypophysectomized rats (23,29). The distribution of immunoreactive β-LPH was in fact found to be identical to that of ACTH, although the immunoreaction for β-LPH was generally weaker than that for ACTH (Figs. 6 and 7). In the human hypothalamus, immunostained neuronal cell bodies were observed in the arcuate nucleus, whereas β-LPH-positive nerve fibers could be detected in a large area of the periventricular nucleus (26). Immunoelectron microscopic localization of β-LPH indicated that, in cell bodies and fibers, immunostaining could be detected only in dense-core vesicles similar to those containing ACTH (Fig. 8). Since in the pituitary gland from several species β-LPH and ACTH have been localized not only in the same cells but also in the same granules (30), it seemed important to determine if these two peptides were also present in the same neurons. Immunostaining of consecutive ultrathin sections through the rat arcuate nucleus

---

FIG. 6. A: Localization of β-LPH in a coronal section through the rat mediobasal hypothalamus. Immunostained cell bodies *(short arrows)* and fibers *(long arrows)* are located in the arcuate nucleus. (V) third ventricle. ×200. **Inset** ×500. **B:** Control section adjacent to that shown in **A.** Immunoabsorption with an excess of purified human β-LPH has completely prevented staining. ×200.

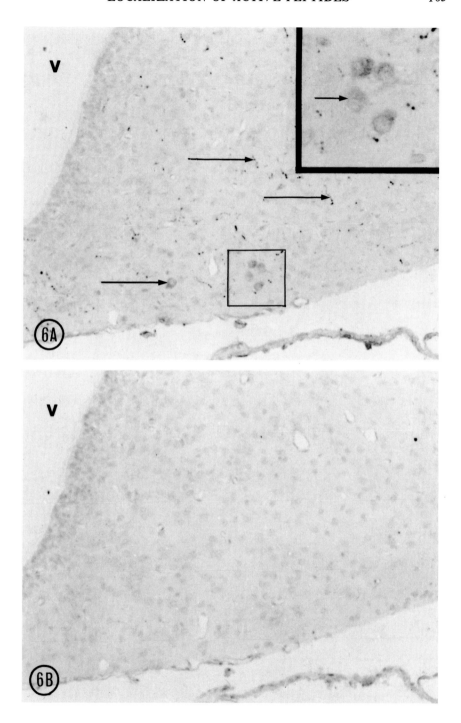

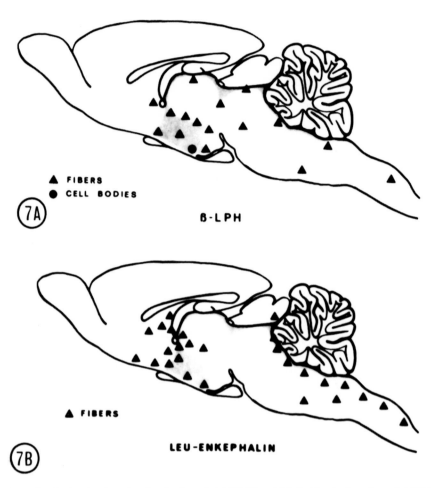

FIG. 7. Rat brain showing the distribution of β-LPH **(A)**, which is identical to that of ACTH, and leu-enkephalin **(B).**

recently established that ACTH and β-LPH are stored in the same dense-core vesicles in both perikarya and fibers (Pelletier, *in preparation*).

Whereas β-LPH has no activity when injected into the brain, there is now convincing evidence that endorphins are involved at the level of the CNS not only as analgesics and modulators of behavior but also in the control of neuroendocrine secretion (3,6,14,15).

The presence of β-endorphin has also been described in the CNS (4,17,18). In preliminary experiments involving use of antibodies to γ-endorphin, which show a very low cross reactivity with β-LPH, it was possible to demonstrate that the pattern of distribution of positive fibers is similar to that of β-LPH

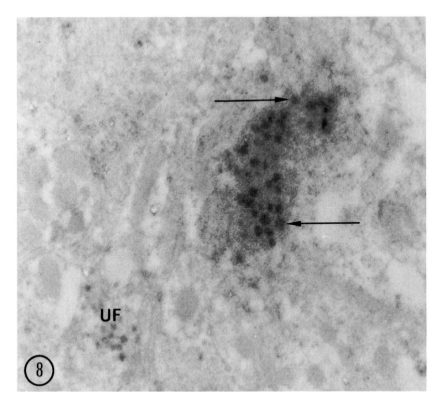

FIG. 8. Ultrastructural localization of β-LPH in the rat hypothalamic periventricular nucleus. A nerve fiber containing positive dense-core vesicles *(arrows)* is present. An unstained fiber (UF) can also be observed in the same section. ×34,000.

and ACTH (Pelletier et al., *in preparation*). Since endorphins were not detected in cell bodies, it is tempting to speculate that the cleavage of β-LPH into endorphins could occur in the axons.

LOCALIZATION OF ENKEPHALINS

After the discovery in the brain of two opioid pentapeptides, leucine-enkephalin (leu-enkephalin) and methionine-enkephalin (met-enkephalin), it was hypothesized that the biosynthetic pathway for met-enkephalin might be: β-LPH → β-endorphin → met-enkephalin. On the other hand, the relation of leu-enkephalin with β-LPH, endorphins, and met-enkephalin has not yet been studied. Recent immunohistochemical data (4) seem to indicate that there are two opiate peptide neuronal systems: the met-enkephalin system and the β-LPH–endorphins system.

In an attempt to clarify the relation between leu-enkephalin, met-enkephalin,

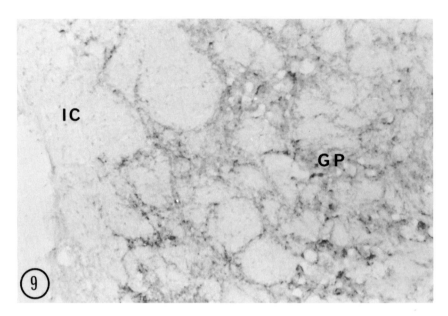

FIG. 9. Localization of leu-enkephalin in the rat striatum. A strong reaction is found in the globus pallidus (GP), whereas the internal capsule (IC) is completely unstained. ×150.

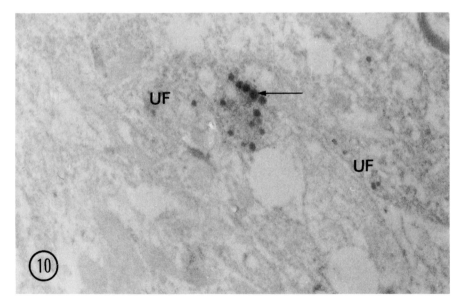

FIG. 10. Ultrastructural localization of leu-enkephalin in the globus pallidus. The immunostaining is localized in dense-core vesicles *(arrow)* of nerve fibers. (UF) unstained fibers. ×22,500.

and the β-LPH–endorphins systems, we performed an immunohistochemical localization of leu-enkephalin with the help of a specific antiserum to leu-en-kephalin (29). The distribution of leu-enkephalin appeared to be similar to that already reported for met-enkephalin (Figs. 7 and 9). At the electron microscopic level, specific immunostaining was observed in the globus pallidus, nucleus para-brachialis, and substantia gelatinosa. In these three regions, a positive reaction was found in the dense-core vesicles of the nerve fibers of endings (Fig. 10). The diameter of the vesicles positive for leu-enkephalin ranged between 70 and 100 nm. These ultrastructural data, similar to those obtained for the other peptides (e.g., α-MSH, ACTH, β-LPH, and substance P), suggest that leu-enkephalin could act as a neurohormone or neuromodulator.

SUMMARY AND CONCLUSION

During the last few years, the application of immunohistochemical techniques for the localization of neuropeptides of biological importance has produced interesting observations leading to some generalizations. It now appears that four peptides—α-MSH, ACTH, β-LPH, and β-endorphin—first discovered in the pituitary gland and now investigated for their effects on the CNS, are present in large amounts in the hypothalamus. Since the neuronal cell bodies containing these peptides, which are distributed in many brain areas, are located in the arcuate nucleus of the hypothalamus, it is tempting to speculate that this hypoth-alamic nucleus could play a key role in the modulation of some functions of the CNS. It seems also well established that the enkephalin system and the β-LPH–ACTH–endorphin system are contained within separate neuronal systems. Our recent immunoelectron microscopic observations clearly indicate that all the neuropeptides so far studied are localized within dense-core vesicles in both neuronal cell bodies and axons. In fact, these systems appear similar to the classical neurosecretory systems involved in the secretion of vasopressin and oxytocin. It may be suggested that these peptides act as local neurohormones and then should belong to a category of biologically active substances distinct from the classical neurotransmitters.

ACKNOWLEDGMENTS

The author is grateful to Dr. M. J. Brownstein who performed hypothalamic deafferentation procedures and to Dr. J. M. Saavedra who supplied the gluta-mate-injected rats. Dr. C. H. Li supplied the antiserum to human β-LPH. Dr. H. Vaudry supplied the antibodies to γ-endorphin. Dr. H. Miller supplied the specific antiserum to leu-enkephalin.

REFERENCES

1. Baba, Y., Matsuo, H., and Schally, A. V. (1971): Structure of the porcine LH- and FSH-releasing hormone. II. Confirmation of the proposed structure by conventional sequential analyses. *Biochem. Biophys. Res. Commun.*, 44:459–467.

2. Bargmann, W. (1954): *Das Zwischenhim Hypophysensystem.* Springer-Verlag, Berlin.
3. Bloom, F., Segal, D., Ling, N., and Guillemin, R. (1976) Endorphins: Profound behavioral effects in rats suggest new etiological factors in mental illness. *Science,* 194:630–632.
4. Bloom, F., Battenberg, E., Rossier, J., Ling, N., and Guillemin, R. (1978): Neurons containing β-endorphin in rat brain exist separately from those containing enkephalin: Immunocytochemical studies. *Proc. Natl. Acad. Sci. USA,* 75:1591–1595.
5. Boler, J., Enzman, F., Folkers, K., Bowers, C. Y., and Schally, A. V. (1969): The identity of chemical and hormonal properties of the thyrotropin-releasing hormone and pyroglutamyl-histidyl proline amide. *Biochem. Biophys. Res. Commun.,* 37:705–710.
6. Bradbury, A. F., Smyth, D. G., and Snell, C. R. (1976): Lipotropin: Precursor to two biologically active peptides. *Biochem. Biophys. Res. Commun.,* 69:950–956.
7. Brazeau, P., Vale, W., Burgus, R., Ling, N., Butcher, M., Rivier, J., and Guillemin, R. (1973): Hypothalamic polypeptide that inhibits the secretion of immunoreactive pituitary growth hormone. *Science,* 179:77–79.
8. Burgus, R., Butcher, M., Ling, N., Monahan, M., Rivier, J., Fellows, R., Amoss, M., Blackwell, R., Vale, W., and Guillemin, R. (1971): Structure moléculaire du facteur hypothalamique (LRF) d'origine ovine contrôlant la sécrétion de l'hormone gonadotrope hypophysaire de lutéinisation. *C R Acad. Sci [D] (Paris),* 273:1611–1613.
9. Burgus, R., Dunn, T. F., Desiderio, D., and Guillemin, R. (1969): Structure moléculaire du facteur hypothalamique TRF d'origine ovine: Mise en évidence par spectrométrie de masse de la séquence PCA-His-Pro-NH². *C R Acad. Sci. [D] (Paris),* 269:1870–1873.
10. Dattu, P. C., and King, M. G. (1977): Effects of melanocyte-stimulating hormone (MSH) and melatonin on passive avoidance and on an emotional response. *Biochem. Behav.,* 6:449–452.
11. Désy, L., and Pelletier, G. (1973): Immunohistochemical localization of α-melanocyte-stimulating hormone (α-MSH) in the human hypothalamus. *Brain Res.,* 154:377–381.
12. De Wied, D., and Gispen, W. H. (1976): Behavioral effects of peptides. In: *Peptides in Neurobiology,* edited by H. Gainer, pp. 397–448. Plenum Press, New York.
13. Dubé, D., Lissitsky, J. C., Leclerc, R., and Pelletier, G. (1978): Localization of α-melanocyte-stimulating hormone in the rat brain and pituitary. *Endocrinology,* 102:1283–1291.
14. Dupont, A., Cusan, L., Labrie, F., Coy, D. H., and Li, C. H. (1976): Stimulation of prolactin release in the rat by intraventricular injection of β-endorphin and methionine-enkephalin. *Biochem. Biophys. Res. Commun.,* 75:76–82.
15. Jacquet, Y. F., and Marks, N. (1976): The C-fragment of β-lipotropin: An endogenous neuroleptic or anti-psychotogen. *Science,* 194:632–635.
16. Krieger, D. T., Liotta, A., and Brownstein, M. J. (1977): Presence of corticotropin in brain of normal and hypophysectomized rats. *Proc. Natl. Acad. Sci. USA,* 74:648–652.
17. Krieger, D. T., Liotta, A., Sudo, T., Palkovits, M., and Brownstein, M. J. (1977): Presence of immunoassayable β-lipotropin in bovine brain and spinal cord: Lack of concordance with ACTH concentrations. *Biochem. Biophys. Res. Commun.,* 76:930–936.
18. Labella, F., Queen, G., and Senyshyn, J. (1977): Lipotropin: Localization by radioimmunoassay of endorphin precursor in pituitary and brain. *Biochem. Biophys. Res. Commun.,* 75:350–352.
19. Larsson, L. I. (1977): Corticotropin-like peptides in central nerves and in endocrine cells of gut and pancreas. Lancet, 2:1321–1323.
20. Leeman, S. E., Mroz, E. A., and Carraway, R. E. (1977): Substance P and neurotensin. In: *Peptides in Neurobiology,* edited by H. Gainer, pp. 99–144. Plenum Press, New York.
21. Moriarty, G. C. (1973): Adenohypophysis: Ultrastructural cytochemistry: A review. *J. Histochem. Cytochem.,* 21:855–894.
22. Oliver, C., Barnea, A., Usategui, R., Mical, R. S., and Porter, J. C. (1976): Localisation et sécrétion de l'α-MSH chez le rat. In: Inserm Report No. 7, pp. 49–53. Inserm, Paris.
23. Pelletier, G. (1979): Immunohistochemical localization of hypothalamic hormones and other peptides in the central nervous system. In: *Central Nervous System: Effects of Hypothalamic Hormones and Other Peptides,* edited by R. Collu, A. Barbeau, T. R. Ducharme and J. G. Rochefort, pp. 331–344. Raven Press, New York.
24. Pelletier, G., and Dubé, D. (1977): Electron microscopic immunohistochemical localization of α-MSH in the rat brain. *Am. J. Anat.,* 150:201–205.
25. Pelletier, G., Dubé, D., and Puviani, R. (1977): Somatostatin: Electron microscope immunohistochemical localization in secretory neurons of rat hypothalamus. *Science,* 196:1469–1470.

26. Pelletier, G., Désy, L., Lissitszky, J. C., Labrie, F., and Li, C. H. (1978): Immunohistochemical localization of β-LPH in the human hypothalamus. *Life Sci.* 22:1799–1804.
27. Pelletier, G., Labrie, F., Arimura, A., and Schally, A. V. (1974): Electron microscopic immunohistochemical localization of growth hormone release inhibiting hormone (somatostatin) in the rat median eminence. *Am. J. Anat.,* 140:445–450.
28. Pelletier, G., Labrie, F., Puviani, R., Arimura, A., and Schally, A. V. (1974): Immunohistochemical localization of luteinizing hormone-releasing hormone in the rat median eminence. *Endocrinology,* 95:314–317.
29. Pelletier, G., Leclerc, R., and Dubé, D. (1979): Morphological basis of neuroendocrine functions in the hypothalamus. In: *Clinical Neuroendocrinology,* edited by G. Tolis and F. Labrie. Raven Press, New York *(in press).*
30. Pelletier, G., Leclerc, R., Labrie, F., Côté, J., Chretien, M., and Lis, M. (1977): Immunohistochemical localization of β-lipotropic hormone in the pituitary gland. *Endocrinology,* 100:770–776.
31. Sandman, C. A., George, J., McCanne, T. R., Nolan, J. P., Kaswan, J., and Kastin, A. J. (1977): MSH/ACTH[4-10] influences: Behavioral and physiological measures of attention. *J. Clin. Endocrinol. Metab.,* 44:884–891.
32. Scharrer, E. (1928): Die Lichtempfindlichkert blinder Elutzen I. Untersuchungen ùler das Zwischenhun der Fische. *Z. Vergluch. Physiol.,* 7:1–38.
33. Scharer, E., and Scharrer, B. (1954): Hormones produced by neurosecretory cells. *Recent Prog. Horm. Res.,* 10:183–240.
34. Sternberger, L. A. (1974): *Immunocytochemistry.* Prentice-Hall, Englewood Cliffs, N.J.
35. Usategui, R., Oliver, C., Vaudry, H., Lombardi, G., Rozenberg, I., and Mourne, A. M. (1976): Immunoreactive α-MSH and ACTH levels in rat plasma and pituitary. *Endocrinology,* 98:189–196.
36. Van Riezen, H., Rigter, H., and De Wied, D. (1977): Possible significance of ACTH fragments for human mental performance. *Behav. Biol.,* 20:311–324.
37. Watson, S. J., Barchas, J. P., and Li, C. H. (1977): β-Lipotropin: Localization of cells and axons in rat brain by immunocytochemistry. *Proc. Natl. Acad. Sci. USA,* 74:5155–5158.

The Endocrine Functions of the Brain,
edited by Marcella Motta.
Raven Press, New York © 1980

9

Cellular Biochemistry of Brain Peptides: Biosynthesis, Degradation, Packaging, Transport, and Release

Jeffrey F. McKelvy, Jean-Louis Charli*, Patricia Joseph-Bravo*, Thomas Sherman, and Catherine Loudes

Neuroendocrine Program, Departments of Psychiatry and Biochemistry, University of Pittsburgh School of Medicine, Western Psychiatric Institute and Clinic, Pittsburgh, Pennsylvania 15261

This volume seeks to examine the endocrine functions of the brain, a topic which can now be viewed in two ways: (a) from a "classical" neuroendocrinological view, more or less consistent with long-held views on brain–endocrine interactions, in which an increasingly detailed understanding of the hypothalamic modulation of adenohypophysial secretory activity is emerging from studies utilizing chemically defined hypophysiotropic substances; and (b) from a contemporary view, characterized by a great deal of uncertainty, in which a body of information is accumulating which implies a much closer relationship between peptide-secreting cells found in diverse tissues than has heretofore been appreciated. As part of this contemporary view, it is necessary to consider the meaning of delivery of adenohypophysial hormones to the brain due to bidirectional flow in the hypophysial portal system (108); the possible biosynthesis of pituitary hormones [e.g., growth hormone (110) and ACTH (72)] and gastrointestinal hormones (e.g., cholecystokinin) by neurons in the brain; and the possible existence of common precursor polypeptides for a diversity of hormonal substances (75) which precursors may be processed differently by neural and endocrine tissue. It is clear that an understanding of the endocrine function of the brain requires biochemical information in the form of knowledge of sites of hormone biosynthesis in the central nervous system (CNS) and endocrine systems, specific cleavage sites in polypeptide chains, the properties of enzymes catalyzing the hydrolysis of peptide bonds in high- and low-molecular-weight peptides, and the interaction

* Present address: Inst. Invest. Biomedicas, Universidad Nacional Autonoma de Mexico, Mexico City, Mexico.

of peptides with plasma and cell organellar membranes. With this view in mind, we reviewed the literature on the biochemical studies of brain peptides. It must be stated that this review is not encyclopedic; rather, we discuss existing data in terms of our views on important biochemical problems related to the endocrine function of the brain.

BIOSYNTHESIS OF BRAIN PEPTIDES

Studies on the biosynthesis of brain peptides are of potential importance to understanding the points of regulation of a physiological process in which cells secreting a given peptide participate. Thus if a functional demand is placed on a given peptide-secreting neuronal subsystem, stimulation of the cells could be reflected in a primary stimulation of peptide biosynthesis, and the system would return to the steady state by the operation of regulatory elements exerted at the level of the biosynthetic process. Other models, however, could of course be visualized in which primary stimulatory and regulatory responses were elicited at the level of the secretion process, with alterations in the rate of peptide biosynthesis reflecting only a compensatory restoration of a (large) store of peptide. A significant difference between these two possibilities is that primary regulation at the level of biosynthesis could operate via direct stimulation or inhibition of gene action. This would implicate action at the level of the genetic mechanism in the immediate operation of the nervous system, a feature which would have profound implications for basic and clinical research in neurobiology. Thus it is necessary to characterize the biosynthetic process.

Another point can now be made with regard to the importance of peptide biosynthetic studies in the nervous system—that such studies comprise the most definitive evidence for the existence of "peptidergic" neurons in any locus. This is a consideration of importance currently because of the wide tissue distribution observed for "brain" and "gut" peptides and because of the reported presence of pituitary hormones such as prolactin (34), α-MSH (27), growth hormone (110), and ACTH (67) in mammalian brain. When interpreting these data, the following additional observations must be kept in mind: Bidirectional flow of pituitary hormones in the hypophysial portal system has been reported to occur (108), and labeled ACTH injected into the pituitary was found to be able to migrate into a number of brain regions (90); stimulation of secretion from neural lobes incubated *in vitro* can be accompanied by the incorporation of markers for the extracellular space into neurosecretory neurons by reverse exocytosis (94). These observations, coupled with the uncertainty of antibody cross reactivity which attends the use of immunocytochemical and radioimmunoassay methods, lend great importance to the application of biosynthetic studies to localize sites of elaboration of biologically active peptides. An ultimate example of the application of a biosynthetic approach is afforded by studies carried out by Agarwal and co-workers (102), who employed oligodeoxynucleotide probes to isolate specific messenger RNAs (mRNA) for gastrin and cholecystokinin, both of which were reported to be present in the gut and the brain. These workers found that gastrin mRNA was present in gut but not in brain, whereas cholecystokinin mRNA was present in both tissues. The sensitivity of the mRNA isolation method is sufficient to have detected the reported levels of gastrin found in brain. It is clear that further application of molecular biological methods to studies on brain peptides will yield much valuable information.

In the sections to follow, the extant experimental evidence regarding the biosynthesis of biologically active peptides of defined structure found in the vertebrate CNS are reviewed.

Biosynthesis of Neurohypophysial Hormones and Neurophysins

The studies of Sachs and co-workers carried out during the 1960s and early 1970s (124,125) represent the first biochemical investigations of brain neuropeptide biosynthesis and, in fact, still constitute the most rigorous body of biochemical work on neurohypophysial hormone biosynthesis. In these pioneering studies, Sachs provided a biochemical basis for the firm establishment of the model of neurosecretion of the posterior pituitary principles proposed by Bargmann and Scharrer (6), and in addition made a novel finding on a basic aspect of protein biosynthesis, i.e., the existence of a precursor form (125) for a secreted peptide. Sachs' chief contributions were to: (a) demonstrate that biosynthetic studies on vasopressin required the application of extensive purification procedures in order to be able to isolate radiochemically pure peptide, a finding of great importance to contemporary studies on the biosynthesis of biologically active peptides in neural tissue; (b) demonstrate that vasopressin was synthesized only when the somata of magnocellular neurosecretory neurons were present, and show the subcellular distribution of newly synthesized neurohypophysial principles; and (c) establish a close relationship between the biosynthesis of vasopressin and neurophysin and propose that they shared a common biosynthetic precursor. This was a novel idea at the time of its enunciation, and it has come to assume a central position in present-day studies on protein and peptide biosynthesis. Although Sachs' studies (124,125) contributed much to an elucidation of the cellular biochemistry of neurosecretion, they dealt less completely with aspects of the regulation of neurohypophysial hormones and neurophysin biosynthesis. Although the rate of vasopressin labeling was shown to be increased by osmotic stimulation (124), it was not demonstrated that this was due to increased *de novo* biosynthesis. In other studies carried out on organ-cultured guinea pig mediobasal hypothalamus, inhibition of RNA synthesis resulted in a progressive decline in vasopressin biosynthesis, with a half-time of approximately 28 hr (112). It was suggested that this was the approximate half-life of mRNA for vasopressin, and that transcriptional control was exerted on hormone biosynthesis. However, and as acknowledged by the authors, this half-time is actually a resultant time for the restitution of a number of RNA species directly or indirectly involved in vasopressin biosynthesis. Thus although the suggestion of transcriptional control of vasopressin biosynthesis is a stimulating one, it has not yet been critically demonstrated, and the question of the nature of the regulation of neurohypophysial hormone biosynthesis is an open one.

Recently a welcome addition to Sachs' work (124,125) has come in the form of studies aimed at directly identifying precursors to neurohypophysial hormones and neurophysins. This is an important avenue of exploration since it offers the possibility of defining the biosynthetic relationships between the neurohypophysial hormones and the neurophysins.

Mendelson and Walter (89) carried out *in vitro* labeling experiments with [35S]L-methionine on blocks of guinea pig mediobasal hypothalamus, and used 13.7% acid–urea polyacrylamide gel electrophoresis to examine labeled proteins formed in short-term incubates. They observed [35S]-labeled species which migrated in the acid-urea gels with mobilities corresponding to those of vasopressin and neurophysin as well as proteins of intermediate electrophoretic mobility. Water deprivation of animals prior to *in vitro* incubation, addition of inhibitors of cytoribosomal protein synthesis, use of a pulse-chase paradigm, use of an inhibitor of proteolysis, and observation of cross reactivity with nonspecific antibodies to rat neurophysin led these authors (89) to conclude that labeled species of intermediate electrophoretic mobility, and of molecular weights 13,700 and 28,000, gave rise to labeled neurophysin and vasopressin. Other studies from this laboratory (137) were carried out in the dog by *in vivo* ventricular perfusion and *in vitro* hypothalamic incubation under conditions which precluded *de novo* peptide bond synthesis. Under these conditions, there was a greater amount of labeled neurophysin-like proteins and labeled vasopressin in *in vitro* incubated tissue, suggesting that after the incorporation of isotope *in vivo* processing events occurred *in vitro*.

Other studies on neurophysin biosynthesis, directed at the identification of biosynthetic precursors, were carried out in the rat by Gainer and co-workers (20,35,36). In initial experiments (35) they injected [35S]L-cysteine adjacent to the supraoptic nucleus and, as a function of time after injection, sampled supraoptic nucleus, median eminence, and neural lobe using the Palkovits punch technique for radioactive proteins as assayed by acid-urea polyacrylamide gel electrophoresis. They observed rapid incorporation into a 20,000 molecular weight species and a progressive decline in the radioactivity in this species concomitant with the appearance of a labeled species of molecular weight 12,000 which had neurophysin-like properties. In subsequent work (20,36), more detailed electrophoretic analysis, examination of the diabetes insipidus rat, and use of immunoprecipitation using a nonspecific anti-rat neurophysin antibody revealed the following: (a) A labeled "precursor species" in the supraoptic nucleus exists in a 20,000 molecular weight pI 6.1 form for the vasopressin neurophysin and a 20,000 molecular weight and pI 5.4 form for oxytocin neurophysin, whereas labeled species of "intermediate" kinetic character exist in the form of 17,000 molecular weight and pI 5.1 for the oxytocin neurophysin and pI 5.6 for the vasopressin neurophysin, and labeled "product" species exist in the form of

12,000 molecular weight and pIs 4.6 and 4.8 for the oxytocin and vasopressin neurophysins, respectively. (b) The putative precursors and intermediates bound anti-rat neurophysin antibodies. (c) K^+ stimulated release from *in vitro* incubated neural lobes containing [^{35}S]L-cysteine-labeled species synthesized *in vivo* revealed that neurophysins and several other labeled species were released in a Ca^{2+}-dependent manner. Thus these studies represent the groundwork for the demonstration of a precursor molecule in neurohypophysial hormone biosynthesis.

Recent studies from our own laboratory directed at identifying neurohypophysial precursor molecules were carried out in cell-free mRNA translation systems (87). We found that the primary translation product from rat and mouse hypothalamic mRNA recognized by anti-rat neurophysin and antivasopressin antisera has a molecular weight of approximately 18,000. This is in good agreement with the *in vivo* observations of Gainer and colleagues (20,35,36). Much further work remains to be done; however, the direct demonstration of separate precursor molecules for vasopressin and oxytocin must be attempted at the level of cell-free translation, and the primary sequences of putative precursor molecules must be established. With this kind of background information, many interesting questions could then be addressed: the fate and possible roles of the "rest of" the precursor molecule, the biochemical nature of the processing steps occurring in the neurosecretory granules (e.g., are these reactions subject to metabolic regulation?), and whether transcriptional or translational control is exerted on the biosynthesis of the precursor. Answers to at least some of these questions should be forthcoming in the next 1 or 2 years.

Biosynthesis of Hypothalamic Releasing Hormones

After 8 years of effort, relatively little is known about hypothalamic releasing hormone biosynthesis. On the other hand, we now have a full appreciation of the considerable technical problems which have held up progress in this most important area. Moreover, during the past year we have seen the emergence of new tools with which to handle these problems, so that an acceleration of progress can be expected.

The pioneering work of Reichlin and his collaborators (92) initiated studies on hypothalamic releasing hormone biosynthesis in 1971. In these studies fragments of rat hypothalamus were incubated in Krebs–Ringer–bicarbonate-buffered medium in the presence of radioactive amino acid precursors. Methanolic extracts of the tissue were subjected, individually, to such separation systems as thin-layer chromatography, electrophoresis, carboxymethylcellulose chromatography, and gel filtration, where a radioactive species whose mobility corresponded to that of synthetic thyrotropin releasing hormone (TRH) could be observed. Also in 1971, Guillemin (43) reported on the ability of rat hypothalamic tissue to incorporate [^{3}H]L-proline into a compound with the chromatographic properties of TRH in a cycloheximide-insensitive process. Subsequent work from Reichlin's laboratory (93) proposed modes of regulating TRH biosynthesis by monoamines and thyroid hormones, and set forth a claim for a "TRH synthe-tase," a soluble, enzymatic RNA-independent system for the biosynthesis of the tripeptide. For the most part, these studies were based on a simple purification methodology, e.g., using [^{14}C]L-proline as a precursor, terminating the reaction by addition of methanol followed by cellulose acetate electrophoresis of the methanolic supernatant with or without prior charcoal treatment of samples.

In 1974 we reported our experience with isotope studies of TRH biosynthesis and described the multiplicity of labeled peptide species formed after incubation of guinea pig hypothalamic organ cultures with [^{3}H]L-proline (84). In the guinea pig system, for example, a multistep sequential purification scheme was required to achieve adequate radiochemical purity of labeled TRH. During the course of the purification, 99.97 to 99.98% of the crude homogenate radioactivity had to be eliminated. These studies demonstrated several important features of the investigation of TRH biosynthesis: (a) Sequential purification is mandatory in labeling experiments in order to remove radioactive species (derived from precursor [^{3}H]L-proline and from the metabolizing tissue) whose mobility matches that of standard synthetic TRH in many separation systems. (b) A multistep purification procedure must be used, emphasizing high performance liquid chromatography and requiring the use of carrier synthetic TRH and purification to a point of constant specific activity (counts per minute per unit of biological or immunological activity). (c) The putative pure biosynthetically derived TRH of constant specific activity must be further tested for purity by derivatization, with evidence provided for the coincidence of chromatographic properties of the biosynthetic derivative with those of derivatives prepared from synthetic TRH. Appropriate derivatives can be prepared by dinitrophenylation and its reversal by thiolysis, butanolysis, and enzymatic deamidation (85).

It has been generally concluded that the simple purification methodology used in the earliest studies of TRH biosynthesis rendered the subjects of these studies open to reinvestigation. Our studies, utilizing the above-mentioned approach to releasing hormone biosynthetic studies, showed that in rat hypothalamic homogenates the biosynthesis of TRH and luteinizing hormone releasing hormone (LHRH) is diminished when inhibitors of ribosomal protein synthesis are present (87). This implies the likely derivation of these small peptides from a higher-molecular-weight precursor. Attempts are currently being made to isolate such precursors.

Several reports are in the literature on the biosynthesis of LHRH. These studies, however, have not utilized rigorous purification methodologies and so, as discussed above, cannot be adequately evaluated.

Biosynthesis of ACTH-Related Peptides

Several peptides and proteins related to ACTH and found in the pituitary have been detected in brain by radioimmunoassay, bioassay, or both. These include 31K ACTH (big ACTH, the presumed common precursor for ACTH and β-lipotropin, or pro-opiocortin), ACTH, α-MSH, β-lipotropin (β-LPH), and β-endorphin (72). Met- and leu-enkephalins, originally isolated from brain, are either low in or absent from the pituitary. These pentapeptides have been reported to be synthesized *de novo* in the myenteric plexus (130) and in cultured mouse spinal cord cells (87) by a ribosomal mechanism. Because, as mentioned before, it has been claimed that bidirectional flow may occur in the hypophysial portal system, it is possible that the presence in brain of ACTH-related peptides other than the enkephalins is due to their delivery to this site by the portal system. However, recent studies by Krieger and her colleagues (72) indicate that dispersed bovine brain cells are capable of *de novo* synthesis of 31K ACTH, ACTH, and β-LPH. At the present writing, it is not known whether the enkephalin pentapeptides are derived from β-endorphin or indeed from a β-LPH precursor. Although it has been claimed on the basis of immunocytochemical observations that β-endorphin and enkephalins are present in different cell populations in the CNS (18), these are indirect observations. Somewhat more direct evidence on this matter is afforded by recent observations that striatal extracts contain proteins which, on tryptic digestion, yield opioid peptides that do not exhibit the chromatographic properties of known LPH fragments (71). Moreover, a new pentadecapeptide has been isolated from porcine hypothalamus which contains the leu-enkephalin sequence (58). Recently sequence analysis of a cloned cDNA for bovine pro-opiocortin has provided the amino acid sequence for this precursor (97). Inspection of the sequence reveals that the precursor protein is composed of several repetitive units separated by pairs of basic amino acid residues (97). Although such a structure implies the production of physiologically active molecules by the action of trypsin-like enzymes, it is still possible that other enzymes may exist in certain neurons which give rise to either further cleavage of tryptic peptides or to entirely novel cleavages, resulting in the ultimate production of enkephalins from pro-opiocortin. Biosynthetic studies in CNS tissue involving isolation and sequencing of peptides derived from a pulse-chase paradigm of enkephalin biosynthesis are needed to provide information on this point.

Biosynthesis of Other Brain Peptides

At the present time no major studies on the biosynthesis by neural tissue of other neuropeptides [e.g., somatostatin, substance P, neurotensin, or vasoactive intestinal polypeptide (VIP)] have been reported. As noted early in the chapter, Agarwal and his group (102) showed that, although brain has been reported to contain gastrin-like immunoreactivity, there is no mRNA for gastrin there whereas there is mRNA in brain cholecystokinin (CCK). This suggests that the observed gastrin immunoreactivity is probably due to the cross reactivity of brain CCK with antigastrin antibodies or to delivery of gastrin to the brain.

Recent studies implicate carnosine as a neurotransmitter in the primary olfactory pathway (76). Studies on the biosynthesis of carnosine carried out by Margolis and co-workers (54), showed that the dipeptide is synthesized by soluble enzymes and therefore comprises a synthetase mechanism. If carnosine is conclusively shown to be a neurotransmitter or a synaptically active molecule, it seems that the nervous system is capable of utilizing peptides derived in diverse ways for information processing, and the fascinating problem of possible differences in the regulation of neuropeptide action exerted on peptides of differing biosynthetic origin is presented.

DEGRADATION OF BRAIN PEPTIDES

Most neuropeptides are rapidly degraded when incubated with brain homogenates (77,78). Several kinds of peptidase activity are inferred to exist based on the cleavage sites so far identified. However, with only a couple of exceptions *(vide infra),* the enzymes catalyzing these reactions have not yet been purified and characterized with respect to specificity. Thus at the present time, the role of peptidases in the physiology of neuropeptides is not clear.

Degradation of TRH

Redding and Schally (119) were the first to report the inactivation of TRH in plasma. Inactivating enzymes for TRH are also present in other organs, e.g., liver, kidney, and brain. In studies with TRH incubated in plasma or serum, the first mechanism revealed was the action of a deamidase with no further degradation (96), suggesting that the free acid TRH-OH was the main degradation product. However, other workers (59,134) demonstrated further degradation of TRH. With [H³]L-proline-labeled TRH, Knigge and Schock (59) were able to find no more than 1 to 5% of the free acid of TRH, the major labeled product being proline. They proposed that removal of the amido group was followed by breakage of the peptide bond between His and Pro. Recently a third activity was detected in rat serum: An enzyme which degrades TRH into pyroglutamic acid and His-Pro-NH₂ was partially purified (134).

Brain tissue degrades TRH through similar pathways. A soluble enzyme responsible for deamidation and a membrane-bound peptidase capable of splitting the His-Pro bond are present (9,12). The latter activity seems to be subsequent to the action of the deamidase (12). The existence of the soluble deamidase has been further corroborated by Taylor and Dixon (133) in freeze-dried porcine hypothalamus and in supernatants obtained after centrifugation of rat hypothalamic homogenates at $100,000 \times g$. Indirect evidence indicates that the brain deamidase differs from that in serum (10,86). Hersh and McKelvy (47) showed that this enzyme can also cleave the Pro^9-Gly^{10}-NH_2 bond of LHRH, and they suggest that the enzyme is similar to the postproline cleavage enzyme of kidney (63). The enzyme was purified to homogeneity from rat brain (123), but its specificity has not yet been investigated. Using partially purified bovine brain deamidase, we (McKelvy, Hersh, and Charli, *unpublished observations*) and Tate

(132) suggested that the enzyme has a rather broad specificity, requiring as a minimum an N-blocked amino acid prior to the proline.

Finally, attack at the N-terminus of the molecule was also reported by Marks (77). This pyroglutamyl peptidase seems to be present in the soluble fraction and has been partially purified from hamster hypothalamic homogenates (115). This enzyme has characteristics (susceptibility to inhibitors) quite different from those of the serum enzyme (134).

As in the case of LHRH, synaptosomal fractions contain only a small proportion (15%) of the total enzymatic activity degrading TRH, with high activity associated with the synaptosomal membrane (57). It remains to be shown if that activity is essentially the same membrane-bound enzyme described by Bauer and Lipmann (12) and suggested by the work of Taylor and Dixon (133) and McKelvy et al. (88).

Serum degrading activity seems to be correlated with the thyroid status of the animal (10), but contradictory results were found in man (8). Rats treated with propylthiouracil or thyroxine (T_4) show a significant change in enzymatic activity (10). When protein synthesis was inhibited, the increase in enzymatic activity by T_4 was prevented (10). Neary et al. (98) found that the TRH degrading activity of rat plasma increased from undetectable activity to high levels during the maturation of the rat, and that daily administration of triiodothyronine (T_3) to rats for 8 to 26 days resulted in a twofold increase in plasma TRH degrading activity. These groups suggested that serum proteases could be an important factor regulating the hypothalamo-hypophysial-thyroid axis. It is not known if the same findings with regard to serum TRH degrading activity and thyroid status hold true for hypophysial portal blood. It now seems clear, however, that direct interaction of factors influencing the thyroid status of the animal (T_3, T_4, TSH) with the pyroglutamate amino peptidase can now be excluded (134).

Degradation of LHRH

Peptidases able to degrade the LHRH molecule are present in all brain regions, the pituitary, liver, kidney (62), and serum (118). The action of a neutral endopeptidase cleaving the Tyr^5-Gly^6 or Gly^6-Leu^7 bonds (60,81), similar to the cleavage of bradykinin at the Phe^5-Ser^6 bond (22), was suggested. The resulting peptides could be further degraded by amino- and carboxypeptidase action. Removal of glycineamide was also observed but at a lower rate, whereas N-terminal degradation of the pyroglutamyl residue was not detected (81). The internal cleavage was confirmed by further studies on degradation of LHRH analogs containing D-amino acids at the Gly^6 position and showing reduced degradation, compared to LHRH (61). Bauer (11) suggested the existence of three enzymes with LHRH-degrading activity with cleavage of the Gly^6-Leu^7 bond, the initial step in LHRH degradation, followed by cleavage of Pro^9-Gly^{10}-NH_2. Partial purification of brain homogenates by DEAE chromatography (11) or hydroxylapatite chromatography (47) yields two enzymatic activities, one that converts LHRH to the 1–9 fragment by splitting the Pro^9-Gly^{10}-NH_2 bond, and another not yet characterized. Bauer (11) proposed that the final step of degradation is an attack at the N-terminus, leading to the formation of pyroglutamic acid, a step also suggested by other workers (118) who showed that injected LHRH gave rise to Pyroglu and Pyroglu-His as major products in urine. In addition, Fridkin et al. (33) reported preliminary evidence for the presence of a pituitary enzyme able to open the N-terminal Pyroglutamyl ring. Study of the subcellular distribution of peptidases showed that the synaptosomes contained only a small proportion (10%) of the total enzymatic activity (56).

Two groups have partially purified a neutral endopeptidase degrading LHRH: the enzyme, isolated by Marks (79) using myelin basic protein as a substrate, inactivates LHRH and has properties similar to those of cathepsin. Akopyan et al. (3) showed that the enzyme, isolated using LHRH as substrate, cleaves at the Tyr^5-Gly^6 and the Gly^6-Leu^7 bonds and is also able to cleave somatostatin to the left of one or more of the phenylalanine residues, and substance P at bonds Gln^6-Phe^7 and Phe^7-Phe^8. There is evidence that the hypothalamic enzymes responsible for LHRH degradation are subject to physiological regulation. Griffiths and Hooper (40) showed that soluble enzymatic activity was decreased by orchiectomy and that this effect could be reversed by testosterone injections. The same was observed after ovariectomy and estradiol injection (41). However, under conditions which permit one to calculate kinetic constants, Loudes et al. (73) found that the specific activity of this enzyme(s) was not modified after castration.

The activity of L-cysteine arylamidase is competitively inhibited by LHRH and other C-terminal amides (65). Because of this competition, Kuhl and Taubert (65,66) used these enzymes as an indirect study of LHRH degradation under steroid and gonadotropic influence. They propose that hypothalamic arylamidase is an integral part of an LH short-loop feedback mechanism. At the moment, further work is needed to elucidate the role of this enzyme in LHRH degradation, since LHRH has not yet been demonstrated to be its substrate.

Degradation of Somatostatin

From *in vitro* studies Marks and co-workers (82,83) suggested preferential cleavage of the Trp^8-Lys^9 bond by rat brain extracts and to a lesser extent the bonds adjacent to the Phe residues. Ala and Cys are slowly released, suggesting that attack at the ends of the molecule is not the primary mechanism of inactivation. More evidence for internal cleavage has been obtained by the use of N-blocked analogs which still are processed to release internal residues. Partial purification of the endopeptidase shows properties akin to the one degrading substance P and LHRH. The site of cleavage by this partially purified neutral endopeptidase has not yet been determined, but the enzyme probably cleaves prior to one or more of the Phe residues of somatostatin (2). Purified lysosomal cathepsin D from brain or hypothalamus cleaves somatostatin at the Phe[6]-Phe[7] and Trp[8]-Lys[9] bonds, with release of trace amounts of Lys (2,15).

Degradation of Substance P

Substance P is degraded by a soluble enzyme that has the same properties as the neutral endopeptidase already mentioned with regard to LHRH and somatostatin degradation. Release of breakdown products is consistent with cleavage of Phe[7]–Phe[8] or Gln[6]–Phe[7] bonds in addition to release of Arg by an aminopeptidase, and Met–NH$_2$ by a C-terminal cleaving enzyme (3,16). Substance P is also processed by the lysosomal cathepsin D isolated from calf brain (15) or bovine hypothalamus (3); the brain enzyme cleaves the Phe[7]–Phe[8] bond, and the hypothalamic one cleaves the Pro[4]–Gln[5] or the Gln[5]–Gln[6] bond.

Recently it was shown that substance P is also cleaved by postproline-cleaving enzyme partially purified from bovine brain, giving rise to a N-terminal tetrapeptide and a C-terminal heptapeptide through cleavage of the Pro[4]–Gln[5] bond (19). The two products of degradation seem to have different biological activity, and the peptide may be a precursor of two peptides with different biological activities (19).

Degradation of Enkephalins and β-Endorphin

Brain homogenates or derived supernatants readily cleave the Tyr[1]–Gly[2] bond of enkephalins by the action of aminopeptidases (29,45,80). Met-enkephalin is further processed by a carboxypeptidase yielding Met and Phe and by a slow-acting dipeptidase giving Gly–Gly as intermediate product (80).

Enzymes present in membrane fractions are also able to rapidly process the enkephalins (91); in particular, leu-enkephalin-hydrolyzing activity has been found in synaptosomal membranes at high specific activity (69).

The N-terminus of β-endorphin is more slowly degraded than that of enkephalins (42,80). Intramolecular interactions between the N-terminal part and other portions of the molecule may be responsible for this enhanced stability (4,5,53). The C-terminus of β-endorphin is also resistant to the action of carboxypeptidases, probably because of the presence of two Lys residues in tandem (37).

The conformation of β-endorphin renders it vulnerable to attack by endopeptidases at the Thr[16]–Leu[17]–Phe[18]–Lys[19]–Asn[20] region. Incubation of β-endorphin with cathepsin D gives rise to γ-endorphin by cleavage of the Leu–Phe bond (14); under mild conditions, treatment with renin at pH 4.0 also gives rise to γ-endorphin; chymotrypsin (pH 7.4) and trypsin also cleaved the Phe[18]–Lys[19] and Lys[19]–Asn[20] bonds, respectively. Brain membrane-bound proteases cleaved β-endorphin at pH 7.4 in the presence of bacitracin to give γ-endorphin and small amounts of met-enkephalin (4). Further study of these enzymes is of the greatest importance in terms of their possible physiological regulation and thus their ability to regulate the concentrations of these important peptides.

As can be seen from the literature cited above, considerable work has been done to identify the mode of peptide degradation. However, we feel that reproducibility of these cleavage sites is not in itself sufficient proof for documentation of the specificity of the phenomenon. Other criteria must be fulfilled, one of which is the consideration of their subcellular distribution: Do the peptides, *in vivo,* contact the peptidases? If so, what are the mechanisms controlling this? Or do some of the soluble activities detected *in vitro* originate from other compartments broken during homogenization? If, for example, the peptides are compartmentalized in vesicles and secreted as granules *(vide infra),* a peptidase present at a lysosomal compartment will have a different role than the one present in the extracellular space or at the membrane of the target cell.

Attempts to localize the peptidases have been few, and some evidence points to a lysosomal origin of a "renin-like" peptidase that transforms angiotensinogen. In this case, as well as in the case of the internal cleavage of substance P, there are two mechanisms by which the breakdown of neuropeptide occurs at the same bond, suggesting that the degradation of the peptide depends on its localization with respect to one (neutral pH) or the other (acid pH) enzyme.

Measuring the disappearance of immunoreactive TRH and LHRH (57), it was observed that the peptidases were mainly in the soluble fraction, with only 10 to 15% present at the synaptosomal level. Some activity responsible for TRH degradation was present in the membrane of synaptosomes, but this was not characterized.

Enzyme activity responsible for enkephalin degradation seems to be confined to the extracellular space (69). It has been suggested that the aminopeptidase acting in enkephalin breakdown comes from the blood vessels present in the CNS, and the enkephalin degrading activity reported in synaptosomal fractions (126) could be due only to contamination by the vascular elements.

In order to firmly define the localization of such enzyme and their involvement in peptide metabolism, their purification becomes of eminent importance. This is because antisera can be prepared against the purified enzyme and used for accurate quantification of the enzyme for studies on enzyme turnover under functional demand and for localization of the enzymes by immunocytochemistry. Although this task is arduous owing to difficulties in purifying enzymes and to the apparent multiplicity of activities involved, it must be accomplished in order to obtain the type of information desired.

SUBCELLULAR DISPOSITION OF BRAIN PEPTIDES

Although LHRH, TRH, and somatostatin were first isolated from hypothalamic preparations, they have now been localized in other brain areas by radioimmunoassay and immunocytochemical techniques. As mentioned previously, peptides thought to be confined to the adenohypophysis have now been localized also in brain areas. For a detailed account of regional distribution, see Hökfelt (49) and Chapter 1. This extrahypothalamic distribution of releasing hormones (107) has prompted several investigators to study their role in other CNS areas as putative neurotransmitters or neuromodulators (114,120). Furthermore, peptides and monoamine neurotransmitters have been shown to coexist within the same neuron [substance P and serotonin (23) and somatostatin and norepinephrine (50)]. This finding is of particular interest since, because of putative synaptic actions of these peptides, their concomitant storage with monoamines suggests that more than one type of chemical agent may operate at a given synapse.

The nature of extrahypothalamic immunoreactive TRH has been investigated in several studies; gel filtration, ion exchange, and thin-layer chromatography, as well as degradation by plasma, have been used to confirm the identity of immunoreactive material as authentic TRH in brain extracts (55). However, another study (139), employing an immunoaffinity adsorbant to isolate TRH, followed by chromatography of material eluted from the adsorbant, found that a substantial proportion of CNS TRH did not cochromatograph with authentic TRH, with a resultant claim that most extrahypothalamic TRH was not authentic TRH. This claim must be taken with caution, however, due to the fact that the authors failed to take their TRH standard through the entire extraction procedure. The question can be answered only by rigorous chemical analysis. For example, Vale (135) actually demonstrated the identity of brain and pancreatic somatostatin by amino acid sequencing.

The subcellular distribution in brain of several of these peptides seems to be largely confined to nerve endings. At this locus there is evidence pointing to their localization within vesicles, which in some cases is corroborated by the use of electron microscopic immunocytochemical techniques showing immunoreactive granules (113,131). This has been well documented for TRH (7,138), LHRH (7,116,127), somatostatin (30), VIP (38), substance P (28,51), and enkephalins (128).

If we assume that this vesicular compartmentalization is a generalized phenomenon for all secretory peptides and, in turn, that this suggests possible biosynthesis in those cells where they have been localized, it seems important not only to detect the presence of the peptide in a brain region but also its subcellular localization. This is nicely exemplified by the finding that angiotensinogen, the precursor form of angiotensin whose topographical distribution has been described (70), seems to be mainly present in the extracellular space. Only 3% of the hormone was present in vesicles, and it was shown to be due to nonspecific uptake (95). However, it should be emphasized that the detection of the peptide in vesicles at the nerve-ending level is still not conclusive proof for biosynthesis in the cell, since the vesicle could enter the cell by a pinocytotic mechanism due to a neighboring neuron having released it into the extracellular space. This process has been observed in the case of substance P neurons (24) where the cells in spinal sensory ganglia project their axons to the spinal cord and release granules to the extracellular space from which the granules move into the blood. These granules are also observed in Schwann cells and fibroblasts.

The subsynaptosomal localization of TRH and LHRH has also been studied. In the hypothalamus LHRH is found mainly in subsynaptosomal particles which contain dense-core granules (111). On the other hand, it is not clear if TRH is a component of hypothalamic nerve endings or if it is sequestered within neurons of the hypothalamus in labile particles which have not yet been isolated.

Studies on the axonal transport of neuropeptides are in their infancy. The principle reason for this is that at present the complete projections of neuronal subsystems utilizing peptides are just beginning to be elucidated.

The majority of axonal transport studies involving peptidergic neurons have been carried out on the hypothalamo-neurohypophysial system (HNS), which has proved to be an excellent model for study of the general mechanism of peptide and granule transport in neurosecretory cells. Several recent reviews treat this topic in detail (100,106).

Classically, the neurohypophysial hormones originate in sites of protein synthesis in paraventricular and supraoptic nuclei and are released from the neural lobe after having progressed through four identifiable stages of transport: (a) compartmentalization into granules at the Golgi stage (140); (b) initiation of axonal transport; (c) axonal transport proper; and (d) cessation of transport at the neuronal ending.

Studies on the transport process in the HNS took on an added dimension once it became clear that transport served not only to supply the neural lobe with hormone but as a mechanism to permit intragranular processing of prohormone species into the individual neurohormones and their related neurophysins (35,36). In [^{35}S]L-cysteine labeling studies, Gainer and co-workers (35) demonstrated posttranslational modification during axonal transport of a 20,000-dalton precursor into a 12,000-dalton labeled neurophysin. The continued elucidation of the extent of coupling between transport and posttranslational processing will prove to be a major area of interest in the coming years, since the possibility exists that regulatory events may occur at the organellar level.

Postulates as to the biochemical mechanism of axoplasmic transport vary as extensively as the systems in which they have been studied. Many of the originally believed dissimilarities between the mechanism of transport in the peripheral nervous system and the HNS were recently discounted (106), permitting the axoplasmic transport process to be studied as a general characteristic of all neurons.

In brief, although current models of axoplasmic transport abound, the transport filament hypothesis as proposed by Ochs (193,105,106) and the continuous axonal smooth endoplasmic reticulum (SER) model as proposed by Droz et al. (26) have gained the most acceptance. The transport filament model stems from the sliding filament theory of muscle contraction and proposes a microtubular-based mechanism which would have transport filaments, coupled to the material to be transported, progressing along the microtubule system by means of cross bridges. The model appears consistent with the demonstrated effects of mitotic blocking agents on axoplasmic flow, and the system's requirement for energy fits the known dependence of transport on oxidative metabolism (104).

Three-dimensional electron microscopic reconstruction studies of SER visualizes it as a continuous intra-axonal compartment connecting the perikaryon and the axon terminus, providing a vehicle for the fast transport of material down the axon, independent of microtubules[26].

The question of whether microtubules are involved in the transport mechanism is problematic (21). Studies with the cytotoxic agents colchicine and vinblastine demonstrate that, although clearly reducing the amount of material transported to the neural lobe (32,101), these agents do not necessarily act by depolymerizing the microtubules (48) but may in fact be acting by disruption of the axoplasmic SER. Models of axoplasmic flow based on microtubules clearly cannot be supported solely by the colchicine studies.

In summary, the actual pathway and mechanism(s) of axonal transport are not yet clear, but, as they become so, application of this knowledge to neuropeptide-secreting neurons may reveal important information about the regulation of neuropeptide metabolism due to the already observed processing of neuropeptide precursors during axonal transport.

RELEASE OF BRAIN PEPTIDES

When studying the release of hypothalamic peptides, considerable work by different research groups has been oriented toward characterization of the neurotransmitters involved in the release of hypothalamic releasing hormones and other neuropeptides (64). The majority of the evidence comes from pharmacological experiments *in vivo*, where the blood concentrations of pituitary hormones have been measured. In these circumstances it is difficult to distinguish the level at which the interaction occurs and whether the effect observed is a direct or a mediated one; for example, in the case of TRH modulation of TSH release, any neurotransmitter could be involved in regulating TSH secretion at one or more of the following sites: (a) relay along the multisynaptic pathways which converge on the hypothalamus; (b) synaptic connections with the dendrites or cell body of the neurosecretory neuron containing TRH; (c) at axoaxonic or other functional connections with the neurosecretory nerve terminal; (d) at the pituitary level, either directly or by modulating the effect of TRH; (e) by regulating the activity of a hypothalamic release inhibiting hormone (e.g., somatostatin) which could also influence TSH release by any of the mechanisms in (a) through (d). Furthermore, there is no reason why a specific neurotransmitter should not be involved in both excitatory and inhibitory pathways. Thus the complexity of potential interactions explains the controversial results which have arisen from studies *in vivo* (68,117).

Attempts have been made to exploit *in vitro* preparations consisting of incubates of hypothalamic fragments (56,121), slices (25), synaptosomes (13,136), or hypothalamo-neurohypophysial systems (129). Some of these systems respond to depolarizing concentrations of potassium in a calcium-dependent manner, criteria that have been widely accepted as an index of functional integrity of *in vitro* preparations. Although by these methods it has been possible to better characterize the possible site of action of a given neurotransmitter upon the release of a particular releasing hormone, many of the problems in interpretation associated with *in vivo* studies still exist with these preparations. It remains to be studied if the release is linked to intracellular activities such as the transformation of a prohormone or translocation of peptides from storage to active pools, and to specify feedback mechanisms which may occur at these levels. Thus in our view the most meaningful studies involving release will take into account experimentally knowledge of the biosynthetic process, especially processing reactions. Recent work demonstrated a concomitant release of ACTH and β-endorphin from the pituitary after stress stimulation (44). Because of the existence of a common precursor to these peptides and several other biologically active peptides, it would be of interest to see if they are released concomitantly and what their target organs are. Another example in this regard issues from the work of Gainer and colleagues (36) who found that, after *in vivo* labeling of the neurohypophysial system with [^{35}S]cysteine, subsequent *in vitro* release studies with neural lobes gave rise to the release of a number of [^{35}S]-labeled peptides, in addition to neurohypophysial hormones and neurophysins. Thus appropriate studies on release could address the important question as to whether various products of precursor polypeptide processing play physiological roles, either by communicating the secretion of a given hormone to other physiological systems or by acting on a given target tissue in concert with the other products of processing.

Theories concerning the biochemical mechanism of neurosecretion, based largely on studies carried out on the neurohypophysial system, support the view that the process of exocytosis is the principal means by which neurosecretory material is released into the extracellular space. However, and as mentioned above, Chan-Palay and Palay (24) observed the release from neurons of intact granules containing substance P-like immunoreactivity. This provocative observation awaits confirmation but could have important implications for the study of neuropeptide release in tissues not organized in a neurohemal fashion. An additional cautionary note with regard to the universality of a classical exocytotic mechanism for neuropeptide release can be made on the basis of the reported release of parathyroid hormone from a nongranular pool (74). Finally, even in the well studied neurohypophysial system, it was observed by electron microscopic immunocytochemistry that extragranular reaction product for neurophysin can be observed with neurohypophysial neurons (A. Silverman, *personal communication*). At present, there is no definitive evidence regarding the mechanism of exocytosis. However, most theories postulate that the limiting membrane of the neurosecretory granule fuses with the plasmalemma membrane, and a gap, or opening, develops at the site of membrane fusion through which the soluble granule contents may pass. Several recent reviews (94,99) addressed this question, so only a few additional points are mentioned here.

The exact molecular nature of the relationship between the granule membrane and plasma membrane just prior to the initiation of membrane fusion is unclear but could involve the participation of microtubules (31,122), actin and myosin (17), and specific phospholipids (46,52). Whether any of these structural constituents constitute a receptor for granule–plasma membrane is yet to be determined.

REUPTAKE OF BRAIN PEPTIDES

Uptake is one of the proposed neuronal mechanisms by which active substances (e.g., biogenic amines) are removed from their membrane sites of action (i.e., synaptic receptors), in addition to the degradation of such substances by specific enzymes present in the extracellular medium (i.e., synaptic cleft). The physiological mechanism(s) by which neuronal peptide action is terminated is not known at this time; as mentioned above, the role of peptidases in regulating the physiological actions of neuropeptides is also unclear. The possibility that carrier-mediated reuptake mechanisms exist in neural tissue for biologically active peptides is supported by early studies by Udenfriend's laboratory (1). These workers found an energy-dependent, carrier-mediated transport system for carnosine, but not homocarnosine, in rodent brain slices *in vitro* (1). Recent studies examined the possible uptake of TRH (111) and α-MSH, arginine, vasopressin, and MSH release inhibitory factor (39) by brain synaptosome preparations. In neither of these studies was evidence obtained for peptide transport. Studies in our laboratory in which the uptake of [³H]TRH into cerebellar slices was assessed revealed the existence of a carrier-mediated transport process for this peptide (109). Based on the (scanty) experimental evidence obtained to date, it may be that the synaptosome is an inappropriate model for peptide transport studies. Much further work needs to be done in this area, as it is of great potential importance to peptide neurobiology.

ACKNOWLEDGMENTS

The authors wish to acknowledge support from the National Science Foundation (NSF GB-4043), Research Career Development Award (AM-00331) from the National Institutes of Health (J.F.M.), and National Institutes of Health National Service Award GM 07062 from the NIGMS (T.S.). The authors express their gratitude for the skillful secretarial assistance of Ms. Barbara Lewis.

REFERENCES

1. Abraham, D., Pisano, J. J., and Udenfriend, S. (1963): Uptake of carnosine and homocarnosine by rat brain slices. *Arch. Biochem. Biophys.,* 104:160–165.
2. Akopyan, T. N., Arutunyan, A. A., Lajtha, A., and Galoyan, A. A. (1978): Acid proteinase

of hypothalamus: Purification, some properties and action on somatostatin and substance P. *Neurochem. Res.,* 3:89–99.

3. Akopyan, T. N., Arutunyan, A. A., Oganisyan, A. I., Lajtha, A., and Galoyan, A. A. (1979): Breakdown of hypothalamic peptides by hypothalamic neutral endopeptidase. *J. Neurochem.,* 32:629–631.

4. Austen, B. M., and Smyth, D. G. (1977): Specific cleavage of lipoprotein C-fragment by endopeptidases: Evidence for a preferred conformation. *Biochem. Biophys. Res. Commun.,* 77:86–94.

5. Austen, B. M., and Smyth, D. G. (1977): The NH_2 terminus of C fragment is resistant to the action of aminopeptidases. *Biochem. Biophys. Res. Commun.,* 76:477–482.

6. Bargmann, W., and Scharrer, E. (1951): The site of origin of the hormones of the posterior pituitary. *Am. Sci.,* 39:255–259.

7. Barnea, A., Ben-Jonathan, N., Colston, C., Johnston, J. M., and Porter, J. C. (1975): Differential sub-cellular compartmentalization of thyrotopin releasing hormone (TRH) and gonadotropin releasing hormone (LRH) in hypothalamic tissue. *Proc. Natl. Acad. Sci. USA,* 72:3153–3156.

8. Bassiri, R. M., and Utiger, R. D. (1972): Serum inactivation of the immunological and biological activity of TRH. *Endocrinology,* 91:657–665.

9. Bauer, K. (1974): Degradation of TRH: Its inhibition by pyroglu-his-OCH_3 and the effect of the inhibitor in attempts to study the biosynthesis of TRH. In: *Lipmann Symposium: Energy, Biosynthesis and Regulation in Molecular Biology,* pp. 57–73. De Gruyter, Berlin.

10. Bauer, K. (1976): Regulation of degradation of TRH by thyroid hormones. *Nature,* 259:591–593.

11. Bauer, K. (1978): Degradation of thyroliberin: Possible physiological role of neuropeptide-degrading enzyme. In: *Biologie Cellulaire des Processus Neurosecretoires Hypothalamiques,* edited by J. D. Vincent and C. Kordon, pp. 478–486. Colloques Internationaux du CNRS No. 280. CNRS Press, Paris.

12. Bauer, K., and Lipmann, F. (1976): Attempts towards the biosynthesis of the TRH and studies on its breakdown in hypothalamic tissue preparations. *Endocrinology,* 99:230–240.

13. Bennett, G. W., Edwardson, J. A., Holland, D., Jeffcoate, S. L., and White, N. (1975): Release of immunoreactive LHRH and TRH from hypothalamic synaptosomes. *Nature,* 257:323–325.

14. Benuck, M., Grynbaum, A., Cooper, T. B., and Marks, N. (1978): Conversion of lipotropic peptides by purified cathepsin D of human pituitary: Release of γ-endorphin by cleavage of the leu[77]-phe[78] bond. *Neurosci. Lett.,* 10:3–9.

15. Benuck, M., Grynbaum, A., and Marks, N. (1977): Cleavage of substance P and somatostatin by lysosomal cathepsin D purified by affinity chromatography. *Brain. Res.,* 113:181–185.

16. Benuck, M., and Marks, N. (1975): Enzymatic inactivation of substance P by a partially purified enzyme from rat brain. *Biochem. Biophys. Res. Commun.,* 65:150–153.

17. Berl, S., Puszkin, S., and Nicklas, W. J. (1973): Actomyosin-like protein in brain. *Science,* 179:441–446.

18. Bloom, F., Battenberg, E., Rossier, J., Ling, N., and Guillemin, R. (1978): Neurons containing β-endorphin in rat brain exist separately from those containing enkephalin: Immunocytochemical studies. *Proc. Natl. Acad. Sci. USA,* 75:1591–1595.

19. Blumberg, S., Teichberg, V. I., Charli, J. L., Hersh, L., and McKelvy, J. (1979): Cleavage of substance P to an N-terminal tetrapeptide and a C-terminal heptapeptide by a postproline cleaving enzyme from bovine brain. *Fed. Proc.,* 38:350.

20. Brownstein, M., and Gainer, H. (1977): Neurophysin biosynthesis in normal rats and in rats with hereditary diabetes insipidus. *Proc. Natl. Acad. Sci. USA,* 74:4046–4049.

21. Byers, M. R. (1974): Structural correlates of rapid axonal transport: Evidence that microtubules may not be directly involved. *Brain Res.,* 75:97–113.

22. Camargo, A., Shapanka, R., and Greene, L. (1973): Preparation, assay and partial characterization of a neutral endopeptidase from rabbit brain. *Biochemistry,* 12:1838–1844.

23. Chan-Palay, V., Jonsson, G., and Palay, S. L. (1978): Serotonin and substance P coexist in neurons of the rat's central nervous system. *Proc. Natl. Acad. Sci. USA,* 75:1852–1856.

24. Chan-Palay, V., and Palay, S. L. (1977): Ultrastructural identification of substance P cells and their processes in rat sensory ganglia and their terminals in the spinal cord by immunocytochemistry. *Proc. Natl. Acad. Sci. USA,* 74:4050–4054.

25. Charli, J. L., Joseph-Bravo, P., Palacios, J. M., and Kordon, C. (1978): Histamine-induced release of thyrotropin releasing hormone from hypothalamic slices. *Eur. J. Pharmacol.,* 52:401–403.

26. Droz, B., Rambourg, A., and Koenig, H. L. (1975): The smooth endoplasmic reticulum: Structure and role in the renewal of axonal membrane and synaptic vesicles by fast axonal transport. *Brain Res.,* 93:1–13.
27. Dube, D., Lissitzky, J. C., Leclerc, R., and Pelletier, G. (1978): Localization of α-melanocyte-stimulating hormone in rat brain and pituitary. *Endocrinology,* 102:1283–1291.
28. Duffy, M. J., Mulhall, D., and Powell, D. (1975): Subcellular distribution of substance P in bovine hypothalamus and substantia nigra. *J. Neurochem.,* 25:305–307.
29. Dupont, A., Lusan, L., Garon, M., Alvarado-Urbina, G., and Labrie, F. (1977): Extremely rapid degradation of ³H-methionine-enkephaline by various rat tissues in vivo and in vitro. *Life Sci.,* 21:908–913.
30. Epelbaum, J., Brazeau, P., Tsang, D., Brawer, J., and Martin, J. B. (1977): Subcellular distribution of radioimmunoassayable somatostatin in rat brain. *Brain Res.,* 126:309–383.
31. Feit, H., Dutton, G. R., Barondes, S. H., and Shelanski, M. L. (1971): Microtubule protein. *J. Cell. Biol.,* 51:138–147.
32. Flament-Durand, J., Couck, A-M, and Dustin, P. (1975): Studies on the transport of secretory granules in the magnocellular hypothalamic neurons of the rat. II. Action of vincristine on axonal flow and neurotubules in the paraventricular and supraoptic nuclei. *Cell Tissue Res.,* 164:1–9.
33. Fridkin, N., Hazum, E., Baram, T., Lindner, H. R., and Koch, Y. (1977): Hypothalamic and pituitary LRF degrading enzymes: Characterization, purification and physiological role. In: *Peptides,* edited by M. Goodman and J. Merenhofen pp. 193–196. Wiley, New York.
34. Fuxe, K., Hökfelt, T., Eneroth, P., Gustafsson, J. A., and Skett, P. (1977): Prolactin: Localization in nerve terminals of the rat hypothalamus. *Science,* 196:899–900.
35. Gainer, H., Sarne, Y., and Brownstein, M. (1977): Neurophysin biosynthesis: Conversion of a putative precursor during axonal transport. *Science,* 195:1354–1356.
36. Gainer, H., Sarne, Y., and Brownstein, M. (1977): Biosynthesis and axonal transport of rat neurohypophysial proteins and peptides. *J. Cell Biol.,* 73:366.
37. Geisow, M. T., and Smyth, D. G. (1977): Lipotropin C fragment has a terminal sequence with high intrinsic resistance to the action of exopeptidase. *Biochem. Biophys. Res. Commun.,* 75:625–629.
38. Giachetti, A., Said, S. I., Reynolds, R. C., and Koniges, F. C. (1977): Vasoactive intestinal polypeptide in brain: Localization in and release from isolated nerve terminals. *Proc. Natl. Acad. Sci. USA,* 74:3424–3428.
39. Greenberg, R., Whalley, C. E., Jourdikian, F., Mendelson, I., Walter, R., Nikolics, K., Coy, D. H., Schally, A. V., and Kastin, A. J. (1976): Peptides readily penetrate the blood-brain barrier; uptake by synaptosomes is passive. *Pharmacol. Biochem. Behav.,* 5:151–158.
40. Griffiths, E. C., and Hooper, K. C. (1973): The effects of orchidectomy and testosterone propionate injection on peptidase activity in the male rat hypothalamus. *Acta Endocrinol. (Kbh),* 72:1–10.
41. Griffiths, E. C., Hooper, K. C., Jeffcoate, S. L., and Holland, D. T. (1975): The effects of gonadectomy and gonadal steroids on the activity of hypothalamic peptidases inactivating luteinizing hormone releasing hormone (LHRH). *Brain Res.,* 88:384–392.
42. Grynbaum, A., Kastin, A. J., Coy, D. H., and Marks, N. (1977): Breakdown of enkephalin and endorphin analogs by brain extracts. *Brain Res. Bull.,* 2:479–484.
43. Guillemin, R. (1971): In vitro synthesis of thyrotropin releasing factor. *Program First Meet. Neurosci. Soc.,* p. 70.
44. Guillemin, R., Vargo, T., Rossier, J., Minick, S., Ling, N., Rivier, C., Vale, W., and Bloom, F. (1977): β-Endorphin and adrenocorticotropin are secreted concomitantly by the pituitary gland. *Science,* 197:1367–1369.
45. Hambrook, T. M., Morgan, B. A., Rance, M. T., and Smith, C. F. C. (1976): Mode of deactivation of the enkephalins by rat and human plasma and rat brain homogenates. *Nature,* 262:782–783.
46. Hawthorne, J. N., and Bleasdale, J. E. (1975): Phosphatidic acid metabolism, calcium ions and transmitter release from electrically stimulated synaptosomes. *Mol. Cell. Biochem.,* 8:83–87.
47. Hersh, L., and McKelvy, J. (1979): Enzymes involved in the degradation of thyrotropin releasing hormone (TRH) and luteinizing hormone releasing hormone in bovine brain. *Brain Res.,* 168:553–564.
48. Hindelang-Gertner, C., Stoeckel, M. E., Porte, A., and Stutinsky, F. (1976): Colchicine effects

on neurosecretory neurons and other hypothalamic and hypophysial cells, with special reference to change in the cytoplasmic membranes. *Cell Tissue Res.*, 170:17–41.

49. Hökfelt, T. (1979): Peptidergic neural pathways. In: *Brain Peptides: The New Endocrinology*, edited by A. Gotto, pp. 5–25. Elsevier, Amsterdam.

50. Hökfelt, T., Elfovin, L. G., Elde, K., Schultzger, M., Goldstein, M., and Luft, R. (1977): Occurrence of somatostatin-like immunoreactivity in some peripheral sympathetic noradrenergic neurons. *Proc. Natl. Acad. Sci. USA*, 75:2587–2591.

51. Hökfelt, T., Myerson, B., Nilsson, G., Pernow, B., and Sachs, C. (1976): Immunohistochemical evidence for substance P-containing nerve endings in the human cortex. *Brain Res.*, 104:181–186.

52. Hokin, L. E. (1976): Functional activity in glands and synaptic tissue and the turnover of phosphatidylinositol. *Ann. NY Acad. Sci.*, 695–709.

53. Hollosi, M., Kajtar, M., and Graf, L. (1977): Studies on the conformation of β endorphin and its constituent fragments in water and trifluoroethanol by CD spectroscopy. *FEBS Lett.*, 74:185–189.

54. Horinishi, H., Grillo, M., and Margolis, F. (1978): Purification and characterization of carnosine synthetase from mouse olfactory bulbs. *J. Neurochem.*, 31:909–919.

55. Jeffcoate, S. L., and White, N. (1975): Studies on the nature of mammalian hypothalamic TRH using immunochemical, chromatographic and enzymatic techniques. *Endocrinology*, 65:83–93.

56. Joseph-Bravo, P., Charli, J. L., Palacios, J. M., and Kordon, C. (1979): Effect of neurotransmitters on the in vivo release of immunoreactive-TRH from rat mediobasal hypothalamus. *Endocrinology*, 104:801–806.

57. Joseph-Bravo, P., Loudes, C., Charli, J. L., and Kordon, C. (1979): Subcellular distribution of brain peptidases degrading LHRH and TRH. *Brain Res.*, 166:321–329.

58. Kangawa, K., Matsuo, H., and Igarashi, M. (1979). αNeo-endorphin: A "big" leu-enkephalin with potent opiate activity from porcine hypothalami. *Biochem. Biophys. Res. Commun.*, 86:153–160.

59. Knigge, K. M., and Schock, D. (1975): Characteristics of the plasma TRH degrading enzyme. *Neuroendocrinology*, 19:277–290.

60. Koch, Y., Baram, T., Chobsieng, P., and Fridkin, M. (1974): Enzymatic degradation of LHRH by hypothalamic tissue. *Biochem. Biophys. Res. Commun.*, 61:95–103.

61. Koch, Y., Baram, T., Hazum, E., and Fridkin, M. (1977): Resistance to enzyme degradation of LHRH and analogues possessing increased biological activity. *Biochem. Biophys. Res. Commun.*, 74:488–491.

62. Kochman, K., Kerdelhue, B., Zor, U., and Jutisz, M. (1975): Studies of enzymatic degradation of luteinizing hormone-releasing hormone by different tissues. *FEBS Lett.*, 50:190–194.

63. Koida, M., and Walter, R. (1976): Post-proline cleaving enzyme: Purification of this endopeptidase by affinity chromatography. *J. Biol. Chem.*, 251:7593–7599.

64. Kordon, C., Enjalbert, A., Hery, M., Joseph-Bravo, P., Rotsztejn, W. H., and Ruberg, M. (1979): Interactions between neurohormones and neurotransmitters. In: *Handbook of the Hypothalamus*, edited by P. Morgane. Dekker, New York *(in press)*.

65. Kuhl, H., and Taubert, H. D. (1975): Inactivation of LHRH by ray hypothalamic L-cysteine arylamidases. *Acta Endocrinol. (Kbh)*, 78:634–645.

66. Kuhl, H., and Taubert, H. D. (1975): Short-loop feedback mechanism of luteinizing hormone: LH stimulates hypothalamic L-cysteine arylamidase to inactivate LHRH in the rat hypothalamus. *Acta Endocrinol. (Kbh)*, 78:649–663.

67. Krieger, D. T., Liotta, A., and Brownstein, M. J. (1977): Presence of corticotropin in brain of normal and hypophysectomized rats. *Proc. Natl. Acad. Sci. USA*, 74:648–652.

68. Krulich, L., Giachetti, A., Marcholowska-koy, A., Hefco, E., and Jameson, H. E. (1977): On the role of the central noradrenergic and dopaminergic systems in the regulation of TSH secretion in the rat. *Endocrinology*, 100:496–505.

69. Lane, A. C., Rance, M. J., and Walter, D. S. (1977): Subcellular localization of leucine-enkephalin hydrolysing activity in rat brain. *Nature*, 269:75–77.

70. Leivicki, J. A., Fallon, J. H., and Prentz, M. P. (1979): Regional distribution of angiotensinogen in rat brain. *Brain Res.*, 158:359–371.

71. Lewis, R., Stein, S., Gerber, L., Rubinstein, M., and Udenfriend, S. (1978): High molecular weight opioid-containing proteins in striatum. *Proc. Natl. Acad. Sci. USA*, 75:4021–4023.

72. Liotta, A., Gildersleeve, D., Brownstein, M., and Krieger, D. (1979): Evidence for brain synthesis of immunoreactive ACTH and β-endorphin-like activity. *Proc. Natl. Acad. Sci. USA,* 76:1448–1452.

73. Loudes, C., Joseph-Bravo, P., Leblanc, P., and Kordon, C. (1978): Specific activity of LHRH and TRH degrading enzymes in various tissues of normal and castrated male rats. *Biochem. Biophys. Res. Commun.,* 83:921–926.

74. MacGregor, R. R., Hamilton, J. W., and Cohn, D. V. (1975): The by-pass of tissue hormone stores during the secretion of newly synthesized parathyroid hormone. *Endocrinology,* 97:178–188.

75. Mains, R. E., Eipper, B. A., and Ling, N. (1977): Common precursor to corticotrophins and endorphins. *Proc. Natl. Acad. Sci. USA,* 74:3014–3018.

76. Margolis, F., and Grillo, M. (1977): The role of carnosine in the primary olfactory pathway. *Neurochem. Res.,* 2:507–519.

77. Marks, N. (1976): Biodegradation of hormonally active peptides in the central nervous system. In: *Subcellular Mechanisms in Reproductive Neuroendocrinology,* edited by F. Naftolin, K. Ryan, and J. Davies, pp. 129–148. Elsevier, Amsterdam.

78. Marks, N. (1977): Conversion and inactivation of neuropeptides. In: *Neurobiology of Peptides,* edited by H. Gainer, pp. 221–258. Plenum Press, New York.

79. Marks, N. (1977): Specificity of breakdown based on the inactivation of active proteins and peptides by brain proteolytic enzymes. In: *Intracellular Protein Catabolism, Vol. II,* edited by V. Turk and N. Marks, pp. 85–102. Plenum Press, New York.

80. Marks, N., Grynbaum, A., and Neidle, A. (1977): On the degradation of enkephalin and endorphins by rat and mouse brain extracts. *Biochem. Biophys. Res. Commun.,* 74:1552–1559.

81. Marks, N., and Stern, F. (1974): Enzymatic mechanisms for the inactivation of LHRH. *Biochem. Biophys. Res. Commun.,* 61:1458–1464.

82. Marks, N., and Stern, F. (1975): Inactivation of somatostatin (GH-RIH) and its analogs by crude and partially purified rat brain extracts. *FEBS Lett.,* 55:220–224.

83. Marks, N., Stern, F., and Benuck, M. (1976): Correlation between biological potency and biodegradation of a somatostatin analogue. *Nature,* 261:511–512.

84. McKelvy, J. F. (1974): Biochemical neuroendocrinology. I. Biosynthesis of thyrotropin releasing hormone (TRH) by organ cultures of mammalian hypothamalus. *Brain Res.,* 65:489–502.

85. McKelvy, J. F. (1978): Biosynthesis of brain peptides. In: *Hypothalamic Peptide Hormones and Pituitary Regulation,* edited by J. C. Porter, pp. 77–98. Plenum Press, New York.

86. McKelvy, J. F., LeBlanc, P., Loudes, C., Perrie, S., Grimm-Jorgensen, Y., and Kordon, C. (1976): The use of bacitracin as an inhibitor of the degradation of TRH and LHRH. *Biochem. Biophys. Res. Commun.,* 73:507–515.

87. McKelvy, J. F., Lin, C. J., Chan, L., Joseph-Bravo, P., Charli, J. L., Pacheco, M., Neale, J., and Barker, J. (1979): Biosynthesis of brain peptides. In: *Brain Peptides, The New Endocrinology,* edited by A. Gotto, pp. 183–196. Elsevier, Amsterdam.

88. McKelvy, J. F., Sheridan, M. N., Joseph-Bravo, S., Phelps, C., and Perrie, S. (1975): Biosynthesis of TRH in organ cultures of guinea pig median eminence. *Endocrinology,* 97:908–918.

89. Mendelson, I., and Walter, R. (1976): On the biosynthesis of putative neurophysin-vasopressin precursors in the hypothalamo-neurohypophysial gland of the guinea pig. In: *Hypothalamic Hormones,* edited by H. Voelter and D. Gupta. Verlag Chemie, Weinheim *(in press).*

90. Mezey, E., Palkovits, M., deKloet, E., Verhoef, J., and deWied, D. (1978): Evidence for pituitary-brain transport of a behaviorally potent ACTH analog. *Life Sci.,* 22:831–838.

91. Miller, R. J., Chang, K. J., Cuatrecasas, P., and Wilkinson, S. (1977): The metabolic stability of the enkephalins. *Biochem. Biophys. Res. Commun.,* 74:1311–1317.

92. Mitnick, M., and Reichlin, S. (1971): Biosynthesis of TRH by rat hypothalamic tissue in vitro. *Science,* 172:1241–1243.

93. Mitnick, M., and Reichlin, S. (1972): Enzymatic synthesis of thyrotropin releasing hormone. *Endocrinology,* 91:1145–1153.

94. Morris, J. F., Nordmann, J. J., and Dyball, R. E. J. (1978): Structure/function correlation in mammalian neurosecretion. *Int. Rev. Exp. Pathol.,* 18:1–95.

95. Morris, B. J., and Reid, I. A. (1978): The distribution of angiotensinogen in dog brain studied by cell fractionation. *Endocrinology,* 103:492–500.

96. Nair, R., Redding, T., and Schally, A. (1971): Site of inactivation of TRH by human plasma. *Biochemistry,* 19:3621–3627.

97. Nakanishi, S., Inoue, A., Kita, T., Nakamura, M., Chang, A., Cohen, S., and Numa, S. (1979): Nucleotide sequence of a cloned cDNA for bovine corticotropin-β-lipotropin precursor. *Nature* 278:423–427.

98. Neary, J. T., Kieffer, J. D., Nakamura, C., Moier, H., Soodak, M., and Maloof, F. (1978): The developmental pattern of TRH-degrading activity in the plasma of rats. *Endocrinology,* 103:1849–1854.

99. Nordmann, J. J. (1978): Hormone release and membrane retrieval in neurosecretion. In: *Cell Biology of Hypothalamic Neurosecretion,* edited by J. D. Vincent and C. Kordon, pp. 619–636. CNRS Press, Paris.

100. Norström, A. (1975): Axonal transport and turnover of neurohypophyseal proteins in the rat. *Ann. NY Acad. Sci.,* 248:46–63.

101. Norström, A., Hansson, H. A., and Sjöstrand, J. (1971): Effects of colchicine on axonal transport and ultrastructure of the hypothalamo-neurohypophyseal system of the rat. *Z. Zellforsch.,* 113:271–293.

102. Noyes, B. E., Mevarech, M., Stein, R., and Agarwal, K. (1979): Detection and partial sequence analysis of gastrin mRNA using an oligodeoxynucleotide probe. *Proc. Natl. Acad. Sci. USA (in press).*

103. Ochs, S. (1971): Characteristics and a model for fast axoplasmic transport in nerve. *J. Neurobiol.,* 2:331–345.

104. Ochs, S. (1972): Fast transport of materials in mammalian nerve fibers. *Science,* 176:252–260.

105. Ochs, S. (1974): Systems of material transport in nerve fibers (axoplasmic transport) related to nerve function and trophic control. *Ann. NY Acad. Sci.,* 228:202–253.

106. Ochs, S. (1977): Axoplasmic transport in peripheral nerve and hypothalamoneurohypophyseal systems. In: *Hypothalamic Peptide Hormones and Pituitary Regulation,* edited by J. C. Porter, pp. 13–40. Plenum Press, New York.

107. Oliver, C., Eskay, R. L., Ben-Jonathan, N., and Porter, J. C. (1974): Distribution and concentration of TRH in the rat brain. *Endocrinology,* 95:540–546.

108. Oliver, C., Mical, R., and Porter, J. C. (1977): Hypothalamic-pituitary vasculature: Evidence for retrograde blood flow in the pituitary stalk. *Endocrinology,* 101:598–604.

109. Pacheco, M., Woodward, D., and McKelvy, J. F. (1978): Uptake of [³H]-TRH by rat cerebellar slices. In: *Abstracts, 8th Annual Meeting, Society for Neuroscience,* Vol. 4, p. 1304.

110. Pacold, S. T., Kirsteins, L., Hojvat, S., and Lawrence, A. M. (1978): Biologically active pituitary hormones in the rat brain amygdaloid nucleus. *Science,* 199:804–805.

111. Parker, C. R., Neaves, W. B., Barnea, A., and Porter, J. C. (1977): Studies on the uptake of [³H]-thyrotropin releasing hormone and its metabolites by synaptosome preparations of the rat brain. *Endocrinology,* 101:66–71.

112. Pearson, D., Shainberg, A., Malamed, S., and Sachs, H. (1976): The hypothalamic-neurohypophysial complex in organ culture: Effects of metabolic inhibitors, biologic and pharmacologic agents. *Endocrinology,* 96:994–1003.

113. Pelletier, G., Leclerc, R., and Dupont, A. (1977): Electron microscope immunohistochemical localization of substance P in the central nervous system of the rat. *J. Histochem. Cytochem.,* 25:1373–1375.

114. Prange, A. J., Breese, G. R., Jahnke, G. D., Cooper, B. R., Cott, J. M., Wilson, I. C., Lipton, M. A., and Plotnikoff, N. P. (1975): Parameters of alteration of pentobarbital response by hypothalamic polypeptides. *Neuropsychobiology,* 1:121–129.

115. Prasad, C., and Peterkovsky, A. (1976): Demonstration of pyroglytamyl peptidase and amidase activities toward TRH in hamster hypothalamus extracts. *J. Biol. Chem.,* 251:3229–3234.

116. Ramirez, B. D., Gautron, J. P., Epelbaum, J., Pattou, E., Lamora, A., and Kordon, C. (1975): Distribution of LHRH in subcellular fractions of the basomedial hypothalamus. *Mol. Cell. Endocrinol.,* 3:399–403.

117. Ranta, T., Mannisto, P., and Tuomisto, J. (1977): Evidence for dopaminergic control of thyrotropin secretion in the rat. *J. Endocrinol.,* 72:329–335.

118. Redding, T. W., Kasten, A. J., Gonzalez-Barcena, D., Coy, D. H., Coy, E. J., Schalch, D. S., and Schally, A. V. (1973): The half life, metabolism and excretion of tritiated LRRH in man. *J. Clin. Endocrinol. Metab.,* 37:662–663.

119. Redding, T. W., and Schally, A. V. (1969): Studies on inactivation of TRH. *Proc. Soc. Exp. Biol. Med.,* 131:415–418.

120. Renaud, L. P., Martin, J. B., and Brazeau, P. (1975): Depressant action of TRH, LHRH and somatostatin on activity of central neurons. *Nature,* 255:233–235.
121. Rotsztejn, W. H., Charli, J. L., Pattou, E., Epelbaum, J., and Kordon, C. (1976): In vitro release of luteinizing hormone releasing hormone (LHRH) from rat mediobasal hypothalamus: Effects of potassium, calcium and dopamine. *Endocrinology,* 99:1663–1668.
122. Rufener, C., Orci, L., Nordmann, J., and Rouiller, C. H. (1972): Effect of vincristine on rat neurohypophysis in vitro. *Gen. Comp. Endocrinol.,* 18:621–630.
123. Rupnow, J., Taylor, W., and Dixon, J. (1979): Purification and characterization of a thyrotropin releasing hormone deamidase from rat brain. *Biochemistry (in press).*
124. Sachs, H., Fawcett, C. P., Takabatake, Y., and Portanova, R. (1969): Biosynthesis and release of vasopressin and neurophysin. *Recent Prog. Horm. Res.,* 25:447–491.
125. Sachs, H., and Takabatake, Y. (1964): Evidence for a precursor in vasopressin biosynthesis. *Endocrinology,* 75:943–948.
126. Shaw, S. G., and Cook, W. F. (1978): Localization and characterization of aminopeptidases in the CNS and the hydrolysis of enkephalin. *Nature,* 274:816–817.
127. Shin, S. H., Morris, A., Snyder, J., Hymer, W. C., and Milligan, J. V. (1974): Subcellular localization of LHRH in the rat hypothalamus. *Neuroendocrinology,* 16:191–201.
128. Simantov, R., Snowman, A. M., and Snyder, S. H. (1976): A morphine-like factor "enkephalin" in rat brain: Subcellular localization. *Brain Res.,* 107:650–657.
129. Sladek, C. D., and Knigge, K. M. (1977): Cholinergic stimulation of vasopressin release from the rat hypothalamo-neurohypophysial system in organ culture. *Endocrinology,* 101:411–420.
130. Sosa, R., McKnight, A., Hughes, J., and Kosterlitz, H. (1977): Incorporation of labelled amino acids into the enkephalins. *FEBS Lett.,* 84:195–198.
131. Styne, D. M., Goldsmith, P. C., Burstein, L. R., Kaplan, J. L., and Grumbach, M. M. (1977): Immunoreactive somatostatin and luteinizing hormone releasing hormone in median eminence synaptosomes of the rat: Detection by immunohistochemistry and quantification by radioimmunoassay. *Endocrinology,* 101:1099–1103.
132. Tate, S. (1978): Purification and properties of a brain thyrotropin releasing factor (TRF) deamidase. *Fed. Proc.,* 37:1780.
133. Taylor, W. L., and Dixon, J. E. (1976): The inhibition of TRH deamidation in porcine hypothalamic tissue. *Biochem. Biophys. Acta,* 444:428–435.
134. Taylor, W., and Dixon, J. (1978): Characterization of a pyroglutamate aminopeptidase from rat serum that degrades TRH. *J. Biol. Chem.,* 19:6934–6940.
135. Vale, W. (1979): Structure/function relations of hypothalamic hormones. In: *Brain Peptides: The New Endocrinology,* edited by A. Gotto. Elsevier, Amsterdam *(in press).*
136. Walberg, J., Eskay, R. L., Barnea, A., Reynolds, R. C., and Porter, J. C. (1977): Release of LHRH and TRH from a synaptosome enriched fraction of hypothalamic homogenates. *Endocrinology,* 100:814–822.
137. Walter, R., Audhya, T. K., Schlesinger, D. H., Shin, S., Saito, S., and Sachs, H. (1977): Biosynthesis of neurophysin proteins in the dog and their isolation. *Endocrinology,* 100:162–174.
138. Winokur, A., Davis, R., and Utiger, R. D. (1977): Subcellular distribution of TRH in rat brain and hypothalamus. *Brain Res.,* 120:623–634.
139. Youngblood, W. H., Humm, J., and Kizer, J. S. (1978): TRH-like immunoreactivity in urine, serum and extrahypothalamic brain: Nonidentity with synthetic pyruglu-his-pro-NH₂ (TRH). *Brain Res.,* 163:101–110.
140. Zambrano, D., and DeRobertis, C. (1966): The secretory cycle of synaptic neurons in the rat: A structural-functional correlation. *Z. Zellforsch.,* 73:414–431.

The Endocrine Functions of the Brain,
edited by Marcella Motta.
Raven Press, New York © 1980

10

Relationships of Some Releasing-Hormone-Producing Neuron Systems to the Ventricles of the Brain

Karl M. Knigge, Carol Bennett-Clarke, Barbara Burchanowski, Shirley A. Joseph, Mary A. Romagnano, and Ludwig A. Sternberger

Department of Anatomy, University of Rochester, School of Medicine and Dentistry, Rochester, New York 14642

The ventricular cerebrospinal fluid (CSF) constitutes a large and important compartment of the fluid environment of the brain, and much attention has been focused on the physiology of its formation and absorption (12,37). The CSF is in anatomical continuity with the extracellular space of the brain, and bidirectional exchanges take place on a regional basis. For more than three decades morphologists have provided evidence which indicates that many neurons communicate with the ventricular CSF by direct contact of cell body or processes. Numerous studies at the light and electron microscopic level verified the presence of a variety of neuronal processes and terminals which end in or are bathed by ventricular CSF. Furthermore, entire networks of neurons have been identified within the ventricular cavities (11). The ependymal lining of the ventricles has been studied extensively and in many areas found to be secretory or specialized for active transport.

The central neuronal systems associated with control of the pituitary gland have been the object of much study. They synthesize a series of neuropeptides which eventually are delivered to the pituitary and regulate the secretion of its tropic hormones. The isolation and chemical synthesis of some of the hypothalamic peptides led rapidly to the generation of antisera with which the immunocytochemist has finally been able to visualize these releasing-hormone-producing neurons. Beginning with the initial report of Barry and Dubois (7) on luteinizing hormone releasing hormone (LHRH) neurons, immunocytochemists provided new insights into the organization of these cells. One of the most immediate and remarkable results of these studies is the demonstration that hypothalamic neurons responsible for the synthesis and activity of releasing

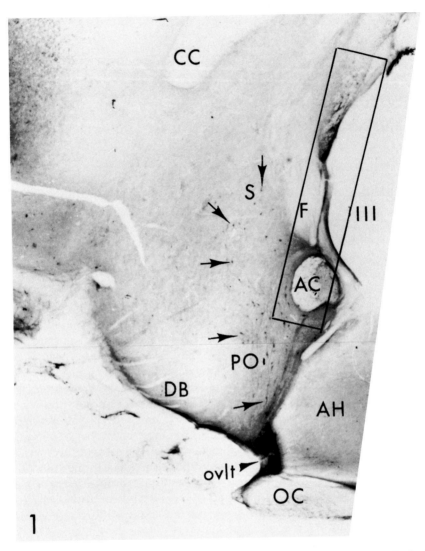

FIG. 1. Parasagittal section of the preoptic–septal region of mouse brain showing the distribution of some immunoreactive LHRH neurons in this area. The brain was prepared by perfusion with Zamboni's solution and sectioned with a Vibratome at 100 μm. Sections were stained immunocytochemically for LHRH using the unlabeled antibody method of Sternberger. Arrows identify LHRH neurons and indicate the approximate limits of this field of cells. (AC) anterior commissure. (AH) anterior hypothalamus. (CC) corpus callosum. (DB) band of Broca. (F) fornix column. (OC) optic chiasm. (ovlt) organum vasculosum laminae terminalis. (PO) preoptic area. (S) septum. (III) third ventricle. (From Burchanowski et al., *in preparation*.)

peptides to the pituitary gland project to many areas of the brain in addition to the median eminence. Immunocytochemical studies also provided further evidence for the relationship between these neuronal systems and the CSF.

Figures 1 through 3 illustrate a projection of fibers from the preoptic pool of LHRH neurons to the anterior wall of the third ventricle. Figure 1 presents a low-power image of this area for anatomical orientation. It is of interest to note how high in the septum some of these neurons are located. Figure 2 represents an enlarged photomontage illustrating the projections from some of these neurons over the anterior commissure, between (and through) the descending fibers of the columns of the fornix to the wall of the ventricle. They ascend along the wall and, in the thalamic recess of the third ventricle, develop a remarkable plexus of fibers, many of which appear to terminate in the ventricle (Fig. 3).

Figure 4 is a frontal section of a rat brain at the level of the optic chiasm and suprachiasmatic nucleus. The periventricular zone of the medial preoptic area at this level contains a near-maximal concentration of somatostatin-immunoreactive neurons. Perikarya and fibers appear to be in contact with the ventricular cavity. Figures 5 through 10 illustrate some of these relationships. Beaded fibers, oriented perpendicular to the ventricular wall, can be traced to the edge, and frequently beyond the edge, of the ependymal lining (Figs. 5 and 10). Somatostatin neurons appear generally to be bipolar, with both processes containing somatostatin immunoreactive staining product for distances of several hundred micrometers from the cell body. Their morphological appearance in the region of the cell body does not provide any clues with respect to the identification of axon and dendrite. A considerable number of somatostatin neurons appear to be in communication with the ventricle via one of their processes (Figs. 7 through 10); alternately, the cell body directly contacts the ventricular lumen (Figs. 5 and 6).

The morphological evidence presented in figs. 1 through 10 contribute additional support for the concept of a close structural and probably functional relationship between certain central neuron systems and the ventricular CSF. Of the two examples cited here, the morphological details of the preoptic LHRH projection to the ventricle suggests delivery and release of hormone into CSF. The morphological details of the somatostatin neuron contacts with CSF are open to other interpretations; the processes of these cells which are in contact with CSF may be dendritic and specialized to serve as a sensor. Such a sensor component in magnocellular neurons of the supraoptico-hypophysial systems was proposed by Rodriguez and Heller (49,50) and generalized for other systems by Oksche et al. (40), Vigh and Vigh-Teichmann (62), and others. The ventricular CSF serves to: (a) remove biologically active or metabolically inactivated molecules from the central nervous system (CNS); (b) distribute within the CNS biologically active substances of neural or extraneural origin; or (c) deliver peptides of neural origin to "peripheral" organs such as the adenohypophysis. Tentative anatomical evidence for axonal transport and delivery of LHRH and other

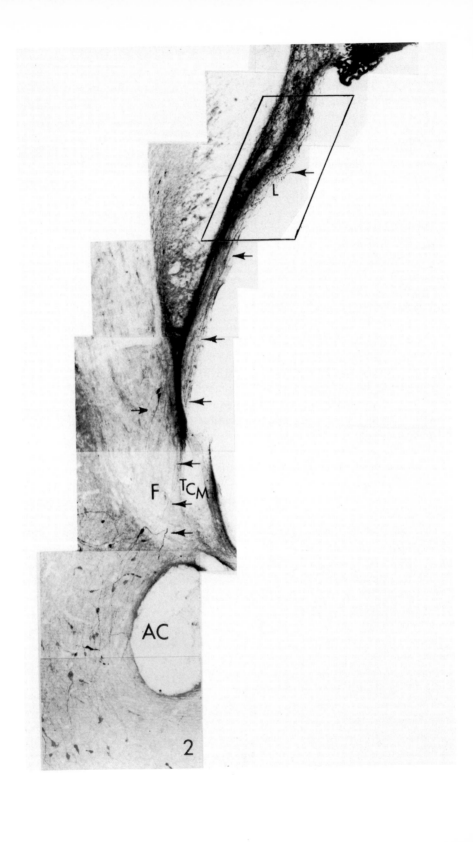

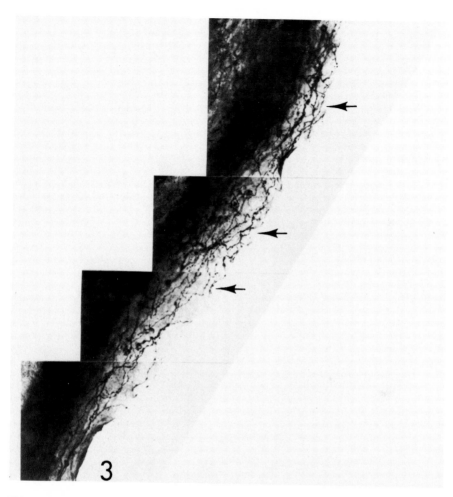

FIG. 3. Photomontage enlargement of the region of the ventricular wall outlined in Fig. 2. The LHRH-immunoreactive fibers form a dense network with many fibers appearing to terminate in the ventricle *(arrows)*. (From Burchanowski et al., *in preparation.*)

FIG. 2. Photomontage enlargement of the region of the brain outline in Fig. 1. LHRH-immunoreactive neurons from a portion of this preoptic field are arched around the anterior commissure with many processes oriented in a dorsoventral direction. Horizontally oriented fibers can be traced caudally into the thalamus and rostrally into forebrain areas. Fibers which project dorsally *(arrows)* interdigitate with those of the fornix columns (F), reach the ventricular wall, and form a conspicuous plexus. Additional details of these terminals are seen in Fig. 3. None of these fibers from the preoptic LHRH field appear to join the medial corticohypothalamic tract (TCM). (AC) anterior commissure. (From Burchanowski et al., *in preparation.*)

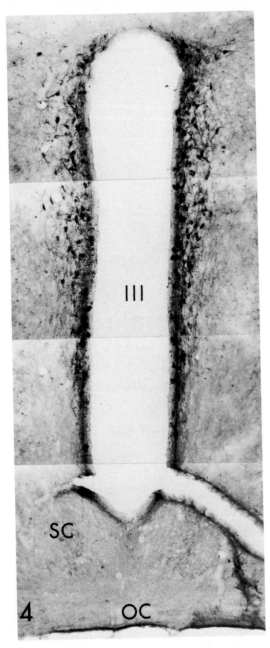

FIG. 4. Frontal section of a rat brain at the level of the optic chiasm and suprachiasmatic nucleus. The brain was prepared by perfusion with Bouin's solution and sectioned with a Vibratome at 30 μm. Sections were stained immunocytochemically for somatostatin using "Charlie-8" antisera (S. A. Joseph) and the unlabeled antibody enzyme method of Sternberger. Somatostatin-immunoreactive neurons are abundant in the periventricular zone: (OC) optic chiasm. (SC) suprachiasmatic nucleus. (III) third ventricle. (From Bennett-Clarke et al., *in preparation.*)

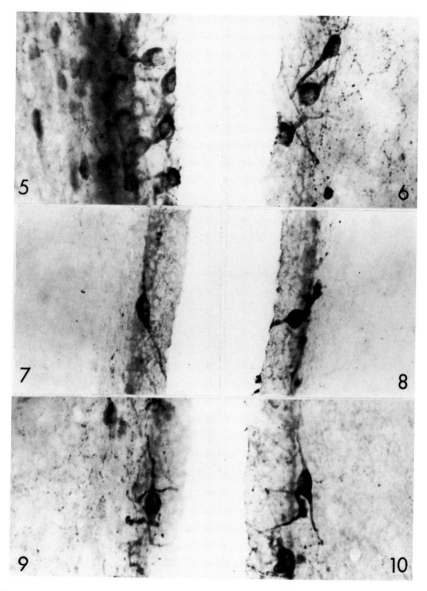

FIG. 5–10. Photomicrographs of somatostatin neurons along the wall of the third ventricle illustrating several ways in which these cells appear to be directly in contact with CSF of the ventricle. See text for description. (From Bennett-Clarke et al., *in preparation.*)

neuropeptides to CSF is supported by considerable evidence indicating the presence of these bioactive molecules in ventricular fluid. A partial list of central peptides which have been detected in CSF includes thyrotropin releasing hormone (TRH) (21,29,54), LHRH (26,38,51), somatostatin (41), vasopressin (13,19), angiotensin (15,20,24,47), neurophysin (48), sleep factor (39,42,43), enkephalins (3–5,52), and endorphins (22,56,59,60). The question of whether all these neuropeptides are present in ventricular CSF as a result of active axonal delivery cannot be answered at present. The brain parenchyma may contribute as much as 40% to CSF formation by continuous bulk flow of the extracellular fluid. This "lymphatic-like" circulation to the CSF may represent a vehicle for removing these peptides from the sites where they are acting as neurotransmitters. Current studies on catecholamines in CSF (27,46,63,66) appears predicated on the view that the metabolites in CSF represent washout from the parenchyma of the brain. Direct axonal projections to the ventricle for these transmitters was also described, however; Lorenz and Richards (36), Aghajanian and Gallager (2), and Chan-Palay (9) described serotonin projections ascending from midbrain raphe nuclei which distribute widely to the third and lateral ventricles.

The median eminence of the hypothalamus represents one of several unique "circumventricular organs" of the brain where special anatomical arrangements bring central neurons into virtually barrier-free contact with the peripheral vasculature. In median eminence, additionally, the ventricular ependyma are modified to become a direct structural interface between CSF and blood of the pituitary portal capillary plexus. Detailed anatomical and physiological studies on the transport of hormones and other substances from CSF to pituitary portal blood were previously reviewed (25,30–33). Neuropeptides such as LHRH and TRH, when infused or injected into the ventricular CSF, gain access to the median eminence, are transported to portal blood, remain biologically active, and influence secretion of their respective pituitary target cells (25,30–33). Endogenous neuropeptides in CSF are presumably afforded the same opportunity of being delivered to the pituitary via this route. Future studies must describe the mechanisms by which this form of delivery is controlled as well as the extent of its physiological role in regulating pituitary secretion.

In addition to peptides of central origin, CSF appears to contain substances of peripheral origin. Among those detected in CSF are growth hormone (28,53), TSH (28), ACTH (6), LH (17), prolactin (8,10,23,35,65), β-MSH (55,57), arginine vasotocin (16,44,45), vasoactive intestinal peptide (14), and melatonin (1, 17,18,34,58,61,64). Since the majority of these substances are normally excluded by the blood–brain barriers of the central vasculature and choroid plexus, it is necessary to postulate other routes of entry. The circumventricular organs appear to be likely candidates for this function. Relatively little experimental data are available, however, to present this possibility as more than a hypothesis. The close proximity of the LHRH and somatostatin neuron pools to the ventricle, together with the present evidence of apparent direct contact of cells and processes with CSF, may offer encouragement to explore this further.

ACKNOWLEDGMENTS

Supported by USPHS grants 1 R01 AM-22029 to K. M. Knigge and 5 R01 HD07926 to S. A. Joseph. B. Burchanowski is a USPHS Postdoctoral Fellow (1F32 AM-05995).

REFERENCES

1. Arendt, J., Wetterberg, L., Heyden, T., Sizonenko, P. C., and Paunier, L. (1977): Radioimmunoassay of melatonin: Human serum and cerebrospinal fluid. *Horm. Res.,* 8:65–75.
2. Aghajanian, G. K., and Gallager, D. W. (1975): Raphe origin of serotonergic nerves terminating in the cerebral ventricles. *Brain Res.,* 88:221–231.
3. Akil, H., Richardson, D. E., Hughes, J., and Barchas, J. D. (1978): Enkephalin-like material elevated in ventricular cerebrospinal fluid of pain patients after analgesic focal stimulation. *Science,* 201:463–465.
4. Akil, H., Watson, S. J., Berger, P. A., and Barchas, J. D. (1978): Endorphins, β-LPH and ACTH: Biochemical, pharmacological and anatomical studies. *Adv. Biochem. Psychopharmacol.,* 18:125–137.
5. Akil, H., Watson, S. J., Sullivan, S., and Barchas, J. D. (1978): Enkephalin-like material in normal human CSF: Measurement and levels. *Life Sci.,* 23:121–125.
6. Allen, J. P., Kendall, J. W., McGilvra, R., and Vancura, C. (1974): Immunoreactive ACTH in cerebrospinal fluid. *J. Clin. Endocrinol. Metab.,* 38:586–593.
7. Barry, J., and Dubois, M. P. (1973): Etude en immunofluorescence des structures hypothalamiques a competence gonadotrope. *Ann. Endocrinol. (Paris),* 34:735–742.
8. Bjerkenstedt, L., Eneroth, P., Harnryd, C., and Sedvall, G. (1977): Effects of melperone and thiothixene on prolactin levels in cerebrospinal fluid and plasma of psychotic women. *Arch. Psychiatr. Nervenkr.,* 224:281–293.
9. Chan-Palay, V. (1977): Indoleamine neurons and their processes in the normal rat brain and in chronic diet-induced thiamine deficiency demonstrated by uptake of ^{3}H-serotonin. *J. Comp. Neurol.,* 176:467–494.
10. Clemens, J. A., and Sawyer, B. D. (1974): Identification of prolactin in cerebrospinal fluid. *Exp. Brain Res.,* 21:399–402.
11. Coates, P. W. (1973): Supraependymal cells in the recesses of the monkey third ventricle. *Am. J. Anat.,* 136:533–539.
12. Davson, H. (1970): *Physiology of the Cerebrospinal Fluid.* Little Brown, Boston.
13. Dogterom, J., Van Wimersma Greidanus, T. B., and Swabb, D. F. (1977): Evidence for the release of vasopressin and oxytocin into cerebrospinal fluid: Measurements in plasma and CSF of intact and hypophysectomized rats. *Neuroendocrinology,* 24:108–118.
14. Fahrenkrug, J., Schaffalitzky De Muckadell, O. B., and Fahrenkrug, A. (1977): Vasoactive intestinal polypeptide (VIP) in human cerebrospinal fluid. *Brain Res.,* 124:581–584.
15. Finkielman, S., Fisher-Ferraro, C., Diaz, A., Goldstein, D. J., and Nahmod, V. E. (1972): A pressor substance in the cerebrospinal fluid of normotensive and hypertensive patients. *Proc. Natl. Acad. Sci. USA,* 69:3341–3344.
16. Goldstein, R., and Pavel, S. (1977): Vasotocin release into the cerebrospinal fluid of cats induced by luteinizing hormone releasing hormone, thyrotrophin releasing hormone and growth hormone release-inhibiting hormone. *J. Endocrinol.,* 75:175–176.
17. Hedlund, L., Lischko, M. M., Kesler, D. J., and Garverick, H. A. (1977): Examination of calf cerebrospinal fluid and plasma for the presence of luteinizing hormone. *J. Endocrinol.,* 73:531–532.

18. Hedlund, L., Lischko, M. M., Rollag, M. D., and Niswender, G. D. (1977): Melatonin: Daily cycle in plasma and cerebrospinal fluid of calves. *Science,* 195:686–687.
19. Heller, H., Hasan, S. H., and Saifi, A. Q. (1968): Antidiuretic activity in the cerebrospinal fluid. *J. Endocrinol.,* 41:273–280.
20. Hutchinson, J. S., Csicsmann, J., Korner, P. I., and Johnston, C. I. (1978): Characterization of immunoreactive angiotensin in canine cerebrospinal fluid as des-aspi-angiotensin II. *Clin. Sci. Mol. Med.,* 54:147–151.
21. Ishikawa, H. (1973): Study on the existence of TRH in the cerebrospinal fluid in humans. *Biochem. Biophys. Res. Commun.,* 54:1203–1209.
22. Jeffcoate, W. J., Rees, L. H., McLoughlin, L., Ratter, S. J., Hope, J., Lowry, P. J., and Besser, G. M. (1978): Beta-endorphin in human cerebrospinal fluid. *Lancet,* 2:119–121.
23. Jimerson, D. C., Post, R. M., Skyler, J., and Bunney, W. E. (1976): Prolactin in cerebrospinal fluid and dopamine function in man. *J. Pharm. Pharmacol.,* 28:845–847.
24. Johnson, A. K., and Epstein, A. N. (1975): The cerebral ventricles as the avenue for the dipsogenic action of intracranial angiotensin. *Brain Res.,* 86:399–418.
25. Joseph, S. A., and Knigge, K. M. (1978): Anatomy of the endocrine hypothalamus. In: *The Hypothalamus,* edited by S. Reichlin, R. J. Baldessarini, and J. B. Martin, pp. 15–48. Raven Press, New York.
26. Joseph, S. A., Sorrentino, S., and Sundberg, D. K. (1975): Releasing hormones, LRF and TRF, in cerebrospinal fluid of the third ventricle. In: *Brain-Endocrine Interaction. II. The Ventricular System in Neuroendocrine Mechanisms,* edited by K. M. Knigge, D. E. Scott, H. Kobayashi, and S. Ishii, pp. 306–312. Karger, Basel.
27. Karoum, F., Bunney, W., Jr., Gillin, J. C., Jimerson, D., Van Kammen, D., and Wyatt, R. J. (1977): Effect of probenecid on the concentration of the lumbar cerebrospinal fluid acidic metabolites of tyramine, octopamine, dopamine and norepinephrine. *Biochem. Pharmacol.,* 26:629–632.
28. Kendall, J. W., Seaich, J. L., and Allen, J. P. (1975): Pituitary-CSF relationships in man. In: *Brain-Endocrine Interaction. II. The Ventricular System in Neuroendocrine Mechanisms,* edited by K. M. Knigge, D. E. Scott, H. Kobayashi, and S. Ishii, pp. 313–323. Karger, Basel.
29. Knigge, K. M., and Joseph, S. A. (1974): Thyrotropin releasing factor (TRF) in cerebrospinal fluid of the third ventricle of rat. *Acta Endocrinol. (Kbh),* 76:209–213.
30. Knigge, K. M., Joseph, S. A., Hoffman, G. E., Arimura, A., and Sternberger, L. (1978): Organization of LRF and SRIF neurons in the endocrine hypothalamus. In: *The Hypothalamus,* edited by S. Reichlin, R. J. Baldessarini, and J. B. Martin, pp. 49–68. Raven Press, New York.
31. Knigge, K. M., Joseph, S. A., Scott, D. E., and Jacobs, J. J. (1971): Observations on the architecture of the arcuate-median eminence region after deafferentation, with reference to the organization of hypothalamic RF-producing elements. In: *The Neuroendocrinology of Human Reproduction,* edited by H. C. Mack and A. I. Sherman, pp. 6–22. Thomas, Springfield, Ill.
32. Knigge, K. M., Joseph, S. A., Sladek, J. R., Notter, M. F., Morris, D. K., Sundberg, M. A., Holzwarth, M. A., Hoffman, G. E., and O'Brien, L. (1976): Uptake and transport activity of the median eminence of the hypothalamus. *Int. Rev. Cytol.,* 45:383–408.
33. Knigge, K. M., and Silverman, A. J. (1975): Anatomy of the endocrine hypothalamus. In: *Handbook of Physiology, Vol. 4: Endocrinology,* edited by E. Knobil and W. Sawyer, pp. 1–32. American Physiological Society, Washington, D.C.
34. Kovács, L., Trentini, G. P., and Mess, B. (1975): Melatonin content of cat cerebrospinal fluid and blood following intravenous injection of melatonin as measured by Xenopus laevis skin melanophore test. *Acta Physiol. Acad. Sci. Hung.,* 46:33–36.
35. Login, I. S., and Macleod, R. M. (1977): Prolactin in human and rat serum and cerebrospinal fluid. *Brain Res.,* 132:477–483.
36. Lorenz, H. P., and Richards, J. G. (1973): Distribution of indolealkylamine nerve terminals in the ventricles of the rat brain. *Z. Zellforsch.,* 144:511–522.
37. Milhorat, T. H. (1976): Structure and function of the choroid plexus and other sites of cerebrospinal fluid formation. *Int. Rev. Cytol.,* 47:225.
38. Morris, M., Tandy, B., Sundberg, D. K., and Knigge, K. M. (1975): Modification of brain and CSF LHRH following deafferentation. *Neuroendocrinology,* 18:131–135.
39. Nagasaki, H., Iriki, M., Inoue, S., and Uchizono, K. (1974): The presence of a sleep-promoting material in the brain of sleep deprived rats. *Proc. Jpn. Acad.,* 50:241–246.

40. Oksche, A., Oehmke, H. J., and Hortwig, H. G. (1974): A concept of neuroendocrine cell complexes. In: *Neurosecretion. The Final Common Pathway,* edited by F. Knowles and L. Vollrath, pp. 154–164. Springer-Verlag, Heidelberg.

41. Patel, C. Y., Krishna, R., and Reichlin, S. (1977): Somatostatin in human cerebrospinal fluid. *N. Engl. J. Med.,* 296:529–533.

42. Pappenheimer, J. R., Koski, G., Fencl, V., Karnovsky, M. L., and Krueger, J. (1975): Extraction of sleep-promoting factor S from cerebrospinal fluid from brains of sleep-deprived animals. *J. Neurophysiol.,* 38:1299–1311.

43. Pappenheimer, J. R., Miller, T. B., and Goodrich, C. A. (1967): Sleep-promoting effects of cerebrospinal fluid from sleep-deprived goats. *Proc. Natl. Acad. Sci. USA,* 58:513–517.

44. Pavel, S. (1970): Tentative identification of arginine vasotocin in human cerebrospinal fluid. *J. Clin. Endocrinol. Metab.,* 31:369–371.

45. Pavel, S. (1973): Arginine vasotocin release into cerebrospinal fluid of cats induced by melatonin. *Nature,* 246:183–184.

46. Perlow, M., Ebert, M. H., Gordon, E. K., Ziegler, M. G., Lake, C. R., and Chase, T. N. (1978): The circadian variation of catecholamine metabolism in the subhuman primate. *Brain Res.,* 139:101–113.

47. Reid, I. A., and Ramsay, D. J. (1975): The effects of intracerebroventricular administration of renin on drinking and blood pressure. *Endocrinology,* 97:536–542.

48. Robinson, A. G., and Zimmerman, E. A. (1973): Cerebrospinal fluid and ependymal neurophysin. *J. Clin. Invest.,* 52:1260–1267.

49. Rodriguez, E. M. (1976): The cerebrospinal fluid as a pathway in neuroendocrine integration. *J. Endocrinol.,* 71:407–443.

50. Rodriguez, E. M., and Heller, H. (1970): Antidiuretic activity and ultrastructure of the toad choroid plexus. *J. Endocrinol.,* 46:83–91.

51. Rolandi, E., Barreca, T., Perria, C., Olivieri, V., Masturzo, P., Gianrossi, R., and Polleri, A. (1975): Presence of gonadotropin releasing hormone (GNRH) in the fluid of the third ventricle in humans. *Boll. Soc. Ital. Biol. Sper.,* 51:762–765.

52. Sarne, Y., Azov, R., and Weissman, B. A. (1978): A stable enkephalin-like immunoreactive substance in human CSF. *Brain Res.,* 151:399–403.

53. Schaub, C., Bluet-Pajot, M. T., Szikla, G., Lornet, C., and Talairach, J. (1977): Distribution of growth hormone and thyroid-stimulating hormone in cerebrospinal fluid and pathological compartments of the central nervous system. *J. Neurol. Sci.,* 31:123–131.

54. Shambaugh, G. E., Wilber, J. R., Montoya, E., Ruder, H., and Blonsky, E. R. (1975): Thyrotropin-releasing hormone (TRH): Measurement in human spinal fluid. *J. Clin. Endocrinol. Metab.,* 41:131–134.

55. Shuster, S., Smith, A., Plummer, N., Thody, A., and Clark, F. (1977): Immunoreactive beta-melanocyte-stimulating hormone in cerebrospinal fluid and plasma in hypopituitarism: Evidence for an extrapituitary origin. *Br. Med. J.,* 1:1318–1319.

56. Sjolund, B., Terenius, L., and Ericksson, M. (1977): Increased cerebrospinal fluid levels of endorphins after electro-acupuncture. *Acta Physiol. Scand.,* 100:382–384.

57. Smith, A. G., and Shuster, S. (1976): Immunoreactive beta-melanocyte-stimulating hormone in cerebrospinal fluid. *Lancet,* 1:1321–1322.

58. Smith, I., Mullen, P. E., Silman, R. E., Snedden, W., and Wilson, B. W. (1976): Absolute identification of melatonin in human plasma and cerebrospinal fluid. *Nature,* 260:716–718.

59. Terenius, L., and Wahlstrom, A. (1975): Morphine-like ligand for opiate receptors in human CSF. *Life Sci.,* 16:1759–1764.

60. Terenius, L., and Wahlstrom, A. (1978): Physiological and clinical relevance of endorphins. In: *Centrally Acting Peptides,* edited by J. Hughes, pp. 161–178. University Park Press, Baltimore.

61. Vaughan, G. M., McDonald, S. D., Jordan, R. M., Allen, J. P., Bohmfalk, G. L., AbouSamra, M., and Story, J. L. (1978): Melatonin concentration in human blood and cerebrospinal fluid: Relationship to stress. *J. Clin. Endocrinol. Metab.,* 47:220–223.

62. Vigh, B., and Vigh-Teichmann, I. (1973): Comparative ultrastructure of the cerebrospinal fluid contacting neurons. *Int. Rev. Cytol.,* 35:189–251.

63. Wightman, R. M., Plotsky, P. M., Strope, E., Delcore, R., Jr., and Adams, R. N. (1977): Liquid chromatographic monitoring of CSF metabolites. *Brain Res.,* 131:345–349.

64. Wilson, B. W., Snedden, W., Silman, R. E., Smith, I., and Mullen, P. (1977): A gas

chromatography-mass spectrometry method for the quantitative analysis of melatonin in plasma and cerebrospinal fluid. *Anal. Biochem.,* 81:283–291.

65. Wode-Helgodt, B., Eneroth, P., Fyro, B., Gullberg, B., and Sedvall, G. (1977): Effect of chlorpromazine treatment on prolactin levels in cerebrospinal fluid and plasma of psychotic patients. *Acta Psychiatr. Scand.,* 56:280–293.

66. Ziegler, M. G., Lake, C. R., Foppen, F. H., Shoulson, I., and Kopin, I. J. (1976): Norepinephrine in cerebrospinal fluid. *Brain Res.,* 108:436–440.

The Endocrine Functions of the Brain,
edited by Marcella Motta.
Raven Press, New York © 1980

11

Mechanism of Action of Hypothalamic Hormones and Interaction with Peripheral Hormones at the Pituitary Level

Fernand Labrie, Martin Godbout, Lisette Lagacé, Jocelyne
Massicotte, Louise Ferland, Nicholas Barden, Jacques Drouin,
Jérôme Lépine, Jean-Claude Lissitzky, Vincent Raymond, Pierre
Borgeat, Michèle Beaulieu, and Raymonde Veilleux

*Medical Research Council Group in Molecular Endocrinology, Le Centre Hospitalier de
l'Université Laval, Quebec, Quebec G1V 4G2, Canada*

The rate of secretion of the six main anterior pituitary hormones is controlled by neurohormones released from the hypothalamus and transported to their adenohypophysial site of action by a short portal blood system (69). The secretion of LH, FSH, and ACTH is thought to be exclusively under positive control, whereas that of GH, TSH, and prolactin results from the balance of action of inhibitory and stimulatory neurohormones. The overall influence of the hypothalamus on GH and TSH secretion is stimulatory, whereas it is inhibitory on prolactin secretion. It is only recently that the concept of neurohormonal control of adenohypophysial function could be translated into biochemical and chemical terms. The discovery of hypothalamic hormones and the relative ease of synthesis of three hypothalamic peptides—thyrotropin releasing hormone (TRH), luteinizing hormone releasing hormone (LHRH), and somatostatin— and their analogs opened new possibilities for studying their mechanism of action and led to a rapid increase in our knowledge of the physiology of the hypothalamo-pituitary complex.

Although peripheral hormones have long been known to play a major role in the control of adenohypophysial activity in man and experimental animals, *in vivo* approaches could not dissociate between hypothalamic and pituitary sites of action. This area of research has been much facilitated by the development of the pituitary cell culture system (51,76). In fact, adenohypophysial cells in primary culture have been extremely useful, not only for assessing the biological activity of analogs of TRH, LHRH, and somatostatin (7,48,49,51) but also for determining the characteristics of interaction between hypothalamic and peripheral hormones at the adenohypophysial level (25,27–29).

This chapter summarizes the evidence obtained so far on the effect of three synthetic hypothalamic hormones—TRH, LHRH, and somatostatin—as well as of one catecholamine, dopamine, on cyclic AMP accumulation in anterior pituitary gland. Since the characteristics of TRH binding and the properties of cyclic AMP-dependent adenohypophysial protein kinase and some of its substrates were described in recent reviews (47,50), these aspects are not included in the present discussion.

Knowing that LHRH stimulates the secretion of LH and FSH (11,51), the divergence frequently observed *in vivo* between the rate of secretion of the two gonadotropins can be best explained by differential effects of gonadal steroids at the pituitary level on the secretion of these two hormones. Emphasis is thus placed on the specific effects of estrogens, progesterone, and androgens on basal and LHRH-induced secretion of LH and FSH in anterior pituitary cells in culture. Data describing the effects of "inhibin" of testicular and ovarian origin at the pituitary level on gonadotropin secretion is also presented. A combined *in vivo* and *in vitro* approach is then used to study the site of action and the characteristics of the action of estrogens in the control of prolactin secretion. A close correlation is found between changes of prolactin responsiveness to TRH and the level of receptors for the neurohormone.

Since estrogens are known to be potent stimulators of prolactin secretion, the interaction of estrogens with dopaminergic action is then studied at the pituitary level *in vitro* and *in vivo*. Estrogens were found to act directly at the pituitary level and, more surprisingly, to have potent antidopaminergic activity on prolactin secretion. Finally, data are presented on the distribution and control of secretion of β-lipotropin and β-endorphin-like peptides in rat anterior pituitary gland.

STIMULATORY EFFECT OF LHRH AND TRH ON PITUITARY CYCLIC AMP ACCUMULATION

The observation that theophylline, an inhibitor of cyclic nucleotide phosphodiesterase, and cyclic AMP derivatives (51,66) have a stimulatory effect on LH release, as well as the potentiation by theophylline of the effect of a crude preparation of FSH-releasing hormone on FSH release (42), suggested that cyclic AMP plays a role in the control of gonadotropin secretion. Definite proof that the adenylate cyclase system is a mediator of the action of LHRH had to be obtained, however, by measuring adenohypophysial adenylate cyclase activity or cyclic AMP concentration under the influence of the pure neurohormone.

It is now well known that addition of LHRH leads to stimulation of cyclic AMP accumulation in rat anterior pituitary gland *in vitro* (11,12,43,57,61). The concentration of LHRH required for half-maximal stimulation of cyclic AMP accumulation is 0.1 to 1.0 ng/ml or 0.1 to 1 nM LHRH. When LHRH analogs having a spectrum of biological activity ranging between 0.001% and 500 to 1,000% of the activity of LHRH itself were used, the same close parallelism between stimulation of cyclic AMP accumulation and both LH and FSH release was found under all experimental conditions (12). That LHRH exerts its action by activating adenylate cyclase and not by inhibiting cyclic nucleotide phosphodiesterase is indicated by the observation that a similar effect of the neurohormone is observed in the presence or absence of theophylline (11).

The possibility of developing a contraceptive method based on inhibitory LHRH analogs led to the synthesis of many such substances, some of which are potent inhibitors of LHRH action *in vivo* (32) and *in vitro* (52). The availability of such LHRH antagonists offered the possibility of investigating the correlation between their inhibitory effect on LHRH-induced cyclic AMP accumulation and LH and FSH release.

As an example, Fig. 1 shows the inhibitory effect of increasing concentrations of [D-Phe², D-Leu⁶]LHRH on cyclic AMP accumulation and LH and FSH release in rat anterior pituitary gland *in vitro*. The close correlation observed between inhibition of LHRH-induced cyclic AMP accumulation and LH and FSH release adds strong support to the concept of an obligatory role of the

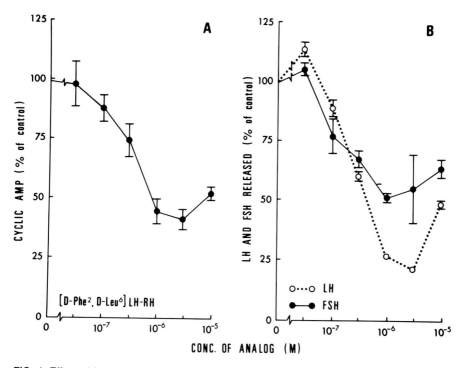

FIG. 1. Effect of increasing concentrations of [D-Phe², D-Leu⁶]LHRH on 3 nM LHRH-induced cyclic AMP accumulation **(A)** and LH and FSH **(B)** release in male rat hemipituitaries *in vitro.*

adenylate cyclase system as mediator of LHRH action in the anterior pituitary gland.

As additional direct evidence for a stimulatory effect of LHRH on pituitary adenylate cyclase activity, the neurohormone stimulates cyclic AMP formation in rat anterior pituitary homogenate (22) and membrane fractions (57). A stimulatory effect of LHRH on adenylate cyclase activity has also been reported in homogenate from the ventral lobe of the pituitary of the dogfish (23).

Since gonadotrophs represent about 5% of the total cell population in the anterior pituitary gland, it is not surprising that addition of LHRH leads to only 100 to 300% stimulation (over control) of anterior pituitary cyclic AMP concentration (11,12,51,60,61). In order to induce a significant increase of total cyclic AMP accumulation, LHRH must then stimulate specific cyclic AMP formation at least 20- to 60-fold in gonadotrophs.

We recently found (29) that estrogens increase the sensitivity of LH responsiveness to LHRH by a direct action at the pituitary level, and androgens have the opposite effect. Such a gonadal-hormone-induced change of pituitary responsiveness to LHRH may explain why pituitaries obtained from male rats show a consistent increase of pituitary cyclic AMP levels under the influence of LHRH (11,12,47,50,51,60,61) whereas no significant effect could be observed using female rat pituitaries (P. Borgeat, M. Beaulieu, and F. Labrie, *unpublished observations*). The higher sensitivity to LHRH in female animals is expected to require lower changes of cyclic AMP levels to induce LH release, whereas higher changes of the intracellular cyclic AMP concentration are likely to be needed in male pituitaries.

Suggestions against an obligatory role of cyclic AMP as mediator of LHRH action pertain to the findings that nonspecific agents leading to changes of total pituitary cyclic AMP accumulation (e.g., theophylline, prostaglandins or inhibitors of their synthesis, cyclic AMP derivatives, and cholera toxin) did not always lead to parallel changes of LH release and cyclic AMP concentration (61,72). Since it is now clear that prostaglandins are not involved in LHRH action at the level of the anterior pituitary gland (26,28,48,58) and, as mentioned earlier, gonadotrophs represent only 5% of the total cell population in the anterior pituitary gland, it is not surprising that the changes of cyclic AMP levels observed with the above-mentioned compounds take place in cell types other than gonadotrophs. In fact, somatotrophs represent approximately 50% of the total adenohypophysial cell population and are highly sensitive to all the substances tested in the above-mentioned studies (4,28,47–50). All these negative attempts to correlate changes of cyclic AMP levels with alterations of LH release can be explained by the lack of specificity of the substances used which did not take into account the heterogeneity of the pituitary cell population. In fact, although the above-mentioned nonspecific compounds could also be acting in other cell types, their action in somatotrophs could by itself explain all the reported changes of cyclic AMP levels which were not accompanied by specific effects on LH secretion (60,61,72).

Although the changes of cyclic AMP levels were of relatively small magnitude, a significant increase (30% over control) was measured after 15 min of incubation with TRH, whereas a maximal effect at 50% over control was found after 2 hr of incubation (47,50). As found previously with LHRH for LH and FSH release, the changes of cyclic AMP levels induced by TRH were accompanied by parallel changes of TSH release. Since the experiments were performed in the presence of 5 mM theophylline, it is likely that the observed changes of cyclic AMP concentrations are secondary to parallel modifications of adenylate cyclase activity rather than to inhibition of cyclic nucleotide phosphodiesterase.

INHIBITORY EFFECT OF SOMATOSTATIN AND DOPAMINE ON PITUITARY CYCLIC AMP ACCUMULATION

Since we had found that a purified fraction of growth hormone releasing hormone (GHRH) led to marked stimulation of pituitary cyclic AMP accumulation and GH release (14), it was of interest to study the effect of somatostatin on pituitary cyclic AMP accumulation. It was then found that somatostatin led to rapid inhibition of cyclic AMP accumulation in anterior pituitary gland *in vitro* (13,43), and this inhibitory effect was accompanied by marked inhibition of GH and TSH release (13).

Since GH- and TSH-secreting cells account for 50 to 70% of the total adenohypophysial cell population in adult male rats, the 50% inhibition of cyclic AMP accumulation in total pituitary tissue suggests almost complete inhibition of cyclic AMP accumulation in the GH- and TSH-secreting cells. The inhibitory effect of somatostatin is observed under basal and prostaglandin $E_2(PGE_2)$- or theophylline-induced conditions, thus suggesting an inhibitory action of somatostatin on adenylate cyclase activity.

The correlation observed between inhibition of cyclic AMP levels and GH release was further demonstrated by an experiment performed in pituitary cells in primary culture (data not shown). We then found that the approximately 10-fold increase of cyclic AMP levels induced by 10^{-5} M PGE_2 is 60% inhibited by somatostatin at an ED_{50} value of 0.3 nM. Under the same experimental conditions, GH release is 90 to 95% inhibited at maximal concentrations of somatostatin. It has also been observed that the inhibitory effect of somatostatin on cyclic AMP levels and GH release is measured at the same ED_{50} value (0.3 nM). The absence of a significant effect of somatostatin on basal cyclic AMP levels in cells in culture in the presence of an approximately 50% inhibitory effect on basal GH release can probably be explained by the presence of fibroblasts in the culture. A similar inhibitory effect of somatostatin on PGE_1-induced adenylate cyclase activity was also observed in rat anterior pituitary gland homogenate, half-maximal inhibition ($p < 0.01$) being observed at 15 nM somatostatin. In addition to its intrinsic interest, this system could be advantageous as a model for studying the mechanisms of action of peptides having opposite effects on cyclic AMP accumulation.

Much evidence obtained in the rat indicates that dopamine (DA) secreted by the tuberoinfundibular system is the main factor involved in the control of prolactin secretion (10,56,71,75). According to these data, DA released from nerve endings in the median eminence is transported to the pituitary prolactin-secreting cells by the hypothalamo-adenohypophysial portal blood system. In support of such a physiological role of DA at the pituitary level on prolactin secretion, DA was recently measured in portal blood (8), and a typical dopaminergic receptor has been characterized in anterior pituitary gland (15–18,21,46).

The first suggestive evidence that cyclic AMP may play a role in the control of prolactin secretion originated from the observations that a cyclic AMP derivative (53) or theophylline (53,64,79) stimulated prolactin release. These data obtained with theophylline and cyclic AMP derivatives suggested that the cyclic nucleotide has a stimulatory role in the control of prolactin secretion.

More convincing evidence to support the idea that cyclic AMP has a role in the action of dopamine on prolactin secretion had to be obtained, however, by measuring adenohypophysial adenylate cyclase activity or cyclic AMP concentration under the influence of the catecholamine. As illustrated in Fig. 2,

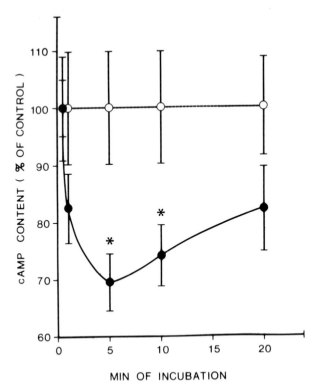

FIG. 2. Effect of dopamine (100 nM) on cyclic AMP accumulation in male rat anterior pituitaries. The experiment was performed as described by Borgeat et al. (11). (O - - - O) control; ●—●, 100 nM.

addition of 100 nM DA to male rat hemipituitaries led to rapid inhibition of cyclic AMP accumulation, a maximal effect (30% inhibition) being obtained as early as 5 min after addition of the catecholamine. Thus although DA is known to stimulate adenylate cyclase activity at the level of the striatum (44,45), its effect at the adenohypophysial level in intact cells is inhibitory.

The data presented so far clearly show that two stimulatory hypothalamic hormones, TRH and LHRH, lead to parallel stimulation of cyclic AMP accumulation and specific hormone release, and one inhibitory peptide, somatostatin, and a catecholamine, DA, lead to parallel inhibition of cyclic AMP accumulation and hormone release. Such findings strongly suggest that changes of adenylate cyclase activity are involved in the mechanism of action of these three peptides and DA in the anterior pituitary gland.

INTERACTIONS BETWEEN LHRH, SEX STEROIDS, AND INHIBIN IN THE CONTROL OF LH AND FSH SECRETION

Although the influence of the hypothalamus on the secretion of both gonadotropins is probably exerted exclusively through LHRH, it is well recognized that gonadal steroids can have a marked influence on LH and FSH secretion. The recent observation that LHRH can potentiate the LH response to subsequent injection of the neurohormone (1,19,34) illustrates that it is almost impossible to distinguish between hypothalamic and pituitary sites of steroid action under *in vivo* conditions. In fact, a stimulatory effect of gonadal steroids on LHRH secretion should lead to an increased LH responsiveness to the neurohormone (in the absence of any direct effect of the steroid at the pituitary level), and the opposite situation should follow the inhibitory effect of a steroid on LHRH secretion.

As shown in Fig. 3, preincubation of male rat anterior pituitary cells for 40 hr in medium containing 10^{-8} M estradiol (E_2) increased the LH responsiveness to LHRH. The LHRH concentration required to produce half-maximal stimulation (ED_{50}) of LH release is decreased by E_2 pretreatment from 2.30 ± 0.03 to 1.20 ± 0.01 nM ($p < 0.01$). It can also be seen (Fig. 3A) that preincubation with E_2 increased the basal LH release from 120 ± 8 ng LH-RP-1/ml/4 hr to 205 ± 10 ng/ml/4 hr ($p < 0.01$). Moreover, in this and similar experiments performed with adenohypophysial cells obtained from male and female animals (29), the maximal LH response to LHRH is slightly but not significantly increased. E_2 pretreatment increased the basal FSH release and the maximal response of the hormone to LHRH (Fig. 3B). Similar effects were previously obtained in anterior pituitary cells obtained from female rats (29).

This stimulatory effect of E_2 at the adenohypophysial level may well be at least partly responsible for the increased LH and FSH sensitivity to LHRH observed at proestrus in the rat (33,39) and during the preovulatory period in the human (63,82).

On the other hand, pretreatment with 10^{-8} M testosterone led to marked

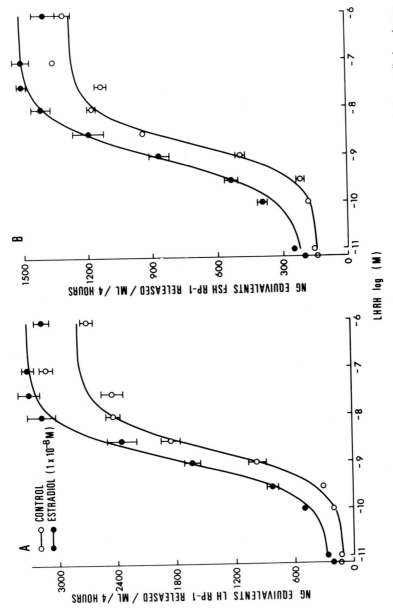

FIG. 3. Effect of increasing concentrations of LHRH on LH **(A)** and FSH **(B)** release by anterior pituitary cells in primary culture preincubated for 40 hr in the presence of 10^{-8} M estradiol or control medium. Anterior pituitary cells were obtained from adult male rats. The response to LHRH was performed during a 4-hr period after preincubation in the presence or absence of the estrogen. The results are presented as the mean ± SEM of data obtained from triplicate determinations.

inhibition of the LH responsiveness to LHRH, the LHRH ED_{50} being increased from 1 to 3 nM in the presence of the androgen ($p < 0.01$, data not shown). We also observed that the androgen did not affect basal LH release but slightly decreased the maximal response to the neurohormone. In contrast with the LH data, testosterone did not significantly affect the LHRH ED_{50} (1 nM) for FSH release. However, the spontaneous and the maximal release of FSH were slightly (30 to 40%) but consistently increased after androgen pretreatment ($p < 0.01$).

These data indicate that androgens have not only specific but also opposite effects at the pituitary level on LH and FSH secretion. In fact, pretreatment of pituitary cells with androgens can markedly inhibit the LH response to LHRH, whereas the effect on FSH secretion is stimulatory. Qualitatively similar results were obtained when anterior pituitary cells obtained from male or female rats were used. These findings can offer an explanation for the observations in rat (74) and man (73) of a greater sensitivity of LH than FSH release to the inhibitory action of androgen administration *in vivo*.

The data summarized above show differential and specific effects of sex steroids on LH and FSH secretion: Whereas estrogens stimulate basal and LH-induced secretion of LH and FSH, androgens and progesterone (in the presence of estrogens) inhibit LH but stimulate FSH secretion. It thus appears that the action of the three classes of sex steroids on FSH secretion at the adenohypophysial level is exclusively stimulatory. These data provide some support to the concept first proposed by McCullagh (59) of an inhibitory substance of testicular origin which could be involved in the specific inhibition of FSH secretion.

Incubation of female rat anterior pituitary cells for 72 hr in the presence of increasing concentrations of Sertoli cell culture medium (days 5 to 8 in culture) led to a maximal 45% inhibition of spontaneous FSH release whereas basal LH release was not affected (Fig. 4). It can be seen, however, that the LHRH-induced release of both gonadotropins was inhibited by Sertoli cell culture medium.

That porcine follicular fluid (treated with dextran-coated charcoal to remove endogenous steroids) exerts the same specific effects on spontaneous gonadotropin secretion is illustrated in Fig. 5. It can be seen that porcine follicular fluid, in analogy with Sertoli cell culture medium, has no effect on spontaneous LH release although it leads to an approximately 70% inhibition of spontaneous FSH secretion. It can also be seen that the inhibitory effect of porcine follicular fluid is much less specific when LHRH-stimulated gonadotropin secretion is studied instead of spontaneous release (Fig. 5). In fact, although LHRH-induced FSH secretion is inhibited to a greater degree than that of LH, significant inhibition of LHRH-induced LH release can also be observed in the presence of follicular fluid. "Inhibin" leads to an increase of the LHRH ED_{50} value for LH release from 0.3 to 1 nM, and the maximal response to the neurohormone is 25% reduced ($p < 0.01$). A similar decrease in the sensitivity of the FSH response to LHRH is also observed in the presence of porcine follicular fluid,

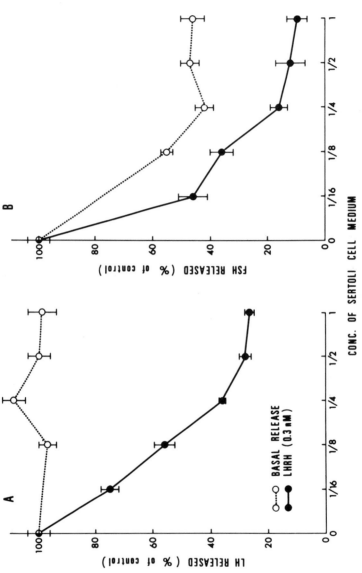

FIG. 4. Effect of increasing concentrations of Sertoli cell culture medium (days 5–8 in culture, 35-day-old animals, 1.5 mg protein/7.5 ml culture medium) on basal and 0.3 nM LHRH-induced LH (**A**) and FSH (**B**) release. The response to LHRH was performed during a 4-hr period after a 72-hr preincubation in the presence of the indicated concentrations of Sertoli cell culture medium. The results are presented as percent of control (mean ± SEM of triplicate determinations). Hormone release in control cells under basal and LHRH-induced conditions was: 25 ± 2 and 710 ± 21 ng/ml (LH) and 20 ± 2 and 110 ± 5 ng/ml (FSH), respectively.

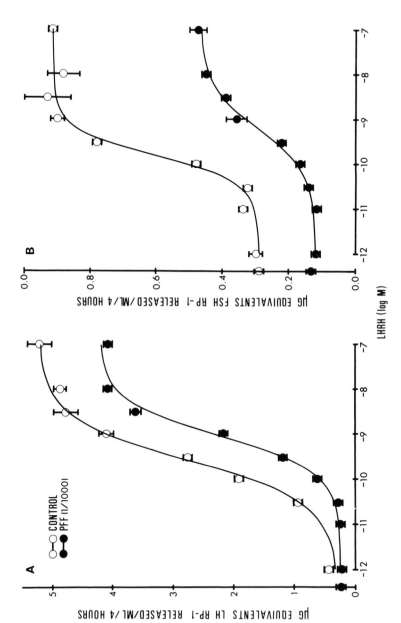

FIG. 5. Effect of porcine follicular fluid on LH **(A)** and FSH **(B)** dose-response curves to LHRH in anterior pituitary cells in culture. Cells were incubated for 40 hr in the presence or absence of procine follicular fluid (PFF) at a 1:1,000 dilution; the LHRH response was performed during a 4-hr period. The results are presented as the mean ± SEM of triplicate determinations.

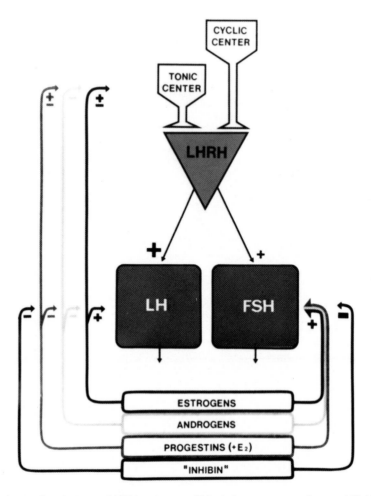

FIG. 6. Interactions between LHRH, estrogens (E₂), androgens, progestins, and "inhibin" in the control of LH and FSH secretion in the rat.

whereas the maximal FSH response to LHRH is 50% reduced. It should be mentioned that identical results were obtained when anterior pituitary cells were prepared from animals ovariectomized 3 weeks previously. Although the concentration of porcine follicular fluid used in this experiment (1:1,000) was maximal, significant inhibition of LHRH-induced LH and FSH release was observed at a 1:50,000 dilution.

The present data indicate that, like estradiol, androgens, and progesterone, the substance(s) of rat Sertoli cell and porcine follicular fluid origin exert specific and differential effects on LH and FSH secretion by a direct action at the anterior pituitary level (Fig. 6). These findings suggest that testicular and ovarian "inhibin" could interact with sex steroids and LHRH in the differential control of LH and FSH secretion and explain the changes in the ratio of LH and FSH secretion that are frequently observed in man (36,40) and experimental animals (34).

INTERACTIONS BETWEEN SEX STEROIDS AND DOPAMINE IN THE CONTROL OF PROLACTIN SECRETION AT THE PITUITARY LEVEL

In vivo treatment with estrogens leads to stimulation of prolactin secretion in man (37,81) and rats (2,20,24,38). At least part of this stimulatory effect of estrogens is likely to be due to a direct action at the pituitary level on prolactin secretion (55,62,67). Recently we found that 17β-estradiol not only stimulates basal and TRH-induced prolactin secretion in rat anterior pituitary cells in primary culture but, somewhat surprisingly, could reverse almost completely the inhibitory effect of DA agonists on prolactin release (17,67). This chapter extends these findings and investigates in more detail the antidopaminergic action of estrogens and their interaction with progestins and androgens on the pituitary DA receptor that controls prolactin secretion.

The interest of such studies is strengthened by the recent observation that the antidopaminergic action of estrogens, first observed at the anterior pituitary level (46,67), also takes place in the central nervous system. In fact, estrogen treatment decreases the circling behavior induced by apomorphine administration in rats having a unilateral lesion of the entopedoncular nucleus (5) and inhibits the apomorphine-induced accumulation of acetylcholine in rat striatum (31). Moreover, clinical studies have recently shown that estrogens have a beneficial effect on L-DOPA- and neuroleptic-induced dyskinesias (6). It is thus hoped that the pituitary cell culture system can be used as a model for other less accessible brain dopaminergic systems.

A detailed analysis of the inhibitory effect of estrogens on the activity of the DA receptor is presented in Fig. 7. It can be seen that 2-bromo-α-ergocryptine (CB-154) led to maximal (70%) inhibition of prolactin release at an ED_{50} value of approximately 3 nM in the presence and absence of 10 nM TRH in control cells. However, preincubation for 5 days with 17β-estradiol led to slight stimulation (approximately 20%) of spontaneous prolactin release whereas the maximal response to TRH was increased by 70%. The most dramatic effect of estrogen treatment was observed in the presence of CB-154: The 70% inhibition of prolactin release induced by the DA agonist in control cells was reduced to 20% in 17β-estradiol-treated cells.

Since progestins and androgens exert antiestrogenic activity at the uterine level, we next studied the possibility of a similar effect on prolactin secretion in rat anterior pituitary cells in culture. Although preincubation for 10 days with 10 nM progesterone alone had no effect on prolactin release, the stimulatory effect of 17β-estradiol was 40 to 50% reversed by the progestin in the presence and absence of the dopamine agonist dihydroergocornine (Fig. 8). 5α-Dihydro-

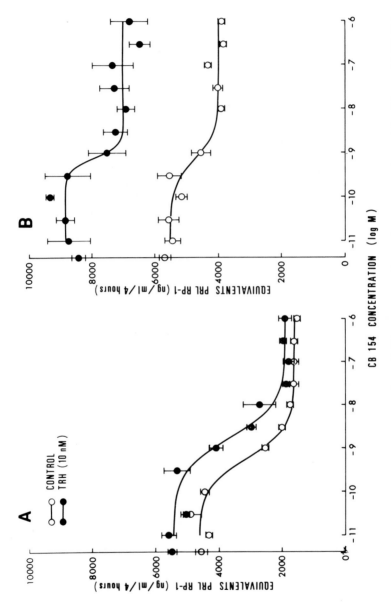

FIG. 7. Effect of 17β-estradiol on the prolactin (PRL) response to increasing concentrations of the DA agonist CB-154 in rat adenohypophysial cells in culture. The cells were preincubated for 5 days in the presence **(B)** or absence **(A)** of 1 nM 17β-estradiol before a 4 hr incubation in the presence or absence of 10 nM TRH and the indicated concentrations of CB-154.

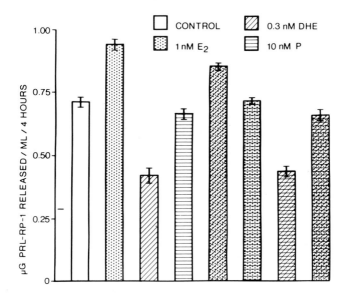

FIG. 8. Effect of preincubation for 10 days with 17β-estradiol (E$_2$; 1 nM) or progesterone (P; 10 nM) alone or in combination on spontaneous prolactin (PRL) release in the presence or absence of dihydroergocornine (DHE; 0.3 nM). Prolactin release was measured during a 4-hr incubation.

testosterone exerts antiestrogenic effects almost superimposable to those observed with progesterone.

Following our *in vitro* data showing a potent antidopaminergic effect of estrogens on prolactin secretion, it then became of interest to investigate if such a potent activity of estrogens occurs under *in vivo* conditions. The present study was facilitated by our recent findings that the endogenous inhibitory dopaminergic influence on prolactin secretion can be eliminated by the administration of opiates, thus making it possible to study the effect of exogenous dopaminergic agents without interference by endogenous dopamine.

The subcutaneous administration of 100 or 400 μg DA completely prevented the increase of plasma prolactin levels following morphine injection in rats ovariectomized 2 weeks previously. Treatment with estradiol benzoate (20 μg/day) for 7 days (Fig. 9B) led to stimulation of basal plasma prolactin levels from 14 $\pm$ 1 to 56 $\pm$ 8 ng/ml and to a marked increase of the maximal plasma prolactin response to morphine, from 215 $\pm$ 60 to 2,175 $\pm$ 390 ng/ml plasma. The most interesting finding, however, was that the 100 and 400 μg doses of DA, which could maintain plasma prolactin levels at undetectable levels after morphine injection in control rats, led to only 40% and 85% inhibition of prolactin levels, respectively, in animals treated with estrogens.

These studies clearly demonstrate that estrogens have potent antidopaminergic activity on prolactin secretion, not only in anterior pituitary cells in culture but also *in vivo*, the effect being qualitatively similar in female and male animals.

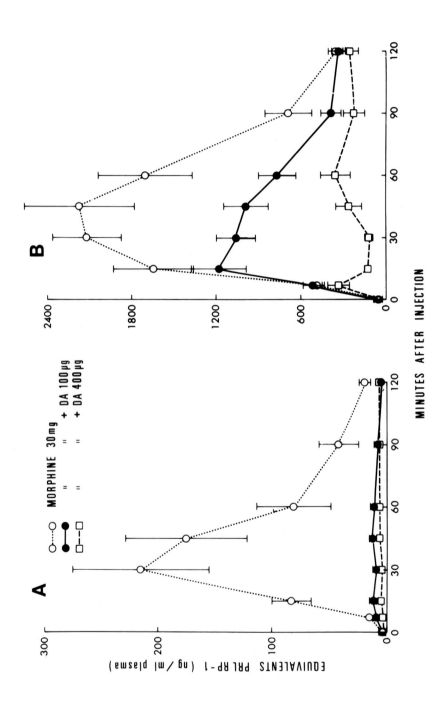

MINUTES AFTER INJECTION

Legend (Panel A):
MORPHINE 30 mg — ○
" " + DA 100 μg — ●
" " + DA 400 μg — □

Y-axis (left plot): EQUIVALENTS PRL RP-1 (ng/ml plasma) — 100, 200, 300

Y-axis (right plot, B): 600, 1200, 1800, 2400

X-axis: 0, 30, 60, 90, 120

As reflected by an increase of the ED_{50} value of DA agonists, the *in vitro* effect of estrogens was due to a decreased sensitivity of prolactin release to DA action at the anterior pituitary level. Such findings indicate that higher concentrations of DA in the hypothalamo-hypophysial portal blood system are likely to be required to inhibit prolactin secretion under conditions of high estrogenic influence. The almost complete reversal of the inhibitory effect of low doses of DA by estrogen treatment clearly indicates an important interaction between estrogens and dopamine at the adenohypophysial level.

PARALLEL RELEASE OF ACTH, β-ENDORPHIN, α-MSH, AND β-MSH-LIKE IMMUNOREACTIVITIES IN ANTERIOR PITUITARY CELLS IN CULTURE

Since rat anterior pituitary cells in primary culture proved to be a precise system to study the control of adenohypophysial hormone secretion (27,30, 51,67,76), we took advantage of the availability of specific radioimmunoassays (RIAs) for ACTH, β-lipotropin (β-LPH), β-endorphin (β-LPH$_{61-91}$), β-MSH, and α-MSH to study changes in the release of the corresponding peptides under conditions of inhibited (with the glucocorticoids) or stimulated [with purified corticotropin releasing factor (CRF), $N^6,O^{2'}$-dibutyryl cyclic AMP (dbcAMP), or theophylline] release. Separation by gel filtration was also performed in preliminary experiments to assess the forms of immunoreactive material. Some of these data have appeared in abstract form (68).

Since not only β-endorphin but also larger peptides containing the β-endorphin amino acid sequence (31K precursor and β-LPH) cross react in the β-endorphin RIA system used (54), we first characterized the β-endorphin immunoreactive components present in pituitary secretion products after their separation by gel filtration. The main secretion products from rat anterior pituitary cells in culture measured in the β-endorphin RIA system comigrate with β-LPH and β-endorphin (Fig. 10A). The major peak of β-MSH immunoreactivity comigrates with γ-LPH, with a significant amount of immunoreactive material at the position of β-LPH. α-MSH immunoreactivity elutes exclusively at the position of α-MSH itself whereas that of ACTH is equally distributed between 4.5 and 13K ACTH (Fig. 10B).

FIG. 9. Effect of estrogen treatment on the inhibitory effect of dopamine (DA) on prolactin (PRL) release in the female rat. Adult Sprague–Dawley rats ovariectomized 2 weeks previously were injected subcutaneously (s.c.) with estradiol benzoate (10 μg b.i.d.) for 7 days or the vehicle alone (0.2 ml 0.1% gelatin in 0.9% NaCl) before insertion of a catheter into the right superior vena cava under anesthesia (Surital, 50 mg/kg i.p.). Two days later undisturbed, freely moving animals were injected with morphine sulfate (30 mg s.c.) alone or in combination with DA (100 or 400 μg s.c.). Blood samples (0.7 ml) were then withdrawn at the indicated time intervals for measurement of plasma prolactin concentration. Data are expressed as the mean ± SEM of duplicate determinations of samples obtained from 8 to 10 animals per group.

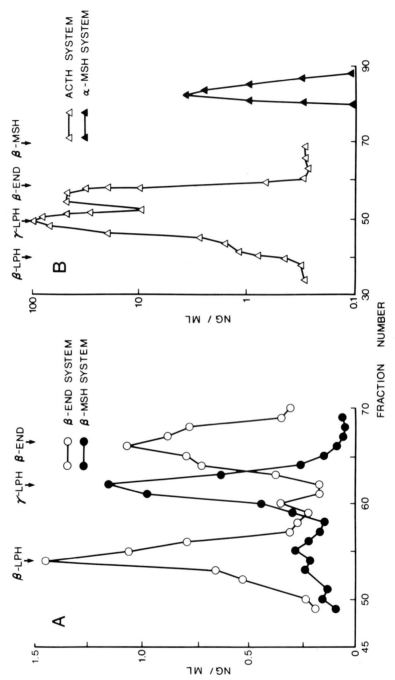

FIG. 10. Gel filtration [G-75 (**A**) or G-50 (**B**) Sephadex] of rat pituitary cell culture medium. **A:** Immunoreactivity in the β-endorphin (END) and β-MSH RIA systems. **B:** Immunoreactivity in the ACTH and α-MSH RIA systems. β-LPH, γ_o-LPH, and β-endorphin were used as markers.

Since theophylline, a cyclic nucleotide phosphodiesterase inhibitor, and cyclic AMP derivatives stimulate ACTH release in intact and cultured pituitaries (35,77), we studied the effect of increasing concentrations of dbcAMP on the release of ACTH, β-endorphin + β-LPH, β-MSH, and α-MSH immunoreactivities. It can be clearly seen in Fig. 11 that increasing concentrations of the cyclic AMP derivative led to progressive and parallel stimulation of ACTH, β-endorphin + β-LPH, α-MSH, and β-MSH immunoreactivities. As found with the CRF fractions, a 24-hr preincubation with dexamethasone led to 20 to 60% inhibition of spontaneous as well as dbcAMP-induced peptide release. Time-course experiments showed that the inhibitory effect of the steroid was already maximal after an 8-hr preincubation with the steroid (data not shown). A similar parallelism was observed when anterior pituitary cells were incubated in the presence of 1 mM 8Br-cAMP or increasing concentrations of theophylline (data not shown).

The availability of four well characterized and specific RIA systems (ACTH, β-endorphin, β-MSH, and α-MSH) coupled to gel filtration permitted identification of the corresponding immunoreactive components secreted in rat anterior pituitary cells in culture under basal as well as stimulated and inhibited conditions of release. It could thus be clearly shown that all the above-mentioned immunoreactive components are released in a parallel fashion under all experimental conditions, thus indicating that acute changes of their secretion rate are not accompanied by altered activity of the endopeptidases responsible for their processing.

In agreement with the observations of Vale et al. (78), the present data show that the β-endorphin-like immunoreactivity present in the incubation medium is apparently distributed in approximately equal amounts between β-LPH and β-endorphin. Allen et al. (3) observed β-endorphin immunoreactive material in culture medium from AtT-20/D-16v mouse pituitary tumor cells comigrating at the positions of the 31K-precursor, β-LPH, and β-endorphin, the β-LPH peak being predominant.

Recently Guillemin et al. (41) demonstrated that β-endorphin and ACTH immunoreactive components were secreted concomitantly in the rat in response to acute stress or long-term adrenalectomy. However, interpretation of *in vivo* studies in rodents is complicated by the likelihood of different control mechanisms for ACTH and β-LPH secretion in the intermediate and anterior lobes and by the finding of different processing of β-LPH and ACTH in the two pituitary lobes (54,70).

Although an inhibitory effect of glucocorticoids on ACTH secretion has been observed (9,65,80), it is of interest that the steroid inhibited to the same extent spontaneous as well as stimulated ACTH and β-endorphin + β-LPH release induced by natural and synthetic substances, thus suggesting that the steroid exerts its effect at a step following cyclic AMP formation. Such a site of action of the synthetic glucocorticoid is analogous to the stimulatory effect of estradiol on LH and FSH release induced by cyclic AMP derivatives and LHRH (30).

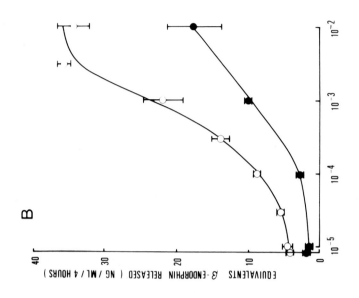

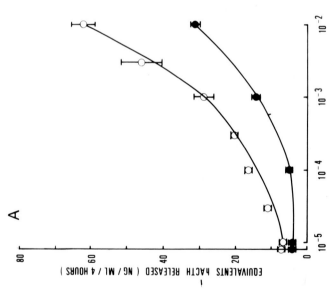

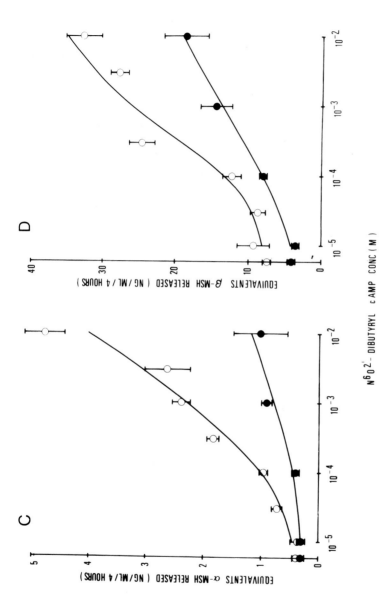

FIG. 11. Effect of increasing concentrations of N^6, $O^{2'}$-dibutyryl cyclic AMP (dbcAMP) on the release of ACTH (**A**), β-endorphin + β-LPH (**B**), α-MSH (**C**), and β-MSH (**D**) immunoreactivities in rat anterior pituitary cells in culture. Cells were preincubated for 24 hr in DMEM containing DCC-adsorbed sera in the presence or absence of 10 nM dexamethasone before a 4-hr incubation with the indicated concentrations of dbcAMP. Results are presented as the mean ± SEM of triplicate determinations. (○—○), control; (●—●), dexamethasone.

REFERENCES

1. Aiyer, B. S., Chiappa, S. A., Fink, G., and Greig, F. J. (1973): A priming effect of luteinizing hormone releasing factor on the anterior pituitary gland in the female rat. *J. Physiol. (Lond),* 234:81P–82P.
2. Ajika, K., Krulich, L., Fawcett, C. P., and McCann, S. M. (1972): Effects of estrogen on plasma and pituitary gonadotropins and prolactin on hypothalamic releasing and inhibitory factors. *Neuroendocrinology,* 9:304–315.
3. Allen, R. G., Hekbert, E., Hinman, M., Shibuya, H., and Pert, C. B. (1978): Coordinate control of corticotropin, β-lipotropin and β-endorphin release in mouse pituitary cell cultures. *Proc. Natl. Acad. Sci. USA,* 75:4972–4976.
4. Barden, N., Bergeron, L., and Betteridge, A. (1976): Effects of prostaglandin synthetase inhibitors and prostaglandin precursors on anterior pituitary cyclic AMP and hormone secretion. In: *Prostaglandin and Thromboxane Research,* pp. 341–344. Raven Press, New York.
5. Bédard, P., Dankova, J., Boucher, R., and Langelier, P. (1978): Effect of estrogens on apomorphine-induced circling behavior in the rat. *Can. J. Physiol. Pharmacol.,* 56:538–541.
6. Bédard, P., Langelier, P., and Villeneuve, A. (1977): Estrogens and the extra-pyramidal system. *Lancet,* 1:1367.
7. Bélanger, A., Labrie, F., Borgeat, P., Savary, M., Côté, J., Drouin, J., Schally, A. V., Coy, D. H., Coy, E. J., Immer, H., Sestanj, K., Nelson, V., and Götz, M. (1974): Inhibition of growth hormone and thyrotropin release by growth hormone-release inhibiting hormone. *Mol. Cell. Endocrinol.,* 1:329–339.
8. Ben-Jonathan, N., Oliver, C., Weiner, H. J., Mical, R. S., and Porter, J. C. (1977): Dopamine in hypophyseal portal plasma of the rat during the estrous cycle and throughout pregnancy. *Endocrinology,* 100:452–458.
9. Berthold, K., Arimura, A., and Schally, A. V. (1970): Effect of 6-dehydro-16-methylene-hydrocortisone and dexamethasone on the release of ACTH from rat pituitaries in vitro. *Acta Endocrinol. (Kbh),* 63:431–443.
10. Bishop, W., Fawcett, C. P., Krulich, L., and McCann, S. M. (1972): Acute and chronic effects of hypothalamic lesions on the release of FSH, LH and prolactin in intact and castrated rats. *Endocrinology,* 91:643–656.
11. Borgeat, P., Chavancy, G., Dupont, A., Labrie, F., Arimura, A., and Schally, A. V. (1972): Stimulation of adenosine $3',5'$-cyclic monophosphate accumulation in anterior pituitary gland in vitro by synthetic luteinizing hormone-releasing hormone/follicle-stimulating hormone-releasing hormone (LHRH/FSH-RH). *Proc. Natl. Acad. Sci. USA,* 69:2677–2681.
12. Borgeat, P., Labrie, F., Côté, J., Ruel, F., Schally, A. V., Coy, D. H., Coy, E. J., and Yanaihara, N. (1974): Parallel stimulation of cyclic AMP accumulation and LH and FSH release by analogs of LHRH in vitro. *Mol. Cell. Endocrinol.,* 1:7–20.
13. Borgeat, P., Labrie, F., Drouin, J., Bélanger A., Immer, I., Sestanj, K., Nelson, V., Gotz, M., Schally, A. V., Coy, D. H., and Coy, E. J. (1974): Inhibition of adenosine $3',5'$-monophosphate accumulation in anterior pituitary gland in vitro by growth hormone release-inhibiting hormone. *Biochem. Biophys. Res. Commun.,* 56:1052–1059.
14. Borgeat, P., Labrie, F., Poirier, G., Chavancy, G., and Schally, A. V. (1973): Stimulation of adenosine $3',5'$-cyclic monophosphate accumulation in anterior pituitary gland by purified growth hormone-releasing hormone. *Trans. Assoc. Am. Physicians,* 86:284–299.
15. Brown, G. M., Seeman, P., and Lee, T. (1976): Dopamine neuroleptics receptors in basal hypothalamus and pituitary. *Endocrinology,* 99:1407–1410.
16. Calabro, M. A., and MacLeod, R. M. (1978): Binding of dopamine to bovine anterior pituitary gland membranes. *Neuroendocrinology,* 25:32–46.
17. Caron, M. G., Beaulieu, M., Raymond, V., Gagné, B., Drouin, J., Lefkowitz, R. J., and Labrie, F. (1978): Dopaminergic receptors in the anterior pituitary gland: Correlation of [³H]dihydroergocryptine binding with the dopaminergic control of prolactin release. *J. Biol. Chem.,* 254:2244–2253.
18. Caron, M. G., Raymond, V., Lefkowitz, R. J., and Labrie, F. (1977): Identification of dopaminergic receptor in anterior pituitary: Correlation with the dopaminergic control of prolactin release. *Fed. Proc.,* 36:278.
19. Castro-Vasquez, A., and McCann, S. M. (1975): Cyclic variations in the increased responsiveness of the pituitary to luteinizing hormone releasing hormone (LHRH) indicated by LHRH. *Endocrinology,* 97:13–19.

20. Chen, L., and Meites, J. (1970): Effects of estrogen and progesterone on serum and pituitary prolactin levels in ovariectomized rats. *J. Endocrinol.*, 86:503–505.
21. Creese, I., Schneider, R., and Snyder, S. H. (1977): [³H]Spiroperidol labels dopamine receptor in pituitary and brain. *Eur. J. Pharmacol.*, 46:377–381.
22. Deery, D. J., and Howell, S. L. (1973): Rat anterior pituitary adenyl cyclase activity: GTP requirement of prostaglandin E_1 and E_2 and synthetic luteinizing hormone-releasing hormone activation. *Biochim. Biophys. Acta*, 329:17–22.
23. Deery, D. J., and Jones, A. C. (1975): Effects of hypothalamic extracts, neurotransmitters and synthetic hypothalamic releasing hormones on adenylyl cyclase activity in the lobes of the pituitary of the dogfish (Scylrorhinus canicula L). *J. Endocrinol.*, 64:49–57.
24. De Léan, A., Garon, M., Kelly, P. A., and Labrie, F. (1977): Changes in pituitary thyrotropin-releasing hormone receptor levels and prolactin responses to TRH during the rat estrous cycle. *Endocrinology*, 100;1505–1510.
25. Drouin, J., De Léan, A., Rainville, R., Lachance, R., and Labrie, F. (1976): Characteristics of the interaction between TRH and somatostatin for thyrotropin and prolactin release. *Endocrinology*, 98:514–521.
26. Drouin, J., Ferland, L., Bernard, J., and Labrie, F. (1976): Site of the in vivo stimulatory effect of prostaglandins on LH release. *Prostaglandins*, 11:367–376.
27. Drouin, J., and Labrie, F. (1976): Selective effect of androgens on LH and FSH release in anterior pituitary cells in culture. *Endocrinology*, 98:1528–1534.
28. Drouin, J., and Labrie, F. (1976): Specificity of the stimulatory effect of prostaglandins on hormone release in anterior pituitary cells in culture. *Prostaglandins*, 11:355–366.
29. Drouin, J., Lagacé, L., and Labrie, F. (1976): Estradiol-induced increase of the LH responsiveness to LHRH in anterior pituitary cells in culture. *Endocrinology*, 99:1477–1481.
30. Drouin, J., Lavoie, M., and Labrie, F. (1978): Effect of gonadal steroids on the LH and FSH response to 8-Br cyclic AMP in anterior pituitary cells in culture. *Endocrinology*, 102:358–361.
31. Euvrard, C., Labrie, F., and Boissier, J. R. (1978): Antagonism between estrogens and dopamine in the rat striatum. In: *Proc. 4th Int. Catecholamine Symposium*, p. 21. Pergamon Press, Oxford.
32. Ferland, L., Labrie, F., Coy, D. H., Coy, E. J., and Schally, A. V. (1975): Inhibitory activity of four analogs of luteinizing hormone-releasing horome in vivo. *Fertil. Steril.*, 26:889–893.
33. Ferland, L., Borgeat, P., Labrie, F., Bernard, J., De Léan, A., and Raynaud, J. P. (1975): Changes in pituitary sensitivity to LHRH during the estrous cycle. *Mol. Cell. Endocrinol.*, 2:107–115.
34. Ferland, L., Drouin, J., and Labrie, F. (1976): Role of sex steroids on LH and FSH secretion in the rat. In: *Hypothalamus and Endocrine Functions*, edited by F. Labrie, J. Meites, and G. Pelletier, pp. 191–209. Plenum Press, New York.
35. Fleischer, H., Donald, R. A., and Butcher, R. W. (1969): Involvement of adenosine $3',5'$-monophosphate in release of ACTH. *Am. J. Physiol.*, 5:1287–1291.
36. Franchimont, P., Chari, S., Hagelstein, M. T., and Duraiswami, S. (1975): Existence of follicle-stimulating hormone inhibiting factor "inhibin" in bull seminal plasma. *Nature*, 257:402–404.
37. Frantz, A. G., Kleinberg, D. L., and Noel, G. L. (1972): Studies on prolactin in man. *Recent Prog. Horm. Res.*, 28:527–590.
38. Fuxe, K., Hökfelt, T., and Nilsson, O. (1969): Castration, sex hormones and tuberoinfundibular dopamine neurons. *Neuroendocrinology*, 5:107–120.
39. Gordon, J. H., and Reichlin, S. (1974): Changes in pituitary responsiveness to luteinizing hormone-releasing factor during the estrous cycle. *Endocrinology*, 94:974–978.
40. Grumbach, M., Roth, J. C., Kaplan, S. L., and Kelch, P. (1974): Hypothalamic-pituitary regulation of puberty: evidence and concepts derived from clinical research. In: *The Control of the Onset of Puberty*, edited by M. Grumbach, G. Grave, and F. E. Mayer, pp. 115–166. Wiley, New York.
41. Guillemin, R., Vargo, T., Rossier, J., Minick, S., Ling, N., Rivier, C., Vale, W., and Bloom, F. (1977): β-Endorphin and adrenocorticotropin are secreted concomitantly by the pituitary gland. *Science*, 197:1367–1369.
42. Jutisz, M., and De la Llosa, P. M. (1970): Requirement of Ca^{++} and Mg^{++} ions for the in vitro release of follicle-stimulating hormone from rat pituitary gland and its subsequent biosynthesis. *Endocrinology*, 86:761–768.
43. Kaneko, T., Saito, S., Oka, H., Oda, T., and Yanaihara, N. (1973): Effects of synthetic LHRH

and its analogs on rat anterior pituitary cyclic AMP and LH and FSH release. *Metabolism*, 22:77–78.

44. Kebabian, J. W. (1977): Biochemical regulation and physiological significance of cyclic nucleotides in the nervous system. *Adv. Cyclic Nucleotide Res.*, 8:421–508.

45. Kebabian, J. W., Petzold, G. L., and Greengard, P. (1973): Dopamine sensitive adenylate cyclase in caudate nucleus of rat brain and its similarity to the dopamine receptor. *Proc. Natl. Acad. Sci. USA*, 69:2145–2149.

46. Labrie, F., Beaulieu, M., Caron, M. G., and Raymond, V. (1978): The adenohypophyseal dopamine receptor: specificity and modulation of its activity by estradiol. In: *Progress in Prolactin Physiology and Pathology*, edited by C. Robyn and M. Harter, pp. 121–136. Elsevier-North Holland, Amsterdam.

47. Labrie, F., Borgeat, P., Lemay, A., Lemaire, S., Barden, N., Drouin, J., Lemaire, I., Jolicoeur, P., and Bélanger, A. (1975): Role of cyclic AMP in the action of hypothalamic regulatory hormones. *Adv. Cyclic Nucleotide Res.*, 5:787–801.

48. Labrie, F., De Léan, A., Drouin, J., Barden, N., Ferland, L., Borgeat, P., Beaulieu, M., and Morin, O. (1976): New aspects of the mechanism of action of hypothalamic regulatory hormones. In: *Hypothalamus and Endocrine Functions*, edited by F. Labrie, J. Meites, and G. Pelletier, pp. 147–169. Plenum Press, New York.

49. Labrie, F., Pelletier, G., Borgeat, P., Drouin, J., Ferland, L., and Bélanger, A. (1976): Mode of action of hypothalamic regulatory hormones. In: *Frontiers in Neuroendocrinology*, Vol. 4, edited by W. F. Ganong and L. Martini, pp. 63–94. Raven Press, New York.

50. Labrie, F., Pelletier, G., Borgeat, P., Drouin, J., Savary, M., Côté, J., and Ferland, L. (1975): Aspects of the mechanism of action of hypothalamic hormone (LHRH). In: *Gonadotropins and Gonadal Functions*, Vol. 1, edited by J. A. Thomas and R. L. Singhal, pp. 77–127. University Park Press, Baltimore.

51. Labrie, F., Pelletier, G., Lemay, A., Borgeat, P., Barden, N., Dupont, A., Savary, M., Côté, J., and Boucher, R. (1973): Control of protein synthesis in anterior pituitary gland. In: *Karolinska Symposium on Protein Synthesis in Reproductive Tissue*, edited by E. Diczfalusy, pp. 301–340. Bogtrykkeriert Forum, Copenhagen.

52. Labrie, F., Savary, M., Coy, D. H., Coy, E. J., and Schally, A. V. (1976): Inhibition of LH release by analogs of LH-releasing hormone (LHRH) in vitro. *Endocrinology*, 98:289–294.

53. Lemay, A., and Labrie, F. (1972): Calcium-dependent stimulation of prolactin release in rat anterior pituitary in vitro by N^6-monobutyryl adenosine $3',5'$-monophosphate. *FEBS Lett.*, 20:7–10.

54. Lissitzky, J. C., Morin, O., Dupont, A., Labrie, F., Seidah, N. G., Chretien, M., Lis, M., and Coy, D. H. (1978): Content of β-LPH and its fragments (including endorphins) in anterior and intermediate lobes of the bovine pituitary gland. *Life Sci.*, 22:1715–1722.

55. Lu, K. H., Koch, Y., and Meites, J. (1971): Direct inhibition by ergocornine of pituitary prolactin release. *Endocrinology*, 89:229–233.

56. MacLeod, R. M., and Lehmeyer, J. E. (1974): Restoration of prolactin synthesis and release by the administration of monoaminergic blocking agents to pituitary tumor-bearing rats. *Cancer Res.*, 34:345–350.

57. Makino, T. (1973): Study of the intracellular mechanism of LH release in the anterior pituitary. *Am. J. Obstet. Gynecol.*, 115:606–614.

58. McCann, S. R., Ojeda, P. G., Harms, J. E., Wheaton, D. K., Sundberg, K. D., and Fawcett, G. P. (1976): Role of prostaglandins (PGs) in the control of adenohypophyseal hormone secretion. In: *Hypothalamus and Endocrine Functions*, edited by F. Labrie, G. Pelletier, and J. Meites, pp. 21–36. Plenum Press, New York.

59. McCullagh, D. R. (1932): Dual endocrine activity of the testis. *Science*, 76:19–20.

60. Naor, F., Koch, Y., Bauminger, S., and Zor, U. (1975): Action of luteinizing hormone and synthesis of prostaglandins in the pituitary gland. *Prostaglandins*, 9:211–219.

61. Naor, F., Koch, Y., Chobsieng, P., and Zor, U. (1975): Pituitary cyclic AMP production and mechanism of luteinizing hormone release. *FEBS Lett.*, 58:318–321.

62. Nicoll, C. S., and Meites, J. (1964): Prolactin secretion "in vitro": Effects of gonadal and adrenal corticol steroids. *Proc. Soc. Exp. Biol. Med.*, 117:579–583.

63. Nillius, S. J., and Wide, L. (1971): Induction of a midcycle-like peak of luteinizing hormone in young women by exogenous estradiol-17β. *J. Obstet. Gynaecol. Br. Commonw.*, 78:822–827.

64. Parsons, J. A., and Nicoll, C. C. (1970): Cations secretion of prolactin and growth hormone in PIF action. *Fed. Proc.,* 29:377.
65. Pollock, J. J., and Labella, F. S. (1966): Inhibition by cortisol of ACTH release from anterior pituitary tissue in vitro. *Can. J. Physiol. Pharmacol.,* 44:549–556.
66. Ratner, A. (1970): Stimulation of luteinizing hormone release in vitro by dibutyryl cyclic AMP and theophylline. *Life Sci.,* 9:1221–1226.
67. Raymond, V., Beaulieu, M., and Labrie, F. (1978): Potent antidopaminergic activity of estradiol at the pituitary level on prolactin release. *Science,* 200:1173–1175.
68. Raymond, V., Ferland, L., Lépine, J., Lissitzky, J. C., Godbout, M., and Labrie, F. (1978): Parallel release of β-endorphin, β-LPH and ACTH in rat anterior pituitary cells in culture. In: *Characteristics and Function of Opioids,* edited by J. M. Van Ree and L. Terenius, pp. 333–334. Elsevier-North Holland, Amsterdam.
69. Schally, A. V., Arimura, A., Bowers, C. Y., Kastin, A. J., Sawano, A. S., and Redding, T. W. (1968): Hypothalamic neurohormones regulating anterior pituitary function. *Recent Prog. Horm. Res.,* 24:497–588.
70. Scott, A. P., Ratcliffe, J. G., Rees, L. H., Landon, J., Bennett, H. P. S., Lowry, P. J., and McMartin, C. (1973): Pituitary peptide. *Nature,* 244:65–69.
71. Shaar, C. J., and Clemens, J. A. (1974): The role of catecholamines in the release of anterior pituitary prolactin in vitro. *Endocrinology,* 95:1202–1212.
72. Sundberg, D. K., Fawcett, C. P., and McCann, S. M. (1976): The involvement of cyclic $3',5'$-cyclic AMP in the release of hormones from the anterior pituitary in vitro. *Proc. Soc. Exp. Biol. Med.,* 151:149–154.
73. Swerdloff, R. S, and Odell, W. D. (1968): Feedback control of male gonadotropin secretion. *Lancet,* 2:683–687.
74. Swerdloff, R. W., Walsh, P. C., and Odell, W. D. (1972): Control of LH and FSH secretion in the male: Evidence that aromatization of androgens to estradiol is not required for inhibition of gonadotropin secretion. *Steroids,* 20:13–22.
75. Takahara, J., Arimura, A., and Schally, A. V. (1974): Suppression of prolactin release by a purified porcine PIF preparation and catecholamines infused into a rat hypophyseal portal vessel. *Endocrinology,* 95:462–465.
76. Vale, W., Grant, G., Amoss, M., Blackwell, R., and Guillemin, R. (1972): Culture of enzymatically dispersed pituitary cells: Functional validation of a method. *J. Clin. Endocrinol. Metab.,* 91:562–572.
77. Vale, W., and Rivier, J. (1977): Substances modulating the secretion of ACTH by cultured anterior pituitary cells. *Fed. Proc.,* 36:2094–2099.
78. Vale, W., Rivier, C., Yang, L., Minick, S., and Guillemin, R. (1978): Effects of purified hypothalamic corticotropin-releasing factor and other substances on the secretion of adreno-corticotropin and β-endorphin-like immunoactivities in vitro. *Endocrinology,* 103:1910–1915.
79. Wakabayashi, K., Date, Y., and Tamaoki, B. (1973): On the mechanism of action of luteinizing hormone-releasing factor and prolactin release inhibiting factor. *Endocrinology,* 92:698–704.
80. Watanabe, H., Nicholson, W. E., and Orth, D. N. (1973): Inhibition of adrenocorticotrophic hormone production by glucocorticoids in mouse pituitary tumor cells. *Endocrinology,* 93:411–416.
81. Yen, S. S. C., Enara, Y., and Siler, T. M. (1974): Augmentation of prolactin secretion by estrogen in hypogonadectomized women. *J. Clin. Invest.,* 53:652–655.
82. Yen, S. S. C., Tsai, C. C., Vandenberg, G., and Rebar, R. (1972): Gonadotropin dynamics in patients with gonadal dysgenesis: A model for the study of gonadotropin regulation. *J. Clin. Endocrinol. Metab.,* 35:897–904.

The Endocrine Functions of the Brain,
edited by Marcella Motta.
Raven Press, New York © 1980

12

Peptide Receptors in the Brain

Robert C. A. Frederickson

Lilly Research Laboratories, Eli Lilly and Company, Indianapolis, Indiana 46206

The idea that drugs act through physicochemical interactions at definite sites in target tissue originated from the works of Langley (138) and of Erlich (68) at the beginning of this century. Erlich gave the name "receptors" to the "side chains" of antigens that recognized chemotherapeutic drugs. This concept of receptors has become the backbone of modern pharmacology and endocrinology and was used for the interpretation of pharmacological data in these disciplines long before the first demonstration and characterization of receptive sites in tissue by direct binding studies. The concept of receptors developed to accommodate two broad categories: the physiological receptor and the drug receptor. The physiological receptor has been defined as a "genetically determined tissue component which has been designed to interact with a naturally-occurring substance, this interaction initiating a series of events culminating in an effect" (64). Drug receptors have been more generally defined as "macromolecules with which a drug interacts to produce its characteristic biological effects" (90).

The demonstration of stereospecific receptors for opiates in the brain (184, 228,243) followed by the discovery of their endogenous ligands, the opioid peptides (115,247), has provided a major advance in our understanding of the receptor concept and drug activity. This has focused our attention on the elementary idea that the brain and other sites do not possess "drug receptors," i.e., sites intended by nature to receive drugs, but rather that the drugs are utilizing physiological receptors intended for an endogenous ligand that the drug resembles structurally. This raises the likelihood that drugs acting by unknown mechanisms may be mimicking or antagonizing the action of an as yet unidentified endogenous ligand, possibly a neurotransmitter or a neurohormone, and thereby providing a means of searching for this new material. An example of this is the search for the endogenous ligand for the benzodiazepine receptor, which may be a new peptide neurotransmitter (152,234). The concept of receptors on the surface of cell membranes as sites of action of peptide hormones derived from many years of studying hormonal effects (102,103). It was not until 1969 that the binding step was measured directly, using iodinated ACTH and angioten-

sin (93,142). The behavioral effects of the peptide hormones and their effects
on the firing rate of neurons in the brain suggested the presence of receptors
for these substances in the brain as well as in the periphery. It is only in the
last decade that we have become aware of the diversity of physiological roles
for peptides.

The secretion of anterior pituitary peptide hormones is regulated by the release
of hypothalamic peptide hormones into the capillaries of the portal system in
the median eminence, which conduct them to their anterior pituitary target
cells. For example, thyrotropin releasing hormone (TRH) stimulates thyrotropin
(TSH) and prolactin (PRL) secretion, luteinizing hormone releasing hormone
(LHRH) releases luteinizing hormone (LH), and follicle stimulating hormone
(FSH), and somatostatin inhibit growth hormone (GH) and TSH release. Thus,
there must be peptide receptors for each of the hypothalamic release promoting
and inhibiting hormones in the anterior pituitary and peptide receptors for
each of the anterior pituitary hormones in the respective target tissues. And
indeed, the above hypothalamic hormones and other peptide hormones are also
found in extrahypothalamic regions, where evidence is building that they act
as neurotransmitters or neuromodulators, requiring the presence of peptide neurotransmitter receptors in these various brain regions. The regions with peptide
neurotransmitter receptors include the hypothalamus, where, for example, the
neurotransmitter candidate enkephalin pentapeptides may control the release
of the hypothalamic peptide hormones, which in turn regulate pituitary hormone
secretion. Clearly, the term peptide receptors refers to a diverse group of sites
that subserve an equally diverse set of functions. Therefore, when we speak of
peptide receptors we may refer to hormone receptors or neurotransmitter receptors, to sites in the periphery or in the hypothalamus, or to sites in other brain
regions. Peptide receptors, furthermore, may be found in systems that subserve
neuroendocrine regulation and in systems subserving nonendocrine-related function. Covering all these aspects of peptide receptors would be beyond the scope
of this chapter; many of these aspects have been the subject of numerous review
papers over the last decade (34,47,84,122,194,206,242).

This chapter will concentrate on peptide receptors in brain subserving neuroendocrine regulation and other functions, with emphasis on neurotransmitter-neu-
romodulator roles. I would first like to give a brief overview of peptide receptors
in general, and their functions and properties, before examining specific receptor
types in more detail.

GENERAL PROPERTIES OF PEPTIDE RECEPTORS

Receptors for peptide hormones and neurotransmitters are generally considered to be macromolecular components, usually high molecular weight proteins,
of the plasma membrane of cells. The first step in the action of a peptide hormone
is the binding to these receptors. This phase of receptor activation can be studied
by measuring the binding of radiolabeled peptides to particular tissue prepara-

tions, which process should be rapid, reversible, saturable, and of high affinity and specificity. The success of this reaction depends on the availability of labeled ligands of very high specific activity, which allows the use of concentrations low enough to minimize nonspecific binding, which may be further reduced by rapid washing procedures. Of course, functional receptor activation requires such receptor binding (which is quantified in terms of affinity and numbers of receptor sites) to be followed by the effector event, which results in the alteration of the state of the target cell and which is quantitated in terms of the efficacy (or intrinsic activity) of the ligand.

It is apparent, therefore, that the radiolabeled ligand studies mentioned above can define only binding sites that may or may not represent the physiologically functional receptors of interest. There are ways of overcoming this weakness in the technique. The use of intact dispersed cells rather than cell homogenates or purified membrane fractions may permit correlation between hormone binding and biological responses (129,157). Another approach is to determine whether the addition of a series of unlabeled ligands to the binding assay displaces the labeled ligand with relative potencies that are proportional to their relative biological potencies *in vivo* (261).

Some of the biological responses that may follow the peptide-receptor interaction are: (a) increase or decrease of hormone or transmitter secretion; (b) stimulation or inhibition of muscle contraction; or (c) depolarization or hyperpolarization of neuronal membranes. The effector event leading to such response might be calcium mobilization or a change in membrane permeability to sodium, potassium, or chloride ions. In earlier studies of hormone action this sequence was shown to be usually mediated by stimulation of adenylate cyclase, with formation of cyclic AMP, which acted as a second messenger (205). More recent evidence, together with the recognition that peptides probably function as neurotransmitters as well as hormones, indicates that the effector event may also be mediated by an inhibition of adenylate cyclase (128) or even a direct action on membrane sodium permeability (222,270,271).

GENERAL MODEL OF RECEPTOR-EFFECTOR ACTIVATION

The model discussed here is based mainly on α-adrenoceptor studies rather than peptide hormone receptor studies because of the greater information available on the former systems. This is mainly due to the more widespread availability of such systems for study and the availability of a wide variety of agonists and antagonists with which it is possible to examine adrenoreceptor function. The process of cell fusion has been developed whereby cell membrane components from two different cell types can be intermixed (230). Schramm and colleagues (217) employed this fusion process to demonstrate that the catecholamine receptors of turkey erythrocytes, with their adenylate cyclase inactivated by N-ethyl-maleimide or heat, can activate the adenylate cyclase of mouse erythroleukemia cells, which possess no catecholamine receptors. They showed further

$$\text{Ant} \longrightarrow \text{R} \Longrightarrow \text{Ant} \cdot \text{R} \xrightarrow{\quad} \text{E}$$

$$\text{Ag} \longrightarrow \text{R} \Longrightarrow \text{Ag} \cdot \text{R}_\text{A} \longrightarrow \text{E} \Longrightarrow \text{Ag} \cdot \text{R} \cdot \text{E}_{\text{PA}}$$

$$\downarrow \text{N}$$

$$\text{Ag} + \text{R} + \text{E}_\text{A}$$

FIG. 1. Agonist **(Ag)** reacts with receptor **(R)** to produce the activated complex **Ag R**$_\text{A}$ in which the receptor has been converted to a higher-affinity form. This activated agonist-receptor complex is recognized by the adenylate cyclase **(E)** with which it interacts to produce the potentially active agonist-receptor-enzyme complex **(Ag R E**$_{\text{PA}}$**)**. Guanine or other nucleotide **(N)** reacts with this complex to dissociate it, with release of free agonist, free low-affinity receptor and activated adenylate cyclase **(E**$_\text{A}$**)**. Antagonist **(Ant)** also binds to the receptor but does not produce the conformational change that activates the ligand-receptor complex to allow it to interact with adenylate cyclase.

that the matching of a receptor to a heterologous adenylate cyclase system readily occurs with a variety of different cells and that the same cell may contribute adenylate cyclase to couple with a foreign receptor, or the receptor to couple with a foreign adenylate cyclase. They conclude that the receptor is a unit independent of the enzyme and that the mechanism for coupling between receptors and adenylate cyclase may be universal for all eukaryotic cells. They suggest, furthermore, that the change that occurs in the receptor upon binding of the hormone may be universal for hormone receptors, which probably have a common chemical structure differing only in the confined area that binds the hormone (217). These findings, together with the knowledge that antagonists bind receptors but do not activate the effectors and that guanine nucleotides, or other nucleotides at higher concentrations, are required for activation of adenylate cyclase by catecholamines, and yet inhibit agonist, but not antagonist, binding, have been explained by a "dynamic receptor affinity model for activation of adenylate cyclase" (143). A somewhat simplified version of this model is presented in Fig. 1.

RECEPTORS FOR SPECIFIC PEPTIDES

Besides the hypothalamic and anterior pituitary peptide hormones already mentioned there are also the peptide hormones that are produced in the hypothalamus and released from the posterior pituitary (the hypothalamoneurohypophysial neurosecretory system), such as oxytocin, vasopressin, and neurophysin. There are, furthermore, the gastrointestinal peptides, such as gastrin and vasoactive intestinal peptide (VIP) and many others, such as angiotensin, substance P, enkephalins, endorphins, and neurotensin. These have all been found to be distributed in the central nervous system as well as in peripheral sites, and evidence is growing that many, if not all, of these function in the central nervous system as neurotransmitters or neuromodulators (6,65,176,232). The remainder of this review will discuss the available information concerning the receptors in the brain for these peptides (see Table 2), beginning with the receptors for enkephalins and endorphins (opioid receptors) because these are the most extensively studied and best characterized; the opioid peptides, furthermore, may serve in most of the roles discussed earlier for peptides.

Opioid Peptides

At the outset we must clarify some terminology. The term endorphin (from *endo*genous m*orphine*) refers to all endogenous peptides with morphine-like activity, including met-enkephalin, leu-enkephalin and β-endorphin. The receptors for these peptides were originally studied as the "opiate receptors" and were first demonstrated in brain about 6 years ago by three independent groups using either [^{3}H]naloxone (184), [^{3}H]dihydromorphine (243), or [^{3}H]etorphine (228) as the binding ligand. These "opiate receptors" have been the subject of numerous reviews both before (90,226,233) and subsequent to (160,227,246,254) the discovery of the endogenous opioid peptides, their natural ligands. The term opiate refers to substances derived from opium, whereas the term opioid refers to all substances with opiate-like pharmacological properties.

On the basis of the extensive pharmacology and structure-activity data for opiates, both from *in vivo* studies and studies with tissues, such as guinea pig ileum and mouse vas deferens *in vitro,* the existence of specific receptors was assumed long before they were demonstrated in the brain with labeled ligands. The successful demonstration of the latter began with the suggestion by Goldstein et al. (92) to use the stereospecificity of the opiates to reveal the true receptor. Stereospecific receptors were defined as being measured by the proportion of labeled ligand binding that was prevented by an excess of unlabeled levorphanol, but not its inactive *enan*tiomer, dextrorphan. In these experiments, however, only 2% of the binding to mouse brain homogenate appeared to be stereospecific. The use of labeled ligands of very high specific radioactivity, which allowed the use of very low concentrations of ligand, and also the rapid but thorough washing of the membrane preparation to reduce nonspecific binding, were refinements that allowed the subsequent groups (184,228,243) to clearly demonstrate stereospecific binding as a much larger proportion of total binding.

Properties of the Opiate Receptor

Stereospecific binding of opiates is not observed in non-nervous tissue but is localized to synaptic membranes prepared from the crude mitochondrial pellet of nervous tissues such as brain or myenteric plexus of guinea pig ileum (183). These receptors probably occur at both presynaptic and postsynaptic neuronal sites (5,130,137,189,270,271). Sodium ions decrease agonist binding but enhance antagonist binding, providing a means to distinguish between such ligands and prompting suggestions of separate receptive sites for agonists versus antagonists, or changes in conformational state of the same site (227,254). Stereospecific binding sites for the opiates have been demonstrated in every vertebrate species studied, but not in invertebrates (181). High-affinity opiate receptors have also been demonstrated in a cell line of nervous origin, a mouse neuroblastoma x rat glioma hybrid (NG 108–15), with specificity for a series of ligands similar to that of synaptic plasma membranes (86,127). The ontogenetic development of opiate receptors in the brain of rat and guinea pig has been studied by several groups (40,45). The rate of increase of opiate binding in the rat is greatest (three- to fourfold) between the midfetal stage and 3 weeks postpartum, then becomes more gradual (about twofold) until adulthood (10 to 20 weeks). The changes are due to increases in numbers of receptors rather than affinity.

Stereospecific opiate binding is saturable and saturation occurs at about 0.25 pmol drug bound per mg of protein in whole brain homogenate, which is equivalent to about 12 to 15 pmoles per g wet weight of brain tissue (227). Evidence for participation of protein in the binding site is provided by the high lability to proteolytic enzymes and sulfhydryl reagents (177,228,243). The receptors also appear to be disrupted by phospholipase A_2, but are not affected by phospholipase C, ribonuclease, deoxyribonuclease, or neuraminidase (177). Cerebroside sulfate will bind opiates in a stereospecific fashion, but there is some question as to what relevance this has to the actual opiate receptors (147,160). A correlation has been observed in several studies between the relative binding affinities and relative analgesic potencies of a large number of different ligands (46,184, 235,261). The stereospecificity and saturability of the high-affinity binding sites and the good correlation of affinity with analgesic potency for a large number of opiates provides evidence that the binding studies are identifying pharmacologically relevant receptors. And now there is also evidence for their physiological relevance, which we will discuss.

Endogenous Peptide Ligands

The discovery of opioid peptides in the brain (115,247) and the growing evidence that the enkephalins (116) are neurotransmitters in the brain (72) places the "opiate receptors" in a new light. Thus, the "opiate receptors" appear to be physiological receptors for endogenous opioid peptide ligands. These endogenous ligands include met-enkephalin, leu-enkephalin, and β-endorphin, for which there is convincing evidence of physiological roles in brain. There is little evidence for such a role for α-endorphin or γ-endorphin (146). Thus, there are multiple ligands and possibly more than one receptor type even for one ligand. Since none of the binding studies yet has criteria for distinguishing these, it is clear that the binding studies to date may be examining heterogeneous populations of receptors. The one unifying aspect of all these receptors is that they recognize opioids; since all natural ligands identified to date are peptides, I prefer to refer to these receptors from now on as opioid peptide receptors. Both met- and leu-enkephalin bind the opioid receptors with affinities comparable to that of morphine (17,30,225), as determined by their ability to inhibit the binding of [^{3}H]dihydromorphine or [^{3}H]naloxone.

A difficulty arises in measuring the affinity of the enkephalins for the receptors at 25° or 37°C because of rapid enzymatic degradation (225). This degradation is minimized by incubating samples at 0°C or by adding bacitracin (50 μg/ml) to incubations at higher temperatures (225). The binding of the enkephalins is reduced (12- to 20-fold) in the presence of sodium and is slightly enhanced in the presence of manganese (225), consistent with roles as agonist ligands. Binding studies have also been done with [^{3}H]met-enkephalin as labeled ligand (222), and Scatchard analysis (213) revealed two binding sites with dissociation constants of 1.8 and 5.8 nM. The maximal number of high-affinity binding sites for [^{3}H]met-enkephalin in whole rat brain minus cerebellum is about 30 pmoles per g brain (222).

Multiple Opioid Receptors

Martin (153) earlier suggested that there may be more than one opiate receptor; more recently he and his colleagues (88,154) have proposed three receptors—the mu, the kappa, and the sigma receptor—on the basis of pharmacological studies in chronic spinal dog.

Studies of the binding characteristics of the enkephalins have also provided evidence for the existence of multiple opioid receptors (89,148,222,245,246). Kosterlitz and colleagues (148), for example, have reported that leu-enkephalin and met-enkephalin are more effective at inhibiting the binding of [^{3}H]-leu-enkephalin than of [^{3}H]naloxone whereas morphine and naloxone are more effective at inhibiting [^{3}H]naloxone binding. β-Endorphin, on the other hand, was equally effective versus [^{3}H]leu-enkephalin and [^{3}H]naloxone binding. Snyder and colleagues (222) similarly reported that the enkephalins had lower IC$_{50}$'s (concentration reducing labeled ligand binding by 50%) versus [^{3}H]met-enkephalin than versus [^{3}H]dihydromorphine or [^{3}H]naloxone. Morphine, naloxone, and other opiates had the reverse preference and β-endorphin was equally effective versus all three [^{3}H]ligands. Terenius (245) obtained similar results, which suggested the existence of three kinds of opioid binding sites. Kosterlitz and colleagues (89), furthermore, have reported that the number of binding sites for enkephalins, determined by Scatchard analysis, is greater than the number determined for dihydromorphine.

The above data are interpreted as support for the hypothesis of multiple opioid peptide receptors in the vertebrate brain.

Evidence for this multiple receptor concept has also derived from studies of isolated vas deferens from mouse and ileum from guinea pig. These tissues have been shown to possess opioid receptors very similar to those in the brain (131). In the guinea pig ileum, met-enkephalin, β-endorphin, and morphine are roughly equipotent, whereas in the mouse vas deferens, met-enkephalin is up to 60 times more potent than normorphine and β-endorphin (77,148,258). The pA$_2$ value (215) of naloxone versus met-enkephalin in the mouse vas deferens is different from that versus normorphine, indicating that the two ligands are acting preferentially on two different populations of receptors in this tissue (77,148). Kosterlitz and colleagues (148) have proposed that the receptor preferred by normorphine may be the mu receptor and have suggested that the receptor preferred by enkephalin be called the delta receptor. The guinea pig ileum apparently contains only or predominantly the mu receptor. How these receptor types identified in peripheral tissues relate to the proposed multiple receptor types in the brain is not yet clear.

Regional Distribution of Opioid Peptide Receptors in the Brain

Even before the discovery of the endogenous peptide ligands, the distribution in different brain regions of receptors for these materials was mapped by several groups of investigators using labeled opiate ligands in several species, including man, monkey, and rat (106,134,184). These receptors are widely distributed throughout the brain but are not uniform in number between different areas, indicating multiple hormonal and/or transmitter roles with differences in contribution to neuronal activity in different areas subserving different functions. The distribution of [³H]etorphine binding in human brain obtained at autopsy is shown in Table 1 (106). Of particular interest is the high level of binding associated with regions of the limbic system, which probably play a role in regulating emotional phenomena. Opiates are known to influence the emotional response to pain more than its perception. The limbic system is also one of the areas with the highest concentrations of enkephalins. Indeed, the distribution of the opioid peptides in general is closely correlated to the distribution of opioid receptors (15,66,109,210,223,224,267). Autoradiographic studies have allowed localization of receptor binding in intact animals, and the distribution observed with this technique agrees well with the results of the *in vitro* binding studies (3,4,182). Of particular interest are the relatively high levels of both receptors and opioid peptides in the hypothalamus. Immunohistochemical studies revealed that many hypothalamic nuclei contain groups of enkephalin cell bodies (109). These include the preoptic periventricular nucleus, the medial preoptic nucleus, the paraventricular nucleus, the ventromedial nucleus, the dorsal and ventral premammillary nuclei, the perifornical area, and the arcuate nucleus. Furthermore, nearly all hypothalamic nuclei appear to contain moderate to high concentrations of enkephalin fibers and terminals. In particular, immunofluorescence localizations revealed enkephalin-positive nerve terminals within the external layer of the median eminence. These findings suggest that this opioid peptide has a role in neuroendocrine regulation and there is functional evidence for this.

Role of Hypothalamic Opioid Peptides and Receptors in Neuroendocrine Regulation

The presence of an enkephalinergic interneuronal system in the hypothalamus regulating the descending control of growth hormone and prolactin release from

TABLE 1. *Distribution of [³H]etorphine binding in human brain*[a]

High Binding (0.44–0.23 pmole/mg protein)	
Olfactory trigone[b]	Centromedian nucleus of thalamus[b]
Amygdala[b]	Preoptic area and supraoptic nucleus[b]
Septal nuclei[b]	Cingulate gyrus[b]
Supraorbital gyrus of frontal lobe[b]	Dorsomedian nucleus of thalamus[b]
Parahippocampal gyrus[b]	Frontal lobe cortex[b]
Periventricular gray matter[b]	Pulvinar of thalamus
Temporal lobe[b]	

Moderate Binding (0.21–0.15 pmole/mg protein)	
Caudate nucleus	Olfactory bulb
Parietal lobe cortex	Periaqueductal gray
Hypothalamus[b]	Putamen
Ventral anterior nucleus of thalamus	Ventral posterolateral nucleus of thalamus

Low Binding (0.12–0.07 pmole/mg protein)	
Occipital lobe cortex	Cerebellar cortex
Corpora quadrigemina	Pretectum
Hippocampus[b]	Substantia nigra
Globus pallidus	Area postrema

Very Low Binding (0.05–0 pmole/mg protein)	
Mammillary bodies	Olives
Medullary sensory nuclei	Dentate nucleus of cerebellum
Cerebral white matter	Tegmentum of mid pons
Posterolateral nucleus of thalamus	Pineal gland
Red nucleus	Pituitary gland

[a] Adapted from Hiller et al., ref. 106, with permission.
[b] Indicates components of the limbic system or regions associated with the limbic system.

the anterior pituitary has been postulated (78), and evidence for this has been obtained (42,94,136,203,220). The partially metabolically protected analogs of the enkephalins, (D-ala²-met⁵)- and (D-ala²-leu⁵)-enkephalinamide, as well as morphine sulfate, at doses in the range of 1 to 20 mg/kg subcutaneously, caused significant dose-dependent elevations of serum GH and PRL (220). These effects were antagonized by naloxone in a dose-dependent fashion but naloxone was more potent at antagonizing morphine than either of the enkephalins. Indeed, naloxone alone, in naive animals, inhibited the release of these hormones and the dose response curve for this inhibitory effect was coincident with its curve for antagonism of the opioid peptides, suggesting that its direct effect was due to antagonism of endogenous opioids. Several lines of evidence suggested that the effects described are the result of a central action of the opioid agonists and antagonist. Neither morphine, the enkephalins, nor naloxone have a direct action on isolated pituitary (94,203,220) and, furthermore, in the intact animal the compounds are active after intracerebral administration (42,136,203). An enkephalin analog has been reported to increase serum GH and PRL in man, also (256).

The above findings suggest that opioid peptides are released from interneurons in the hypothalamus to serve the physiological role of regulating the release of hypothalamic factors, probably growth hormone releasing hormone (GHRH) and dopamine, which control the secretion of GH and PRL as depicted in Fig. 2. In support of this proposed mechanism, endorphins have been recently demonstrated to decrease the turnover of dopamine in the median eminence of the rat (57). The effect on GH is presumed to be via GHRH, since opioids still stimulate GH release when somatostatin is neutralized by excess somatostatin antiserum (62). The PRL and GH responses are not equally sensitive to the opioids, and other differences between the two systems have also been reported (136). That these differences may be due to different opioid systems acting on different opioid receptors receives support from structure activity studies using a series of different ligands (C. J. Sharr, unpublished observation). Studies with the opioid antagonist, naloxone, have, furthermore, provided evidence for a physiological role for endogenous opioids in stress- and suckling-induced release of prolactin (136,254). Other studies with opioid agonists and antagonists have suggested roles for the endogenous opioid peptides in the endocrine events leading to sexual maturation (14) and to sexual activity after maturation (158,178).

Electrophysiological and Behavioral Effects of Opioid Receptor Activation

The technique of microiontophoresis provides a means of examining the effects of activation of receptors on neurons in the brain of intact animals. The opioid peptides are unique among neurally-active peptides in that the full array of pharmacological tools (many potent and metabolically stable agonists, potent and specific antagonists, and inactive stereoisomers) is available to allow convincing demonstration of the results of activation of the "genuine" receptors. The effects on neuronal activity of activation of opioid receptors were studied with the microiontophoretic technique before the discovery of the endogenous ligands, using morphine as activator (18,51,212). The characterization of the opioid

---

FIG. 2. Schematic representation of proposed roles of hypothalamic enkephalinergic **(ENK)** interneurons providing stimulatory effect on GH and PRL release from anterior pituitary. The opioid peptides appear to at least partly stimulate PRL release through inhibition of dopamine **(DA)** release. DA is certainly capable of exerting a direct inhibitory effect in the anterior pituitary after release into the portal system, although there is some controversy whether it may act partly through stimulation of the release of an unknown prolactin inhibiting factor (219). It is not known whether enkephalinergic neurons have also a postsynaptic interaction with DA cell bodies in the hypothalamus, as has been demonstrated in the locus coeruleus and A_2 catecholaminergic region (189). The opioid peptides apparently stimulate GH secondary to stimulation of GHRH rather than to inhibition of somatostatin (60). Since the opioid peptides are inhibitory to neurons it is postulated that they may stimulate GHRH by a disinhibitory mechanism, as is reported to occur in the hippocampus (272). Thus, there may be two types of enkephalinergic receptor in the basal hypothalamus (types A and B), each associated with different groups of neurons related to PRL and GH release, respectively (there is some evidence for this; *see text*). It should be emphasized that aspects of this proposed scheme are still hypothetical.

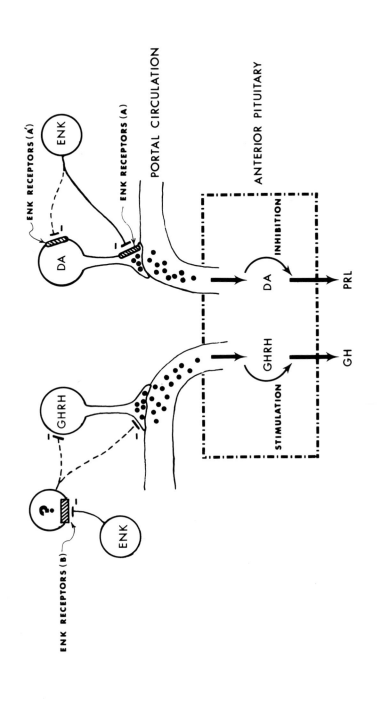

receptors and their regional distribution in the brain, together with the regional distribution of the endogenous peptide ligands, has greatly facilitated the design and interpretation of such experiments. The investigations of the effects of opiates and opioid peptides on single-unit activity in the brain has been the subject of several recent reviews (72,169,272). The opiates and opioid peptides are predominently inhibitory on neurons in brain regions where stereospecific receptors have been demonstrated (72,74–76,169,272). The majority of these depressant actions could be prevented or reduced by the narcotic antagonist naloxone. A smaller proportion of nonspecific excitatory actions were also seen but these were more frequent with morphine than with the opioid peptides, and were more frequent in areas without significant levels of stereospecific opioid receptors than in areas with high levels of such binding sites (74–76). Furthermore, the Phe[1]-analog of enkephalin (H-Phe-Gly-Gly-Phe-Met-OH), which is inactive as an analgesic and on receptors in mouse vas deferens (74), produced no naloxone-reversible depressions of single units (74-76), thus providing evidence of a correlation between the electrophysiological effects and behavioral effects. Although the bulk of evidence suggested that the enkephalins may be inhibitory transmitters in specified brain regions, apparent exceptions to this general rule were the naloxone-sensitive excitation of Renshaw cells in feline spinal cord (48) and of pyramidal cells in hippocampus (105,168). Subsequent experiments revealed, however, that the excitations of pyramidal cells in hippocampus were actually secondary to naloxone-sensitive inhibition of hippocampal basket cells (272).

Apparently, these spontaneously active gabaergic interneurons tonically depress pyramidal cell discharge. Thus, inhibition of the basket cell firing disinhibits the pyramidal cells, resulting in an increase in their discharge rate. It is not known at this time whether or not the excitations in spinal cord are also due to such a disinhibitory mechanism.

The receptors in the region of periaqueductal gray (PAG) matter (106,134, 180,223) are of particular interest because they may mediate a portion of the analgesic response to opiates and opioid alkaloids. Enkephalin levels are high in this region, in correlation with the receptors (223), and focal electrical stimulation (155) or microinjection of opioids (265) in this area produces naloxone-reversible analgesia. Nociceptive stimuli modulate the firing of neurons in this area, and the surrounding reticular tegmentum and the basal and nociceptive-stimuli conditioned activity of these neurons can be inhibited or accelerated by systemically or microiontophoretically administered opioids (76,85,100,156). The above findings can be explained by assuming an inhibitory enkephalinergic interneuron in the region of the PAG, which regulates the activity of a second inhibitory interneuron, which, in turn, inhibits the discharge of a neuron whose axons leave the PAG and activate raphespinal neurons to ultimately inhibit nociception (75,76,149). Thus, the opioid-induced excitations in the PAG (85) could be disinhibitions secondary to inhibition of inhibitory interneurons, as suggested for the mechanism of opioid activation of hippocampal pyramidal cells (272). The above scheme best explains all the available information but is still hypothetical. It has been suggested that the importance of the PAG opioid system may vary between species (4) and, furthermore, other brain areas besides the PAG have also been implicated as playing a role in nociception and analgesia (265). Opioid receptors and opioid peptides have also been demonstrated in brain regions not implicated in nociception or analgesia; the opioids depress cell firing in these regions, as in the regions related to nociception (74, 75,272). Thus, the opioids and their receptors probably have behavioral roles beyond that of pain perception. Frenk et al. (79) have reported that enkephalins produce seizure activity by acting on receptors that differ in both properties and location from those that mediate the analgesic activity of these peptides. The opioids, furthermore, have been reported to produce seizure-like activity in the hippocampus (168). Some of the behavioral effects of the opioid peptides other than analgesia have been the subject of several recent review articles (16,218). Some of these effects include grooming, hyperactivity, immobility, and rigidity, all of which are antagonizable by naloxone. These peptides have also shown nonopiate-like effects on active and passive avoidance behavior (218).

Mechanisms of Opioid Receptor Activity

NG108-15 hybrid cells derived from fusion of mouse neuroblastoma clone N18TG-2 with rat glioma clone C6BU-1 are richly endowed with opioid receptors, apparently coupled to adenylate cyclase (127). The result of binding of opiates or opioid peptides to these receptors is inhibition of adenylate cyclase in homogenates and inhibition of cyclic AMP accumulation in intact cells (127,128,248). The opioids do not inhibit adenylate cyclase of the glioma parent, which lacks opioid receptors (127,128). The effect on adenylate cyclase is antagonized by naloxone and the dissociation constant determined for naloxone in direct binding studies agrees closely with dissociation constants determined for antagonism of opioid inhibition of adenylate cyclase (128). Morphine has been shown to inhibit prostaglandin E_1 stimulation of adenylate cyclase activity in rat brain homogenate (44). Thus, opioid peptides may be neurotransmitters and/or hormones that regulate neuronal activity by suppression of the activation of adenylate cyclase.

Electrophysiological studies have suggested a possible consequence in neuronal membranes of inhibition of adenylate cyclase by activation of opioid receptors. Zieglgansberger and associates (270,271) have recorded intracellularly from neurons in spinal cord of cats; they observed that opioids applied microiontophoretically depress basal and excitatory transmitter-induced firing of these neurons without hyperpolarizing the cells. They suggest that opioids may act by impairing the Na^+ influx triggered at the postsynaptic membrane by excitatory neurotransmitters, such as glutamate and acetylcholine. There is, however, no evidence as yet directly correlating inhibition of adenylate cyclase with this impairment of Na^+ influx. Other authors (126,170), furthermore, have reported that the result of activation of opioid receptors in myenteric plexus of guinea pig ileum is a hyperpolarization of neurons.

Substance P

Substance P (SP), although discovered some 43 years before the enkephalins, also remains putative as a neurotransmitter, and its receptors are far less well characterized than are the opioid receptors. SP was first extracted from equine brain and intestine by Von Euler and Gaddum in 1931 (255) as a material characterized by hypotensive and smooth muscle stimulant properties. Leeman and coworkers (35,36), some 35 to 40 years later, serendipitously found a "sialogen" in bovine hypothalamic extracts, which they purified and realized had the properties of SP, and subsequently sequenced and synthesized. Studer et al. (240) subsequently purified and sequenced a material isolated from equine intestine, using the original methodology (255), which turned out to be identical to the hypothalamic substance identified by Leeman and coworkers.

This peptide, still referred to as SP, has the sequence: H-Arg-Pro-Lys-Pro-Gln-Gln-Phe-Phe-Gly-Leu-Met-NH$_2$. Studies with crude SP before its purification and identification indicated that mammalian spinal dorsal root contains a larger amount of SP than does the ventral root (179). This finding led Lembeck (144) to propose that it may be an excitatory transmitter of primary sensory neurons. Since the identification of SP, much work has been done with synthetic material that lends support to this proposal. This and the earlier work has been extensively reviewed over the last 4 years (6,29,65,141,175,176).

The differential distribution of SP in the central nervous system has been studied using both bioassay and radioimmunoassay (23,125,179). Exceptionally high levels have been found in substantia nigra, interpeduncular nucleus, and several hypothalamic nuclei. Levels in whole rat brain are approximately 50 pmol/g wet weight of tissue, ranging from about 10 pmoles/g in cerebellum to about 1,800 pmoles/g in substantia nigra. Immunohistochemical studies by Hokfelt and colleagues (65,110,111) revealed the presence of SP in neuronal cell bodies, fibers, and nerve terminals in various hypothalamic nuclei. SP fibers were absent from the external layer of the median eminence, suggesting that there is no neuroendocrine terminal system containing SP in rodent hypothalamus capable of affecting anterior pituitary function via the portal vessels.

SP does, however, influence GH and PRL release in rats, presumably secondarily to effects on somatostatin and opioid peptides at the level of the hypothalamus (39). Extrahypothalamic cell bodies have been seen in the amygdala, nucleus interstitialis stria terminals, medial habenular nucleus, interpeduncular nucleus, periaqueductal central gray, dorsal tegmental nucleus, commissural nucleus, and nuclei raphe magnus and pallidus. Terminals were seen in the amygdala, nucleus interstitialis stria terminalis, lateral septal nucleus, zona reticulata of substantia nigra, interpeduncular nucleus, periaqueductal central gray, nucleus parabrachialis dorsalis, part of nucleus of spinal trigeminal tract, nucleus of solitary tract, and commissural nucleus. Some neuronal pathways probably utilizing SP as neurotransmitter are the habenulo-interpeduncular tract, a striatonigral pathway, a descending projection from the raphe nuclei to the spinal cord, and the pathway from dorsal spinal ganglion to dorsal horn of spinal cord (65,110,113,120,124,162,176). The peroxidase-antiperoxidase technique of sternberger (238) has been utilized to demonstrate at the electron microscope level that SP is contained in synaptic vesicles in axon terminals (189,190). In these studies it was demonstrated that axon terminals containing vesicles labeled for SP, and also terminals containing enkephalin, synapse with dendrites of catecholaminergic neurons in locus ceruleus and the A_2 region of rat brain (189). As a potential neurotransmitter, SP should be released from nerve terminals under the appropriate conditions and this has been demonstrated for several neural sites, including substantia nigra, hypothalamus, spinal cord, and even sensory neurons in culture (118,119,121,163,173,214). Several of these studies, furthermore, provide evidence that GABA and opioid peptides may regulate the release of SP (119,121,163).

After neuronal release, fulfillment of synaptic transmission or modulation requires receptor activation. Receptors for SP have not been nearly as well characterized as have the opioid receptors. Indeed, there has been only one report of a successful demonstration of SP receptors (165). Nakata et al. (165) observed specific saturable binding of [^{3}H]SP to synaptic membranes from rabbit brain. The apparent maximal number of binding sites in brain stem was 95.7 fmoles/mg protein and the dissociation constant was 2.74 nM. A study of the regional distribution of specific binding revealed the greatest binding in diencephalon, with decreasing levels in the following order: corpus striatum, mesencephalon, dorsal spinal cord, ventral spinal cord, hippocampus, cortex, and pons-medulla. This distribution of binding capacity correlated reasonably well with the distribution of SP itself. Maximum binding affinity appeared to reside not in the parent SP molecule but in smaller C-terminal fragments. The 3-11, 4-11 and 7-11 fragments were less potent than SP in competing with [^{3}H]SP binding, but the 5-11 and 6-11 fragments were 42 and three times as potent, respectively. Studies on rat spinal motoneurons revealed that the C-terminal amino acid sequence is also essential for the motoneuron-depolarizing activity of SP, the 5-11 and 6-11 fragments being more active than SP itself (174). The hypotensive and ileum-contracting properties of SP analogs roughly parallel their motoneuron depolarizing activities (29,266). Two other linear undecapeptides with similar C-terminal amino acid residues, eledoisin and physalaemin, have pharmacological activity similar to SP in many systems (29), but these did not compete well in the binding studies. Eledoisin had only 0.05% the potency of SP and physalaemin was essentially inactive. The above data are very suggestive that the SP receptor has been identified, but they should be considered with caution, since they have not been replicated (232). Lembeck et al. (145) recently reported that brain lipid, possibly phosphatidylserine, binds SP with a very high capacity by a pH dependent process. Since SP would be highly bound at physiological pH the authors suggest that this may be the storage form of SP in the brain. Phosphatidylserine, however, is a major phospholipid in neural membranes and they suggest, therefore, that it may also be related to the membrane receptors for SP.

A number of electrophysiological studies in various regions of the central nervous system where SP and receptors reportedly occur have been undertaken to examine the neuronal effects of SP receptor activation. Low concentrations of SP depolarize motoneurons in isolated frog and rat spinal cord (174,175). This appears to be due to a direct postsynaptic action of SP, which is 1,000 to 9,000 times more potent than glutamate. Baclofen (β-(4-chlorophenyl)-GABA) was reported to antagonize this depolarizing action of SP but does not appear to be a very specific antagonist in most systems (8,49,187,211). Microiontophoretic SP, furthermore, selectively excited nociceptive neurons in laminae IV to VI (104) and laminae I to III (198) of dorsal horn of cat. These results supported the concept of SP as an excitatory transmitter at synapses in dorsal horn of cord associated with nociception. SP has also been reported to depolarize neurons in the interpeduncular nucleus in an isolated guinea pig brain stem preparation (171). In accord with the *in vitro* data, microiontophoretic SP excites neurons in the interpeduncular nucleus of intact anesthetized rat (211). SP has been shown to excite neurons in other SP-containing areas as well, such as mesencephalic reticular formation (257), substantia nigra (49,257), locus ceruleus (99), and cerebral cortex (188). Thus, SP appears to function as an excitatory neurotransmitter in the various brain regions where it occurs and probably acts by a direct depolarization secondary to activation of postsynaptic receptors. There is evidence that the effects of SP, like those of other putative neurotransmitters, may be mediated by cyclic AMP (60,166).

SP has many pharmacological effects, such as spasmogenic activity on smooth muscle, hypotensive activity, sedative effects, diuresis, and induction of salivary secretion (29). Placed directly into the substantia nigra, SP produced retrograde amnesia for a passive avoidance task in rats (117). Intracerebral SP caused drinking in pigeons but depressed angiotensin-induced drinking in rats (71). The physiological roles these pharmacological actions may reflect remain to be established. There have been several reports that analgesic activity occurred after low doses of SP were given intracerebrally or systemically (73,151,236,239). This analgesic activity could be antagonized by naloxone, indicating an interaction with an endogenous opioid peptide system. Indeed, the distribution of SP in the brain is similar to that of the enkephalin (65,66,112). Frederickson et al. (73) reported a biphasic effect of intracerebral SP on nociception: low doses produced analgesia, whereas higher doses were ineffective. These higher doses of SP, however, produced analgesia when they were given to mice pretreated with baclofen and produced hyperalgesia when given to mice pretreated with naloxone. They suggested that the analgesia may have been caused by the release of endogenous opioids and raised the possibility that there may be more than one receptor type for SP. There is some support for this from electrophysiological studies at the single cell level. Davies and Dray (50) reported that microiontophoretically-applied SP had naloxone-reversible, morphine-like effects on some spinal neurons, but on other spinal neurons it also had nonmorphine-like effects. SP, moreover, is reported to have both pre- and postsynaptic actions at Mauthnerfiber-giant fiber synapses in the hatchetfish (237). The presence and properties of these receptors for SP in the brain remain to be established; the availability of inactive stereoisomers and specific antagonists would greatly facilitate this endeavor.

Angiotensin

Angiotensin II (AII), an octapeptide (H-Asp-Arg-Val-Tyr-Ile-His-Pro-Phe-OH) that is the active form of angiotensin, is produced via several precursors. Renin, a proteolytic enzyme secreted into the bloodstream by the juxtaglomerular cells in arterioles of the kidney, converts an α_2-globulin (angiotensinogen) produced in the liver to the inactive decapeptide, angiotensin I (AII-His-Leu-OH). Angiotensin I is converted to the active AII by converting enzyme, which occurs in the highest concentrations in lung but occurs also in other sites, such as brain.

The physiological mechanisms for maintaining body fluid balance include thirst, which stimulates water intake; the secretion of vasopressin, which helps prevent water loss; and the secretion of aldosterone, which helps prevent sodium depletion. These mechanisms are mediated by the actions of angiotensin on the brain, although AII apparently does not readily cross the blood-brain barrier (BBB). There are two means by which this may be accomplished. AII in the peripheral circulation may produce central effects by action on the circumventricular organs [subformical organ (SFO); organum vasculosum (OV) of lamina terminalis; median eminence; area postrema; pineal; subcommissural organ; and infundibular recess] where the BBB is weak or absent. Of these sites, the SFO and OV seem the most sensitive to the dipsogenic action of AII. The other possibility is that the effects may be mediated in the brain by AII endogenous to the brain. Indeed, all components of the renin angiotensin system are reported to occur in the brain, where they are referred to as the isorenin-angiotensin system (see Chapter 16). AII is formed in biologically active concentrations when exogenous renin is injected into the cerebral ventricles. AII produces drinking behavior, an increase in blood pressure, and release of vasopressin when injected directly into the cerebrospinal fluid, from which it would not have as ready access to the circumventricular sites as after systemic administration. However, it is not yet totally clear whether intravenous and intraventricular AII act on the same or a different set of receptor sites. The question of whether or not there is a physiologically functional brain isorenin-angiotensin system mediating blood pressure regulation and body fluid balance remains under debate. The above questions have been the subject of several recent reviews (81,82, 185,199).

Peripherally, AII has a potent constricting effect on vascular and nonvascular smooth muscle, stimulates the release of aldosterone from the adrenal cortex, and potentiates the activity of sympathetic nerve endings. Characteristics of AII receptors in various peripheral systems have been recently reviewed (55). Such binding sites are located on the plasma membrane and there appear to be two classes of sites. In adrenal cortex there are high-affinity sites with a calculated dissociation constant (K_D = dissociation rate constant/association rate constant) of K_D = 0.3 nM, which comprise 25 to 33% of the sites, and lower-affinity sites with K_D = 4 nM, which make up the remainder (59). A dispersed canine adrenal cell system has been used to correlate the binding process with the physiological response of aldosterone production (59). These studies demonstrated the biological significance of the AII binding sites of the adrenal glomerulosa cell, confirming their identity as peptide hormone receptors.

Similar results have been obtained for AII receptors in brain membranes. These receptors have been characterized by their binding properties *in vitro* and their biological effects both *in vitro* and *in vivo*. Bennet and Snyder (9) and Sirett et al. (231) demonstrated specific, reversible, saturable, high-affinity binding of [125I]AII to membranes from rat and calf brain. Degradation of peptide was prevented by adding glucagon to the final incubation medium and a proteolytic enzyme inhibitor in preincubation and incubation media (9) or by the addition of EDTA to the incubation medium (231). The dissociation binding constant of this high-affinity binding was 0.2 nM at 37°C in one study (9) and 0.9 nM at 22°C in the other (231). Binding was associated with particulate matter and was concentrated in the crude microsomal fraction. The biological relevance of these binding sites was examined by competition studies with analogs and fragments of AII (9). These various peptides competed for binding sites with potencies that correlated with their *in vivo* biological potencies and also with their binding potencies in bovine adrenal cortex. Angiotensin I, the 3-8 hexapeptide, and 4-8 pentapeptide were weaker than AII whereas angiotensin III (desAsp1-AII) was slightly more potent than AII. Several AII antagonists, such as Sar1-leu8-AII, were also somewhat more potent than AII. In calf brain, AII binding was restricted almost exclusively to the cerebellar cortex (220 fmoles/g) and deep nuclei (35 fmoles/g), but small amounts were also found in the choroid plexus of fourth ventricle (12.1 fmoles/g) and the superior colliculus (7.7 fmoles/g). Binding was observed in all areas examined in rat brain but was highest in septum, thalamus, hypothalamus, midbrain, and brainstem. The highest binding of all tissues occurred in the lateral septum and the highest binding in the brainstem was associated with the area postrema. These areas of high binding are for the most part areas believed to mediate the central effects of AII. The role of the very high levels of AII binding in calf cerebellar cortex is not yet clear.

In more recent studies, Scatchard analysis indicated two components of binding in calf cerebellar membranes (10,11). With [125I]Sar1-Leu8-AII as ligand there was a high-affinity site with a dissociation constant of 0.03 nM and a low-affinity component with a dissociation constant of 0.4 nM. The apparent maximal number of binding sites for the high- and low-affinity components were 0.44 and 2.2 pmoles/g, respectively. Two components, although of lower affinity (6.9 and 22 nM), were also seen for binding in bovine adrenal cortex, whereas only a single component of specific saturable binding (1.5 nM; 18.8 pmoles/g) was observed in rabbit uterine membranes. It was also found in these studies that AII receptor binding in calf cerebellum and bovine adrenal cortex are regulated by sodium ions, but the influence of sodium does not effectively differentiate agonist and antagonist binding. At physiological (150 mM) sodium ion concentration, both types of ligands saturate with demonstrable high- and low-affinity components. Reduction to 10 mM sodium causes loss of detectable high-affinity binding sites and the appearance of an even lower-affinity site than that observed at 150 mM sodium.

Localized groups of neurons with functional receptors for AII have also been identified, using the techniques of electrophysiological recording and microiontophoresis. In one of the initial studies, microelectrodes were used to record intracellularly from organ-cultured canine supraoptic nucleus cells (208). Superfusion of the explant with AII induced neuronal spiking in a dose-dependent fashion. The specificity of this response was demonstrated by the selective ability of AII antagonists, such as Cys^8-AII and Sar^1-$Ileu^8$-AII, to inhibit AII-induced spiking but not the similar effects of glutamate or nicotine. It was concluded that there are specific AII membrane receptors on supraoptic nucleus neurons with probable physiological significance, such as stimulation of vasopressin secretion. There remained a question, however, as to whether the origin of AII intended for these receptors was circulating plasma, cerebrospinal fluid, or nerve terminals synapsing in the supraoptic nucleus. Felix and coworkers (69,70,186) have shown that surface application of AII to the SFO in anesthetized cats elicits an increase in neuronal firing, similar to the findings described above for supraoptic nucleus, and they followed this with microiontophoretic studies. AII and also some fragments accelerated the firing rate of single units in the SFO, and this could be antagonized by the AII antagonist, saralasin. Saralasin itself produced inhibition of firing of some cells; this was speculated to be due to antagonism of endogenous AII. The authors concluded that there are specific AII responsive neurons in the SFO but acknowledged that neither the function of these neurons nor the source of the AII intended to activate them has been established. There is evidence, however, that the subfornical organ (SFO) participates in the control of drinking behavior in mammals by a mechanism involving AII (229). Microiontophoretic experiments have also revealed that AII excites a high proportion of neurons in the medial preoptic area, many of which are also stimulated by acetylcholine chloride (97). Antagonism by saralasin provided evidence of the specificity of a proportion (60%) of these excitatory responses to AII. There was a distribution of responsive cells between the preoptic area and more dorsal areas not bordering the third ventricle. Within the preoptic area, directly adjacent to the third ventricle, 66% of the cells were excited by

AII, whereas few cells in the nucleus of the anterior commissure responded to AII. These results are consistent with evidence identifying the region of the anterior third ventricle in general as an important site for the dipsogenic and pressor actions of AII (26,108) and more specifically, the medial preoptic area itself for the dipsogenic effects (2).

In summary, there is evidence that AII acts in the brain to elicit drinking behavior, to increase blood pressure, to release vasopressin, and to release ACTH; periventricular sites are implicated in these responses. For example, the subfornical organ, preoptic region, and region of the anterior third ventricle have been proposed as receptive sites for the drinking response; the area postrema, the subnucleus medialis in cats, and the anterior third ventricle in rats have been proposed for the pressor response; and the supraoptic nucleus has been proposed for the release of vasopressin. Direct ligand binding studies and microiontophoretic studies have provided evidence for the presence of specific receptors in these areas, but a strict correlation with function in each case has not been established, nor has the source of the endogenous AII intended for each receptive site been established. Assays of AII in brain have led to conflicting results concerning its presence and distribution, but immunohistochemical studies demonstrating a wide distribution in brain have led some to propose that AII may reach receptive sites in the central nervous system by both vascular and neuronal channels (37,38).

Thyrotropin Releasing Hormone

About two decades ago, extracts were prepared from hypothalamus that stimulated the secretion of thyrotropin (98,221). The active principle was determined to be a tripeptide, thyrotropin releasing hormone (TRH), with the structure pyroglutamyl-histidyl-prolinamide (27,164). This peptide is secreted from the hypothalamus and acts on the anterior pituitary gland to stimulate the release of thyrotropin and possibly of prolactin (13,259). Radiolabeled TRH binds to sites in membrane fractions of pituitary gland that appear to be specific receptors mediating the actions of TRH on thyrotropin release (95,96,135). The membrane receptors for TRH in pituitary tissue are not fixed in number. Thyroid hormones and TRH itself decrease the number of TRH receptors on pituitary cells, without altering the affinity of the receptors for TRH (107,180). Hydrocortisone increases the number of specific TRH binding sites on pituitary cells (241). Estrogen treatment induces parallel increases in PRL secretion and TRH receptor levels in rat pituitary (52). Indeed, TRH receptor levels in rat pituitary vary with the estrus cycle (53), a two- to threefold difference being observed between the levels at diestrus II (minimum) and those at proestrus (maximum).

TRH appears to have effects on behavior and mood in animals and man, in addition to and independent of the actions on pituitary endocrine function discussed above. Low doses will potentiate the central stimulatory activity of L-dopa in hypophysectomized, as well as in normal, mice (193); it has also been observed to antagonize barbiturate and ethanol narcosis (20,195). Intravenous TRH, furthermore, has been reported to elevate mood in both normal and depressed women (196,260).

TRH has been measured by radioimmunoassay in rat brain, which contains a total of 10 to 20 ng of TRH-like activity (24,172,264). It occurs in most areas of the brain, although levels are very low in cerebellum. The highest levels occur in hypothalamus, which may account for about one-third of the total in the brain, but significant levels also occur in extrahypothalamic areas, such as thalamus, brainstem, and preoptic and septal areas. The highest level of TRH (38.4 ng/mg tissue) was found in the median eminence (24). These findings and the localization of TRH in nerve terminals (7,263) indicate that it may have physiological role as a neurotransmitter in brain.

In support of a neurotransmitter role in the brain, saturable binding of [^{3}H]-TRH to sites in rat brain membranes has been demonstrated (28). The characteristics of this binding to brain membranes resembles the binding to pituitary membranes. Saturable binding in whole brain amounts to 3.3 fmol/mg of tissue, compared to 5.8 fmoles/mg of tissue in pituitary. High- and low-affinity sites have been defined in the brain membranes, as in pituitary. The dissociation constants for the high- and low-affinity binding sites are similar in all brain regions examined except for the cerebellum in which high-affinity binding was not detected. In cerebral cortex, hypothalamus, hippocampus, and midbrain the high-affinity K_D ranged from 32 to 52 nM and the number of sites from 100 to 190 fmoles/mg of protein. The high-affinity K_D was similar in corpus striatum and pons-medulla oblongata (38 and 27 nM, respectively), but there were fewer numbers of sites in these regions (60 and 40 fmoles/mg of protein, respectively). The K_D of the low-affinity site ranged from 0.9 to 9 μM with 30 to 46 pmoles/mg of protein, except in the pons-medulla oblongata and cerebellum, where the number of sites was about one-fifth the level in other sites. For both high- and low-affinity binding the greatest percentage of total sites occurred in the P_2 subcellular fractions, which contain both mitochondria and synaptosomes. Increased potassium (25 and 100 mM) or sodium (100 mM) in the buffer inhibited TRH binding in brain and pituitary but not in liver. The specificity of the binding to brain membranes was shown by the relative potency of optical isomers of TRH and other tripeptide analogs to compete with [^{3}H]-TRH for binding sites. The data support the concept of a physiological function for TRH in the brain, probably as a neurotransmitter.

Reflecting the results of receptor activation, the microiontophoretic application of TRH to neurons in various brain regions produced marked short-term changes in neuronal excitability. Such studies have revealed an inhibitory effect of TRH on neurons in the hypothalamus (63,200) and other brain regions as well (201). Winokur and Beckman (262) reported that hypothalamic and septal neurons responded similarly to microiontophoretic TRH, with 31 of 46 cells in these regions decreasing their firing rate, whereas none of the 12 cells tested in the cerebral cortex was responsive to TRH. None of the cells tested in the septal or hypothalamic regions was excited by TRH, nor were excitatory responses of cortical neurons to acetylcholine potentiated by TRH, as has been previously reported (268). The septal region takes on special significance as the possible site for the central stimulatory activity of TRH. TRH (24) and TRH receptors (28) occur in relatively high levels in the septum, and septal neurons are inhibited by the microiontophoretic application of TRH (262). More recently, the septum has been shown to be the brain site where TRH acts in the smallest amounts (as low as 5 ng) to antagonize pentobarbital narcosis (123).

Vasoactive Intestinal Peptide

Since the original isolation of vasoactive intestinal polypeptide (VIP) from pig small intestine (207), high concentrations of this octacosapeptide (H-His-Ser-Asp-Ala-Val-Phe-Thr-Asp-Asn-Tyr-Thr-Arg-Leu-Arg-Lys-Gln-Met-Ala-Val-Lys-Lys-Tyr-Leu-Asn-Ser-Ileu-Leu-Asn-NH$_2$) have been detected by radio-immunoassay throughout the gastrointestinal tract and central nervous system (12,25,67,87). Immunohistochemical studies, furthermore, revealed VIP-positive cell bodies and terminals in brain (80,140). The highest concentration of VIP in rat brain was found in the cerebral hemispheres, particularly occipital and parietal cortex (12,25). The brain stem, posterior hypothalamus, and pineal gland contained lower amounts, whereas it was not detectable in cerebellum or neurohypophysis. Similar distributions were found in pig and human brain, with the exception that in the human the highest levels were detected in the median eminence (25,209). Further support for its potential role as a neurotransmitter in the brain comes from its localization in vesicles in nerve terminals and the demonstration of a calcium-dependent, potassium-evoked release from central nervous system tissue (12,67,87). The hypothalamic nerve endings containing VIP apparently originate from cell bodies located both within and outside the mediobasal hypothalamus (12).

The specific saturable binding of [^{125}I]VIP has been demonstrated in whole brain membranes from guinea pig (204). Scatchard analysis of the inhibition of binding by cold VIP (at 37°C) revealed the presence of a high-affinity component with a K_D of 36 nM and a maximal binding capacity of 4 pmoles/mg of protein as well as a low-affinity component with a K_D of 285 nM and a maximal binding capacity of 20 pmoles/mg protein. Sodium and potassium, at concentrations greater than 20 mM, inhibited binding, as did calcium and magnesium at concentrations as low as 2 and 5 mM, respectively. Nucleoside triphosphates and diphosphates also inhibited binding. VIP and secretin were the only peptides examined that inhibited binding, and secretin was 200 times less potent than VIP. Neither the parent peptide glucagon nor bombesin, substance P, somatostatin, leu-enkephalin, or the C-terminal octapeptide of pancreozymin inhibited VIP binding. These properties of the VIP receptor in brain are similar to the properties described for VIP receptors in the periphery. It is interesting that VIP, but not the peptides mentioned above, which are relatively inactive at the brain VIP receptor, activates an adenylate cyclase system in the same guinea pig brain membrane preparation (54).

VIP has many powerful actions in the periphery, including systemic vasodilation, stimulation of myocardial contractility, glycogenolysis, lipolysis, stimulation of insulin secretion, inhibition of gastric acid secretion, stimulation of alkaline pancreatic juice flow, and stimulation of small intestinal cAMP and juice secretion; in the brain its functions are unknown. Nevertheless, the demonstration that the same synaptic membrane preparation possesses specific binding sites for VIP and also an adenylate cyclase effector system responsive to VIP, with similar substrate specificity and a guanine nucleotide regulatory site, adds strong support for a physiological neurotransmitter role for this polypeptide in mammalian brain.

Neurotensin

Neurotensin is a tridecapeptide recently isolated from bovine hypothalamic extracts (31), which has the sequence H-Glu-Leu-Tyr-Glu-Asn-Lys-Pro-Arg-Arg-Pro-Tyr-Ileu-Leu-OH (32). Peripherally administered neurotensin produces hypotension, hyperglycemia, pain sensation, and secretion of ACTH, LH, and FSH, among other effects (33). Administered intracerebroventricularly, neurotensin enhances barbiturate effects and produces marked hypothermic and analgesic effects (41,167).

[125I]Neurotensin binds saturably, reversibly, and with high affinity to membrane preparations from rat and calf brain (250). There appears to be only a single population of binding sites, with a K_D of 3.7 nM and a maximal binding capacity of 3.1 pmoles/g for cerebral cortex. The localization of neurotensin itself in rat central nervous system has been studied with immunohistochemical techniques (252). This study revealed the presence of immunoreactive material in cell bodies and processes in the brain and in cells of the anterior pituitary. The material showed a widespread distribution in the brain, with notable densities in the substantia gelatinosa of spinal cord and trigeminal nucleus, central amygdaloid nucleus, anterior pituitary, median eminence, and preoptic and basal hypothalamic areas. There are also marked variations in regional distribution of [125I]neurotensin binding in the brain. The lowest levels of binding are seen in cerebellum and pons-medulla oblongata, and the highest levels occur in cerebral cortex and hypothalamus. High levels of binding are also observed in the thalamus and midbrain, and intermediate levels are seen in the hippocampus and striatum. Thus, the hypothalamus is enriched in both neurotensin and its binding sites, whereas the cerebellar cortex has the lowest levels of both (253). The cerebral cortex has substantial binding sites but little endogenous neurotensin, which is similar to the situation for putative monoamine transmitters in this region.

To date there has been only one study in which an effect of neurotensin applied by microiontophoresis onto neurons in the brain has been demonstrated

(269). In this study neurotensin caused a rapid, reversible inhibition of firing in 13 of 35 cells tested in the vicinity of the locus coeruleus in rat.

Other Peptides

Many other peptides originally discovered to have a peripheral hormonal role in pituitary, gut, or elsewhere have been found to occur in the brain as well. The evidence for a central neurotransmitter role for most of these is not as extensive as for the peptides already discussed above but is sufficient in several cases to require mention here.

Somatostatin or growth hormone release-inhibiting factor is a tetradecapeptide (H-Ala-Gly-Cys-Lys-Asn-Phe-Phe-Try-Lys-Thr-Phe-Thr-Ser-Cys-OH) that was isolated from ovine hypothalamus (19). It was subsequently shown to be distributed widely in the central nervous system, in extrahypothalamic as well as hypothalamic regions, and also in pancreas, gut, and the thyroid (150,191). It has been suggested to be a neurotransmitter in the nervous system, a hormone in the hypophysial portal circulation, and a local (paracrine) effector in gut and pancreas (150,191). In nervous tissue somatostatin is present in cell bodies and nerve terminals and, indeed appears to occur together with norepinephrine in some neurons (150). Using [^{125}I]somatostatin as ligand, functional receptors have been defined in rat pituitary cells in culture (216), but specific binding of somatostatin to plasma membranes in other regions has not yet been reported. There is evidence, however, for an interaction of somatostatin with rat brain opioid receptors (197,244), although in neuroblastoma x glioma hybrid cells it appears that the somatostatin receptors are separate from the opioid receptors (249). Evidence for receptive sites in various brain regions has been provided by several electrophysiologic studies (58,201). A depressant action of microiontophoretic somatostatin was observed (201) on neurons in cerebellar cortex (55% of neurons tested) and in cerebral cortex and hypothalamus (approximately 80% of neurons tested in both areas). When applied to pyramidal cells in rat hippocampal slices *in vitro,* somatostatin had an excitatory effect on spike activity accompanied by a depolarization of the neuron (58). It is not clear if this effect might be the result of a disinhibition, as was demonstrated for the excitatory effects of endorphins on hippocampol pyramidal neurons (272). The function of somatostatin in the brain is not known, nor is it clear whether the neuronal effects mentioned above are physiological or pharmacological. Intracerebral somatostatin, however, results in an increase in monoamine turnover in various brain regions (83), and behavioral responses to intracerebral somatostatin have also been reported (43,192,202), including an analgesic effect (101).

The adenohypophysial hormone adrenocorticotropic hormone (ACTH) is found not only in the pituitary but also in the brain and gastrointestinal tract, and its distribution in the latter sites is not altered by hypophysectomy (132,139). Specific binding sites for ACTH in the brain have not yet been demonstrated, but ACTH and various fragments and analogs do have potent behavioral effects

TABLE 2. *Summary of brain peptides reviewed*

Peptide [a]	Location of receptors [b]	References [c]
1. Opioid peptides Met- and Leu-enkephalin H-Tyr-Gly-Phe-Met-OH, H-Tyr-Gly-Gly-Phe-Leu-OH β-Endorphin H-Tyr-Gly-Gly-Phe-Met-Thr-Ser-Glu-Lys-Ser-Gln-Thr- -Pro-Leu-Val-Thr-Leu-Phe-Lys-Asn-Ala-Ile-Ile-Lys-Asn- -Ala-Tyr-Lys-Lys-Gly-Gly-OH (human)	See Table 1	3,4,15,66,106,107,109, 134,182,184,210, 223,224,267
2. Substance P H-Arg-Pro-Lys-Pro-Gln-Gln-Phe-Phe-Gly-Leu-Met-NH₂	Diencephalon, corpus striatum, mesencephalon, spinal cord, hip- pocampus, cortex, brainstem	23,65,110,111,125,145, 165,179,232
3. Angiotensin II H-Asp-Arg-Val-Tyr-Ile-His-Pro-Phe-OH (human)	Adrenal cortex, septum, thalamus, hypothalamus, midbrain, brain- stem, cerebellum	9,10,11,37,38,55,59, 231
4. Thyrotropin releasing hormone pGlu-His-Pro-NH₂	Pituitary, cerebral cortex, hypothala- mus, hippocampus, midbrain, cor- pus striatum, brainstem	7,24,28,53,95,96,107, 135,172,180,241, 263,264
5. Vasoactive intestinal peptide H-His-Ser-Asp-Ala-Val-Phe-Thr-Asp-Asn-Tyr-Thr-Arg-Leu- -Arg-Lys-Gln-Met-Ala-Val-Lys-Lys-Tyr-Leu-Asn-Ser-Ileu- -Leu-Asn-NH₂	Whole brain	12,25,67,80,87,140, 204,209
6. Neurotensin H-Glu-Leu-Tyr-Glu-Asn-Lys-Pro-Arg-Arg-Pro-Tyr-Ileu-Leu-OH	Cerebral cortex, hypothalamus, thal- amus, midbrain, hippocampus, corpus striatum, cerebellum, brainstem	250,251,252
7. Somatostatin H-Ala-Gly-Cys-Lys-Asn-Phe-Phe-Trp-Lys-Thr-Phe-Thr-Ser-Cys-OH	Pituitary	150,191,197,216,244, 249
8. Bombesin PGlu-Gln-Arg-Leu-Gly-Asn-Gln-Trp-Ala-Val-Gly-His-Leu-Met-NH₂	Whole brain	21,161

[a] Receptors in brain have not yet been demonstrated for adrenocorticotrophic hormone; however, see references 132 and 139.
[b] Regions where binding of labeled ligands to specific sites has been reported (listed in approximate order of relative density of binding sites).
[c] Regarding the presence and regional distribution of the peptide and/or its receptors (binding sites for labeled ligand).

(56). Bombesin is a tetradecapeptide originally isolated from frog skin (1); bombesin-like activity has since been found in mammalian brain (21). Bombesin is 10^4 times more potent than neurotensin in lowering body temperature in rats after intracisternal administration, making it one of the most potent neuroactive peptides yet reported (22). High-affinity ($K_D = 1$ nM) saturable binding of a radiolabeled tyrosine analog of bombesin to rat membranes has been reported (161).

We have discussed several of the more prominent peptide neurotransmitter candidates in the brain (see Table 2 for summary). There are many others for which the evidence is less complete, and of which time and space do not permit a discussion here.

CONCLUSIONS

The great diversity of biological roles for peptides has only begun to be appreciated over the last decade. The various peptides originally found in peripheral organs such as the pituitary and gut and in hypothalamic extracts have been demonstrated over the last few years to occur throughout the central nervous system. The radioimmunoassay and immunocytochemical techniques have been critical to this demonstration and have shown these materials to be distributed not in a randomized or generalized fashion but with regional specificity for each peptide, which appears in many cases to correlate with the distribution of specific receptors. In most cases the specific functional implications of these systems are unknown. Nevertheless, these materials certainly must function as hormones, neurotransmitters, or neuromodulators, and such roles require specific receptors for each peptide in the appropriate brain regions. Such receptors have been demonstrated for many of the putative peptide neurotransmitters and the data have been reviewed here. The data are still preliminary but they provide support for the various proposed roles for peptides in the brain. The lack of specific antagonists for most of these substances, other than the opioid peptides and angiotensin II, has slowed progress. In many cases there is uncertainty as to the origin of the natural ligand intended for the demonstrated receptors, i.e., neural, vascular, or ventricular.

Immunohistochemical studies have provided dramatic evidence for a neuronal source and a neurotransmitter role for many of the peptide candidates in the brain.

Many of the peptides discussed have potent behavioral effects after administration into the circulation or ventricular fluids, however, and there is evidence for a pituitary-brain transport of an ACTH analog (159). There is, furthermore, evidence for a physiological role in the regulation of behavior for ACTH released into the ventricles. A recent study reported data suggesting that the increased grooming behavior in rats induced by a novel environment is due to release of ACTH into the ventricular system (61). It seemed the pituitary was the major source for this ACTH, although a contribution from cerebral ACTH-containing neurons was not discounted. Indeed, the possibility of peptides serving neuroendocrine roles, with both source and target within the brain is intriguing and probable. One specific example of this kind of role for brain peptides may be provided by β-endorphin.

β-Endorphin is localized in a midline periventricular-periaqueductal tract distinct from enkephalin-containing neuronal systems (15). Electrical stimulation of the periaqueductal-periventricular gray matter produces analgesia, which can be reversed by naloxone (155). It has now been reported that such stimulation to provide pain relief in human patients results in significant increases in ventricular β-endorphin (114). This raises the possibility that whereas the enkephalins appear to be neurotransmitters, β-endorphin may be released into the ventricular system to serve as a central hormone modulating neuronal excitability of brain regions accessible from this source. A role as a neuronal modulator has also been proposed for substance P (133). The report that peptides and monoamines may occur in the same nerve terminals (150) raises the possibility that one and the same neuron may release both a neurotransmitter and a neuromodulator.

In summary, the demonstration of peptides and their receptors distributed throughout the brain has initiated an extensive study of the new endocrinology of the brain. The elucidation of how these materials mediate and regulate the activity and functions of the brain promises a profound advance in our understanding of normal and diseased mental states and the treatment of the latter.

REFERENCES

1. Anastasi, A., Erspamer, V., and Bucci, M. (1972): Isolation and amino acid sequences of alytesin and bombesin, two analogous active tetradecapeptides from the skin of European discoglossid frogs. *Arch. Biochem. Biophys.,* 148:443–446.
2. Assaf, S. Y., and Mogenson, G. J. (1976): Evidence that the preoptic region is a receptive site for the dipsogenic effects of angiotensin II. *Biochem. Behav.,* 5:697–699.
3. Atweh, S. F., and Kuhar, M. J. (1977): Autoradiographic localization of opiate receptors in rat brain. I. Spinal cord and medulla. *Brain Res.,* 124:53–67.
4. Atweh, S. F., and Kuhar, M. J. (1977): Autoradiographic localization of opioid receptors in rat brain. II. The brain stem. *Brain Res.,* 129:1–12.
5. Atweh, S. F., Murrin, L. C., and Kuhar, M. J. (1977): Presynaptic localization of opiate receptors in the vagal and accessory optic systems: An autoradiographic study. *Neuropharmacology,* 17:65–71.
6. Barker, J. L. (1976): Peptides: Roles in neuronal excitability. *Physiol. Rev.,* 56:435–452.
7. Barnea, A., Ben-Jonathan, N., Colston, C., Johnston, J. M., and Porter, J. C. (1975): Differential sub-cellular compartmentalization of thyrotropin releasing hormone (TRH) and gonadotropin releasing hormone (LRH) in hypothalamic tissue. *Proc. Natl. Acad. Sci. U.S.A.,* 72:3153–3157.
8. Ben-Ari, Y., and Henry, J. L. (1976): Effects of the para-chlorophenyl derivative of GABA on spinal neurons in the rat. *J. Physiol.,* 259:46–47P.
9. Bennett, Jr., J. P., and Snyder, S. H. (1976): Angiotensin II binding to mammalian brain membranes. *J. Biol. Chem.,* 251:7423–7430.
10. Bennett, J. P., and Snyder, S. H. (1980): Receptor binding interactions of the angiotensin II antagonist, ^{125}I-sarcosine^1-leucine^8-angiotensin II, with mammalian brain and peripheral tissues. *J. Biol. Chem. (in press).*
11. Bennett, J. P., and Snyder, S. H. (1980): Regulation of receptor binding interactions of ^{125}I-angiotensin II and ^{125}I-sarcosine^1-leucine^8-angiotensin II, an angiotensin antagonist, by sodium ion. *J. Biol. Chem. (in press).*

12. Besson, J., Rotsztejn, W., Laburthe, M., Epelbaum, J., Beaudet, A., Kordon, C., and Rosselin, G. (1979): Vasoactive intestinal peptide (VIP): Brain distribution, subcellular localization and effect of deafferentation of the hypothalamus in male rats. *Brain Res.,* 165:79–85.
13. Blackwell, R. E., and Guillemin, R. (1973): Hypothalamic control of adenohypophysial secretions. *Annu. Rev. Physiol.,* 35:357–390.
14. Blank, M. S., Panerai, A. E., and Friesen, H. G. (1979): Opioid peptides modulate luteinizing hormone secretion during sexual maturation. *Science,* 203:1129–1131.
15. Bloom, F., Battenberg, E., Rossier, J., Ling, N., and Guillemin, R. (1978): Neurons containing β-endorphin in rat brain exist separately from those containing enkephalin: Immunocytochemical studies. *Proc. Natl. Acad. Sci. U.S.A.,* 75:1591–1595.
16. Bohus, B., and Gispen, W. H. (1978): The role of endorphins in behavior. In: *Characteristics and Functions of Opioids,* edited by J. Van Ree and L. Terenius, pp. 367–376. Elsevier, Amsterdam.
17. Bradbury, A. F., Smith, D. G., Snell, C. R., Birdsall, N. J. M., and Hulme, E. C. (1976): C-fragment of lipotropin has a high affinity for brain opiate receptors. *Nature,* 260:793–795.
18. Bramwell, G. J., and Bradley, P. B. (1974): Actions and interactions of narcotic agonists and antagonists on brain stem neurons. *Brain Res.,* 73:167–170.
19. Brazeau, P., Vale, W., Burgus, R., Ling, N., Butcher, M., Rivier, J., and Guillemin, R. (1973): Hypothalamic polypeptide that inhibits the secretion of immunoreactive pituitary growth hormone. *Science,* 179:77–79.
20. Breese, G. R., Cott, J. M., Cooper, B. R., Prange, A. J., Jr., and Lipton, M. A. (1974): Antagonism of ethanol narcosis by thyrotropin releasing hormone. *Life Sci.,* 14:1053–1063.
21. Brown, M. J., Rivier, J., Kobayashi, R., and Vale, W.: Neurotensin-like peptides: CNS distribution and action. International Gut Hormone Symposium, Lausanne, Switzerland, 1977, *(in press).*
22. Brown, M., Rivier, J., and Vale, W. (1977): Bombesin: Potent effects on thermoregulation in the rat. *Science,* 196:998–1000.
23. Brownstein, M. J., Mroz, E. A., Kizer, J. S., Palkovits, M., and Leeman, S. E. (1976): Regional distribution of substance P in the brain in the rat. *Brain Res.,* 116:229–305.
24. Brownstein, M. J., Palkovits, M., Saavedra, J. M., Bassiri, R. M., and Utiger, R. D. (1974): Thyrotropin-releasing hormone in specific nuclei of rat brain. *Science,* 185:267–269.
25. Bryant, M. G., Bloom, S. R., Polak, J. M., Albuquerque, R. H., Modlin, I., and Pearse, A. G. E. (1976): Possible dual role for vasoactive intestinal peptide as gastrointestinal hormone and neurotransmitter substance. *Lancet,* 1:991–993.
26. Buggy, J., and Fisher, A. E. (1976): Anteroventral third ventricle site of action for angiotensin-induced thirst. *Pharmacol. Biochem. Behav.,* 4:651–660.
27. Burgus, R., Dunn, T. F., Desiderio, D., Ward, D. N., Vale, W., and Guillemin, R. (1970): Characterization of hypothalamic hypophysiotropic TSH-releasing factor (TRF) of ovine origin. *Nature,* 226:321–325.
28. Burt, D. R., and Snyder, S. H. (1975): Thyrotropin releasing hormone (TRH): Apparent receptor binding in rat brain membranes. *Brain Res.,* 93:309–328.
29. Bury, R. W., and Mashford, M. L. (1977): Substance P: Its pharmacology and physiological roles. *Ajebak,* 55:671–735.
30. Buscher, H. H., Hill, R. C., Romer, D., Cardinaux, F., Closse, A., Hauser, D., and Pless, J. (1976): Evidence for analgesic activity of enkephalin in the mouse. *Nature,* 261:423–425.
31. Carraway, R., and Leeman, S. E. (1973): The isolation of a new hypothalamic peptide, neurotensin, from bovine hypothalami. *J. Biol. Chem.,* 248:6854–6861.
32. Carraway, R., and Leeman, S. E. (1975): The amino acid sequence of a hypothalamic peptide, neurotensin. *J. Biol. Chem.,* 250:1907–1911.
33. Carraway, R., and Leeman, S. E. (1975): Structural requirements for the biological activity of neurotensin, a new vasoactive peptide. In: *Peptides: Chemistry, Structure and Biology,* edited by R. Walter and J. Meienhofer, pp. 679–685. Ann Arbor Science Publishers, Ann Arbor.
34. Catt, K. J., and Dufau, M. L. (1977): Peptide hormone receptors. *Annu. Rev. Physiol.,* 39:529–557.
35. Chang, M. M., and Leeman, S. (1970): Isolation of a sialagogic peptide from bovine hypothalamic tissue and its characterization as substance P. *J. Biol. Chem.,* 245:4784–4790.
36. Chang, M. M., Leeman, S. E., and Niall, H. D. (1971): Amino acid sequence of substance P. *Nature,* 232:86–87.

37. Changaris, D. G., Keil, L. C., and Severs, W. B. (1978): Angiotensin II immunohistochemistry of the rat brain. *Neuroendocrinology,* 25:257–274.
38. Changaris, D. G., Severs, W. B., and Keil, L. C. (1978): Localization of angiotensin in rat brain. *J. Histochem. Cytochem.,* 26(7):593–607.
39. Chihara, K., Arimura, A., Coy, D. H., and Schally, A. V. (1978): Studies on the interaction of endorphins, substance P, and endogenous somatostatin on growth hormone and prolactin release in rats. *Endocrinology,* 102:281–290.
40. Clendennin, N. J., Petraitis, M., and Simon, E. J. (1976). Ontological development of opiate receptor in rodent brain. *Brain Res.,* 118:157–160.
41. Clineschmidt, B. V., and McGuffin, J. C. (1977): Neurotensin administered intracisternally inhibits responsiveness of mice to noxious stimuli. *Eur. J. Pharmacol.,* 46:395–396.
42. Cocchi, D., Santagostino, A., Gil-Ad, I., Ferri, S., and Muller, E. (1977): Leu-enkephalin-stimulated growth hormone and prolactin release in the rat: Comparison with the effect of morphine. *Life Sci.,* 20:2041–2046.
43. Cohn, M. L., and Cohn, M. (1975): Barrel rotation induced by somatostatin in the non-lesioned rat. *Brain Res.,* 96:138–141.
44. Collier, H. O. J., and Roy, A. C. (1974): Morphine-like drugs inhibit the stimulation by E prostaglandins of cyclic AMP formation by rat brain homogenate. *Nature,* 248:24–27.
45. Coyle, J. T., and Pert, C. B. (1976): Ontogenetic development of ^{3}H-naloxone binding in rat brain. *Neuropharmacology,* 15:555–560.
46. Creese, I., and Snyder, S. H. (1975): Receptor binding and pharmacological activity of opiates in the guinea pig intestine. *J. Pharmacol. Exp. Ther.,* 194:205–219.
47. Cuatrecasas, P. (1974): Membrane receptors. *Annu. Rev. Biochem.,* 43:169–214.
48. Davies, J., and Dray, A. (1976): Effects of enkephalin and morphine on renshaw cells in feline spinal cord. *Nature,* 262:603–604.
49. Davies, J., and Dray, A. (1976): Substance P in the substantia nigra. *Brain Res.,* 107:623–627.
50. Davies, J., and Dray, A. (1978): Comparative effects of substance P and morphine on spinal neurones possessing stereospecific opiate receptors. In: *Iontophoresis and Transmitter Mechanisms in the Mammalian Central Nervous System,* edited by R. W. Ryall and J. S. Kelly. Elsevier, Amsterdam.
51. Davies, J., and Duggan, A. W. (1974): Opiate agonist-antagonist effects on Renshaw cells and spinal interneurones. *Nature,* 250:70–71.
52. DeLean, A., Ferland, L., Drouin, J., Kelly, P. A., and Labrie, F. (1977): Modulation of pituitary thyrotropin releasing hormone receptor levels by estrogens and thyroid hormones. *Endocrinology,* 100:1496–1504.
53 DeLean, A., Garon, M., Kelly, P. A., and Labrie, F. (1977): Changes of pituitary thyrotropin releasing hormone (TRH) receptor level and prolactin response to TRH during the rat estrous cycle. *Endocrinology,* 100:1505–1510.
54. Deschodt-Lauckman, M., Robberecht, P., and Christophe, J. (1977): Characterization of VIP-sensitive adenylate cyclase in guinea pig brain. *FEBS Lett.,* 83:76–80.
55. Devynck, M.-A., and Meyer, P. (1978): Angiotensin receptors. *Biochem. Pharmacol.,* 27:1–5.
56. DeWied, D. (1977): Peptides and behavior. *Life Sci.,* 20:195–204.
57. Deyo, S. N., Swift, R. M., and Miller, R. J. (1979): Morphine and endorphins modulate dopamine turnover in rat median eminence. *Proc. Natl. Acad. Sci. U.S.A. (in press).*
58. Dodd, J., and Kelly, J. S. (1978): Is somatostatin an excitatory transmitter in the hippocampus? *Nature,* 273:674–675.
59. Douglas, J., Saltman, S., Fredlund, P., Kondo, T., and Catt, K. J. (1976): Receptor binding of angiotensin II and antagonists. Correlation with aldosterone production by isolated canine adrenal glomerulosa cells. *Circ. Res.,* 38:108–112.
60. Duffy, M. J., and Powell, D. (1975): Stimulation of brain adenylate cyclase activity by the undecapeptide substance P and its modulation by the calcium ion. *Biochim. Biophys. Acta,* 385:275–280.
61. Dunn, A. J., Green, E. J., and Isaacson, R. L. (1979): Intracerebral adrenocorticotrophic hormone mediates novelty-induced grooming in the rat. *Science,* 203:281–283.
62. Dupont, A., Cusan, L., Garon, M., Labrie, F., and Li, C. H. (1977): β-Endorphin: Stimulation of growth hormone release *in vivo. Proc. Natl. Acad. Sci. U.S.A.,* 74:358–359.

63. Dyer, R. G., and Dyball, R. E. J. (1974): Evidence for a direct effect of LRF and TRF on single unit activity in the rostral hypothalamus. *Nature,* 252:486–488.
64. Ehrenpreis, S., Fleisch, J. H., and Mittag, T. W. (1969): Approaches to the molecular nature of pharmacological receptors. *Pharmacol. Rev.,* 21:131–181.
65. Elde, R., and Hokfelt, T. (1978): Distribution of hypothalamic hormones and other peptides in the brain. In: *Frontiers in Neuroendocrinology, volume 5,* edited by W. F. Ganong and L. Martini, pp. 1–33. Raven Press, New York.
66. Elde, R. P., Hokfelt, T., Johansson, O., and Terenius, L. (1976): Immunohistochemical studies using antibodies to leucine-enkephalin: Initial observations on the nervous system of the rat. *Neuroscience,* 1:349–351.
67. Emson, P. C., Fahrenkrug, J., Schaffalitsky de Muckadell, O. B., Jessel, T. M., and Iversen, L. L. (1978): Vasoactive intestinal polypeptide (VIP): Vesicular localization and potassium-evoked release from rat hypothalamus. *Brain Res.,* 143:174–178.
68. Erlich, P. (1913): Chemotherapeutics: Scientific principles, methods and results. *Lancet,* II:445.
69. Felix, D., and Akert, K. (1974): The effect of angiotensin II on neurons of the cat subfornical organ. *Brain Res.,* 76:350–353.
70. Felix, D., and Schlegel, W. (1978): Angiotensin receptive neurones in the subfornical organ. Structure-activity relations. *Brain Res.,* 149:107–116.
71. Fitzsimmons, J. T., and Evered, M. D. (1978): Eledoisin, substance P and related peptides: Intracranial dipsogens in the pigeon and antidipsogens in the rat. *Brain Res.,* 150:533–542.
72. Frederickson, R. C. A. (1977): Enkephalin pentapeptides: A review of current evidence for a physiological role in vertebrate neurotransmission. *Life Sci.,* 21:23–42.
73. Frederickson, R. C. A., Burgis, V., Harrell, C. E., and Edwards, J. D. (1978): Dual actions of substance P on nociception: Possible role of endogenous opioids. *Science,* 199:1359–1362.
74. Frederickson, R. C. A., Nickander, R., Smithwick, E. L., Shuman, R., and Norris, F. H. (1976): Pharmacological activity of met-enkephalin and analogues *in vitro* and *in vivo*—depression of single neuronal activity in specified brain regions. In: *Opiates and Endogenous Opioid Peptides,* edited by H. W. Kosterlitz, pp. 239–246. Elsevier, Amsterdam.
75. Frederickson, R. C. A., and Norris, F. H. (1976): Enkephalin-induced depression of single neurons in brain areas with opiate receptors—antagonism by naloxone. *Science,* 194:440–442.
76. Frederickson, R. C. A., and Norris, F. H. (1978): Enkephalins as inhibitory neurotransmitters modulating nociception. In: *Iontophoresis and Transmitter Mechanisms in the Mammalian Central Nervous System,* edited by Ryall and J. S. Kelly, pp. 320–322. Elsevier, Amsterdam.
77. Frederickson, R. C. A., Schirmer, E. W., Grinnan, E. L., Harrell, C. E., and Hewes, C. R. (1976): Human endorphin: Comparison with porcine endorphin, enkephalin and normorphine. *Life Sci.,* 19:1181–1190.
78. Frederickson, R. C. A., and Smithwick, E. L., Jr., (1978): Evidence for tonic activity of enkephalins in brain and development of systemically active analogues with clinical potential. In: *Endorphins in Mental Health Research,* edited by E. Usdin, W. E. Bunney, Jr., and N. Kline, pp. 352–365. MacMillan, New York.
79. Frenk, H., McCarty, B. C., and Liebeskind, J. C. (1978): Different brain areas mediate the analgesic and epileptic properties of enkephalin. *Science,* 200:335–337.
80. Fuxe, K., Hokfelt, T., Said, S. I., and Mutt, V. (1977): Vasoactive intestinal peptide and the nervous system: Immunohistochemical evidence for localization in central and peripheral neurons, particularly intracortical neurons of the cerebral cortex. *Neurosci. Lett.,* 5:241–246.
81. Ganong, W. R. (1977): The renin-angiotensin system and the central nervous system. *Fed. Proc.,* 36:1771–1775.
82. Ganten, D., Fuxe, K., Phillips, M. I., Mann, J. F. E., and Ganten, U. (1978): The brain isorenin-angiotensin system: Biochemistry, localization, and possible role in drinking and blood pressure regulation. In: *Frontiers in Neuroendocrinology, volume 5,* edited by W. R. Ganong and L. Martini, pp. 61–99. Raven Press, New York.
83. Garcia-Sevilla, J. A., Magnusson, T., and Carlsson, A. (1978): Effect of intracerebroventricularly administered somatostatin on brain monoamine turnover. *Brain Res.,* 155:159–164.
84. Gardner, J. D. (1979): Receptors for gastrointestinal hormones. *Prog. Gastroenterol.,* 76:202–214.
85. Gent, J. P., and Wolstencroft, J. H. (1976): Actions of morphine, enkephalin and endorphin on single neurons in the brainstem, including the raphe and periaqueductal gray of the cat. In: *Opiates and Endogenous Opioid Peptides,* edited by W. K. Kosterlitz, pp. 217–224. Elsevier, Amsterdam.

86. Gerber, L. D., Stein, S., Rubinstein, M., Wideman, J., and Udenfriend, S. (1978): Binding assay for opioid peptides with neuroblastoma x glioma hybrid cells: Specificity of the receptor site. *Brain Res.,* 151:117–126.
87. Giachetti, A., Said, S. I., Reynolds, R., and Koniges, F. C. (1977): Vasoactive intestinal polypeptide in brain: Localization and release from isolated nerve terminals. *Proc. Natl. Acad. Sci. U.S.A.,* 74:3424–3428.
88. Gilbert, P. E., and Martin, W. R. (1976): The effects of morphine and nalorphine-like drugs in the nondependent, morphine-dependent and cyclazocine-dependent chronic spinal dog. *J. Pharmacol. Exp. Ther.* 198:66–82.
89. Gillan, M. G. C., Paterson, S. J., and Kosterlitz, H. W. (1978): Further support for the hypothesis of multiple opiate receptors. In: *Characteristics and Functions of Opioids,* edited by J. Van Ree and L. Terenius, pp. 475–476, Elsevier, Amsterdam.
90. Goldstein, A. (1974): Opiate receptors. *Life Sci.,* 14:615–623.
91. Goldstein, A., Aronow, L., and Kalman, S. M. (1969): *Principles of Drug Action.* Hoeber Medical Division, Harper and Row, New York.
92. Goldstein, A., Lowney, K. I., and Pal, B. K. (1971): Stereospecific and nonspecific interactions of the morphine congener levorphanol in subcellular fractions of mouse brain. *Proc. Natl. Acad. Sci. U.S.A.,* 68:1742–1747.
93. Goodfriend, T., and Lih, S-Y. (1969): Angiotensin receptors. *Clin. Res.,* 17:243.
94. Grandison, L., and Guidotti, A. (1977): Regulation of prolactin release by endogenous opiates. *Nature,* 270:357–359.
95. Grant, G., Vale, W., and Guillemin, R. (1972): Interaction of thyrotropin releasing factor with membrane receptors of pituitary cells. *Biochem. Biophys. Res. Commun.,* 46:28–34.
96. Grant, G., Vale, W., and Guillemin, R. (1973): Characteristics of the pituitary binding sites for thyrotropin-releasing factor. *Endocrinology,* 92:1629–1633.
97. Gronan, R. J., and York, D. H. (1978): Effects of angiotensin II and acetylcholine on neurons in the preoptic area. *Brain Res.,* 154:172–177.
98. Guillemin, R., Yamazaki, E., Jutisz, M., and Sakiz, E. (1962): Presence dans un extrait de tissus hypothalamiques d'une substance stimulant la secretion de l'hormone hypophysaire thyreotrope (TSH). Premiere purification par filtration sur gel. *C. R. Acad. Sci. (Paris),* 255:1018–1020.
99. Guyenet, P. G., and Aghajanian, G. K. (1977): Excitation of neurons in the nucleus locus coeruleus by substance P and related peptides. *Brain Res.,* 136:178–184.
100. Haigler, H. J.: (1976): Morphine: Ability to block neuronal activity evoked by a nociceptive stimulus. *Life Sci.,* 19:841–858.
101. Havlicek, V., Rezek, M., Leybin, L., and Friesen, H. (1977): Analgesic effect of cerebroventricular administration of somatostatin (SRIF). *Fed. Proc.,* 36:363.
102. Haynes, R. C., Sutherland, E. W., and Rall, T. W. (1960): The role of cyclic adenylic acid in hormone action. *Recent Prog. Horm. Res.,* 16:121–138.
103. Hechter, O. (1955): Concerning the mechanisms of hormone action. In: *Vitamins and Hormones,* pp. 293–346. Academic Press, New York.
104. Henry, J. L. (1976): Effects of substance P on functionally identified units in cat spinal cord. *Brain Res.,* 114:439–451.
105. Hill, R. G., Mitchell, J. F., and Pepper, C. M. (1976): The excitation and depression of hippocampal neurones by iontophoretically applied enkephalins (rat). *J. Physiol.,* 272:50P.
106. Hiller, J. M., Pearson, J., and Simon, E. J. (1973): Distribution of stereospecific binding of the potent narcotic analgesic etorphine in the human brain: Predominance in the limbic system. *Res. Commun. Chem. Pathol. Pharmacol.,* 6:1052–1062.
107. Hinkle, P. M., and Tashjian, A. H., Jr. (1975): Thyrotropin-releasing hormone regulates the number of its own receptors in the GH3 strain of pituitary cells in culture. *Biochemistry,* 14:3845–3851.
108. Hoffmann, W. E., and Phillips, M. I. (1976): Regional study of cerebral ventricle sensitive sites to angiotensin II. *Brain Res.,* 110:313–330.
109. Hokfelt, T., Elde, R. P., Johnasson, O., Terenius, L., and Stein, L. (1977): Distribution of enkephalin-like immunoreactivity in the rat central nervous system. I. Cell bodies. *Neurosci. Lett.,* 5:25–31.
110. Hokfelt, T., Johansson, O., Kellerth, J.-O., Ljungdahl, A., Nilsson, G., Nygards, A., and Pernow, B. (1977): Immunohistochemical distribution of substance P. In: *Nobel Symposium*

37: Substance P, edited by U. S. von Euler and B. Pernow, pp. 117–145. Raven Press, New York.

111. Hokfelt, T., Kellerth, J. O., Nilsson, G., and Pernow, B. (1975): Substance P: Localization in the central nervous system and in some primary sensory neurons. *Science,* 190:889–890.

112. Hokfelt, T., Ljungdahl, A., Terenius, L., Elde, R., and Nilsson, G. (1977): Immunohistochemical analysis of peptide pathways possibly related to pain and analgesia: Enkephalin and substance P. *Proc. Natl. Acad. Sci. U.S.A.* 74:3081–3085.

113. Hong, J. S., Costa, E., and Yang, H.-Y. T (1976): Effects of habenular lesions on the substance P content of various brain regions. *Brain Res.,* 118:523–525.

114. Hosobuchi, Y., Rossier, J., Bloom, F. E., and Guillemin, R. (1979): Stimulation of human periaqueductal gray for pain relief increases immunoreactive β-endorphin in ventricular fluid. *Science,* 203:279–281.

115. Hughes, J. (1975): Isolation of an endogenous compound from the brain with pharmacological properties similar to morphine. *Brain Res.,* 88:295–308.

116. Hughes, J., Smith, T. W., Kosterlitz, H. W., Fothergill, L. A., Morgan, B. A., and Morris, H. R. (1975): Identification of two related pentapeptides from the brain with potent opiate agonist activity. *Nature,* 258:577–579.

117. Huston, J. P., and Staubli, U. (1978): Retrograde amnesia produced by post-trial injection of substance P into substantia nigra. *Brain Res.,* 159:468–472.

118. Iversen, L. L., Jessell, T., and Kanazawa, I. (1976): Release and metabolism of substance P in rat hypothalamus. *Nature,* 264:81–83.

119. Jessell, T. M. (1978). Substance P release from the rat substantia nigra. *Brain Res.,* 151:469–478.

120. Jessell, T. M., Emson, P. C., Paxinos, G., and Cuello, A. C. (1978): Topographic projections of substance P and GABA pathways in the striato- and pallido-nigral system: A biochemical and immunohistochemical study. *Brain Res.,* 152:487–498.

121. Jessell, T. M., and Iversen, L. L. (1977): Opiate analgesics inhibit substance P release from rat trigeminal nucleus. *Nature,* 268:549–551.

122. Kahn, C. R. (1976): Membrane receptors for hormones and neurotransmitters. *J. Cell Biol.,* 70:261–286.

123. Kalivas, P. W., and Horita, A. (1979). Thyrotropin-releasing hormone: Central site of action in antagonism of pentobarbital narcosis. *Nature,* 278:461–463.

124. Kanazawa, I., Emson, P. C., and Cuello, A. C. (1977): Evidence for the existence of substance P containing fibers in striato-nigral and pallido-nigral pathways in rat brain. *Brain Res.,* 119:447–453.

125. Kanazawa, I., and Jessel, T. (1976): Post mortem changes and regional distribution of substance P in the rat and mouse nervous system. *Brain Res.,* 117:362–367.

126. Katayama, Y., and North, A. (1978): Non-somatic site of action of enkephalin on single myenteric neurons. In: *Characteristics and Function of Opioids,* edited by J. Van Ree and L. Terenius, pp. 105–106. Elsevier, Amsterdam.

127. Klee, W. A., and Nirenberg, M. (1974): A neuroblastoma x glioma hybrid cell line with morphine receptors. *Proc. Natl. Acad. Sci. U.S.A.,* 71:3474–3477.

128. Klee, W. A., and Niremberg, M. (1976): Mode of action of endogenous opiate peptides–the opiate peptide-receptor complex is a potent inhibitor of adenylate cyclase. *Nature,* 263:609–612.

129. Kono, T., and Barham, F. W. (1971): The relationship between the insulin-binding capacity of fat cells and the cellular response to insulin. Studies with intact and trypsin-treated cells. *J. Biol. Chem.,* 246:6210–6216.

130. Kosterlitz, H. W., and Hughes, J. (1975): Some thoughts on the significance of enkephalin, the endogenous ligand. *Life Sci.,* 17:91–96.

131. Kosterlitz, H. W., and Waterfield, A. A. (1975). *In vitro* models in the study of structure-activity relationships of narcotic analgesics. *Annu. Rev. Pharmacol.,* 15:29–47.

132. Krieger, D. T., Liotta, A., Brownstein, M. J. (1977): Presence of corticotropin in brains of normal and hypophysectomized rats. *Proc. Natl. Acad. Sci. U.S.A.,* 74:648–652.

133. Krivoy, W., Kroeger, D., and Zimmerman, E. (1977): Additional evidence for a role of substance P (SP) in modulation of synaptic transmission. In: *Nobel symposium 37: Substance P,* edited by U. S. von Euler and B. Pernow, pp. 187–193. Raven Press, New York.

134. Kuhar, M. J., Pert, C. B., and Snyder, S. H. (1973): Regional distribution of opiate receptor binding in monkey and human brain. *Nature,* 245:447–450.

135. Labrie, F., Barden, N., Poirier, G., and Delean, A. (1972): Binding of thyrotropin-releasing hormone to plasma membranes of bovine anterior pituitary gland. *Proc. Natl. Acad. Sci. U.S.A.,* 69:283–287.
136. Labrie, F., Cusan, L., Dupont, A., Ferland, L., and Lemay, A. (1978): Opioids and anterior pituitary hormone secretion. In: *Characteristics and Functions of Opioids,* edited by J. van Ree and L. Terenius, pp. 333–344. Elsevier, Amsterdam.
137. Lamotte, C., Pert, C. B., and Snyder, S. H. (1976): Opiate receptor binding in the primate spinal cord: Distribution and changes after dorsal root section. *Brain Res.,* 112:607–612.
138. Langley, J. N. (1909): On the contraction of muscle, chiefly in relation to the presence of "receptive" substances. Part IV. The effect of curari and of some other substances on the nicotine response of the sartorius and gastrocnemius muscles of the frog. *J. Physiol. (Lond.),* 39:235.
139. Larsson, L.-I. (1978). Distribution of ACTH-like immunoreactivity in rat brain and gastrointestinal tract. *Histochemistry,* 55:225–233.
140. Larsson, L.-I., Fahrenkrug, J., Schaffalitsky de Muckadell, O. B., Sundler, F., Hakanson, R., and Rehfeld, J. F. (1976): Localization of vasoactive intestinal polypeptide (VIP) to central and peripheral neurons. *Proc. Natl. Acad. Sci. U.S.A.,* 73:3197–3200.
141. Leeman, S. E., and Mroz, E. A. (1974): Minireview. Substance P. *Life Sci.,* 15:2033–2044.
142. Lefkowitz, R. J., Roth, J., Pricer, W., et al. (1970): ACTH receptors in the adrenal: Specific binding of ACTH-I^{125} and its relation to adenyl cyclase. *Proc. Natl. Acad. Sci. U.S.A.,* 65:745–752.
143. Lefkowitz, R. J., and Williams, L. T. (1978): Molecular mechanisms of activation and desensitization of adenylate cyclase coupled beta-adrenergic receptors. In: *Advances in Cyclic Nucleotide Research, vol. 9,* edited by W. J. George and L. J. Ignarro, pp. 1–17. Raven Press, New York.
144. Lembeck, F. (1953): Zur frage der zentralen Ubertragung offerenter impulse. III. Mitteibung. Das Vorkommen und die Bedeutung der Substanz P in den dorsalen Wurzeln des Ruckenmarks. *Naunyn Schmiedebergs Arch. Exp. Pathol. Pharmakol.,* 219:197–213.
145. Lembeck, F., Mayer, N., and Schindler, G. (1978): Substance P: Binding lipids in the brain. *Naunyn Schmiedeberg's Arch. Pharmacol.,* 303:79–86.
146. Ling, N., Burgus, R., and Guillemin, R. (1976): Isolation, primary structure, and synthesis of α-endorphin and β-endorphin, two peptides of hypothalamic-hypophysial origin with morphinomimetic activity. *Proc. Natl. Acad. Sci. U.S.A.,* 73:3942–3946.
147. Loh. H. H., Law, P. Y., Oswald, T., Cho, T. M., and Way, E. L. (1978): Possible involvement of cerebroside sulfate in opiate receptor binding. *Fed. Proc.,* 37:147–152.
148. Lord, J. A. H., Waterfield, A. A., Hughes, J., and Kosterlitz, H. W. (1977): Endogenous opioid peptides: Multiple agonists and receptors. *Nature,* 267:495–499.
149. Lovick, T. A., West, D. C., and Wolstencroft, J. H. (1978): Responses of raphe spinal and other bulbar raphe neurones to stimulation of the periaqueductal gray in the cat. *Neurosci. Lett.,* 8:45–49.
150. Luft, R., Efendic, S., and Hokfelt, T. (1978): Somatostatin—both hormone and neurotransmitter? *Diabetologia,* 14:1–13.
151. Malick, J. B., and Goldstein, J. M. (1978): Analgesic activity of substance P following intracerebral administration in rats. *Life Sci.,* 23:835–844.
152. Marangos, P. J., Paul, S. M., Greenlaw, P., Goodwin, F. K., and Skolnick, P. (1978): Demonstration an endogenous, competitive inhibitor of ^{3}H diazepam in bovine brain. *Life Sci.,* 22:1893–1900.
153. Martin, W. R. (1967): Opioid antagonists. *Pharmacol. Rev.,* 19:463–521.
154. Martin, W. R., Eades, C. G., Thompson, J. A., Huppler, R. E., and Gilbert, P. E. (1976): The effects of morphine- and nalorphine-like drugs in the nondependent and morphine-dependent chronic spinal dog. *J. Pharmacol. Exp. Ther.,* 197:517–532.
155. Mayer, D. J., and Price, D. D. (1976): Central nervous system mechanisms of analgesia. *Pain,* 2:379–404.
156. Mayer, M. L., and Hill, R. C. (1978): The effects of intravenous fentanyl, morphine and naloxone on nociceptive responses of neurones in the rat caudal medulla. *Neuropharmacology,* 17:533–539.
157. Mendelsohn, C., Dufan, M. L., and Catt, K. J. (1975): Gonadotropin binding and stimulation of cyclic AMP and testosterone production in isolated Leydig cells. *J. Biol. Chem.,* 250:8818–8823.

158. Meyerson, B. J., and Terenius, L. (1977): β-Endorphin and male sexual behavior. *Eur. J. Pharmacol.,* 42:191–192.
159. Mezey, E., Palkovits, M., de Kloet, E. R., Verhoef, J., and DeWied, D. (1978): Evidence for pituitary-brain transport of a behaviorally potent ACTH analog. *Life Sci.,* 22:831–838.
160. Miller, R. J., and Dawson, G.: Cellular receptors for opiates and opioid peptides. In: *Cell Surface Reviews,* edited by C. Cotman and G. Poste. Elsevier *(in press).*
161. Moody, T. W., and Pert, C. B. (1978): Characterization of the bombesin receptor in mammalian brain. *Program Eighth Meeting Soc. Neurosci.,* Abstract No. 1301, St. Louis, Missouri.
162. Mroz, E. A., Brownstein, M. J., and Leeman, S. E. (1976): Evidence for substance P in the habenulo-interpeduncular tract. *Brain Res.,* 113:597–599.
163. Mudge, A., Leeman, S. E., and Fischbach, G. D. (1979): Enkephalin inhibits release of substance P from sensory neurons in culture and decreases action potential duration. *Proc. Natl. Acad. Sci. U.S.A.,* 76:526–530.
164. Nair, R. M. G., Barrett, J., Bowers, C. Y., and Schally, A. V. (1970): Structure of porcine thyrotropin releasing hormone. *Biochemistry,* 9:1103–1106.
165. Nakata, Y., Kusak, Y., Segawa, T., Yajima, H., and Kitagawa, K. (1978): Substance P: Regional distribution and specific binding to synaptic membranes in rabbit central nervous system. *Life Sci.,* 22:259–268.
166. Narumi, S., and Maki, Y. (1978): Stimulatory effects of substance P on neurite extension and cyclic AMP levels in cultured neuroblastoma cells. *J. Neurochem.* 30:1321–1326.
167. Nemeroff, C. B., Bissette, G., Prange, A. J., Jr., Loosen, P. T., Barlow, T. S., and Lipton, M. A. (1977): Neurotensin: Central nervous system effects of a hypothalamic peptide. *Brain Res.,* 128:485–496.
168. Nicoll, R. A., Siggins, G. R., Ling, N., Bloom, F. E., and Guillemin, R. (1977): Neuronal actions of endorphins and enkephalins among brain regions: A comparative microiontophoretic study. *Proc. Nat'l Acad. Sci. U.S.A.,* 74:2584–2588.
169. North, A.: Electrophysiology of opiates and opioid peptides. *Life Sci. (in press).*
170. North, R. A., and Tonini, M. (1976). Hyperpolarization by morphine of myenteric neurones. In: *Opiates and Endogenous Opioid Peptides,* edited by H. W. Kosterlitz, pp. 205–212. Elsevier, Amsterdam.
171. Ogata, N. (1979): Substance P causes direct depolarization of neurons of guinea pig interpeduncular nucleus *in vitro. Nature,* 277:480–481.
172. Oliver, C., Eskay, R. L., Ben-Jonathan, N., and Porter, J. C. (1974): Distribution and concentration of TRH in the rat brain. *Endocrinology,* 95:540–546.
173. Otsuka, M., and Konishi, S. (1976): Release of substance P-like immunoreactivity from isolated spinal cord of newborn rat. *Nature,* 264:83–84.
174. Otsuka, M., and Konishi, S. (1976): Substance P and excitatory transmitter of primary sensory neurons. *Cold Spring Harbor Symp. Quant. Biol.,* 40:135–143.
175. Otsuka, M., Konishi, S., and Takahashi, T. (1975): Hypothalamic substance P as a candidate for transmitter of primary afferent neurons. *Fed. Proc.,* 34:1922–1928.
176. Otsuka, M., and Takahashi, T. (1977): Putative peptide neurotransmitters. *Annu. Rev. Pharmacol. Toxicol.,* 17:425–439.
177. Pasternak, G. W., and Snyder, S. H. (1974): Opiate receptor binding: Effects of enzymatic treatment. *Mol. Pharmacol.,* 10:183–193.
178. Pellegrini-Quarantotti, B., Corda, M. G., Paglietti, E., Biggio, G., and Gessa, G. L. (1978): Inhibition of copulatory behavior in male rats by D-ala²-met-enkephalinamide. *Life Sci.,* 23:673–678.
179. Pernow, B. (1953): Studies on substance P. Purification, occurrence and biological actions. *Acta Physiol. Scand.,* 291 (Suppl. 105):1–90.
180. Perrone, M. H., and Hinkle, P. M. (1978): Regulation of pituitary receptors for thyrotropin-releasing hormone by thyroid hormones. *J. Biol. Chem.,* 253:5168–5173.
181. Pert, C. B., Aposhian, D., and Snyder, S. H. (1974): Phylogenetic distribution of opiate receptor binding. *Brain Res.,* 75:356–361.
182. Pert, C. B., Kuhar, M. J., and Snyder, S. H. (1976): Opiate receptor: Autoradiographic localization in rat brain. *Proc. Natl. Acad. Sci. U.S.A.,* 73:3729–3733.
183. Pert, C. B., Snowman, A. M., and Snyder, S. H. (1974): Localization of opiate receptor binding in synaptic membranes of rat brain. *Brain Res.,* 70:184–188.
184. Pert, C. B., and Snyder, S. H. (1973): Opiate receptor: Demonstration in nervous tissue. *Science,* 179:1011–1014.

185. Phillips, M. I. (1978): Angiotensin in the brain. *Neuroendocrinology,* 25:354–377.
186. Phillips, M. I., and Felix, D. (1976): Specific angiotensin II receptive neurons in the cat subfornical organ. *Brain Res.,* 109:531–540.
187. Phillis, J. W. (1976): Is β-(4-chlorophenyl)-GABA a specific antagonist of substance P on cerebral cortical neurons? *Experientia,* 32:593–594.
188. Phillis, J. W., and Limacher, J. J. (1974): Substance P excitation of cerebal cortical Betz cells. *Brain Res.,* 69:158–163.
189. Pickel, V. M., Joh, T. H., Reis, D. J. Leeman, S. E., and Miller, R. J. (1979): Electron microscopic localization of substance P and enkephalin in axon terminals related to dendrites of catecholaminergic neurons. *Brain Res.,* 160:387–400.
190. Pickel, V. M., Reis, D. J., and Leeman, S. E. (1977): Ultrastructural localization of substance P in neurons of rat spinal cord. *Brain Res.,* 122:534–540.
191. Pimstone, B. L., and Berelowitz, M. (1978): Somatostatin-paracrine and neuron modulator peptide in gut and nervous system. *S. Afr. Med. J.,* 7:7–9.
192. Plotnikoff, N. P., Kastin, A. J., and Schally, A. V. (1974): Growth hormone release inhibiting hormone: Neuropharmacological studies. *Pharmacol. Biochem. Behav.,* 2:693–696.
193. Plotnikoff, N. P., Prange, Jr., A. J., Breese, G. R., Anderson, M. A., and Wilson, I. C. (1972): Thyrotropin releasing hormone: Enhancement of dopa activity by a hypothalamic hormone. *Science,* 178:417–418.
194. Posner, B. I. (1975): Polypeptide hormone receptors: Characteristics and applications. *Can. J. Physiol. Pharmacol.,* 53:689–703.
195. Prange, A. J., Jr., Breese, G. R., Cott, J. M., Martin, B. R., Cooper, B. R., Wilson, I. C., and Plotnikoff, N. P. (1974): Thyrotropin releasing hormone: Antagonism of pentobarbital in rodents. *Life Sci.,* 14:447–455.
196. Prange, A. J., Jr., Wilson, I. C., Lara, P. P., Alltop, L. B., and Breese, G. R. (1972): Effects of thyrotropin-releasing hormone in depression. *Lancet,* 2:999–1007.
197. Pugsley, T. A., and Lippmann, W. (1978): Effect of somatostatin analogues and 17-α-dihydroequilin on rat brain opiate receptors. *Res. Commun. Chem. Pathol. Pharmacol.,* 21:153–156.
198. Randic, M., and Miletic, V. (1977): Effect of substance P on cat dorsal horn neurones activated by noxious stimuli. *Brain Res.,* 128:164–169.
199. Reid, I. A. (1977): Is there a brain renin-angiotensin system? *Circ. Res.,* 41:147–153.
200. Renaud, L. P., and Martin, J. B. (1975): Thyrotropin releasing hormone (TRH): Depressant action on central neuronal activity. *Brain Res.,* 86:150–154.
201. Renaud, L. P., Martin, J. B., and Brazeau, P. (1975): Depressant action of TRH, LH-RH and somatostatin on activity of central neurones. *Nature,* 255:233–235.
202. Rezek, M., Havlicek, V., Hughes, K. R., and Friesen, J. (1977): Behavioral and motor excitation and inhibition induced by the administration of small and large doses of somatostatin into the amygdala. *Neuropharmacology,* 16:157–162.
203. Rivier, C., Vale, W., Ling, N., Brown, M., and Guillemin, R. (1977): Stimulation *in vivo* of the secretion of prolactin and growth hormone by β-endorphin. *Endocrinology,* 100:238–241.
204. Robberecht, P., DeNeef, P., Lammens, M., Deschodt-Lauckman, M., and Christophe, J.-P. (1978): Specific binding of vasoactive intestinal peptide to brain membranes from the guinea pig. *Eur. J. Biochem.,* 90:147–154.
205. Robison, G. A., Butcher, R. W., and Sutherland, E. W., editors (1971). *Cyclic AMP.* Academic Press, New York.
206. Roth, J. (1973): Peptide Hormone binding to receptors: A review of direct studies *in vitro. Metabolism,* 22:1059–1073.
207. Said, S. I., and Mutt, V. (1970): Polypeptide with broad biological activity: Isolation from small intestine. *Science,* 169:1217–1218.
208. Sakai, K. K., Marks, B. H., George, J., and Koestner, A. (1974): Specific angiotensin II receptors in organ-cultured canine supraoptic nucleus cells. *Life Sci.,* 14:1337–1344.
209. Samson, W. K., Said, S. I., Graham, J. W., and McCann, S. M. (1979): Localization of vasoactive intestinal polypeptide in the human brain. *IRCS Med. Sci.,* 7:13.
210. Sar, M., Stumpf, W. E., Miller, R. J., Chang, K. W., and Cuatrecasas, P. (1978): Immunohistochemical localization of enkephalin in rat brain and spinal cord. *J. Comp. Neurol.,* 182: 17–38.
211. Sastry, B. R. (1978): Effects of substance P, acetylcholine and stimulation of habenula on rat interpeduncular neuronal activity. *Brain Res.,* 144:404–410.

212. Satoh, M., Zieglgansberger, W., Fries, W., and Herz, A. (1974): Opiate agonist-antagonist interaction at cortical neurons of naive and tolerant/dependent rats. *Brain Res.,* 82:378–382.
213. Scatchard, G. (1949): The attraction of proteins for small molecules and ions. *Ann. N. Y. Acad. Sci.,* 51:660–672.
214. Schenker, C., Mroz, E. A., and Leeman, S. E. (1976): Release of substance P from isolated nerve endings. *Nature,* 264:790–792.
215. Schild, H. O. (1947): pA, a new scale for the measurement of drug antagonism. *Br. J. Pharmacol. Chemother.,* 2:189–206.
216. Schonbrunn, A., and Tashjian, A. H., Jr. (1978): Characterization of functional receptors for somatostatin in rat pituitary cells in culture *J. Biol. Chem.,* 253:6473–6483.
217. Schramm, M., Orly, J., Eimerl, S., and Korner, M. (1977): Coupling of hormone receptors to adenylate cyclase of different cells by cell fusion. *Nature,* 268:310–313.
218. Segal, D. S., Browne, R. G., Arnsten, A., and Derrington, D. C. (1978): Behavioral effects of β-endorphin. In: *Characteristics and Functions of Opioids,* edited by J. Van Ree and L. Terenius, pp. 377–388. Elsevier, Amsterdam.
219. Shaar, C. J., and Clemens, J. A. (1974): The role of catecholamines in the release of anterior pituitary prolactin *in vitro. Endocrinology,* 95:1202–1212.
220. Shaar, C. J., Frederickson, R. C. A., Dininger, N. B., and Jackson, L. (1977): Enkephalin analogues and naloxone modulate the release of growth hormone and prolactin—evidence for regulation by an endogenous opioid peptide in brain. *Life Sci.,* 21:853–860.
221. Shibusawa, K., Saito, S., Nishi, K., Yamamoto, T., Abe, C., and Kawai, T. (1956): Effects of the thyrotropin releasing principal after the section of the pituitary stack. *Jap. J. Endocrinol.,* 3:151.
222. Simantov, R., Childers, S. R., and Snyder, S. H. (1978): The opiate receptor binding interactions of ^{3}H-methionine enkephalin, an opioid peptide. *Eur. J. Pharmacol.,* 47:319–331.
223. Simantov. R., Kuhar, M. J., Pasternak, G. W., and Snyder, S. H. (1976): The regional distribution of a morphine-like factor enkephalin in monkey brain. *Brain Res.,* 106:189–197.
224. Simantov, R., Kuhar, M. J., Uhl, G. R., and Snyder, S. H. (1977): Opioid peptide enkephalin: Immunohistochemical mapping in the rat central nervous system. *Proc. Natl. Acad. Sci. U.S.A.,* 74:2167–2171.
225. Simantov, R., and Snyder, S. H. (1976): Morphine-like peptides, leucine enkephalin and methionine enkephalin: Interactions with the opiate receptor. *Mol. Pharmacol.,* 12:987–998.
226. Simon, E. J. (1973): In search of the opiate receptor. *Am. J. Med. Sci.,* 266:160–168.
227. Simon, E. J., and Hiller, J. M. (1978): The opiate receptors. *Annu. Rev. Pharmacol. Toxicol.,* 18:371–394.
228. Simon, E. J., Hiller, J. M., and Edelman, I. (1973): Stereospecific binding of the potent narcotic analgesic ^{3}H-etorphine to rat brain homogenate. *Proc. Natl. Acad. Sci. U.S.A.,* 70:1947–1949.
229. Simpson, J. B., Mangiapane, M. L., and Dellmann, H.-D. (1978): Central receptor sites for angiotensin-induced drinking: A critical review. *Fed. Proc.,* 37:2676–2682.
230. Singer, S. J. (1975): In: *Cell Membranes,* edited by G. Weissmann and R. Claiborne, pp. 35–44. H. P. Publishing, New York.
231. Sirett, N. E., McLean, A. S., Bray, J. J., and Hubbard, J. I. (1977): Distribution of angiotensin II receptors in rat brain. *Brain Res.,* 122:299–312.
232. Snyder, S. H., and Innis, R. B.: Peptide neurotransmitters. *Annu. Rev. Biochem. (in press).*
233. Snyder, S. H., Pert, C. B., and Pasternak, G. W. (1974): The opiate receptor. *Ann. Intern. Med.,* 81:534–540.
234. Squires, R. F., and Braestrup, C. (1977): Benzodiazepine receptors in rat brain. *Nature,* 266:732.
235. Stahl, K. D., Van Bever, W., Janssen, P., and Simon, E. J. (1977): Receptor affinity and pharmacological potency of a series of narcotic analgesic, antidiahrreal and neuroleptic drugs. *Eur. J. Pharmacol.,* 46:199–205.
236. Starr, M. S., James, T. A., and Gaytten, D. (1978): Behavioral depressant and antinociceptive properties of substance P in the mouse: Possible implication of brain monoamines. *Eur. J. Pharmacol.,* 48:203–212.
237. Steinacker, A., and Highstein, S. M. (1976): Pre- and postsynaptic action of substance P at the mauthner fiber-giant fiber synapse in the hatchetfish. *Brain Res.,* 114:128–133.
238. Sternberger, L. A. (1974): *Immunocytochemistry.* Prentice Hall, New Jersey.
239. Stewart, J. M., Getto, C. J., Neldner, K., Reeve, E. B., Krivoy, W. A., and Zimmerman, E. (1976): Substance P and analgesia. *Nature,* 262:784–785.

240. Studer, R. O., Trzeciak, A., and Lergier, W. (1973): Isolierung und Aminosauresequenz von Substanz paus Pferdedarm. *Helv. Chim. Acta,* 56: 860–866.

241. Tashjian, A. H., Jr., Osborne, R., Maina, D., and Knaian, A. (1977): Hydrocortisone increases the number of receptors for thyrotropin-releasing hormone on pituitary cells in culture. *Biochem. Biophys. Res. Commun.,* 79:333–340.

242. Tell, G. P., Haour, F., and Saez, J. M. (1978): Hormonal regulation of membrane receptors and cell responsiveness: A review. *Metabolism,* 27:1566–1592.

243. Terenius, L. (1973): Characteristics of the "receptor" for narcotic analgesics in synaptic plasma membrane fraction from rat brain. *Acta Pharmacol. Toxicol.,* 33:377–384.

244. Terenius, L. (1976): Somatostatin and ACTH are peptides with partial antagonist-like selectivity for opiate receptors. *Eur. J. Pharmacol.,* 38:211–213.

245. Terenius, L. (1977): Opioid peptides and opiates differ in receptor selectivity. *Psychoneuroendocrinology,* 2:53–58.

246. Terenius, L. (1978): The opioid receptors and their ligands. In: *Nobel Symposium No. 42, Principles for the Central Regulation of the Endocrine System,* edited by K. Fuxe. Plenum Press, New York.

247. Terenius, L., and Wahlstrom, A. (1975): Search for an endogenous ligand for the opiate receptor. *Acta Physiol. Scand.,* 94:74–81

248. Traber, J., Fischer, K., Larzin, S., and Hamprecht, B. (1975): Morphine antagonises action of prostaglandin in neuroblastoma and neuroblastoma x hybrid cells. *Nature,* 253:120–122.

249. Traber, J., Glaser, T., Brandt, M., Klebensberger, W., and Hamprecht, B. (1977): Different receptors for somatostatin and opioids in neuroblastoma x glioma hybrid cells. *FEBS Lett.,* 81:351–354.

250. Uhl, G. R., Bennett, Jr., J. P., and Snyder, S. H. (1977): Neurotensin, a central nervous system peptide: Apparent receptor binding in brain membranes. *Brain Res.,* 130:299–313.

251. Uhl, G. R., Childers, S. R., and Snyder, S. H. (1978): Opioid peptides and the opiate receptor. In: *Frontiers in Neuroendocrinology,* Vol. 5, edited by W. R. Ganong and L. Martini, pp. 289–336. Raven Press, New York.

252. Uhl, G. R., Kuhar, M. J., and Snyder, S. H. (1977): Neurotensin: Immunohistochemical localization in rat central nervous system. *Proc. Natl. Acad. Sci. U.S.A.,* 74:4059–4063.

253. Uhl, G. R., and Snyder, S. H. (1977): Neurotensin receptor binding, regional and subcellular distributions favor transmitter role. *Eur. J. Pharmacol.,* 41:89–91.

254. VanVugt, D. A., Bruni, J. F., and Meites, J. (1978): Naloxone inhibition of stress induced increase in prolactin secretion. *Life Sci.,* 22:85–90.

255. Von Euler, U. S., and Gaddum, J. H. (1931): An unidentified depressor substance in certain tissue extracts. *J. Physiol.,* 72:74–87.

256. von Graffenried, B., del Pozo, E., Roubricek, J., Krebs, E., Poldinger, W., Burnmeister, P., and Kerp, L. (1978): Effects of the synthetic enkephalin analogue FK33–824 in man. *Nature,* 272:729–730.

257. Walker, R. J., Kemp, J. A., Yajima, H., Kitagawa, K., and Woodruff, G. N. (1976): The action of substance P on mesencephalic reticular and substantia nigral neurones of the rat. *Experientia,* 32:214–215.

258. Waterfield, A. A., Smokcum, R. W. J., Hughes, J., Kosterlitz, H. W., and Henderson, G. (1977): *In vitro* pharmacology of the opioid peptides, enkephalins and endorphins. *Eur. J. Pharmacol.,* 43:107–116.

259. Wilber, J. F. (1973): Thyrotropin releasing hormone: Secretion and actions. *Annu. Rev. Med.,* 24:353–364.

260. Wilson, I. C., Prange, Jr., A. J., Lara, P. P., Alltop, L. B., Stikeleather, R. A., and Lipton, M. A. (1973): TRH (Lopremone): Psychobiological responses of normal women. *Arch. Gen. Psychiatry,* 29:15–21.

261. Wilson, R. S., Rogers, M. E., Pert, C. B., and Snyder, S. H. (1975): Homologous N-alkylnorketobemidones. Correlation of receptor binding with analgesic potency. *J. Med. Chem.,* 18:240–242.

262. Winokur, A., and Beckman, A. L. (1978): Effects of thyrotropin releasing hormone, norepinephrine and acetylcholine on the activity of neurons in the hypothalamus, septum and cerebral cortex of the rat. *Brain Res.,* 150:205–209.

263. Winokur, A., Davis, R., and Utiger, R. D. (1977): Subcellular distribution of thyrotropin-releasing hormone (TRH) in rat brain and hypothalamus. *Brain Res.,* 120:423–434.

264. Winokur, A., and Utiger, R. D. (1974): Thyrotropin-releasing hormone: Regional distribution in rat brain. *Science,* 185:265–267.
265. Yaksh, T. L., and Rudy, T. A. (1978): Narcotic analgesics: CNS sites and mechanisms of action as revealed by intracerebral injection techniques. *Pain,* 4:299–359.
266. Yanaihara, N., Yanaihara, C., Hirogashi, M., Sato, H., Hasimoto, T., Iizuka, Y., and Sakagami, M., (1976): Substance P analogs: Synthesis, and biological and immunological properties. In: *Nobel Symposium 37: Substance P,* edited by U. S. von Euler and B. Pernow. Raven Press, New York.
267. Yang, H.-Y., Hong, J. S., and Costa, E. (1977): Regional distribution of Leu and Met-enkephalin in rat brain. *Neuropharmacology,* 16:303–307.
268. Yarbrough, G. G. (1976): TRH potentiates excitatory actions of acetylcholine on cerebral cortical neurons. *Nature,* 263:523–524.
269. Young, II, W. S., Uhl, G. R., and Kuhar, M. J. (1978): Iontophoresis of neurotensin in the area of the locus coeruleus. *Brain Res.,* 150:431–435.
270. Zieglgansberger, W., and Bayerl, H. (1976): The mechanism of inhibition of neuronal activity by opiates in the spinal cord of cat. *Brain Res.,* 115:111–128.
271. Zieglgansberger, W., and Fry, J. P. (1976): Actions of enkephalin on cortical and striatal neurones of naive and morphine tolerant/dependent rats. In: *Opiates and Endogenous Opioid Peptides,* edited by H. W. Kosterlitz, pp. 231–238. Elsevier, Amsterdam.
272. Zieglgansberger, W., Siggins, G., French, E., and Bloom, F. (1978): Effects of opioids on unit activity. In: *Characteristics and Function of Opioids,* edited by J. Van Ree and L. Terenius, pp. 75–86. Elsevier, Amsterdam.

The Endocrine Functions of the Brain,
edited by Marcella Motta.
Raven Press, New York © 1980

13

Role of the Tuberoinfundibular Dopaminergic System in the Control of Prolactin Secretion

Louise Ferland, Fernand Labrie, Lionel Cusan, André Dupont, Jérôme Lépine, Michèle Beaulieu, Francine Denizeau, and André Lemay

Medical Research Council Group in Molecular Endocrinology, Le Centre Hospitalier de l'Université Laval, Quebec, Quebec G1V 4G2, Canada

Secretion of prolactin from the anterior pituitary gland is controlled by stimulatory and inhibitory influences of hypothalamic origin. At least part of the stimulatory hypothalamic influence appears to be mediated by the tripeptide thyrotropin releasing hormone (TRH), which stimulates prolactin secretion in the human and experimental animals *in vivo* (13,60) and *in vitro* (31,94).

Much evidence obtained in the rat strongly suggests that dopamine (DA) secreted by the tuberoinfundibular system is the main inhibitory factor involved in the control of prolactin secretion (9,82,100,102). According to these data, DA released from nerve endings in the median eminence (44,57) is transported to the pituitary prolactin-secreting cells by the hypothalamo-adenohypophysial portal blood system. In support of such a physiological role of DA at the pituitary level on prolactin secretion are the facts that DA was recently measured in portal blood (7,92) and a typical dopaminergic receptor was characterized in the anterior pituitary gland (15,17–19,22,23,65).

Moreover, destruction of the dopaminergic cell bodies and terminals resulted in a marked elevation of plasma prolactin levels (9). It has also been found that the prolactin release inhibiting activity contained in purified hypothalamic extracts could be accounted for by their catecholamine content (102), and preincubation of hypothalamic extracts with aluminum oxide or monoamine oxidase led to a complete loss of prolactin release inhibiting activity (100).

Prolactin, in addition to its well known role in the control of lactation, has an important influence on gonadal function in men and women where an excess of secretion leads to infertility (8,43). More recently this hormone was found to be active at the level of the central nervous system (CNS) (46). Such observations of the multiple functions of prolactin stress the importance of obtaining detailed knowledge about the control of its secretion.

The absence of nerve terminals in the anterior pituitary gland offers the possibility of using the control of prolactin secretion as a model for other less accessible postsynaptic dopaminergic systems of the CNS. In addition, *in vivo* changes of prolactin secretion can be used as an index of DA release from the hypothalamo-tuberoinfundibular system under various experimental conditions, including the role of other biogenic amines, peptides, and sex steroids. Using data obtained with combined *in vitro* and *in vivo* approaches, the present report summarizes recent information on the control of DA release from the hypothalamo-tuberoinfundibular system and the control of its action on prolactin secretion at the pituitary level.

SPECIFICITY OF THE DOPAMINERGIC CONTROL OF PROLACTIN SECRETION

Assay of DA Agonistic Activity

The potency of a series of DA agonists on prolactin release in anterior pituitary cells in culture is illustrated in Fig. 1. As measured by the concentration giving a 50% inhibition of hormone release, the following order of potency was obtained: dihydroergocornine (DHE) (0.3 nM) > apomorphine (2.3 nM) > 2-bromo-α-ergocryptine (CB-154, 3.6 nM) > dopamine (20 nM) > piribedil (100 nM). As previously observed, apomorphine, a prototype of DA agonists (3), was approximately 10 times more potent than DA as inhibitor of prolactin release at an ED_{50} value of 2.3 nM.

Dihydroergocryptine (DHEC) and DHE, two ergot alkaloids thought to act mainly through a dopaminergic mechanism on prolactin secretion (81), were tested in this *in vitro* system. It can be seen in Fig. 1 that DHE was very potent in inhibiting prolactin release at an ED_{50} value of 0.3 nM, and similar potency was found for DHEC. CB-154, a compound used as inhibitor of prolactin secretion in the human (29,104), had a potency slightly lower than that of apomorphine (ED_{50} = 3.6 nM). High concentrations of ergot alkaloids, apomorphine, and catecholamines led to the same maximal inhibition of prolactin release. Previous data (18) showed that the inhibition of prolactin release by catecholamines showed the expected stereoselectivity since (−)epinephrine and (−)norepinephrine were approximately eight times more potent than the corresponding (+)enantiomers.

Assay of Antidopaminergic Activity

The potency of a series of neuroleptics to reverse the inhibition of prolactin release induced by the DA agonist DHE (21) in rat anterior pituitary cells in culture has been studied. The antidopaminergic activity of the various drugs

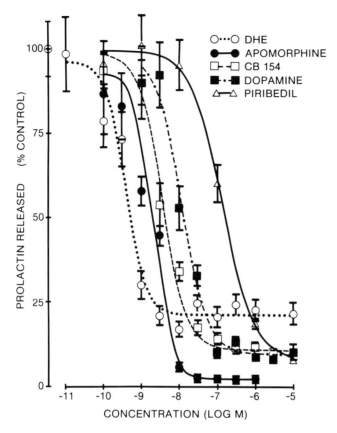

FIG. 1. Effect of increasing concentrations of DA and DA agonists on prolactin (PRL) release in rat anterior pituitary cells in primary culture. Four days after plating, cells were incubated for 3 hr in the presence of the indicated drug concentrations.

is clearly dose-related, and their ability to reverse the action of DHE led to the following order of potency as measured by K_D values: spiroperidol (0.048 nM) > thioproperazine (0.08 nM) > piperacetazine (0.27 nM) > pericyazine (2.9 nM) > pipamperone (149 nM) (data not shown). When assayed alone, those drugs, except spiroperidol, did not show agonistic activity up to 10^{-5} M, thus indicating that they act as pure antagonists on the DA pituitary receptor at least up to the concentration used. It should be mentioned, however, that most neuroleptics do in fact show mixed DA agonist–antagonist activities.

The antidopaminergic activity of 15 other well known neuroleptics on prolactin release was studied and showed a close correlation with their clinical potency. In fact, a close correlation was observed between the clinical potency of the 20 most currently used neuroleptics and their activity on the DA receptor controlling prolactin release in rat anterior pituitary cells in culture ($r = 0.908$, $p < 0.001$; data not shown).

The present data clearly show that changes of prolactin release in rat anterior pituitary cells in primary culture provide a sensitive, precise, specific, and reliable measurement of the agonistic and/or antagonistic activities of dopaminergic drugs. This system is apparently free of the limitations accompanying the use of the DA receptor and DA-sensitive adenyl cyclase assays as screening tests for antiparkinsonian, antihyperprolactinemic, and antischizophrenic drugs. Previous data using rat hemipituitaries clearly showed a direct inhibitory effect of DA agonists on prolactin release (21,81). However, as shown for the assay of luteinizing hormone releasing hormone (LHRH) analogs (68) and study of the feedback action of steroids (31,32,93), the pituitary cell culture system is much more precise.

Since the control of prolactin release is typically dopaminergic, the present findings of a close correlation between reversal of the inhibitory effect of a DA agonist on prolactin release and the clinical potency of a large series of neuroleptics strongly support the suggestion that these drugs are acting in schizophrenic patients through inhibition of the DA receptor.

Since the anterior pituitary gland does not appear to bind catecholamines other than those having dopaminergic activity (18), interference by other mechanisms is minimized in this system. Moreover, a high degree of precision is achieved and minimal quantities of drugs are required. It is hoped that such a system, in addition to its intrinsic interest and predictive value for the clinical potency of neuroleptics and antiparkinsonian and prolactin-lowering drugs, could be used as a model to study the control of the less accessible dopaminergic pathways involved in other brain functions.

Specificity of the Pituitary Dopaminergic Receptor

Following our studies on the dopaminergic control of prolactin secretion, it became important to examine the correlation between the specificity of the binding of labeled dopaminergic agents to the pituitary dopamine receptor and the specificity of action of the same compounds on prolactin secretion.

In preliminary experiments we demonstrated binding of [^{3}H]DHEC to rat anterior pituitary membranes or whole cells in culture that appears to possess features of dopaminergic specificity. However, due to the very small amount of membrane protein that can be derived from rat anterior pituitary, the relatively low concentration of receptors in these preparations, and the modest specific activity of the labeled ligand, it was believed that the bovine anterior pituitary would be a preferable tissue for carrying out such detailed studies of binding to dopaminergic receptors.

Binding of [^{3}H]DHEC to bovine anterior pituitary membranes displayed a specificity typical of a dopaminergic process. As shown in Fig. 2, agonists competed for [^{3}H]DHEC binding with the following order of potency: apomorphine > dopamine > epinephrine > norepinephrine >> isoproterenol = clonidine. This relative order of potency closely resembles the potency of these

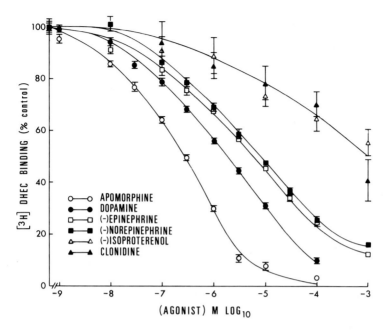

FIG. 2. Competition of various agonists for [³H]DHEC binding to bovine anterior pituitary membranes. Membranes were pretreated at 25°C for 10 min with 0.1% ascorbic acid and 10 μM pargyline. Control specific binding (100%) was 0.185 ± 0.009 pmole/mg ($N = 3$). Results shown are means ± SEM of three experiments determined in triplicate.

agonists in: (a) inhibiting prolactin secretion from rat anterior pituitary (Fig. 1); (b) stimulating the dopamine-sensitive adenylate cyclase (59,62); and (c) competing for [³H]haloperidol (16,98), [³H]dopamine (16,30,55,62,98), and [³H]apomorphine binding (99) in brain tissue.

Ergot alkaloids which act as potent dopaminergic agonists on prolactin secretion (45) are also potent competitors of [³H]DHEC binding. These ergot compounds did in fact compete for binding with a potency that closely parallels their inhibitory effect on prolactin release in anterior pituitary cells in culture (data not shown).

[³H]DHEC binding sites in bovine anterior pituitary displayed marked stereoselectivity toward various neuroleptics and their isomers. Thus (+)butaclamol, which possesses potent pharmacological dopamine-blocking activity (62), was more than 10,000 times more effective than its inactive (−)isomer in competing for binding (18). Accordingly, we have taken as specific binding to the DA receptor sites in these pituitary preparations the amount of [³H]DHEC binding displaceable by 1 to 10 μM (+)butaclamol.

It was also found that [³H]DHEC binding sites exhibit marked stereoselectivity toward other thioxanthene derivatives; α-flupenthixol inhibited binding more potently (1,000 times) than its geometric isomer β-flupenthixol. Similarly, *cis-*

thiothixene competed for binding more potently (75 to 100 times) than *trans*-thiothixene. The characteristics of interaction of these neuroleptics with these binding sites correlate well with their ability to reverse the dopaminergic inhibition of prolactin release and their DA-blocking activity in pharmacological tests.

The present data indicate that the anterior pituitary gland, in addition to its own intrinsic interest, should represent a useful model for detailed study of the mechanisms of dopaminergic action. In fact, changes of [³H]DHEC binding to the dopaminergic receptor can be correlated with an easily accessible and highly precise parameter of biological activity: prolactin release in cells in culture. Such a model of DA action has not been previously available and should be useful for a better understanding of the mechanisms controlling DA receptor-mediated actions.

STIMULATORY EFFECT OF β-ENDORPHIN AND METHIONINE-ENKEPHALIN ON PROLACTIN SECRETION IN THE RAT

Morphine is well known to be a potent stimulus of growth hormone (GH) (41,63) and prolactin (85) release in the rat. The opiate has also been shown to stimulate prolactin secretion in humans (105). Since methionine-enkephalin (met-enkephalin) and β-endorphin bind to the opiate receptor (20,86) and have potent morphine-like activity in various biological assays (20,79), the possibility was raised that the endogenous opioid peptides, in addition to their well known analgesic potency (6,91) and activity as behavior modulators (12), could be involved in the neuroendocrine control of GH and prolactin secretion.

As illustrated in Fig. 3, the intraventricular injection of 0.5 to 25 µg β-endorphin (β-LPH$_{61-91}$) led to a rapid and marked stimulation of prolactin release in unanesthetized freely moving rats. With the 0.5 µg dose, a significant rise was measured as early as 5 min after injection of the peptide and maximal stimulation (approximately seven-fold) was measured after 10 min, with a slow return toward basal plasma hormone levels at later time intervals. The higher doses of β-endorphin (2, 5, and 25 µg) led to a progressive increase of prolactin release, a 30- to 60-fold increase being measured between 20 and 60 min after injection of 25 µg of the peptide.

Met-enkephalin, the NH$_2$-terminal pentapeptide of β-endorphin, was much less potent than β-endorphin for stimulating prolactin release. In fact, at the 500 to 1,000 µg doses, met-enkephalin led to approximately four- and six-fold increases of plasma prolactin levels, respectively.

As mentioned above, the potency of met-enkephalin as stimulator of prolactin release is much lower than that of β-endorphin. In fact, the present data demonstrate that β-endorphin is 2,000 times more potent than met-enkephalin for stimulating prolactin secretion. This difference of biological activity is in marked contrast with the relative affinities of the two peptides for the opiate receptor; met-enkephalin shows a binding affinity for the opiate receptor approximately

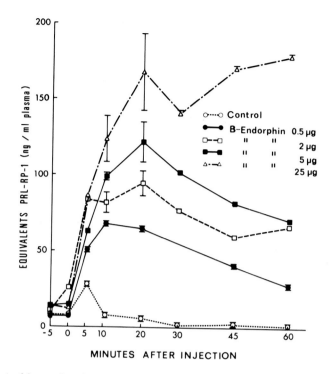

FIG. 3. Effect of increasing doses of β-endorphin on plasma prolactin (PRL) levels in the rat. Male rats bearing intraventricular and intrajugular cannulas were injected intravenously with 0.2 ml of sheep somatostatin antiserum 5 min before the intraventricular injection of the indicated amounts of synthetic β-endorphin. PRL concentrations were measured at the indicated time intervals after administration of β-endorphin to 8 to 10 animals per group. Data are presented as the mean ± SEM.

three times higher than that of β-endorphin (35). These data indicate that the higher potency of β-endorphin is probably due to its higher resistance to degradation. It is of interest, in this connection, to mention that met-enkephalin is rapidly inactivated by plasma and brain tissue. Indeed, 15 sec after intravenous injection of [³H]met-enkephalin, only 5% of total radioactivity comigrated with intact met-enkephalin, whereas 74% of the radioactivity was eluted in the area corresponding to tyrosine (33). The highly potent and long-lasting activity of [D-Ala²]met-enkephalin reported previously (24) indicates the importance of the Tyr–Gly amide bond for action of the degrading enzymes in plasma and various tissues. β-Endorphin and its [D-Ala²] analog displayed similar potency as stimulators of GH and prolactin release when injected intraventricularly, but [D-Ala²]β-endorphin injected intravenously led to an increased duration of action of the peptide relative to the native molecule (67). [D-Ala²]Met-enkephalin and [D-Ala²]met-enkephalin amide were also active on GH and prolactin release after intravenous administration.

ROLE OF ENDORPHINS IN STRESS- AND SUCKLING-INDUCED PROLACTIN RELEASE IN THE RAT

Acute release of prolactin in the rat is well known to be induced by suckling (103) and a variety of stressful stimuli, e.g., ether, surgery, restraint, nicotine injection, exposure to cold or heat, or simple venous puncture (11,61,87). Stress also stimulates serum prolactin levels in the human, the response being greater in women than men (89). Moreover, suckling increases prolactin release in women (95). It was thus of interest to study the possible role of endorphins in the acute release of prolactin induced by stress and suckling. Using the specific opiate antagonist naloxone, the present data provide evidence for such a role of endorphins.

In agreement with previous data (87), it can be seen in Fig. 4 that exposure to ether vapor led to rapid stimulation of plasma prolactin release. A maximal effect was seen at 5 min, with a progressive decrease toward control levels at 30 min. When the opiate antagonist naloxone (10 mg/kg) was injected 10 min

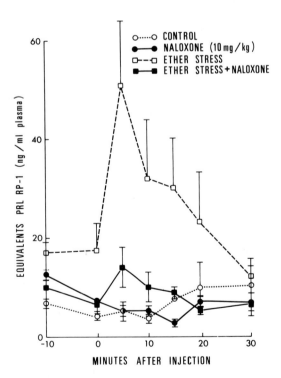

FIG. 4. Effect of naloxone (10 mg/kg) on ether-induced stimulation of plasma prolactin (PRL) levels in the rat. Animals bearing an intrajugular cannula were injected with naloxone 10 min before being exposed to ether vapor for 1 to 2 min. Blood sampling was performed at the indicated time intervals.

before exposure to ether, the stimulation of prolactin release was completely abolished ($p < 0.01$).

A single injection of naloxone (5 mg/kg) 5 min before return of the pups led to 50 to 95% inhibition of the marked rise of plasma prolactin induced by suckling in the rat up to the last time interval studied (90 min) (data not shown). In complementary experiments, where naloxone was injected at -10, 45, and 90 min, plasma prolactin levels were still reduced from 600 ± 95 to 115 ± 40 ng/ml 2 hr after the start of suckling (data not shown).

The present data clearly suggest that endogenous opiate peptides could be involved as mediators of the stimulatory effect of stress and suckling on prolactin release in the rat. Although TRH might be implicated in the effect of stress and suckling on prolactin release, indirect evidence suggests that DA is the main factor involved. The observation that stress elevates plasma prolactin levels in male and female rats except during the afternoon of proestrus or other conditions of high prolactin levels (87) suggests that inhibition of dopaminergic activity is involved in the response of prolactin to stress. It should be mentioned that some workers suggest that serotonin plays a role in the suckling (64) and stress (83) induced release of prolactin.

ROLE OF ENDORPHINS IN THE NOCTURNAL RISE OF PROLACTIN IN THE HUMAN

There are 24-hr studies of plasma prolactin levels in the human which show that this hormone is released episodically and that plasma concentrations of the hormone increase after the onset of sleep. The sleep-related increase in prolactin secretion is dependent on sleep itself and is not related to clock time (90,96). In an attempt to gain a better understanding of the mechanisms involved in the increased release of this hormone during sleep, we studied the effect of naloxone infusion on serum prolactin levels.

Six healthy postmenopausal women took part in this study after giving informed consent. Blood samples (3 ml) were obtained at 20-min intervals through a long brachial intravenous catheter, permitting sampling without disturbing the patient. A 24-hr basal study showed typical nycthemeral secretory profiles. In a subsequent 24-hr study, naloxone was infused continuously between 2300 (11 p.m.) and 0700 (7 a.m.). The marked rise of serum prolactin levels that occurred between 2400 (midnight) and 0700 (7 a.m.) in six women was 45 to 95% inhibited by naloxone infusion (data not shown). As confirmed in other subjects, the inhibition by naloxone of serum prolactin levels is dose-dependent. No apparent change of sleeping pattern was noted during or after naloxone administration.

These data strongly suggest that endorphins are involved as mediators of the nocturnal rise of serum prolactin levels in the human. Coupled with our findings indicating a role of endogenous opiates in the stress- and suckling-induced release of prolactin in the rat (40), the data obtained in the human further support a physiological role of endorphins in the control of prolactin secretion.

ROLE OF DOPAMINE AND SEROTONIN IN THE OPIATE-INDUCED STIMULATION OF PROLACTIN RELEASE IN THE RAT

Changes of DA Turnover

After infusion of met-enkephalin alone (60 μg/1 hr), the catecholamine (CA) stores in the medial palisade zone of the median eminence were increased by about 35%, whereas those in the subependymal layer were reduced by 28%. A trend toward an increase of CA stores in the lateral palisade zone was also noted. Prolactin serum levels were markedly increased (400%) at the same time. In experiments where H44/68 was used in addition, the H44/68-induced CA disappearance was significantly reduced in the medial and lateral palisade zones, whereas there were no significant changes in the H44/68-induced CA disappearance in the subependymal layer. The serum prolactin levels were markedly increased by H44/68 treatment. Prolactin levels were further increased (30%) following met-enkephalin treatment.

Not only met-enkephalin (39) but also β-endorphin and morphine markedly reduced DA turnover within the lateral and medial palisade zones of the median eminence (47). This marked effect on the tuberoinfundibular DA neurons suggests that several of the neuroendocrine actions of opioid peptides and morphine may be mediated via inactivation of these median eminence DA systems. It seems quite likely that the increases of prolactin secretion observed following intraventricular injections of opioid peptides and morphine (34,73) could be mediated, at least in part, via reduced activity in the tuberoinfundibular DA system (39).

Studies with Antidopaminergic Drugs

Following the findings of an opiate-induced inhibition of DA turnover in the tuberoinfundibular neurons, it seemed appropriate to use antidopaminergic drugs as a second approach for measuring the role of DA in the effect of endorphins and opiates on prolactin secretion.

In order to avoid interference by stress or anesthesia, all studies were performed in unanesthetized freely moving rats bearing an intrajugular cannula inserted 2 days previously. A maximal stimulatory effect of morphine on plasma prolactin levels was obtained at a dose of 25 to 100 mg/kg s.c. Maximal plasma prolactin concentrations were measured 15 to 30 min after injection of the opiate with a progressive decrease toward basal levels at later time intervals. No significant change of plasma prolactin levels was seen in animals injected with the vehicle alone.

Before using DA antagonists as an argument for a role of DA in the morphine-induced rise of prolactin secretion, it was useful to determine the dose of neuroleptics giving maximal stimulatory effects on prolactin release. The finding that morphine could not further stimulate prolactin secretion after a maximal dose of an antidopaminergic drug would then indicate that DA is involved in the action of the opiate on prolactin secretion.

That the potent stimulatory effect of morphine on prolactin release is secondary to inhibition of dopaminergic activity was indicated by the observation that the acute response (up to 15 min) of plasma prolactin induced by a maximal dose of morphine (40 mg/kg) was not further increased by simultaneous administration of a high dose of haloperidol (1 mg/kg) (Fig. 5, left). The acute release of prolactin induced by the first injection of morphine is followed by a refractory period since no change of plasma prolactin levels is observed when the same dose of morphine is administered 30 and 60 min later (Fig. 5, right). The presence of this refractory period is further supported by the finding that haloperidol injected 45 min after the opiate leads to marked stimulation of prolactin release, thus suggesting that the rapid decrease of plasma prolactin levels following acute stimulation by morphine is due to a return of inhibitory dopaminergic activity (Fig. 5, right).

Since it was proposed that serotonin plays a role in the stimulation of prolactin secretion induced by stress (51) and suckling (49), and evidence was recently obtained for a role of endorphins in the stress- and suckling-induced rise of prolactin release (40,66,106), we next used an inhibitor, parachlorophenylalanine (PCPA), and a precursor, 5-hydroxytryptophan (5-HTP), of serotonin biosynthesis to study a possible role of serotonin in the stimulatory effect of endorphins on prolactin release.

Inhibition of serotonin biosynthesis with PCPA reduced by 40 to 45% the rise of plasma prolactin levels induced by morphine in the absence (Fig. 6A) or presence (Fig. 6B) of simultaneous treatment with 5-HTP. The inhibitory effect of PCPA on the morphine-induced rise of plasma prolactin was significant at the 30-min interval, whereas that on the effect of morphine plus 5-HTP was significant at all time intervals after 30 min. Treatment with PCPA alone had no significant effect on the already low plasma prolactin levels in control animals. It is of interest that the marked rise of prolactin secretion induced by 5-HTP was superimposable in control and PCPA-treated rats (Fig. 6B), thus indicating that lowering of endogenous serotonin by PCPA does not affect the sensitivity of the serotoninergic response mechanisms.

In order to obtain further support for the results obtained with PCPA, we next studied the effect of methysergide, a serotonin antagonist, on morphine-induced prolactin release. Methysergide, although inactive alone, led to almost complete inhibition of prolactin release following morphine injection.

The present data clearly indicate that the acute release of prolactin induced by morphine can be accounted for by inhibition of the inhibitory hypothalamic dopaminergic influence on prolactin secretion. This is well illustrated by the absence of further stimulation of acute prolactin release by a high dose of haloper

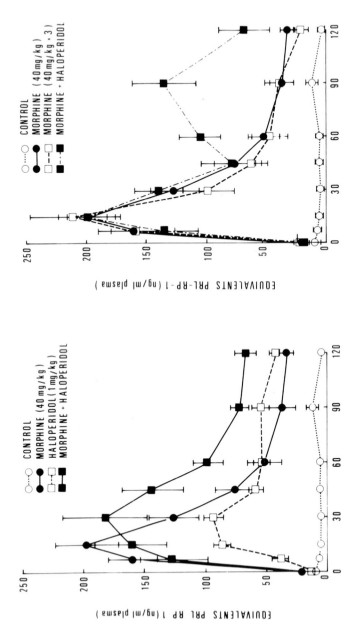

FIG. 5. Effect of a single injection of high doses of morphine, haloperidol, repeated injection of morphine, or a combination of the two drugs on plasma prolactin (PRL) levels in the male rat. **Left:** Morphine (40 mg/kg) was injected as a single dose (●) at time 0. Haloperidol (1 mg/kg) was injected as a single dose (□) at time 0 or in combination with morphine (■) at time 0. **Right:** Morphine (40 mg/kg) was injected as a single dose (●) or given at 0, 30, and 60 min (□). Haloperidol (1 mg/kg) was injected 45 min after morphine (■).

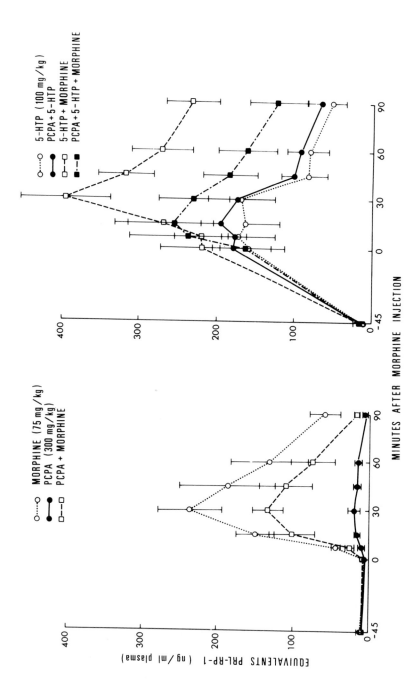

FIG. 6. Effect of morphine, 5-hydroxytryptophan (5-HTP), or parachlorophenylalanine (PCPA) alone or in combination on plasma prolactin (PRL) levels in the rat. Morphine (75 mg/kg s.c.) was injected at time 0; 5-HTP (100 mg/kg s.c.) was injected 45 min before the experiment; and PCPA (300 mg/kg i.p.) was injected 48 and 24 hr before time 0.

idol in animals already treated with morphine (Fig. 5A). The tendency for additive effects of morphine and haloperidol at later time intervals (30 to 120 min) (Fig. 5A) can be explained by the refractoriness of the response to morphine coupled to the relatively long-term action of haloperidol. These data are in agreement with the findings of acute inhibition of dopamine turnover in the medial palisade zone of the median eminence in rats injected intraventricularly with met-enkephalin or β-endorphin (39,47). This effect of opiates is probably due to the activation of presynaptic inhibitory opiate receptors located on tubero-infundibular dopaminergic nerve endings.

Coupled to the previous observations that (a) the prolactin release inhibiting activity contained in hypothalamic extracts could be accounted for by catechol-amines (100,102), (b) DA is present in the hypothalamo-pituitary portal system (7), (c) typical dopaminergic receptors are present in anterior pituitary tissue (18,65), and (d) the control of prolactin release at the anterior pituitary level is typically dopaminergic (65), the present data add strong support for a predominant role of DA in the control of prolactin secretion. In fact, a 5- to 20-fold stimulation of plasma prolactin levels in the male rat after injection of a DA antagonist (or of morphine) indicates that under basal conditions prolactin secretion is 80 to 95% inhibited by DA. It remains possible, however, that part of the action of DA could be mediated by a prolactin releasing factor.

The present observations suggest that presynaptic inhibitory opiate receptors are present on dopaminergic neurons of the tuberoinfundibular system. Since the stimulatory effect of morphine on prolactin secretion is partly prevented after inhibition of serotonin biosynthesis with PCPA, it is also possible that presynaptic stimulatory opiate receptors are present on serotonergic nerve endings in contact with the tuberoinfundibular dopaminergic system. It is also possible that effects of opiates on dopaminergic and serotonergic activity are not direct but are, instead, mediated by other neurotransmitter(s) or neuromodulator(s).

β-LIPOTROPIN AND β-ENDORPHIN-LIKE IMMUNOREACTIVITY IN RAT HYPOTHALAMUS

The discovery that endogenous peptides isolated from brain (58), anterior pituitary gland (14,53,71), or the hypothalamo-pituitary complex (56,74) have the same structure as fragments of the COOH-terminal region of β-lipotropin (β-LPH) already isolated from many species (50,52,70,72,80) suggests that β-LPH may be the precursor of endorphins.

Since the antibodies developed against β-endorphin cross react with β-LPH and the 31K precursor, we studied the distribution of β-endorphin immunoreactivity in bovine hypothalamic extracts after gel filtration. As illustrated in Fig. 7, the main component of the acid extract from bovine hypothalamic tissue measured with the radioimmunoassay (RIA) system specific for the N-terminus of β-LPH (β-LPH$_{1-47}$ system) (75) comigrates with γ-LPH, whereas the second

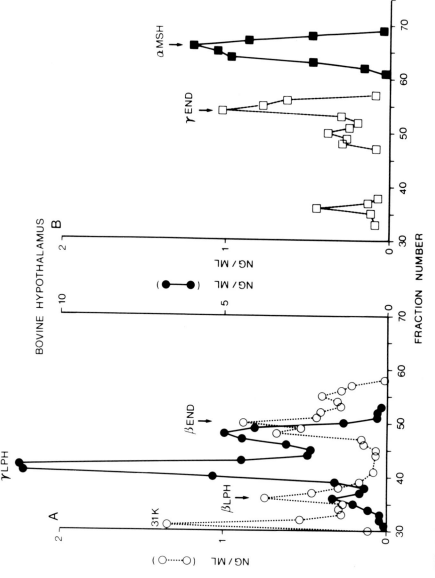

FIG. 7. Chromatography of bovine hypothalamic acid extract. **A:** Immunoreactivity in the β-endorphin (○) and γ-LPH (●) RIA systems. **B:** Immunoreactivity in the γ-endorphin (□) and α-MSH (■) RIAs.

major peak elutes at a position slightly slower than β-endorphin and a minor peak is seen at the position of β-LPH.

When the β-endorphin RIA system was used, the major peaks comigrated with β-endorphin itself, β-LPH, and the 31K precursor, whereas a minor peak was seen at the position of γ-endorphin. When the γ-endorphin RIA system was used, a major peak was seen at the position of γ-endorphin, whereas minor components were seen at the position of β-endorphin and β-LPH. α-MSH immunoreactivity, on the other hand, eluted exclusively at the position of the α-MSH marker. An almost superimposable elution profile was observed with rat hypothalamic extracts.

Combined with our previous findings (75), the present data show that using four RIA systems specific for β-LPH$_{1-47}$, β-endorphin, γ-endorphin, and α-MSH, components of sizes similar to those separated by Sephadex chromatography are present in the extracts from the bovine anterior and intermediate pituitary lobes as well as from the hypothalamus. However, marked differences are seen in the relative amounts of each immunoreactive component, thus indicating different levels of activity of the enzymatic systems responsible for the processing of these peptides.

The finding that β-endorphin is the most potent endogenous opiate-like peptide isolated so far as stimulator of prolactin release (34,35) and the relatively high levels of this peptide in the hypothalamus suggest that β-endorphin could be secreted and acting locally in the physiological control of prolactin secretion.

INTERACTIONS OF THE DOPAMINERGIC TUBEROINFUNDIBULAR SYSTEM WITH SEX STEROIDS

Estrogens are known to be potent stimulators of prolactin secretion in man (60,88,95) and rat (2,26–28). However, these *in vivo* data could not discriminate between pituitary and/or hypothalamic sites of estrogen action. In order to avoid this problem, we recently performed experiments using anterior pituitary cells in primary culture and found that estrogens exert a stimulatory effect on basal and TRH-induced prolactin release by a direct action at the pituitary level (65,93). More surprisingly, estrogens could lead to an almost complete reversal of the inhibitory effect of dopaminergic agents on prolactin release. The increase of plasma prolactin levels following administration of a maximal dose of an antidopaminergic drug was next used to assess the dopaminergic influence on prolactin secretion after sex steroid treatment. As illustrated in Fig. 8A, treatment of adult ovariectomized rats for 10 days with 17β-estradiol led to an eightfold stimulation of the plasma prolactin response to a maximal dose of thioproperazine, a pure and potent dopaminergic antagonist (4). Treatment with testosterone, probably as a consequence of its conversion to estrogens, led to a threefold increase of the prolactin response to the neuroleptic. It is of interest to note that, although inactive alone, 5α-dihydrotestosterone (DHT) and progesterone led to a significant reversal of the stimulatory action of 17β-

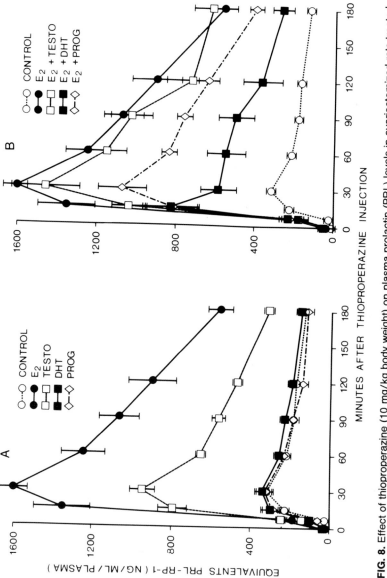

FIG. 8. Effect of thioproperazine (10 mg/kg body weight) on plasma prolactin (PRL) levels in ovariectomized rats treated twice a day for 10 days with various steroids either alone or in combination: estradiol (E₂) (1 µg), testosterone and 5α-dihydrotestosterone (DHT) (250 µg), and progesterone (2 mg). Thioproperazine was injected subcutaneously at time 0 in animals bearing an intrajugular cannula. Blood sampling was performed at the indicated time intervals.

estradiol on the prolactin response whereas combined treatment with testosterone and 17β-estradiol led to a response almost superimposable on that of the estrogen alone (Fig. 8B).

The present data clearly suggest that treatment with 17β-estradiol leads to a marked increase of the dopaminergic inhibitory influence on prolactin secretion. In fact, neutralization of the dopaminergic influence by a neuroleptic drug leads to an eightfold increase of plasma prolactin levels. Since a similar estrogen treatment has been found to decrease the activity of dopamine at the pituitary level *in vivo* in the rat (42), the present data indicate that the rate of release of the DA involved in the control of prolactin secretion is increased more than eightfold under the influence of estrogens. Partial reversal of the stimulatory effect of 17β-estradiol by the association of DHT or progesterone suggests that these two steroids exert antiestrogenic activity at the hypothalamic level. Such data on the effect of sex steroids are in agreement with the observed changes of DA turnover in the hypothalamus in the rat following treatment with sex steroids or at different stages of the estrous cycle (36,48,76). More complete understanding of the effect of sex steroids at the hypothalamic and pituitary levels should be provided by a detailed analysis of the changes of sensitivity to DA occurring at the pituitary level under the same experimental conditions.

α-ADRENERGIC REGULATION OF [³H]DOPAMINE RELEASE IN RAT HYPOTHALAMIC TISSUE *IN VITRO*

In order to obtain more information about the control of DA release in the hypothalamus, the effect of a series of neurotransmitters on the release of [³H]DA was studied in rat hypothalamic slices *in vitro*.

Adult male rats were injected with nialamide (100 mg/kg i.p.) 1 hr prior to decapitation. The brains were then rapidly removed and the hypothalami (2 mm thick, delineated rostrally by the optic chiasm, caudally by the mammillary bodies, and laterally by the hypothalamic scissure) were dissected, cut into slices of 0.225 mm thickness with razor blades or a Sorvall tissue chopper before preincubation in 2 ml of KRBGA (Krebs Ringer bicarbonate buffer containing glucose 1 mg/ml and ascorbic acid 1 mg/ml, pH 7.4) for 5 min at 37°C under an atmosphere of 95% O_2/5% CO_2. The tissue was then incubated for 30 min in fresh KRBGA medium containing 50 nM [³H]DA (2 Ci/mmole). After incubation, the hypothalami [2] were transferred to a Swinnex Millipore filter holder and superfused with KRBGA at a flow rate of 0.5 ml/min essentially as previously described (78). Excess radioactivity was first washed with 15 ml buffer before collection of 2-ml fractions. When high K^+ (53 mM) was used, the concentration of Na^+ was decreased proportionally. Data are expressed as percent of the mean value (counts per minute) of spontaneous [³H] release calculated for the five 2-ml samples collected immediately prior to stimulation.

The stimulatory effects of NE and serotonin are concentration-dependent, and NE is approximately 100 times more potent than serotonin as a stimulator of [³H]DA release (Fig. 9). As observed with high K^+, the norepinephrine (NE)-induced release of [³H]DA depends on the presence of CA^{2+}.

In order to further characterize the specificity of the [³H]DA-releasing action of NE, adrenergic agonists and antagonists were used. Phenylephrine, an α-adrenergic agonist, was almost as potent as NE in stimulating the release of [³H]DA by the hypothalamic tissue, this effect being also concentration-dependent (data not shown). (−)Isoproterenol, a β-adrenergic agonist, had only a very small effect even at 10^{-4} M. Moreover, when the α-adrenergic antagonists phenoxybenzamine and phentolamine (10^{-4} M) were added to the medium at the beginning of the perfusion, the subsequent response to NE or phenylephrine was abolished. When added alone, these antagonist drugs had only a negligible effect on [³H]DA release.

The present data clearly show that NE and serotonin are potent stimulators of preaccumulated [³H]DA release in rat hypothalamic slices, whereas the DA antagonist haloperidol has a small stimulatory effect and a variety of other drugs and neurotransmitters were inactive. Since the stimulatory effect of NE on [³H]DA release was observed at a relatively low concentration (100 nM), it is likely that the effect observed is not due to inhibition of [³H]DA reuptake by DA nerve terminals. In fact, at 100 nM, NE should be taken up specifically by NE nerve terminals (38,101). It thus appears likely that α-adrenergic receptors are present on the tuberoinfundibular DA neurons. This is also supported by the reversal of the NE and phenylephrine effects by the α-adrenergic antagonists phentolamine and phenoxybenzamine.

As mentioned earlier, although no definitive evidence is yet available, convincing data indicate that the tuberoinfundibular DA neurons are directly involved in the control of prolactin secretion (65,82). This is supported, on an anatomical basis, by the observation that short axons originating in cell bodies in the arcuate nucleus have their terminals in the external layer of the median eminence close to the primary capillary plexus of the hypophysial portal system which supplies blood to the anterior pituitary gland (10,77).

The tuberoinfundibular DA system appears to be involved also in the control of LHRH secretion. In fact, DA neurons have been suggested to inhibit (1) or stimulate (97) gonadotropin secretion.

It is thus of great interest to correlate the present *in vitro* findings with pharmacological studies on the control of prolactin and gonadotropin secretion performed *in vivo* (84). Martin et al. (84) recently found that phenoxybenzamine, an α-adrenergic blocker, led to marked stimulation of prolactin release in intact male rats. Stimulation of prolactin secretion by phenoxybenzamine has also been reported in ovariectomized female rats (69) and sheep (25). Our *in vitro* findings of a potent stimulatory effect of NE on [³H]DA release are thus in agreement with the above-mentioned *in vivo* data, and indicate the usefulness of such an *in vitro* system for studying the multiple interactions involved in neuroendocrine control.

The present data indicate that, in addition to its intrinsic interest for more

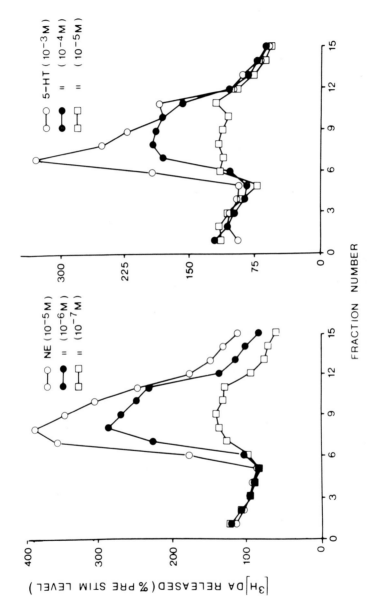

FIG. 9. Effect of increasing concentrations of norepinephrine (NE) **(left)** or serotonin (5-HT) **(right)** on [³H]DA release in rat hypothalamic slices. The indicated concentrations of biogenic amines were present in fractions 6 through 10.

complete knowledge of the control of prolactin secretion, the tuberoinfundibular system can be used as a model for other less accessible dopaminergic systems in the CNS. The antidopaminergic action of estrogens first demonstrated at the anterior pituitary level (93) was recently observed at the striatal level (37). The interest of such studies on the interaction of sex steroids with brain catecholaminergic systems in strengthened by the observations that estrogen administration to male or female patients receiving neuroleptics can facilitate the appearance of parkinsonian symptoms (54). Moreover, treatment with estrogens has been found to improve the symptoms of tardive dyskinesias induced by chronic treatment with L-DOPA or neuroleptics (5). The above-mentioned effects of estrogen treatment in the human are compatible with an antidopaminergic action and open the possibility of clinical applications of sex hormones in neurological as well as psychiatric diseases.

REFERENCES

1. Ahren, K., Fuxe, K., Hamberger, L., and Hökfelt, T. (1971): Turnover changes in the tuberoinfundibular dopamine neurons during the ovarian cycle of the rat. *Endocrinology,* 88:1415–1424.
2. Ajika, A., Krulich, L., Fawcett, C. P., and McCann, S. M. (1972): Effects of estrogen on plasma and pituitary gonadotropins and prolactin and on hypothalamic releasing and inhibitory factors. *Neuroendocrinology,* 9:304–315.
3. Andèn, N. E., Rubenson, A., Fuxe, L., and Hökfelt, T. (1967): Evidence for dopamine receptor stimulation by apomorphine. *J. Pharm. Pharmacol.,* 19:627–629.
4. Beaulieu, M., and Labrie, F. (1980): A precise assay for potential antiparkinsonian and antischizophrenic drugs: Prolactin release in rat anterior pituitary cells in culture. *Mol. Pharmacol. (in press).*
5. Bédard, P., Dankova, J., Boucher, R., and Langelier, P. (1980): Effect of estrogens on apomorphine-induced circling behavior in the rat. *Can. J. Physiol. Pharmacol.,* 56:538–541.
6. Belluzi, J. D., Grant, N., Garsky, V., Sarantakis, D., Wise, C. D., and Stein, L. (1976): Analgesia induced in vivo by central administration of enkephalin in the rat. *Nature,* 260:625–626.
7. Ben-Jonathan, N., Oliver, C., Weiner, H. J., Mical, R. S., and Porter, J. C. (1977): Dopamine in hypophysial portal plasma of the rat during the estrous cycle and throughout pregnancy. *Endocrinology,* 100:452–458.
8. Besser, G. M., Parke, L., Edwards, C. R. W., Forsyth, I. A., and McNeilly, G. (1972): Galactorrhea: Successful treatment with reduction of plasma prolactin levels by bromergocryptine. *Br. Med. J.,* 669–672.
9. Bishop, W., Fawcett, C. P., Krulich, L., and McCann, S. M. (1972): Acute and chronic effects of hypothalamic lesions on the release of FSH, LH and prolactin in intact and castrated rats. *Endocrinology,* 91:643–656.
10. Bjorklund, A., Moore, R. Y., Nobin, A., and Stenevi, V. (1973): The organization of the tubero-hypophyseal and reticulo-infundibular catecholamine neuron systems in the rat brain. *Brain Res.,* 51:171–191.
11. Blake, C. A. (1974): Stimulation of pituitary prolactin and TSH release in lactating and proestrus rats. *Endocrinology,* 94:503–508.
12. Bloom, F., Segal, D., Ling, N., and Guillemin, R. (1976): Endorphins: Profound behavioral effects in rats suggest new etiological factors in mental illness. *Nature,* 194:630–636.
13. Bowers, C. Y., Friesen, H. G., Hwang, P., Guyda, H. J., and Folkers, K. (1971): Prolactin and thyrotropin release in man by synthetic pyroglutamyl-histidyl-prolinamide. *Biochem. Biophys. Res. Commun.,* 45:1033–1041.
14. Bradbury, A. F., Smyth, D. G., and Snell, C. R. (1976): Lipotropin: Precursor of two biologically active peptides. *Biochem. Biophys. Res. Commun.,* 69:950–956.

15. Brown, G. M., Seeman, P., and Lee, T. (1976): Dopamine/neuroleptic receptors in basal hypothalamus and pituitary. *Endocrinology,* 99:1407–1410.
16. Burt, D. R., Creese, I., and Snyder, S. H. (1976): Binding interactions of lysergic acid diethylamide and related agents with dopamine receptors in the brain. *Mol. Pharmacol.,* 12:631–638.
17. Calabro, M. A., and MacLeod, R. M. (1978): Binding of dopamine to bovine anterior pituitary gland membranes. *Neuroendocrinology,* 25:32–46.
18. Caron, M. G., Beaulieu, M., Raymond, V., Gagné, B., Drouin, J., Lefkowitz, R. J., and Labrie, F. (1978): Dopaminergic receptors in the anterior pituitary gland: Correlation of [³H]dihydroergocryptine binding with the dopaminergic control of prolactin release. *J. Biol. Chem.,* 253:2244–2253.
19. Caron, M. G., Raymond, V., Lefkowitz, R. J., and Labrie, F. (1977): Identification of dopaminergic receptors in anterior pituitary: Correlation with the dopaminergic control of prolactin release. *Fed. Proc.,* 36:278.
20. Chang, J. K., Fong, B. T. W., Pert, A., and Pert, C. B. (1976): Opiate receptor affinities and behavioral effects of enkephalin structure-activity relationship of ten synthetic peptide analogs. *Life Sci.,* 18:1473–1482.
21. Clemens, J. A., Shaar, J., Smalstig, E. B., Bach, N. J., and Kornfeld, E. C. (1974): Inhibition of prolactin secretion by ergolines. *Endocrinology,* 94:1171–1176.
22. Creese, I., Schneider, R., and Snyder, S. H. (1977): [³H]Spiroperidol labels dopamine receptor in pituitary and brain. *Eur. J. Pharmacol.,* 4:377–381.
23. Cronin, M. J., Roberts, J. M., and Weiner, R. I. (1978): Dopamine and dihydroergocryptine binding to the anterior pituitary and other brain areas of the rat and sheep. *Endocrinology,* 103:302–309.
24. Cusan, L., Dupont, A., Kledzik, G. S., Labrie, F., Coy, D. H., and Schally, A. V. (1977): Potent prolactin and growth hormone releasing activity of more analogues of met-enkephalin. *Nature,* 268:544–547.
25. Davis, S. L., and Burger, M. L. (1973): Hypothalamic catecholamines effects on plasma levels of prolactin and growth hormone in sheep. *Endocrinology,* 92:303–309.
26. De Léan, A., Ferland, L., Drouin, J., Kelly, P. A., and Labrie, F. (1977): Modulation of pituitary TRH receptor levels by estrogens and thyroid hormones. *Endocrinology,* 100:1496–1504.
27. De Léan, A., Garon, M., Kelly, P. A., and Labrie, F. (1977): Changes in pituitary thyrotropin-releasing hormone receptor level and prolactin response to TRH during the rat estrous cycle. *Endocrinology,* 100:1505–1510.
28. De Léan, A., and Labrie, F. (1977): Sensitizing effect of treatment with estrogens on the TSH response to TRH in male rats. *Am. J. Physiol.,* 2:E235–E239.
29. Del Pozo, E., Varga, L., Schultz, K. D., Kunzig, H. J., Marbach, P., Lopez del Campo, D., and Eppenberger, U. (1975): Pituitary and ovarian response patterns to stimulation in the postpartum and galactorrhea-amenorrhea: The role of prolactin. *Obstet. Gynecol.,* 46:539–543.
30. Donoso, A. O., Banzan, A. M., and Barcaglioni, J. C. (1974): Further evidence of the direct action of L-DOPA on prolactin release. *Neuroendocrinology,* 15:236–239.
31. Drouin, J., De Léan, A., Rainville, D., Lachance, R., and Labrie, F. (1976): Characteristics of the interactions between TRH and somatostatin for the thyrotropin and prolactin release. *Endocrinology,* 98:514–521
32. Drouin, J., and Labrie, F. (1976): Selective effect of androgens on LH and FSH release in anterior pituitary cells in culture. *Edocrinology,* 98:1528–1534.
33. Dupont, A., Cusan, L., Garon, M., Alvarado, G., and Labrie, F. (1977): Extremely rapid degradation of [³H]-methionine-enkephalin by various rat tissues in vivo and in vitro. *Life Sci.,* 21:907–914.
34. Dupont, A., Cusan, L., Labrie, F., Coy, D. H., and Li, C. H. (1977): Stimulation of prolactin release in the rat by intraventricular injection of β-endorphin and methionine-enkephalin. *Biochem. Biophys. Res. Commun.,* 75:76–82.
35. Dupont, A., Cusan, L., Morin, O., Kledzik, G. S., Coy, D. H., Li, C. H., and Labrie, F. (1978): Stimulation of prolactin and growth hormone release by intraventricular injection of met-enkephalin, β-endorphin and endorphin analogues in the rat. In: *Current Studies of Hypothalamic Function 1978, Part I: Hormones,* edited by K. Lederis and W. L. Veale, pp. 151–163. Karger, Basel.
36. Eikenburg, D. C., Ravitz, A. J., Gudelsky, G. A., and Moore, K. E. (1977): Effects of estrogen on prolactin and tuberoinfundibular dopaminergic neurons. *J. Neural Transm.,* 40:235–244.

37. Euvrard, C., Labrie, F., and Boissier, R. J. (1978): Antagonism between estrogens and dopamine in the rat striatum. In: *Catecholamines: Basic and Clinical Frontiers,* edited by E. Usdin, p. 21. Pergamon, Oxford.

38. Farnebo, L. D. (1971): Release of monoamines evoked by field stimulation: Studies on some ionic and metabolic requirements. *Acta Physiol. Scand. [Suppl],* 371:19–27.

39. Ferland, L., Fuxe, K., Eneroth, P., Gustafsson, J. A., and Skett, P. (1977): Effects of methionine-enkephalin on prolactin release and catecholamine levels and turnover in the median eminence. *Eur. J. Pharmacol.,* 43:89–90.

40. Ferland, L., Kledzik, G. S., Cusan, L., and Labrie, F. (1978): Evidence for a role of endorphins in stress- and suckling-induced prolactin release in the rat. *Mol. Cell. Endocrinol.,* 12:267–272.

41. Ferland, L., Labrie, F., Arimura, A., and Schally, A. V. (1977): Stimulated release of hypothalamic growth hormone releasing activity by morphine and pentobarbital. *Mol. Cell. Endocrinol.,* 2:247–252.

42. Ferland, L., Labrie, F., Euvrard, C., and Raynaud, J. P. (1979): Antidopaminergic activity of estrogens on prolactin release at the pituitary level in vivo. *Mol. Cell. Endocrinol.,* 14:199–204.

43. Franks, S., Murray, M. A., Jequier, A. M., Steele, S. J., Nabarro, J. D. N., and Jacobs, H. S. (1975): Incidence and significance of hyperprolactinemia in women with amenorrhea. *Clin. Endocrinol.,* 4:597–607.

44. Fuxe, K. (1964): Cellular localization of monoamines in the median eminence and the infundibular stem of some mammals. *Z. Zellforsch.,* 61:710–724.

45. Fuxe, K., Agnati, L. F., Corrodi, H., Everett, B. J., Hökfelt, T., Lofstrom, A., and Ungerstedt, U. (1975): Action of dopamine receptor agonists in forebrain and hypothalamus, rotational behavior, ovulation and dopamine turnover. *Adv. Neurol.,* 9:223–242.

46. Fuxe, K., Eneroth, P., Gustafsson, J. A., Lofstrom, A., and Skett, P. (1977): Dopamine in the nucleus accumbens: Preferential increase of DA turnover by rat prolactin. *Brain Res.,* 22:177–182.

47. Fuxe, K., Ferland, L., Andersson, K., Eneroth, P., Gustafsson, J. A., and Skett, P. (1978): On the functional role of hypothalamic catecholamine neurons in control of the secretion of hormones from the anterior pituitary, particularly in the control of LH and prolactin secretion. In: *Brain–Endocrine Interaction. III. Neural Hormones and Reproduction,* edited by D. E. Scott, G. P. Kozlowski, and A. Weindl, pp. 172–182. Karger, Basel.

48. Fuxe, K., Hökfelt, T., and Nilsson, O. (1969): Castration, sex hormones and tuberoinfundibular dopamine neurons. *Neuroendocrinology,* 5:107–120.

49. Gallo, R. V., Rabii, J., and Moberg, G. P. (1975): Effect of methysergide, a blocker of serotonin receptors on plasma prolactin levels in lactating and ovariectomized rats. *Endocrinology,* 97:1096–1105.

50. Gilardeau, C., and Chretien, M. (1970): Isolation and characterization of beta-lipolytic hormone from porcine pituitary gland. *Can. J. Biochem.,* 48:1017–1021.

51. Goodman, G., Lawson, D. M., and Galla, R. R. (1976): The effect of neurotransmitter receptor antagonist to an ether-induced prolactin release in ovariectomized estrogen-treated rats. *Proc. Soc. Exp. Biol. Med.,* 153:225–229.

52. Graf, L., Barat, E., Csheh, G., and Ajgo, S. (1973): Amino acid sequence of porcine β-lipotropic hormone. *Biochim. Biophys. Acta,* 229:276–278.

53. Graf, L., Barat, E., and Patthy, A. (1976): Isolation of a COOH-terminal beta-lipotropin fragment (residues 61–91) with morphine-like analgesic activity from porcine pituitary gland. *Acta Biochim. Biophys. Acad. Sci. Hung.,* 11:121–122.

54. Gratton, L. (1960): Neuroleptiques, parkinsonisme et schizophrénie. *Union Med. Can.,* 89:681–694.

55. Greengard, P. (1975): Cyclic nucleotide protein phosphorylation and neuronal function. *Adv. Cyclic Nucleotide Res.,* 585–601.

56. Guillemin, R., Ling, N., and Burgus, R. (1976): Endorphins, peptides d'origine hypothalamique et neurohypophysaire à activité morphinomimétique: Isolement et structure moléculaire de l'α-endorphine. *C R Acad. Sci. [D] (Paris),* 282:783–785.

57. Hökfelt, T. (1967): The possible ultrastructural identification of tuberoinfundibular dopamine-containing nerve endings in the median eminence of the rat. *Brain Res.,* 5:121–123.

58. Hughes, J., Smith, T. W., Kosterlitz, H. W., Fothergill, L. A., Morgan, B. A., and Morris, H. R. (1975): Identification of two related pentapeptides from the brain with potent opiate activity. *Nature,* 258:577–579.

59. Iversen, L. L., Horn, A. S., and Miller, R. J. (1975): Structure-activity relationship for agonist and antagonist drugs at pre- and postsynaptic receptor sites in rat brain. *Psychopharmacol. Bull.*, 11:14–22.

60. Jacobs, L. S., Snyder, P. J., Utiger, R. D., and Daughaday, W. H. (1973): Prolactin response to thyrotropin-releasing hormone in normal subjects. *J. Clin. Endocrinol. Metab.*, 36:1069–1075.

61. Jobin, M., Ferland, L., Côté, J., and Labrie, F. (1975): Effect of cold exposure on hypothalamic TRH activity and plasma levels of TSH and prolactin in the rat. *Neuroendocrinology*, 18:204–214.

62. Kebabian, J. W., Petzold, G. L., and Greengard, P. (1972): Dopamine-sensitive adenylate cyclase in caudate nucleus of rat brain and its similarity to the dopamine receptor. *Proc. Natl. Acad. Sci. USA*, 69:2145–2149.

63. Kokka, N., Garcia, J. F., George, R., and Elliot, H. W. (1972): Growth hormone and ACTH secretion: Evidence for an inverse relationship in rats. *Endocrinology*, 90:735–743.

64. Kordon, C., Blake, C. A., Terkel, J., and Sawyer, C. H. (1974): Participation of serotonin-containing neurons in the suckling-induced rise in plasma prolactin levels in lactating rats. *Neuroendocrinology*, 13:213–223.

65. Labrie, F., Beaulieu, M., Caron, M. G., and Raymond, V. (1978): Adenohypophyseal dopaminergic receptor; specificity and modulation of its activity by estradiol. In: *Progress in Prolactin Physiology and Pathology*, edited by C. Robyn and M. Harter, pp. 121–136. Elsevier, Amsterdam.

66. Labrie, F., Beaulieu, M., Ferland, L., Raymond, V., Di Paolo, T., Caron, M. G., Veilleux, R., Denizeau, F., Euvrard, C., Raynaud, J. P., and Boissier, J. R. (1979): Control of prolactin secretion at the pituitary level: a model for post-synaptic dopaminergic systems. In: *Central Nervous System Effects of Hypothalamic Hormones and Other Peptides*, edited by R. Collu, A. Barbeau, J. R. Ducharme, and J. G. Rochefort, pp. 207–234. Raven Press, New York.

67. Labrie, F., Dupont, A., Cusan, L., Lissitzky, J. C., Lépine, J., Raymond, V., and Coy, D. H. (1979): Effects of endorphins and their analogues on prolactin and growth hormone secretion. In: *Endorphins in Mental Health Research*, edited by E. Usdin, W. Bunney Jr., and N. Kline, pp. 335–343. Macmillan, London.

68. Labrie, F., Savary, M., Coy, D. H., Coy, E. J., and Schally, A. V. (1976): Inhibition of LH release by analogs of LH-releasing hormone (LHRH) in vitro. *Endocrinology*, 98:289–294.

69. Lawson, D. M., and Gala, R. R. (1975): The influence of adrenergic, dopaminergic, cholinergic and serotonergic drugs on plasma prolactin levels in ovariectomized, estrogen-treated rats. *Endocrinology*, 96:313–318.

70. Li, C. H., Barnafi, L., Chretien, M., and Chung, D. (1965): Isolation and amino-acid sequence of β-LPH from sheep pituitary gland. *Nature*, 209:1093–1094.

71. Li, C. H., and Chung, D. (1976): Isolation and structure of an untriakontapeptide with opiate activity from camel pituitary gland. *Proc. Natl. Acad. Sci. USA*, 73:1145–1148.

72. Li, C. H., and Chung, D. (1976): Primary structure of human β-lipotropin. *Nature*, 260:622–624.

73. Lien, E. L., Fenichel, R. L., Garsky, V., Sarantakis, D., and Grant, N. H. (1976): Enkephalin-stimulated prolactin release. *Life Sci.*, 19:837–840.

74. Ling, N., and Guillemin, R. (1976): Morphinomimetic activity of synthetic fragments of beta-lipotropin and analogs. *Proc. Natl. Acad. Sci. USA*, 73:3308–3310.

75. Lissitzky, J. C., Morin, O., Dupont, A., Labrie, F., Serdah, N. G., Chretien, M., and Coy, D. H. (1978): Content of β-LPH and its fragments (including endorphins) in anterior and intermediate lobes of the bovine pituitary gland. *Life Sci.*, 22:1715–1722.

76. Löfstrom, A., Eneroth, P., Gustafsson, J. A., and Skett, P. (1977): Effect of estradiol benzoate on catecholamines turnover in discrete area of median eminence and limbic forebrain and on serum luteinizing hormone follicle-stimulating hormone and prolactin concentration in ovariectomized female rat. *Endocrinology*, 101:1559–1569.

77. Löfstrom, A., Jonsson, G., and Fuxe, K. (1976): Microfluorimetric quantitation of catecholamine fluorescence in rat median eminence. I. Aspects on the distribution of dapamine and noradrenaline nerve terminals. *J. Histochem. Cytochem.*, 24:415–429.

78. Loh, H. H., Brase, D. A., Sampath-Khanna, S., Mar, J. B., Leong-Way, E., and Li, C. H. (1976): β-Endorphin in vitro inhibition of striatal dopamine release. *Nature*, 264:567–568.

79. Loh, H. H., Tseng, L. F., Wei, E. I., and Li, C. H. (1976): β-Endorphin is a potent analgesic agent. *Proc. Natl. Acad. Sci. USA*, 73:2895–2898.

80. Lohmar, P., and Li, C. H. (1967): Isolation of bovine beta-lipotropic hormone. *Biochim. Biophys. Acta,* 147:381–383.
81. MacLeod, R. M. (1969): Influence of norepinephrine and catecholamine-depleting agents on the synthesis and release of prolactin and growth hormone. *Endocrinology,* 85:916–923.
82. MacLeod, R. M., and Lehmeyer, J. E. (1974): Restoration of prolactin synthesis and release by the administration of monoaminergic blocking agents to pituitary tumor-bearing rats. *Cancer Res.,* 34:345–350.
83. Marchlewska-Koy, A., and Krulich, L. (1975): The role of central monoamine in the stress-induced prolactin release in the rat. *Fed. Proc.,* 34:191.
84. Martin, J. B., Durand, D., Gurd, W., Faille, G., Audet, J., and Brazeau, P. (1978): Neuropharmacological regulation of episodic growth hormone and prolactin secretion in the rat. *Endocrinology,* 102:106–113.
85. Meites, J. (1966): Control of mammary growth and lactation. In: *Neuroendocrinology,* Vol. 1, edited by L. Martini and W. F. Ganong, pp. 669–707. Academic Press, New York.
86. Morin, O., Caron, M. G., De Léan, A., and Labrie, F. (1976): Binding of the opiate pentapeptide methionine-enkephalin to a particulate fraction from rat brain. *Biochem. Biophys. Res. Commun.,* 3:940–946.
87. Neill, J. D. (1970): Effect of "stress" on serum prolactin and luteinizing hormone levels during the estrous cycle of the rat. *Endocrinology,* 87:1192–1197.
88. Noel, G. L., Dimond, R. C., Wartofsky, L., Earl, J. M., and Frantz, A. G. (1974): Studies of prolactin and TSH secretion by continuous infusion of small amounts of thyrotropin releasing hormone (TRH). *J. Clin. Endocrinol. Metab.,* 39:6–17.
89. Noel, G. L., Suh, H. K., Stone, G., and Frantz, A. G. (1972): Human prolactin and growth hormone release during surgery and other conditions of stress. *J. Clin. Endocrinol. Metab.,* 35:840–851.
90. Parker, D. C., Rossman, L. G., and Vander Loan, E. F. (1973): Sheep related nycthemeral and briefly episodic variation in human plasma prolactin concentrations. *J. Clin. Endocrinol. Metab.,* 36:1119–1124.
91. Pert, A. (1977): Behavioral pharmacology of D-alanine²-methionine-enkephalin amide and other long-acting opiate peptides. In: *Opiates and Endogenous Opioid Peptides,* edited by H. Kosterlitz, S. Archer, E. J. Simon, and A. Goldstein, pp. 87–94. Elsevier, Amsterdam.
92. Plotsky, P. M., Gibbs, D. M., and Neill, J. D. (1978): Liquid chromatographic-electrochemical measurement of dopamine in hypophyseal stalk blood of rats. *Endocrinology,* 102:1887–1894.
93. Raymond, V., Beaulieu, M., Labrie, F., and Boissier, J. R. (1978): Potent antidopaminergic activity of estradiol at the pituitary level on prolactin release. *Science,* 200:1173–1175.
94. Rivier, C., and Vale, W. (1974): In vivo stimulation of prolactin secretion in the rat by thyrotropin-releasing factor, related peptides and hypothalamic extracts. *Endocrinology,* 95:978–983.
95. Robyn, C., Delvoye, P., Nokin, J., Vekemans, M., Badawi, M., Perez-Lopez, F. R., and L'Hermite, M. (1974): Prolactin and human reproduction. In: *Human Prolactin,* edited by J. L. Pasteels and C. Robyn, pp. 167–182. Excerpta Medica, Amsterdam.
96. Sassin, J. F., Frantz, A. G., Kapen, S., and Weitzman, E. D. (1973): The nocturnal rise of human prolactin is dependent on sleep. *J. Clin. Endocrinol. Metab.,* 37:436–440.
97. Schneider, H. P. G., and McCann, S. M. (1970): Release of LH releasing factor (LRF) into the peripheral circulation of hypophysectomized rats. *Endocrinology,* 87:249–252.
98. Seeman, P., Chau-Wong, M., Tedesco, J., and Wong, K. (1975): Brain receptors for antipsychotic drugs and dopamine: Direct binding assays. *Proc. Natl. Acad. Sci. USA,* 72:4376–4380.
99. Seeman, P., Chau-Wong, M., Tedesco, J., and Wong, K. (1976): Dopamine receptors in human and calf brains, using [³H]apomorphine and an antipsychotic drug. *Proc. Natl. Acad. Sci. USA,* 73:4354–4358.
100. Shaar, C. J., and Clemens, J. A. (1974): The role of catecholamines in the release of anterior pituitary prolactin in vitro. *Endocrinology,* 95:1202–1212.
101. Shaskan, I. G., and Snyder, G. H. (1970): Kinetics of serotonin accumulation into slices from rat brain: Relationship to catecholamine uptake. *J. Pharmacol. Exp. Ther.,* 175:404–415.
102. Takahara, J., Arimura, A., and Schally, A. V. (1974): Suppression of prolactin release by a purified porcine PIF preparation and catecholamines infused into a rat hypophysial portal vessel. *Endocrinology,* 96:462–465.

103. Terkel, J., Blake, C. A., Hoover, V., and Sawyer, C. H. (1973): Pup survival and prolactin levels in nicotine-treated lactating rats. *Proc. Soc. Exp. Biol. Med.,* 143:1131–1135.
104. Thorner, M. O., McNeilly, A. S., Hagan, C., and Besser, G. M. (1974): Long-term treatment of galactorrhea and hypogonadism with bromocryptine. *Br. Med. J.,* 2:419–422.
105. Tolis, G., Hickey, J., and Guyda, H. (1975): Effects of morphine on serum growth hormone, cortisol, prolactin, and thyroid stimulating hormone in man. *J. Clin. Endocrinol. Metab.,* 41:797–800.
106. Van Vugt, D. A., Bruni, J. F., and Meites, J. (1978): Naloxone inhibition of stress-induced increase in prolactin secretion. *Life Sci.,* 22:85–90.

The Endocrine Functions of the Brain,
edited by Marcella Motta.
Raven Press, New York © 1980

14

Role of Extrahypothalamic Centers in Neuroendocrine Integration

Franz Ellendorff and Nahid Parvizi

Institut für Tierzucht and Tierverhalten, FAL, Mariensee, Federal Republic of Germany

Forty years ago Ranson and Magoun (161) reviewed major extrahypothalamic structures connected to the hypothalamus and influencing its function. The communication between the hypothalamus and the pituitary by downward vascular drainage had already been recognized. The extrahypothalamic elements included the amygdala, hippocampus, and mesencephalon. Subsequently, interactions between these structures and the hypothalamus were determined by advanced techniques. Functional links were established between extrahypothalamic areas and hypothalamic and pituitary secretions. These have been reviewed for pituitary gonadotropins (49,50,88,128,179,232), ACTH (15,93,201,202,213), TSH (180,181,232), growth hormone (116,121,130), and posterior pituitary hormones (73,151). It is the purpose of this chapter to discuss recent developments on the influence exerted by the amygdala, hippocampus, and mesencephalon on hypothalamo-pituitary function.

GENERAL MECHANISMS

The limbic system–midbrain circuit (137) possibly represents the largest input to the hypothalamus and encompasses components involved in neuroendocrine integrative mechanisms. A prominent structure of the limbic system is the amygdala, which consists of several subnuclei and conveys its information to the hypothalamus via two major pathways. The stria terminalis originates exclusively in the corticomedial and basolateral area (31). The other major projection system is now generally known as the ventroamygdalofugal pathway (VAF). This pathway has been described as being fan-shaped and is incorporated into the medial forebrain bundle (MFB) (66,67). It might be important for neuroendocrine considerations that the origin of the VAF may be outside the amygdala in the prepyriform cortex (31). The VAF then passes through the basolateral amygdala on its way to other destinations including the hypothalamus. The report that the VAF projection field goes to the lateral hypothalamus (78) may limit the transport of neuroendocrine information. On the other hand, the anterior hypo-thalamic area and the shell of the ventromedial hypothalamus (VMH) receive inputs from the stria terminalis (78). Since lesions in the rostrohypothalamic area result in degenerative patterns in the amygdala, amygdalar-hypothalamic relations must be considered to be reciprocal (31).

Reciprocal amygdalar-hypothalamic relations found ample functional support from neurophysiological experiments as early as 1955 (66,67). Later these studies were expanded (41,135), with the conclusion that the preferred site of functional amygdalar-hypothalamic contact was the outer shell of the ventromedial hypo-thalamic nucleus. Exploration of the amygdalar-VMH relation was repeated (166,168) using techniques of antidromic identification. Cells recorded in the VMH–arcuate region were antidromically invaded from the amygdala, and the response was confined to VMH neurons. The failure of arcuate nucleus neurons to respond to electrical stimulation of the amygdala is consistent with the selective input of the amygdala into the outer shell of the VMH. Only two neurons were invaded by median eminence stimulation, demonstrating the missing link between the VMH and the tuberoinfundibular region.

In most species the preoptic–anterior hypothalamic area (POA/AHA) is con-sidered to be a structure of paramount importance for the regulation of hypo-thalamo-pituitary functions. Bidirectional inhibitory and stimulatory connections between the amygdala and the POA/AHA are known; they involve monosynap-tic as well as multisynaptic connections (44,59,65,146). POA/AHA neurons with established amygdaloid relations may project to the mediobasal hypothala-mus (MBH) monosynaptically or via an undefined number of synapses (44). In one study a small number of "bipolar" cells (10 of 583 cells) in the POA/AHA were directly linked to the amygdala and the arcuate/VMH region (53). In another study "multipolar" cells with one axon in the POA and the other found in amygdaloid structures other than the recording site were recorded from the amygdala (107). Whether "bipolar" or "multipolar" projections truly originate at the cell soma or branch off a common axon seems not to be of great importance. Another feature of amygdalar–hypothalamic relations is the regional specificity of amygdala projections for restricted zones within the POA/AHA and the localization of inhibitory responses to amygdalar and MBH stimu-lations in the ventral part of the POA/AHA (43). All the evidence presented, anatomical and neurophysiological, thus underlines the existence of a close recip-rocal structural and functional organization of an amygdalar-preoptic-hypo-thalamic unit.

The hippocampus may exert control functions over the MBH via its ventral-subicular exit, and further via the fornix and the medial cortico-hypothalamic tract (159,197). Signs of degeneration have also been detected in the dorsal fornix after lesions in the preoptic area and the lateral hypothalamus (158). Analogous to the amygdala projections, the majority of terminations are situated in the outer shell of the ventromedial nucleus of the hypothalamus (197).

Functional connections between the ventral hippocampus and the hypothalamus have been established (155), although two neuroendocrinologically relevant structures, the arcuate nucleus and the supraoptic nucleus, did not seem to contain responsive neurons in this experiment. This does not exclude relations with structures such as the arcuate-median eminence region, since functional connections between hypothalamic nuclei have been established (167). There is also support for a functional ventral hippocampus-arcuate relationship; recording multiunit activity in response to electrical stimulation (64) or single-unit activity (117) was recorded in the rat. Sixty-five percent of median eminence neurons altered their firing pattern in response to dorsal hippocampus stimulation. It is unlikely that dorsal hippocampal-median eminence connections are monosynaptic, since recent neuroanatomical experiments failed to show direct relations between the areas (197).

The septum is not discussed in detail as a part of extrahypothalamic neuroendocrine integration. It should be mentioned, however, as a central structure in amygdala, hippocampus, midbrain, and hypothalamus interactions (29,71, 75,133,157,197).

The midbrain has long been known to be an essential part of neuroendocrine integrative mechanisms. Structures concerned with the regulation of hormone release have been located in a number of mesencephalic structures (24,98). Connections with the MBH via Schutz's dorsal longitudinal fasciculus (137) as well as via the MFB (133) are well established. These connections are not merely morphological but must be considered to be functional connections between the mesencephalon and the preoptic area-anterior hypothalamus (23,46,59). There appears to have been no detailed electroanatomical study of the midbrain-arcuate-median eminence relationship. Nevertheless, a functional link was well established by histofluorescence studies. It is possible to augment the release of norepinephrine (NE) and dopamine (DA) in the hypothalamus and limbic structures when pathways originating in the mesencephalon (ventral-reticular tegmentum) are electrically activated (5,110). More recently (147) 13.8% of 150 POA/AHA neurons were driven antidromically from the MFB, confirming the existence of POA/AHA-MFB connections. Orthodromic inhibitions as well as stimulation of POA/AHA cells were present in the majority of the neurons inhibited by iontophoretically applied NE and DA. This suggests that the aminergic input of the MFB to the POA/AHA is inhibitory, although the authors offer an escape route by interpreting the actions of NE and DA as possible pharmacological effects.

The experiments discussed so far clearly identified mesencephalic afferents and efferents to connect to the POA/AHA-MBH reciprocally. In addition, the ventromedial hypothalamus, amygdala, septum, hippocampus, and midbrain are all interconnected by the MFB. Although it passes mainly through the lateral part of the preoptic area and the hypothalamus, a considerable number of perpendicular collaterals to and from more medial parts (133) ensure intimate exchange of information with the structures concerned with neuroendocrine integration.

INTEGRATION OF THE PITUITARY–GONAD SYSTEM

It is now well established that the amygdala participates in the mechanisms that control gonadotropin secretion. A role of the amygdala on luteinizing hormone releasing hormone (LHRH) and LH secretions can be registered as early as during sexual differentiation, when androgens (or their metabolites) determine the endocrine sex of the brain (68) and modify structural elements of the brain (69,160,210). The functional synaptology related to the amygdala is also affected. There are more cells in males that directly project to the MBH and receive synaptic input from the amygdala than in females (44). Castrated males develop female-type connections, and females treated neonatally with testosterone propionate take an intermediate position. Testosterone or its metabolites thus modify the synaptic input from the amygdala into the POA/AHA. However, it is debatable whether the androgens act directly on the amygdala or close to the POA/AHA by modifying the amygdala inputs. The synaptic pattern changes in the dorsomedial part of the POA, where only a few neurons were observed in a previous study to have connections of nonamygdaloid origin (160). If the development of sexual differentiation is intrinsic to the POA/AHA, there may be some specialization, with neurons that project directly to the MBH and receive input from the amygdala.

Sexual dichotomy of amygdaloid control seems to play a role in the development of puberty. Male rats (165) and ferrets (10) do not need the amygdala to reach puberty at the proper time, independent of whether body growth is retarded by amygdalar destruction. A less clear statement may be made about prepubertal amygdalar-hypothalamic-pituitary relations in the female, since controversial results were obtained when the amygdala or the stria terminalis was destroyed prior to puberty. In some experiments premature puberty was attained after destruction of the amygdala at 18 days of age (55,56) or at 21 days of age when the anterior part of the medial amygdala was destroyed (38). Eliminating the posterior part of the medial amygdala, on the other hand, delayed puberty significantly (38). Transsection of the stria terminalis on day 24 of life again led to advanced vaginal opening and first ovulation (20). The time factor may be another variable. Lesioning of the amygdala of 4-day-old rats causes delayed maturation (164), whereas destruction of the medial or basolateral amygdala at 21 to 22 days of age altered neither the time of vaginal opening nor the subsequent estrous cycle; uterine weight was also unmodified (13).

Little attention has been given to the observation that bilateral destruction of the olfactory stalk mimics the effects of amygdalar destruction, with no change in timing of male puberty but a retardation of female puberty. We mentioned already the close olfactory-amygdalar-hypothalamic relations (93). Is it conceivable in this context that the effects of amygdalar destruction are actually due to destruction of fibers originating in the olfactory system which pass through the cortical and medial amygdala. Changes in estradiol binding to the hypothalamo-preoptic area-amygdala-midbrain system (153,154) could also account for the differences observed. Two observations support this notion: first, within the first 3 weeks of life a specific estradiol binding protein disappears, and, second, an estradiol binding material appears between days 21 and 25; this is associated with pronounced nuclear binding of estradiol. Although we are far from having a precise model that may explain the role of the amygdala during sexual maturation, there is considerable evidence that decisive changes in amygdalar-hypothalamic-pituitary relations take place in the female rat between the third and fourth week of life.

For more than 20 years considerable effort has been invested in elucidating the role of the amygdala in the control of the estrous cycle, gonadotropin secretion, and ovulation. Attention has been focused in particular on the proestrous rat or the rat made persistently estrous by continuous illumination. The responses obtained under various experimental conditions have not been uniform (Table 1). In the persistently estrous animal (or in the proestrous rat in which ovulation is blocked pharmacologically), the induction of ovulation after electrochemical or electrical stimulation indicated that the amygdala may exert a stimulatory role, whereas no ovulation implied no function or inhibition. The medial amygdala was thus stimulated, and ovulation could be induced in 18 of 26 rats (4,214) (Table 1). When the stria terminalis was damaged or transsected, the stimulatory effect was no longer seen (214). Others also damaged the stria terminalis (212) without being able to eliminate the stimulatory effect, possibly because sufficient stria fibers remained intact to let the information pass to the hypophysiotropic area of the hypothalamus. On the other hand, only 2 of 24 rats ovulated when the basolateral or lateral amygdala was stimulated (4,214). In the acute proestrous preparation, electrochemical stimulation induced ovulation when atropine and reserpine had been given to inhibit ovulation (214). Induction of ovulation could be blocked with urethane. It is unlikely that urethane was effective at the ovarian level, since chemical stimulation of the medial amygdala caused 50% of the rats to ovulate. Atropine and reserpine had been given rather early on the day of proestrus [between 900 and 1000 hr (9:00 and 10:00 A.M.)], and urethane was given at noon. Possibly the effectivity of atropine and reserpine to block ovulation had declined relative to urethane.

In other experiments in which the ovulation-blocking agents pentobarbital or reserpine were given on the day of proestrus [at 1330 and 1215 hr, respectively (1:30 and 12:15 P.M.)] amygdalar stimulation also failed to induce ovulation (52). The discrepant results of ether anesthesia under acute conditions (52,82) after amygdalar electrical stimulation on the day of proestrus can perhaps be explained as being due to differences in the depth of anesthesia. The inconsistent results obtained in all the experiments discussed so far point to some kind of amygdalar involvement in the control of ovulation. It is suggested that the role may be a modulatory one. To study this question and to eliminate further confusion by acute studies, we (52) and others (12,26,88) turned to the fully awake proestrous rat chronically implanted with stimulating electrodes in the amygdala. From a total of 31 rats (Table 1) stimulated in the corticomedial

TABLE 1. *Effects of electrical or electrochemical stimulation on ovulation in persistently estrous and proestrous rats*

Area[a]	Stimulus parameters	Coulombs	Ovulation	Note	Ref.
Persistently Estrus Due To Continuous Illumination—Acute					
AMY	25–30 Hz/30–60 min 10–15 volts, train		5/11	Immediately after ether	22
AME	1 mA/10 sec DC/anodal	10	10/14	Ether	214
AME	200 µA/20 sec DC/anodal	4	8/12	Thiopental	4
AME Stria damage	1 mA/10 sec DC/anodal	10	0/8	Ether	214
Stria cut	1 mA/10 sec DC/anodal	10	0/9	Ether	
AME Stria damage	1 mA/10 sec DC/anodal	0	7/10	Ether	212
ABL	1 mA/10 sec DC/anodal	10	2/12	Ether	214
AL	200 µA/20 sec DC/anodal	4	0/12	Thiopental	4
Proestrus—Acute					
AME	1 mA/10 sec DC/anodal	10 10 10	8/11 (5/10) (0/9) 0/10	Atropine Reserpine Urethane Ether	214
AME/ACO	100/µA 150 Hz/0.5 msec 30 sec on/off, 30 min, train		0/9 0/5	Pentobarbital Reserpine	52
AME	100 Hz/0.5 msec 100/300 µA, train 30 min 30 sec on/off, train		10/10	Ether	82

Region	Parameters	Intensity	Ratio	Effect	N
ABL	1 mA/10 sec; DC/anodal	10	3/10	Atropine	214
AL	100 Hz/0.5 msec	10	0/5	Reserpine	82
	100/300 μA, 30 sec on/off train	10	10/17	Ether	

Proestrus—Chronic—Awake

Region	Parameters	Intensity	Ratio	Effect	N
AME/ACO	150 Hz/0.5 msec; 30 sec on/off; 30 min, train; 100 μA		5/5		52
			8/8	Ether	
AME/ACO	20 μA/120 sec; DC/anodal	2.4	4/4	LH surge	26
	50 μA/120 sec; DC/anodal	Bilateral: 4.8; 6	4/4	LH surge Advanced	
AME	100 μA/30 sec; DC/anodal	Bilateral: 12; 3	8/9	LH surge Advanced	12
ACO	dto	3	6/9	LH surge	
ABL	20 μA/120 sec; DC/anodal	2.4	4/4	LH surge; Delayed	26
	50 μA/120 sec	Bilateral: 4.8; 6		LH surge possibly delayed	
ABL	DC/anodal	Bilateral: 12; 3	6/6		12
	100 μA/30 sec; DC/anodal		0/12	No LH surge	
	100 μA/30 sec; DC/cathodal		4/4	LH surge	

[a] ABL = basolateral amygdala. ACO = cortical amygdala. AL = lateral amygdala. AME = medial amygdala. AMY = amygdala. DC = direct current.

amygdala (AME/ACO), 27 ovulated; this seems to eliminate the AME/ACO as a structure inhibitory to LH secretion. What is more interesting is that under appropriate stimulus strength the preovulatory LH surge could be significantly advanced (12,26). Stimulation of the basolateral amygdala, on the other hand, seemed to delay the LH surge or inhibit it. Whether the amygdala is truly necessary for normal ovulation has been questioned in long-term experiments. Regular cycles and ovulations returned after 1 to 2 months, when amygdalar or stria terminalis lesions were performed on the day of proestrus, although the first ovulation on the day of estrus did not take place (20,216). These observations are not limited to the rat. Bilateral destruction of the amygdala in the female rhesus monkey does not inhibit the menstrual cycle or ovulation (191). A different type of approach also restricts the need for the amygdala for ovulation under normal conditions. After repeated stimulation of the amygdala in awake rats over a longer period, only those animals that had been subjected to currents also evoking seizure activities showed disruption of regular cycles (185).

If the amygdala exerts a modulatory action on female hypothalamo-pituitary function, the question must be answered as to how this is brought about. Several investigations have shown close relationships of electrical activity within this system and events associated with pituitary and gonadal hormone secretion (84,89,204). There is ample evidence that steroids are factors which act as modulators within the amygdalar-hypothalamic-pituitary circuit. A detailed map of gonadal steroid distribution within the amygdala is available for several species (3,148,193,231). The interpretation and reliability of data obtained after so-called discrete application of steroids into brain structures was previously discussed; it was shown that some rats showed leukocytic smears after implants of crystalline estradiol into the amygdala (51,106). Furthermore, activity after intracerebral implants of tritiated steroids was detected up to 1.5 mm from the cannula tip (27 G) in rat brains and after microinfusions (2 μl; 28 G) into pig brains 2 to 2.5 mm from the cannula tip (144). Some of the discrepant results shown in Table 2 may thus have their origin in steroid diffusion to other structures. Table 2 summarizes experiments in which steroids were applied to the amygdala to test their effects on plasma LH levels. Obviously, progesterone implants yielded the most consistent results (81,90,152), since all three experiments indicate a stimulatory effect on LH. It is not clear, however, whether progesterone is the active agent or metabolites also come into play. Increases, decreases, and no effects in five altogether different experiments (51,81,90,106,144) leave an unclear picture about the role of estrogen in the amygdala; the preferred retention of estrogen in the amygdala would have implied a more definite answer. It seems surprising that in three experiments (90,106,144) no effects were observed. Possibly the timing of blood collection is crucial, or perhaps the dosage and/ or leakage from the implantation site are responsible for the differences observed. Testosterone did not affect LH levels for 48 hr when microinjected directly into the amygdala of castrated male pigs, but inhibition of LH secretion resulted when crystalline testosterone was left in the amygdala for periods of 7 to 12

TABLE 2. *Effects of steroid implantation or injection into the amygdala on plasma LH levels*

Steroid	Site[a]	Application	Model	Effect on plasma LH	Timing	Ref.
Progesterone	AME	26 G tubing, crystalline plus cocoa butter	OvX, estrogen-primed rat	Increase	After 6 hr	81
	AME/ABL	26 G tubing, crystalline plus cocoa butter	OvX rat	Increase in pituitary content	8 Days after implant	152
	AME	0.35 mm O.D., undiluted crystalline	OvX, estrogen-primed rat	Increase	After 30 hr	90
Estradiol	ACO	27 G tubing, 1:5[b] or undiluted crystalline	OvX rat	No effect	After 3 weeks	106
	AME	26 G tubing, plus cocoa butter crystalline	OvX, estrogen	Increase	After 30 hr	81
Estrone, estradiol	AME/ACO	28 G 1:5	OvX, rat	Decrease	On day 4	51
	AME	0.35 mm O.D., undiluted crystalline	OvX, estrogen-primed rat	No effect	At 6 or 30 hr	90
Estradiol	AMY	6 ng microinjected	Orchidectomized male pig	No effect	At 2, 4, 24, 48 hr	144
2-Hydroxyestradiol	AMY	60 ng microinjected	Orchidectomized male pig	Decrease	Up to 2 hr; 4, 24, 48 hr	143
Testosterone	AMY	27 G tubing, crystalline 1:2	Orchidectomized male pig	Decrease	Over 7–12 days	144
	AMY	60 ng microinjected	Orchidectomized male pig	No effect	Up to 2 hr; 4, 24, 48 hr	144
5 α-DHT	AMY	27 G tubing, crystalline 1:2	Orchidectomized male pig	Increase	12 Days	144
	AMY	60 ng microinjected	Orchidectomized male pig	Increase	Up to 2 hr; 4, 24, 48 hr	144

[a] ABL = basolateral amygdala. ACO = cortical amygdala. AME = medial amygdala. AMY = amygdala. OvX = ovariectomized. O.D. = outer diameter. 5 α-DHT = 5 α-dihydrotestosterone.
[b] Part steroid, five parts cholesterol.

days (144). Testosterone may then have acted after transformation into metabolites (e.g., estrogens), which may be formed by aromatization in limbic structures (61) or in the amygdala (222). In addition, 5α-androstan-17β-ol-3-one (dihydrotestosterone; 5α-DHT) formation also takes place in the amygdala, although to a small degree (184). When 5α-DHT was microinjected or microimplanted into the amygdala of castrated miniature pigs (144), LH levels were elevated. Of particular interest was the use of 2-hydroxylated estradiol (2-OHE$_2$) (143). 2-OHE$_2$ interferes with the normal metabolism of brain catecholamines, competing successfully for a common enzyme (catechol-O-methyltransferase) (95). Alternatively, it has been suggested that 2-OHE$_2$ may affect tyrosine hydroxylase activity (111). Other enzymes of neurotransmitter metabolism—e.g., monoamine oxidase (MAO) and choline acetyltransferase (ChAC)—in the amygdala are affected by estradiol benzoate treatment. Estradiol benzoate inhibited MAO and elevated ChAC in ovariectomized female rats but not in castrated males (113,114).

The normal timing of puberty seems to depend on the intact hippocampus and its efferent fiber connections. At present no uniform hypothesis has evolved (20,37) because delaying effects on the endocrine system could not be dissociated from growth-retarding effects (39). In one instance, however, premature first ovulation was noted despite retarded growth after lesioning of the fimbria, dorsal hippocampus, and stria terminalis (20). Changes in the prepubertal LH-secreting system may not be induced immediately after hippocampal manipulation, since electrical stimulation of this structure did not alter plasma LH levels but did change plasma FSH levels in 27-day-old rats (87). Whether changes in LH levels occur, within a matter of hours or later, or LH is altered at all remains to be established. It is conceivable that some form of timing mechanism, independent of immediate effects, is disturbed by elimination of the prepubertal hippocampus.

In the adult rat, evidence is accumulating that stimulation of the hippocampus leads to inhibition of the preovulatory surge of LH and ovulation (215). Only 2 of 24 and 6 of 10 rats ovulated when the ventral and dorsal hippocampus, respectively, were stimulated electrochemically under acute conditions. This was supported by electrical stimulation in the acute, but not the chronic, preparation (83). When the initial studies (215) were repeated under chronic conditions (26) and with a detailed profile of the preovulatory LH pattern, ovulation and the preovulatory LH surge were blocked in seven of nine proestrous rats by electrochemical stimulation (50 μA, 120 sec, uni- or bilateral, 6 or 12 coulombs) of the dorsal hippocampus. LHRH secretion, on the other hand, was not altered in the proestrous rat within 30 min after electrical stimulation of the dorsal or ventral hippocampus (28). Deviations between various experiments may be explained by differences in stimulus strength.

Whether gonadal steroids are of essential importance for hippocampal-hypothalamic-pituitary secretion is not yet solved. Binding sites for estrogens are negligible in the hippocampus of the rat and the monkey (91,148), although correlations between seizure threshold (204,205), neuronal excitability of the hippocampal-hypothalamic system (105), and circulating estrogen titers have been reported. In contrast, progesterone accumulates in the hippocampus with some preference (115).

As with the amygdala and the hippocampus, it is evident that experimentally induced changes in the midbrain can result in altered hypothalamo-pituitary function and in altered gonadotropin secretion. Early investigators (32) suggested that the mesodiencephalic junction is a "critical area" for the preovulatory surge of LH, but this opinion was contradicted later (145). In both cases, judgments were based on large lesions. Only more discrete localization of electrochemical stimulation (24,198) made it possible to discover a dual role of the midbrain in control of the preovulatory surge of LH and ovulation as well as in the LH surge that occurs in the gonadectomized, estrogen-primed rat.

Electrochemical stimulation of the ventral tegmental area of the raphe nuclei and of the periaqueductal grey matter resulted in inhibition of ovulation, whereas electrochemical stimulation of the dorsal mesencephalic tegmentum and the lateral and inferior periaqueductal region overcame the ovulation blockade induced by continuous illumination (25). The dorsal longitudinal fasciculus and the medial forebrain bundle were shown to carry the information via the hippocampus and further via the corticomedial hypothalamic tract. Similarly, a dual response to midbrain stimulation of preoptic multiunit activity resulted from electrical stimulation of the midbrain raphe nucleus and the dorsal tegmentum (23). Also single-unit response of POA neurons could be inhibitory and stimulatory, with the secondary responses stimulatory and inhibitory, respectively (59). Depending on stimulus frequency, sequential stimulation of the same neuron could cause general excitation or general inhibition of firing rates of the same neuron. The inconsistency of the responses of POA neurons to stimulation from the midbrain has also been noticed by others (46,147). All these observations provided more questions than answers to explain the function of the midbrain in gonadotropin secretion; it must be recalled that the midbrain neurotransmitter systems have been shown to participate intensively in such regulation (100).

A major role of the midbrain-hypothalamic relationship is to convey sensory information that may be modified by gonadal steroids (1,134,178). It has yet to be established whether the accumulation of progesterone (223), and to a lesser degree estrogens (91,148), is related to gonadotropin secretion or to modification of sexual sensory input.

INTEGRATION OF THE PITUITARY-ADRENAL SYSTEM

The brain-pituitary-adrenal axis may be activated or inhibited by a multitude of factors of endogenous or exogenous origin, including hemorrhage, fear, anger, rage, pain, or adverse environmental conditions. To explain the resulting regulatory response of pituitary ACTH secretion, three hypotheses have been offered (72): (a) circulating epinephrine levels regulate ACTH secretion; (b) circulating adrenal cortical hormone levels control ACTH secretion; (c) the hypothalamus acts through the hypophysial portal vessels to determine the release of ACTH.

There is also a fourth hypothesis: Hypothalamic control is dependent on extrahypothalamic integrative mechanisms. Investigations of the extrahypothalamic integration of pituitary ACTH secretion have long been hampered by the lack of specificity of the experimental approaches. Lesions (122) and electrical stimulation (124) of the amygdala have increased ACTH secretion. A dual response mechanism residing within the amygdala-mesencephalon axis has been proposed (162), with a fast-response component inherent in the midbrain. When stimuli of lower strength were applied to the amygdala in later experiments, ACTH was released (126,163), indicating a facilitatory function of the amygdala on ACTH secretion. In more detailed investigations in the rat, facilitatory amygdaloid areas must be distinguished from those that inhibit or delay ACTH secretion (126,199,202). When the basal portion of the basolateral amygdala was stimulated, cortisol increased in 10 of 18 cases and corticosterone in 6 of 18 cases. In four animals corticosterone was decreased. Electrical stimulation in the lateral portion of the basolateral amygdala was followed by increased plasma cortisol levels in six of eight cases; no response was seen in two. After corticomedial amygdala stimulation, all three response types were observed: inhibition, excitation, and no response. It was then noted that the cortisol responses were dependent on the prestimulus cortisol levels. If cortisol was low initially, it was high after stimulation; if it was high initially, the poststimulus levels were low. Finally, most of the stimulations of the anterior amygdala resulted in no plasma cortisol changes. Regionally dependent effects of amygdala stimulation were also noticed by others (63). Cortisol levels increased after basolateral amygdala stimulation, whereas cortisol values tended to decrease when the corticomedial amygdala was stimulated. Effects of amygdala stimulation are not limited to cortisol and corticosterone. Aldosterone can also be stimulated by corticomedial, but not by lateral or basomedial amygdalar stimulation (62). These authors suggest that the effect is due more to stimulation of the renin–angiotensin system than to stimulation of the ACTH system.

Corticosteroid synthesis is one endpoint of brain-pituitary-adrenal cortex relationships. Do corticosteroids exert feedback actions similar to those of gonadal steroids on the amygdala? The question has been a matter of controversy between those investigators favoring the pituitary and those favoring the brain as the feedback site. This was discussed previously (92) with the basic principles of corticosteroid feedback mechanisms. It is recognized that the amygdala, a potent binding site for estrogens, is almost devoid of corticosteroids (194,196,220). Biochemical uptake studies also point to a limited uptake of corticosteroids in the amygdala relative to blood levels (129). On the other hand, a local action of corticosteroids on the amygdala is claimed (86).

Reports that corticosteroid treatment (intraperitoneal) increases the 5-hydroxytryptamine (5-HT) content in the amygdala were unexpected. This effect has been linked to an inhibitory action of 5-HT on corticosteroid feedback

(203). These experiments weakly support a feedback of corticosteroids on the amygdala. ACTH may be of wider importance. A direct effect of ACTH on the amygdala–VMH complex seems to exist (139); in addition, it has been reported that immunoreactive (102) and biologically active (140) ACTH is present in the amygdala of intact and hypophysectomized rats. Whether the "neurogenic" ACTH acts as a neurotransmitter or as a local neuropeptide requires experimental elucidation. The results may help explain its potential role in limbic control of various functions, e.g., circadian rhythmicity, behavior, aggression, fear.

There has been discussion on the possible participation of the hippocampus as a center of extrahypothalamic integration of brain-pituitary-adrenal function. Unlike some parts of the amygdala which are considered to be largely facilitatory for ACTH release, the general notion has been that the hippocampus is inhibitory to corticotropin releasing factor (CRF) and ACTH release. This may be an oversimplification. The conflicting results, recently discussed (213), may be due not only to the different experimental protocols used but also to differences in the questions asked. For example, diurnal rhythms of corticosteroids and stress-induced corticosteroid secretion may be under the control of two distinct systems (17,33,125,213). Ablation or stimulation experiments provide as much evidence for as against the hippocampus as the responsible structure for the control of circadian variations in corticosteroid levels. Reaching a final conclusion may be complicated, since the disappearance of diurnal variations may be only temporary, returning 3 weeks after lesioning (108). Although this has been taken as an indication that the hippocampus may not be necessary for the control of diurnal ACTH/corticosteroid fluctuations, it cannot be excluded that regenerative processes or compensatory mechanisms have taken over. The difficulties faced while attempting to explain in detail the factors which control the stress-induced ACTH/corticosteroid secretion are illustrated by the following two examples. First, it has been noted (85) that electrical stimulation of the hippocampus below the seizure threshold results in inhibition or facilitation of ACTH release, depending on if the experimental situation is stressful. This is somewhat analogous to the experiments already mentioned in which the corticosteroid levels at the beginning of the experiment seem to determine the resulting response of amygdala stimulation (163). In the second example, high-frequency stimulation (120/sec) of the hippocampus failed to induce adrenal responses, whereas low-frequency stimulation (36/sec and less) stimulated the adrenal response (57). Alternative approaches involve electrical stimulation of the hippocampus with simultaneous recording of hypothalamic multiunit activity and measurement of circulating corticosteroids. A biphasic response was observed in the rat (27,200), with facilitation of plasma corticosterone secretion 30 min after electrical stimulation and a depression of plasma corticosterone at 60 min after termination of stimulation. Corresponding multiunit activity was elevated initially, and progressively inhibited later. The results were interpreted carefully, since the authors could not eliminate a feedback of corticosteroids on multiunit activity in the later stages. A possible dual role of the hippocampus, facilitatory and inhibitory, has been suggested. Similarly, correlations between diurnal variations in corticosteroid levels and multiunit activity are known to exist in the pigeon (18). It is interesting that hippocampal multiunit activity occurred out of phase with hypothalamic multiunit activity. The periodicity of multiunit activity could be eliminated by hippocampal destruction (19). Despite these observations it is really not tenable at present to assign a definite role to the hippocampus for either control of circadian or stress-induced release of ACTH/corticosterone on the basis of ablation or stimulation experiments.

The hippocampus has been accepted as a target site of corticosteroids, which have a well defined pattern of distribution within this structure, i.e., in layers CA1 through CA4 and the dentate gyrus (94,127,129,195,219). In addition to a regulatory role in ACTH secretion, they may also have profound effects on behavior (14). Corticosteroids may induce a number of neurochemical and enzymatic changes in the hippocampus (127), but these changes have not been associated with alterations in the hypothalamo-pituitary-adrenal function. Attempts to relate the corticosteroids present in the hippocampus to functional aspects have been numerous (92,127). Recording of hippocampal units has demonstrated changes in action potential activity when corticosteroids are applied. Altering hippocampal neuronal activity by iontophoretically or locally applied corticosteroids has been tried. Either synthetic dexamethasone (132,183,192) or corticosterone sodium succinate (8,192) affected hippocampal firing rates. Neither of these substances produced results identical to those found with natural corticosteroids. When corticosteroids were applied peripherally and units recorded from the freely moving unanesthetized rat, it took much longer for a response to develop; when it did, it was either exclusively inhibitory (149) or almost evenly distributed between inhibited (50%) and excited (40%) neurons (150). Simultaneous monitoring of circulating corticosterone and cortisol along with the recordings led to the conclusion that increasing physiological plasma corticosteroid values progressively increased the percentage of hippocampal neurons responding (35). When these results are compared to earlier experiments, which used corticosteroid implants into the hippocampus to establish feedback responses (16,188), it is obvious that feedback mechanisms of corticosteroids are located within the hippocampus. However, it is not yet possible to recognize what determines inhibition or the increase in CRF-ACTH-corticosteroid secretion. It is conceivable that corticosteroids act on neurons that project directly to CRF-producing neurons or on oligosynaptic or multisynaptic systems with interposed inhibitory or excitatory interneurons. This would enable any kind of response to arrive at areas responsible for CRF secretion.

The mesencephalon is likely to exert a dual control—inhibitory and excitatory—over ACTH secretion. This was noted in earlier presentations (72) and is well illustrated by some recent work.

Increased corticosteroid secretion was observed in the presence of motor activity and restlessness after electrical stimulation of the dorsal tegmentum of the midbrain (60). Electrical recording from hypothalamic units led to the suggestion that stimulatory input from the mesencephalon inhibits anterior hypothalamic neurons but excites medial hypothalamic neurons. Unit activity was inhibited for up to 120 min by cortisol administration. Whether cortisol elevated the threshold of the midbrain to electrical stimulation or affected the response of the hypothalamic neurons could not be established. Inhibition of a stress-induced increase in ACTH and corticosteroids could be induced in the anesthetized dog after stimulation close to the nucleus subceruleus in the ventral ascending noradrenergic system (177). Facilitatory and inhibitory effects of electrical stimulation were also observed (218), depending on the site of stimulation. When stimulated electrically, the locus ceruleus and the lateral ventral tegmental nucleus of Gudden elevated the plasma ACTH, whereas the locus subceruleus and the anteroventral locus ceruleus, as well as the dorsal and ventral tegmental nucleus of Gudden and the raphe, inhibited ACTH release. Since the sensitivity of midbrain neurons to corticosteroids has been established for single neurons (192), corticosteroids may participate in the midbrain control of ACTH secretion.

INTEGRATION OF THE PITUITARY-THYROID SYSTEM

The presence (and possibly the production) of the tripeptide thyroid releasing hormone (TRH) in various extrahypothalamic structures of the brain in a number of species (70,79,80,142,229) and the suppression of TSH after hypothalamic deafferentation (76,77) strongly suggest that the regulatory mechanisms of the pituitary-thyroid system may reside, at least in part, outside the hypothalamus. It is thus surprising that relatively little information is available about extrahypothalamic control of TSH secretion. Although some investigators failed to detect changes in pituitary-thyroid function after amygdalar lesions (101,228), others showed that amygdalar lesions result in atrophic thyroid glands (96) or lead to increased pituitary and decreased plasma TSH levels, as estimated by bioassay, 3 to 16 days after surgery (48). The high concentration of TRH in the amygdala (104)—exceeded only by TRH concentrations in the hypothalamus and the dorsal midbrain—does not necessarily confirm a role in the control of TSH secretion, but is suggestive.

Indirect evidence links the hippocampus to TSH release. Cold exposure increases plasma TSH levels, whereas some other "stressful" environmental situations (e.g., the presence of an observer in the animal room) inhibit cold-induced TSH release (42). If the dental gyrus of the hippocampus is electrically stimulated in such circumstances, TSH release is restored.

More direct evidence about TSH control is available for the mesencephalon, where electrical stimulation of the reticular formation of anesthetized cats was followed by elevated thyroid hormone secretion (2). Possibly mesencephalic noradrenergic and dopaminergic systems participate in the regulation of pituitary-thyroid functions. Systemic administration of α-methyl-p-tyrosine causes depletion of brain mesencephalic norepinephrine and dopamine and a gradual

decrease in cold-induced TSH secretion (103). Furthermore, specific inhibitors
of dopamine-β-hydroxylase (diethyldithiocarbonate and FLA 63) deplete only
central norepinephrine and lead to a striking decrease in serum TSH. Dose-
related rapid inhibition of TSH secretion has also been described following
L-DOPA treatment (103). In addition, thyroidectomy enhances norepinephrine
turnover (30,141) and tyrosine hydroxylase activity (136) in the brainstem of
the male rat. On the basis of these results, it is postulated that the noradrenergic
system is stimulatory, whereas the dopaminergic system has an inhibitory effect
on the pituitary-thyroid system. Recent investigations revealed a number of
effects of TRH at the midbrain level. Intraperitoneal injection of TRH (3 μg/
100 g body weight) caused definite inhibition of mesencephalic reticular formation multiunit activity 30 min after the injection of the tripeptide. On the other
hand, unit activity in the ipsilateral hippocampus was increased beginning at
60 min after treatment when compared to control animals. The effects were
not dependent on the estrous cycle (99). Similarly, TRH iontophoretically applied
to the septum (224), cerebellum, and cerebral cortex (169–171) affected unit
activity. TRH microinjected in amounts of 10 to 20 ng/0.5 μl into the mesencephalon (principally into the reticular formation) evoked behavioral and autonomic changes in the unanesthetized, unrestrained cat. TRH further affected
the electrical activity of mesencephalic neurons. It can therefore be assumed
that TRH acts as a neurotransmitter or neuromodulator in the central nervous
system, and that this action is probably independent of its action as a releasing
hormone (131,174,225,226).

INTEGRATION OF THE GROWTH HORMONE SYSTEM

Of all extrahypothalamic structures considered to be part of the regulatory
mechanisms of growth hormone (GH) secretion, the amygdala is the one most
investigated. Lesions in the medial amygdaloid nuclear complex, but not in
the basolateral or cortical parts, resulted in an increase in bioassayable pituitary
GH and hypothalamic GH releasing hormone (GHRH) content in adult male
deermice (47). Because of a discrepancy between results obtained by radioimmunoassay and bioassay (36,182), the authors were careful to interpret their data
only as an illustration of the role of the medial amygdala in the control of
GH secretion. More detailed studies in which the amygdala was electrically
stimulated gave functional assignments to some of its nuclei (118,123). The
phylogenetically primitive corticomedial portion is inhibitory and the basolateral
part excitatory for pituitary GH secretion. The basolateral amygdala has the
lowest threshold of any brain region for releasing pituitary GH in response to
electrical stimulation. In conscious monkeys electrical stimulation of the posterior part of the amygdala also produces a prompt increase in plasma growth
hormone (5). Subcutaneous administration of GH release inhibiting hormone
(somatostatin) totally blocks the GH release induced by basolateral stimulation

(120). On the basis of these results, it is assumed that different parts of the amygdala selectively control the release of GHRH and somatostatin in the rat (120). Confirmation of these speculations must, however, await definitive methods for determination of GHRH and somatostatin levels immediately after amygdaloid stimulation. The participation of the amygdala in the control of stress-induced inhibition of GH secretion is not conclusive at present. Lesions of the amygdala complex failed to affect stress-induced suppression of plasma GH levels (174).

The hippocampus appears to have a stimulatory effect on GH release. Electrical stimulation of this area induced a nearly threefold increase in GH secretion 10 to 15 min after the start of electrical stimulation in the male rat (118,123). In this study as well as in experiments involving amygdala stimulation (120), the animals were under pentobarbitone anesthesia, although the animals were chronically provided with electrodes and indwelling catheters. Pentobarbitone anesthesia at the same dose has been reported to increase the plasma GH levels 10 min after administration of the drug, but GH levels return to baseline values 20 to 30 min after injection (119). In the experiments mentioned above, electrical stimulation and concomitant blood sampling were performed 20 min after the onset of anesthesia. In this way the increase in GH secretion could be exclusively related to the electrical stimulation. An elevation in GH release was also seen in conscious rhesus monkeys after electrical stimulation of the posterior hippocampus (subicular region) and anterior uncinate gyrus with a rather high stimulus parameter (2 mA; 1 msec duration of each pulse, 40 to 100 Hz) (189). In contrast, electrical stimulation of the anterior hippocampus had no significant effects on GH release (45). Direct microinjection of somatostatin (0.01, 0.1, 1.0, 5.0, and 10.0 μg) into the hippocampus induced a variety of behavioral, locomotor, and electrophysiological changes in the unrestrained freely moving rat (172). The data confirm that the hippocampus is not only a part of the regulatory system for pituitary GH, but it may be a preferential site for somatostatin to exert its behavioral effects (173).

Despite the fact that some data point to correlations between serotonin and dopamine contents of the mesencephalon and diurnal variations in plasma GH levels (112,121,176,186,187), there is little evidence to confirm participation of the mesencephalon in the GH regulatory system. Electrical stimulation or lesions of the locus ceruleus, which depleted hypothalamic norepinephrine to 28% of control values, had no effect on plasma GH levels (58). Local microinjections of 6-OH-dopamine (degenerating catecholaminergic pathways) (11) into the locus ceruleus also failed to produce any significant changes in GH release (58). Likewise, other studies (177) dealing with electrical stimulation of the subceruleus area or the ventral ascending noradrenergic pathway in the male dog did not argue for participation of these areas in GH regulation. Electrical stimulation of the interpeduncular nucleus resulted in an increase in plasma GH levels (118). Thus it can be concluded at present that this nucleus is probably the only midbrain structure involved in the regulation of GH secretion.

OXYTOCIN AND VASOPRESSIN

The hypothalamo-neurohypophysial system (producing and releasing oxytocin and vasopressin) is the most accurately defined of all neuroendocrine control systems (6,34,40,156). Oxytocin secretion has been almost exclusively related to milk ejection, whereas vasopressin secretion has been largely associated with osmotic regulation of body fluids. However, emotional stress has long been known to alter oxytocin- and vasopressin-dependent functions (151). It has been estimated (109) that about one-third of the synaptic boutons of the supraoptic nucleus (NSO) originate from outside the NSO, and of these 13.5% are found in the amygdala, 8.5% in the hippocampus, 32.7% in the brainstem, and the rest elsewhere (230). Indeed, electrical stimulation of the amygdala causes antidiuretic activity in rats (208) and monkeys (74,75). When a temporal pattern was established between vasopressin release and the increase in plasma osmolality, however, vasopressin release and the increase in plasma osmolality ran parallel. Therefore it is at present difficult to decide whether amygdala stimulation first induces an increase in plasma osmolality and then compensates by increased vasopressin release, or vasopressin release is the primary response. Although this may be answered conclusively only by additional experiments, neurophysiological evidence suggests that paraventricular neurons respond to amygdalar stimulation in a matter of milliseconds, probably too fast for osmotic changes to have occurred. The paraventricular nucleus (PVN) neurons (antidromically identified from the neural lobe) as well as transsynaptically activated neurons were responsive to electrical stimulation of the amygdala and the septum. Antidromic PVN cells were largely inhibited, whereas orthodromic cells were largely excited or showed no response (138). Similarly, extrahypothalamic input from the septum to PVN or NSO cells is known (54,97). The phasic firing of presumptive vasopressin neurons, which were identified from the pituitary stalk, could even be abolished by single pulses applied to the septum (54). Whether this indicates that "phase-making" mechanisms for vasopressin neurons reside within extrahypothalamic areas will have to be further investigated. A bidirectional relationship between the magnocellular neurosecretory system and the amygdala is strongly supported by evidence from recent immunohistochemical studies (21,190,221). Vasopressin- or oxytocin-containing fiber systems could be followed into the amygdala and other extrahypothalamic brain structures. It is not yet known, however, if the reciprocal pathways serve as a part of a control system of vasopressin and/or oxytocin secretion or if they perform as neurotransmitters, unrelated to the control system of vasopressin or oxytocin (9).

Morphological and functional connections of the paraventricular supraoptic system with the hippocampus are known (227). Electrical stimulation of the hippocampus results in release of vasopressin and/or oxytocin (7,209).

Mesencephalic participation in the control of oxytocin and vasopressin secretion is beyond dispute, since major pathways of the milk-ejection reflex pass through this area (175,206,207,211). A discrete localization of oxytocin pathways, however, does not seem to be likely, since the results of electrical stimulation (211) and systematic transsection of midbrain structures (217) clearly argue for a very diffusely organized system.

CONCLUSIONS

Current concepts and views about extrahypothalamic integration of hypothalamo-pituitary hormone secretion were discussed. The amygdala, hippocampus, and mesencephalon are connected to the hypothalamus with definite bidirectional links. It seems to be a common phenomenon that integration of hormone secretion by extrahypothalamic structures usually is bimodal, showing inhibitory as well as stimulatory elements that seem to reside in the same extrahypothalamic structure. Obviously there may be some local specificities with inhibitory functions dominating over the stimulatory ones or vice versa. On the other hand, the strength or duration of internal and external variables may alter the modulatory role of each extrahypothalamic structure on the release of pituitary hormone secretion.

ACKNOWLEDGMENTS

The research reported herein was supported by the Deutsche Forschungsgemeinschaft.

REFERENCES

1. Alcaraz, M., Guzmán-Flores, C., Salas, M., and Beyer, C. (1969): Effect of estrogen on the responsivity of hypothalamic and mesencephalic neurons in the female cat. *Brain Res.,* 15:439–446.
2. Amiragova, M. G., and Arkhangelskaya, M. J. (1976): Mechanisms of the effect of the mesencephalic reticular formation on the hypothalamus-hypophysis-thyroid gland system. *Byull. Eksp. Biol. Med.,* 82:916–920.
3. Anderson, C. H. (1975): Localization of cell retaining ^{3}H-estradiol in the forebrain of rabbits. *Anat. Rec.,* 181:287–291.
4. Arai, Y. (1971): Effect of electrochemical stimulation of the amygdala on induction of ovulation in different types of persistent estrous rats and castrated male rats with an ovarian transplant. *Endocrinol. Jpn.,* 18:211–214.
5. Arbuthnott, G. W., Crow, T. J., Fuxe, K., Olson, L., and Ungerstedt, U. (1970): Depletion of catecholamines in vivo induced by electrical stimulation of central monoamine pathways. *Brain Res.,* 24:471–483.
6. Arnauld, E., Dufy, B., and Vincent, J. D. (1975): Hypothalamic supraoptic neurones: Rates and patterns of action potential firing during water deprivation in the unanesthetized monkey. *Brain Res.,* 100:315–325.
7. Aulsebrook, L. H., and Holland, R. C. (1969): Central regulation of oxytocin release with and without vasopressin release. *Am. J. Physiol.,* 216:818–829.
8. Barak, Y. B., Gutnick, M. J., and Feldman, S. (1977): Iontophoretically applied corticosteroids do not affect the firing of hippocampal neurons. *Neuroendocrinology,* 23:249–256.
9. Barker, J. L. (1976): Peptides: Roles in neuronal excitability. *Physiol. Rev.,* 56:438–452.
10. Baum, M. J., and Goldfoot, D. A. (1975): Effect of amygdaloid lesions on gonadal maturation in male and female ferrets. *Am. J. Physiol.,* 228:1646–1651.
11. Bell, L. J., Iversen, L. K., and Uretsky, N. J. (1970): Time course of the effects of 6-

hydroxydopamine and catecholamine-containing neurones in rat hypothalamus and stria terminalis. *Br. J. Pharmacol.*, 38:790–799.

12. Beltramino, C., and Taleisnik, S. (1978): Facilitatory and inhibitory effects of electrochemical stimulation of the amygdala on the release of luteinizing hormone. *Brain Res.*, 144:95–107.

13. Bloch, G. J., and Ganong, W. F. (1971): Lesions of the brain and the onset of puberty in the female rat. *Endocrinology*, 89:898–901.

14. Bohus, B. (1970): Central nervous structures and the effects of ACTH and corticosteroids on avoidance behaviour: A study with intracerebral implantation of corticosteroids in the rat. *Prog. Brain Res.*, 32:171–184.

15. Bohus, B. (1975): The hippocampus and the pituitary-adrenal system hormones. In: *The Hippocampus, Vol. 1: Structure and Development,* edited by R. L. Isaacson and K. H. Pribram, pp. 323–353. Plenum Press, New York.

16. Bohus, B., Nyakas, C., and Lissák, K. (1968): Involvement of suprahypothalamic structures in the hormonal feedback action of corticosteroids. *Acta Physiol. Acad. Sci. Hung.*, 34:1–8.

17. Bouillé, C., and Baylé, J. D. (1973): Effects of limbic stimulations or lesions on basal and stress-induced hypothalamic-pituitary-adrenocortical activity in the pigeon. *Neuroendocrinology,* 13:264–277.

18. Bouillé, C., and Baylé, J. D. (1976): Comparison between hypothalamic, hippocampal and septal multiple unit activity and basal corticotropic function in unrestrained, unanesthetized resting pigeons. *Neuroendocrinology*, 22:164–174.

19. Bouillé, C., and Baylé, J. D. (1978): Comparison between hypothalamic multiple-unit activity and corticotropic function after bilateral destruction of the hippocampus. *Neuroendocrinology,* 25:303–309.

20. Brown-Grant, K., and Raisman, G. (1972): Reproductive function in the rat following selective destruction of afferent fibres to the hypothalamus from the limbic system. *Brain Res.*, 46:23–42.

21. Buijs, R. M., Swaab, D. F., Dogterom, J., and van Leeuwen, F. W. (1978): Intra- and extrahypothalamic vasopressin and oxytocin pathways in the rat. *Cell Tissue Res.*, 186:423–433.

22. Bunn, J. P., and Everett, J. W. (1957): Ovulation in persistent-estrous rats after electrical stimulation of the brain. *Proc. Soc. Exp. Biol. Med.*, 96:369–371.

23. Carrer, H. F., and Sawyer, C. H. (1976): Changes in multiunit spike activity in the rat preoptic area induced by stimulating the midbrain. *Exp. Neurol.*, 52:525–534.

24. Carrer, H. F., and Taleisnik, S. (1970): Effect of mesencephalic stimulation on the release of gonadotrophins. *J. Endocrinol.*, 48:527–539.

25. Carrer, H. F., and Taleisnik, S. (1972): Neural pathways associated with the mesencephalic inhibitory influence on gonadotropin secretion. *Brain Res.*, 38:299–313.

26. Carrillo, A. J., Rabii, J., Carrer, H. F., and Sawyer, C. H. (1977): Modulation of the proestrous surge of luteinizing hormone by electrochemical stimulation of the amygdala and hippocampus in the unanesthetized rat. *Brain Res.*, 128:81–92.

27. Casady, R. L., Branch, B. J., and Taylor, A. N. (1972): Role of electrical seizure activity in the adrenocortical response to hippocampal stimulation in rats. *Anat. Rec.*, 172:285.

28. Chiappa, S. A., Fink, G., and Sherwood, N. M. (1977): Immunoreactive luteinizing hormone releasing factor (LRF) in pituitary stalk plasma from female rats: Effects of stimulating diencephalon, hippocampus and amygdala. *J. Physiol., (Lond)*, 267:625–640.

29. Conrad, L. C. A., and Pfaff, D. W. (1975): Axonal projections of medial preoptic and anterior hypothalamic neurons. *Science*, 190:1112–1114.

30. Constantinidis, J., Geissbühler, F., Gaillard, J. M., Hovaguimian, T., and Tissot, R. (1974): Enhancement of cerebral noradrenaline turnover by thyrotropin-releasing hormone: Evidence by fluorescence histochemistry. *Experientia*, 30:1182–1183.

31. Cowan, W. M., Raisman, G., and Powell, T. P. S. (1965): The connexions of the amygdala. *J. Neurol. Neurosurg. Psychiatry*, 28:137–151.

32. Critchlow, V. (1958): Blockade of ovulation in the rat by mesencephalic lesions. *Endocrinology,* 63:596–610.

33. Critchlow, V. (1963): The role of light in the neuroendocrine system. In: *Advances in Neuroendocrinology,* edited by A. V. Nalbandov, pp. 377–402. University of Illinois Press, Urbana, Ill.

34. Cross, B. A., Dyball, R. E. J., Dyer, R. G., Jones, C. W., Lincoln, D. W., Morris, J. F., and Pickering, B. T. (1975): Endocrine neurons. *Recent Prog. Horm. Res.,* 31:243–286.
35. Dafny, N., Phillips, M. I., Taylor, A. N., and Gilman, S. (1973): Dose effects of cortisol on single unit activity in hypothalamus, reticular formation and hippocampus of freely behaving rats correlated with plasma steroid levels. *Brain Res.,* 59:257–272.
36. Daughaday, W. H., Peak, G. T., Birge, C. A., and Mariz, J. K. (1968): The influence of endocrine factors on the concentration of growth hormone in the rat pituitary. In: *Growth Hormone,* edited by A. Pecile and E. Müller, pp. 238–252. Excerpta Medica, Amsterdam.
37. Döcke, F. (1974): Differential effects of amygdaloid and hippocampal lesions on female puberty. *Neuroendocrinology,* 14:345–350.
38. Döcke, F. (1976): Age-dependent changes in the puberty-controlling function of the medial and cortical amygdaloid nuclei. *Ann. Biol. Anim. Biochem. Biophys.,* 16:423–432.
39. Döcke, F. (1977): A possible mechanism of the puberty-delaying effect of hippocampal lesions in female rats. *Endokrinologie,* 69:258–261.
40. Dreifuss, J. J., Harris, M. C., and Tribollet, E. (1976): Excitation of phasically firing hypothalamic supraoptic neurones by carotid occlusion in rats. *J. Physiol. (Lond),* 257:337–354.
41. Dreifuss, J. J., Murphy, J. T., and Gloor, P. (1968): Contrasting effects of two identified amygdaloid efferent pathways on single hypothalamic neurons. *J. Neurophysiol.,* 31:237–248.
42. Dupont, A., Bastarache, E., Endröczi, E., and Fortier, C. (1972): Effect of hippocampal stimulation on the plasma thyrotropin (TSH) and corticosterone responses to acute cold exposure in the rat. *Can. J. Physiol. Pharmacol.,* 50:364–367.
43. Dyer, R. G., Ellendorff, F., and MacLeod, N. K. (1976): Non-random distribution of cell types in the preoptic and anterior hypothalamic areas. *J. Physiol. (Lond),* 261:495–504.
44. Dyer, R. G., MacLeod, N. K., and Ellendorff, F. (1976): Electrophysiological evidence for sexual dimorphism and synaptic convergence in the preoptic and anterior hypothalamic areas of the rat. *Proc. R. Soc. Lond. [Biol],* 193:421–440.
45. Ehle, A. L., Mason, J. W., and Pennington, L. L. (1977): Plasma growth hormone and cortisol changes following limbic stimulation in conscious monkeys. *Neuroendocrinology,* 23:52–60.
46. Eisenman, J. S. (1974): Unit studies of brainstem projections to the preoptic area and hypothalamus. In: *Recent Studies of Hypothalamic Function,* edited by K. Lederis and K. E. Cooper, pp. 328–340. Karger, Basel.
47. Eleftheriou, B. E., Desjardins, C., Pattison, M. L., Norman, R. L., and Zolovick, A. J. (1969): Effect of amygdaloid lesions on hypothalamic-hypophyseal growth hormone activity. *Neuroendocrinology,* 5:132–139.
48. Eleftheriou, B. E., and Zolovick, A. J. (1968): Effect of amygdaloid lesions on plasma and pituitary thyrotropin levels in the deermouse. *Proc. Soc. Exp. Biol. Med.,* 127:671–674.
49. Ellendorff, F. (1976): Evaluation of extrahypothalamic control of reproductive physiology. *Rev. Physiol. Biochem. Pharmacol.,* 76:103–127.
50. Ellendorff, F. (1978): Extra-hypothalamic centres involved in the control of ovulation. In: *Control of Ovulation,* edited by D. B. Crighton, N. B. Haynes, G. R. Foxcroft, and G. E. Lamming, pp. 7–19. Butterworth, London.
51. Ellendorff, F., Blake, C. A., Colombo, J. A., Whitmoyer, D., and Sawyer, C. H. (1975): Influence of the amygdala on ovulation and gonadotropin release in the female rat. In: *Endocrinology of Sex,* edited by G. Dörner, pp. 335–338. Barth, Leipzig.
52. Ellendorff, F., Colombo, J. A., Blake, C. A., Whitmoyer, D. I., and Sawyer, C. H. (1973): Effects of electrical stimulation of the amygdala on gonadotropin release and ovulation in the rat. *Proc. Soc. Exp. Biol. Med.,* 142:417–420.
53. Ellendorff, F., MacLeod, N. K., and Dyer, R. G. (1976): Bipolar neurones in the rostral hypothalamus. *Brain Res.,* 101:549–553.
54. Ellendorff, F., Poulain, D. A., and Vincent, J. D. (1978): An electrophysiological study of septal input to oxytocin and vasopressin neurones in the supraoptic nucelus of the rat. *J. Physiol. (Lond),* 284:124P.
55. Elwers, M., and Critchlow, V. (1960): Precocious ovarian stimulation following hypothalamic and amygdaloid lesions in rats. *Am. J. Physiol.,* 198:381–385.
56. Elwers, M., and Critchlow, V. (1961): Precocious ovarian stimulation following interruption of the stria terminalis. *Am. J. Physiol.,* 201:281–284.

57. Endröczi, E., and Lissák, K. (1962): Interrelations between paleocortical activity and pituitary-adrenocortical function. *Acta Physiol. Acad. Sci. Hung.,* 21:257–263.
58. Endröczi, E., Marton, I., Radnai, Z., and Biró, I. (1978): Effect of depletion of brain noradrenaline on the plasma FSH and growth hormone levels in ovariectomized rats. *Acta Endocrinol. (Kbh),* 87:55–60.
59. Fenske, M., Ellendorff, F., and Wuttke, W. (1975): Response of medial preoptic neurons to electrical stimulation of the mediobasal hypothalamus, amygdala and mesencephalon in normal, serotonin or catecholamine deprived female rats. *Exp. Brain Res.,* 22:495–507.
60. Filaretov, A. A. (1976): The afferent input and functional organization of the hypothalamus in reactions regulating pituitary-adreno-cortical activity. *Brain Res.,* 107:39–54.
61. Flores, F., Naftolin, F., and Ryan, K. J. (1973): Aromatization of androstenedione and testosterone by rhesus monkey hypothalamus and limbic system. *Neuroendocrinology,* 11:177–182.
62. Frankel, R. J., Jenkins, J. S., Wright, J. J., and Khan, M. U. A. (1976): Effect of brain stimulation on aldosterone secretion in the rhesus monkey (Macaca mulatta). *J. Endocrinol.,* 71:383–391.
63. Frankel, R. J., Jenkins, J. S., and Wright, J. J. (1978): Pituitary-adrenal response to stimulation of the limbic system and lateral hypothalamus in the rhesus monkey (Macaca mulatta). *Acta Endocrinol. (Kbh),* 88:209–216.
64. Gallo, R. V., Johnson, J. H., Goldman, B. D., Whitmoyer, D. I., and Sawyer, C. H. (1971): Effects of electrochemical stimulation of the ventral hippocampus on hypothalamic electrical activity and pituitary gonadotropin secretion in female rats. *Endocrinology,* 89:704–713.
65. Gardner, C. R., and Phillips, S. W. (1977): The influence of amygdala on the basal septum and preoptic area of the rat. *Exp. Brain Res.,* 29:249–263.
66. Gloor, P. (1955): Electrophysiological studies on the connections of the amygdaloid nucleus in the cat. I. The neuronal organization of the amygdaloid projection system. *Electroencephalogr. Clin. Neurophysiol.,* 7:223–242.
67. Gloor, P. (1955): Electrophysiological studies on the connections of the amygdaloid nucleus in the cat. II. The electrophysiological properties of the amygdaloid projection system. *Electroencephalogr. Clin. Neurophysiol.,* 7:243–264.
68. Gorski, R. A. (1971): Gonadal hormones and the perinatal development of neuroendocrine function. In: *Frontiers in Neuroendocrinology,* Vol. 2, edited by L. Martini and W. F. Ganong, pp. 237–290. Oxford University Press, New York.
69. Greenough, W. T., Carter, C. S., Steerman, C., and DeVoogd, T. J. (1977): Sex differences in dendritic patterns in hamster preoptic area. *Brain Res.,* 126:63–72.
70. Guansing, A. R., and Murk, L. M. (1976): Distribution of thyrotropin-releasing hormone in human brain. *Horm. Metab. Res.,* 8:493–494.
71. Hagino, N., Kosaras, B., and Flerkó, B. (1977): Septal projection to the arcuate nucleus of the hypothalamus. *Acta Biol. Acad. Sci. Hung.,* 28:235–238.
72. Harris, G. W., and George, R. (1969): Neurohumoral control of the adenohypophysis and the regulation of the secretion of TSH, ACTH and growth hormone. In: *The Hypothalamus,* edited by W. Haymaker, E. Anderson, and W. J. H. Nauta, pp. 326–388. Thomas, Springfield, Ill.
73. Hayward, J. N. (1977): Functional and morphological aspects of hypothalamic neurons. *Physiol. Rev.,* 57:574–658.
74. Hayward, J. N., Morgas, K., Pavasuthipaisit, K., Perez-Lopez, F. R., and Sofroniew, M. V. (1977): Temporal patterns of vasopressin release following electrical stimulation of the amygdala and the neuroendocrine pathway in the monkey. *Neuroendocrinology,* 23:61–75.
75. Hayward, J. N., and Smith, W. K. (1964): Antidiuretic response to electrical stimulation in brain stem of the monkey. *Am. J. Physiol.,* 206:15–20.
76. Hefco, E., Krulich, L., and Aschenbrenner, J. E. (1975): Effect of hypothalamic deafferentation on the secretion of thyrotropin in resting conditions in the rat. *Endocrinology,* 97:1226–1233.
77. Hefco, E., Krulich, L., and Aschenbrenner, J. E. (1975): Effect of hypothalamic deafferentation on the secretion of thyrotropin during thyroid blockade and exposure to cold in the rat. *Endocrinology,* 97:1234–1240.
78. Heimer, L., and Nauta, W. J. H. (1969): The hypothalamic distribution of the stria terminalis in the rat. *Brain. Res.,* 13:284–297.

79. Hökfelt, T., Fuxe, K., Johansson, O., Jeffcoate, S., and White, N. (1975): Distribution of thyrotropin-releasing hormone (TRH) in the central nervous system as revealed with immunohistochemistry. *Eur. J. Pharmacol.,* 34:389–392.
80. Jackson, J. M. D., and Reichlin, S. (1974): Thyrotropin-releasing hormone (TRH): Distribution in hypothalamic and extrahypothalamic brain tissues of mammalian and submammalian chordates. *Endocrinology,* 95:854–862.
81. Kalra, P. S., and McCann, S. M. (1975): The stimulatory effect of gonadotropin release of implants of estradiol or progesterone in certain sites in the central nervous system. *Neuroendocrinology,* 19:289–302.
82. Kawakami, M., and Kimura, F. (1975): Inhibition of ovulation in the rat by electrical stimulation of the lateral amygdala. *Endocrinol. Jpn.,* 22:61–65.
83. Kawakami, M., Kimura, F., and Wakabayashi, K. (1972): Electrical stimulation of the hippocampus under the chronic preparation and changes of LH, FSH and prolactin levels in serum and pituitary. *Endocrinol. Jpn.,* 19:85–96.
84. Kawakami, M., and Kubo, K. (1971): Neuro-correlate of limbic-hypothalamo-pituitary-gonadal axis in the rat: Change in limbic-hypothalamic unit activity induced by vaginal and electrical stimulation. *Neuroendocrinology,* 7:65–89.
85. Kawakami, M., Seto, K., Kimura, F., and Yanase, M. (1971): Difference in the buffer action between the limbic structures and the hypothalamus to the immobilization stress in rabbits. In: *Influence of Hormones on the Nervous System,* edited by D. H. Ford, pp. 107–120. Karger, Basel.
86. Kawakami, M., Seto, K., and Yoshida, K. (1968): Influence of corticosterone implantation in limbic structure upon biosynthesis of adrenocortical steroid. *Neuroendocrinology,* 3:349–354.
87. Kawakami, M., and Terasawa, E. (1972): Electrical stimulation of the brain on gonadotropin secretion in the female prepubertal rat. *Endocrinol. Jpn.,* 19:335–347.
88. Kawakami, M., and Terasawa, E. (1974): Role of limbic forebrain structures on reproductive cycles. In: *Biological Rhythms in Neuroendocrine Activity,* edited by M. Kawakami, pp. 197–220. Igaku Shoin, Tokyo.
89. Kawakami, M., Terasawa, E., and Ibuki, T. (1970): Changes in multiple unit activity of the brain during the estrous cycle. *Neuroendocrinology,* 6:30–48.
90. Kawakami, M., Yoshioka, E., Konda, N., Arita, J., and Visessuvan, S. (1978): Data on the sites of stimulatory feedback action of gonadal steroids indispensable for luteinizing hormone release in the rat. *Endocrinology,* 102:791–798.
91. Keefer, D. A., and Stumpf, W. E. (1975): Atlas of estrogen-concentrating cells in the central nervous system of the squirrel monkey. *J. Comp. Neurol.,* 160:419–441.
92. Kendall, J. W. (1971): Feedback control of adrenocorticotropic hormone secretion. In: *Frontiers in Neuroendocrinology,* Vol. 2, edited by L. Martini and W. F. Ganong, pp. 177–207. Oxford University Press, New York.
93. Kling, A. (1964): Effects of rhinencephalic lesions on endocrine and somatic development in the rat. *Am. J. Physiol.,* 206:1395–1400.
94. Knizley, H., Jr. (1972): The hippocampus and septal area as primary target sites for corticosterone. *J. Neurochem.,* 19:2737–2745.
95. Knuppen, R., Lubrich, W., Haupt, O., Ammerlahn, U., and Breuer, H. (1969): Wechselwirkungen zwischen Östrogenen und Catecholaminen. I. Beeinflussung der enzymatischen Methylierung von Catecholaminen durch Östrogene und vice versa. *Hoppe Seylers Z. Physiol. Chem.,* 350:1067–1075.
96. Koikegami, H., Fuse, S., Yokoyama, T., Watanabe, T., and Watanabe, H. (1955): Contributions to the comparative anatomy of the amygdaloid nuclei of mammals with some experiments of their destruction or stimulation. *Folia Psychiatr. Neurol. Jpn.,* 8:336–343.
97. Koizumi, K., and Yamashita, H. (1972): Studies of antidromically identified neurosecretory cells of the hypothalamus by intracellular and extracellular recording. *J. Physiol. (Lond),* 221:683–706.
98. Korányi, L., and Guzmán-Flores (1973): Pituitary-adrenocortical hormone influences on multiple units in the brainstem and forebrain structures. In: *Hormones and Brain Function,* edited by K. Lissák, pp. 427–436. Plenum Press, New York.
99. Korányi, L., Whitmoyer, D. I., and Sawyer, C. H. (1977): Effect of thyrotropin-releasing

hormone, luteinizing hormone-releasing hormone and somatostatin on neuronal activity of brain stem reticular formation and hippocampus in the female rat. *Exp. Neurol.,* 57:807–816.

100. Kordon, C. (1978): The role of neurotransmitters in the secretion of pituitary gonadotrophins and prolactin. In: *Control of Ovulation,* edited by D. B. Crighton, N. B. Haynes, G. R. Foxcroft, and G. E. Lamming, pp. 21–28. Butterworth, London.

101. Kovács, S., Sándor, A., Vértes, Z., and Vértes, M. (1965): The effect of lesions and stimulation of the amygdala on pituitary-thyroid function. *Acta Physiol. Acad. Sci. Hung.,* 27:221–235.

102. Krieger, D. T., Liotta, A., and Brownstein, M. J. (1977): Presence of corticotropin in limbic system of normal and hypophysectomized rats. *Brain Res.,* 128:575–579.

103. Krulich, L., Giachetti, A., Marchlewska-Koj, A., Hefco, E., and Jameson, H. E. (1977): On the role of the central noradrenergic and dopaminergic systems in the regulation of TSH secretion in the rat. *Endocrinology,* 100:496–505.

104. Kubek, M. J., Lorincz, M. A., and Wilber, J. F. (1977): The identification of thyrotropin releasing hormone (TRH) in hypothalamic and extrahypothalamic loci of the human nervous system. *Brain Res.,* 126:196–200.

105. Kubo, K., Gorski, R. A., and Kawakami, M. (1975): Effects of estrogen on neuronal excitability in the hippocampal-septal-hypothalamic system. *Neuroendocrinology,* 18:176–191.

106. Lawton, I. E., and Sawyer, C. H. (1970): Role of amygdala in regulating LH secretion in the adult female rat. *Am. J. Physiol.,* 218:622–626.

107. Le Gal La Salle, G. (1976): Antidromic identification of amygdaloid multipolar neurones. *Brain Res.,* 118:479–481.

108. Lengvári, I., and Halász, B. (1973): Evidence for a diurnal fluctuation in plasma corticosterone levels after fornix transection in the rat. *Neuroendocrinology,* 11:191–196.

109. Léranth, C., Záborszky, L., Marton, J., and Palkovits, M. (1975): Studies on the supraoptic nuclei in the rat. I. Synapses. *Exp. Brain Res.,* 22:509–523.

110. Lichtensteiger, W. (1975): Extrahypothalamic effects on anterior pituitary function and possible cholinergic dopaminergic interactions. In: *Anatomical Neuroendocrinology,* edited by W. E. Stumpf and L. D. Grant, pp. 433–434. Karger, Basel.

111. Lloyd, T., and Weisz, J. (1978): Direct inhibition of tyrosine hydroxylase activity by catechol estrogens. *J. Biol. Chem.,* 253:4841–4843.

112. Locatelli, V., Panerai, A. E., Cocchi, D., Gil-Ad, I., Mantegazza, P., Secchi, C., and Müller, E. E. (1978): Drug-induced changes of brain serotoninergic tone and insulin-induced growth hormone release in the dog. *Neuroendocrinology,* 25:84–104.

113. Luine, V. N., Khylchevskaya, R. I., and McEwen, B. S. (1975): Effect of gonadal hormones on enzyme activities in brain and pituitary of male and female rats. *Brain Res.,* 86:283–292.

114. Luine, V. N., Khylchevskaya, R. I., and McEwen, B. S. (1975): Effect of gonadal steroids on activities of monoamine oxidase and choline acetylase in rat brain. *Brain Res.,* 86:293–306.

115. Luttge, W. G., and Wallis, C. J. (1973): In vitro accumulation and saturation of ^{3}H-progestins in selected brain regions and in the adenohypophysis, uterus and pineal of the female rat. *Steroids,* 22:493–502.

116. MacLaren, N. K., Cornblath, M., and Raiti, S. (1974): Human growth hormone. *Am. J. Dis. Child.,* 127:906–908.

117. Mandelbrod, I., and Feldman, S. (1972): Effects of sensory and hippocampal stimulation on unit activity in the median eminence of the rat hypothalamus. *Physiol. Behav.,* 9:565–572.

118. Martin, J. B. (1972): Plasma growth hormone (GH) response to hypothalamic or extrahypothalamic electrical stimulation. *Endocrinology,* 91:107–115.

119. Martin, J. B. (1973): Studies on the mechanism of pentobarbital-induced GH release in the rat. *Neuroendocrinology,* 13:339–350.

120. Martin, J. B. (1974): Inhibitory effect of somatostatin (SRIF) on the release of growth hormone (GH) induced in the rat by electrical stimulation. *Endocrinology,* 94:497–502.

121. Martin, J. B. (1976): Brain regulation of growth hormone secretion. In: *Frontiers in Neuroendocrinology,* Vol. 4, edited by L. Martini and W. F. Ganong, pp. 129–168. Raven Press, New York.

122. Martin, J. B., Endröczi, E., and Bata, G. (1958): Effects of the removal of amygdalic nuclei on the secretion of adrenal cortical hormones. *Acta Physiol. Acad. Sci. Hung.,* 14:131–134.

123. Martin, J. B., Kontor, J., and Mead, P. (1973): Plasma GH responses to hypothalamic,

hippocampal and amygdaloid electrical stimulation: Effects of variation in stimulus parameters and treatment with α-methyl-p-tyrosine (α-MT). *Endocrinology,* 92:1354–1361.

124. Mason, J. W. (1959): Plasma-17-hydroxycorticosteroid levels during electrical stimulation of the amygdaloid complex in conscious monkeys. *Am. J. Physiol.,* 196:44–48.

125. Mason, J. W. (1968): A review of psychoendocrine research on the pituitary-adrenal cortical system. *Psychosom. Med.,* 30:576–607.

126. Matheson, G. K., Branch, B. J., and Taylor, A. N. (1971): Effects of amygdaloid stimulation on pituitary adrenal activity in conscious cats. *Brain Res.,* 32:151–167.

127. McEwen, B. S., Gerlach, J. L., and Micco, D. J. (1975): Putative glucocorticoid receptors in hippocampus and other regions of the rat brain. In: *The Hippocampus, Vol. 1: Structure and Development,* edited by R. L. Isaacson and K. H. Pribram, pp. 285–322. Plenum Press, New York.

128. McEwen, B. S., and Pfaff, D. W. (1973): Chemical and physiological approaches to neuroendocrine mechanisms: attempts at integration. In: *Frontiers in Neuroendocrinology,* Vol. 3, edited by W. F. Ganong and L. Martini, pp. 267–335. Oxford University Press, New York.

129. McEwen, B. S., Weiss, J. M., and Schwartz, L. S. (1969): Uptake of corticosterone by rat brain and its concentration by certain limbic structures. *Brain Res.,* 16:227–241.

130. Merimee, T. J., and Rabin, D. (1973): A survey of growth hormone secretion and action. *Metabolism,* 22:1235–1249.

131. Meyers, R. D., Metcalf, G., and Rice, J. C. (1977): Identification by microinjection of TRH-sensitive sites in the cat's brain stem that mediate respiratory, temperature and other autonomic changes. *Brain Res.,* 126:105–115.

132. Michal, E. K. (1974): Dexamethasone inhibits multi-unit activity in the rat hippocampus. *Brain Res.,* 65:180–183.

133. Millhouse, O. E. (1969): A golgi study of the descending medial forebrain bundle. *Brain Res.,* 15:341–363.

134. Morin, L. P., and Feder, H. H. (1974): Inhibition of lordosis behavior in ovariectomized guinea pigs by mesencephalic implants of progesterone. *Brain Res.,* 70:71–80.

135. Murphy, J. T., and Renaud, L. P. (1969): Mechanisms of inhibition in the ventromedial nucleus of the hypothalamus. *J. Neurophysiol.,* 32:85–102.

136. Nakahara, T., Uchimura, H., Hirano, M., Saito, M., and Ito, M. (1976): Effects of gonadectomy and thyroidectomy on the tyrosine hydroxylase activity in individual hypothalamic nuclei and lower brain stem catecholaminergic cell groups of the rat. *Brain Res.,* 117:351–356.

137. Nauta, W. J. H. (1960): Some neural pathways related to the limbic system. In: *Electrical Studies on the Unanesthetized Brain,* edited by E. R. Ramly and D. S. O'Doherty, pp. 1–16. Hoover, New York.

138. Negoro, H., Visessuwan, S., and Holland, R. C. (1973): Inhibition and excitation of units in paraventricular nucleus after stimulation of the septum, amygdala and neurohypophysis. *Brain Res.,* 57:479–483.

139. Nicolescu-Catargi, A., Faure, J. M. A., and Vincent, J. D. (1972): Influence de l'hormone corticotrope sur les circuits amygdalo-ventro-médians chez le lapin libre éveillé. *J. Physiol. (Paris),* 65:278 A.

140. Pacold, S. T., Kirsteins, L., Hojvat, S., Lawrence, A. M., and Hagen, T. C. (1978): Biologically active pituitary hormones in the rat brain amygdaloid nucleus. *Science,* 199:804–806.

141. Parker, L. N. (1972): The turnover of norepinephrine in the brain stems of dysthyroid rats. *J. Neurochem.,* 19:1611–1613.

142. Parker, C. R., Neaves, W. B., Barnea, A., and Porter, J. C. (1977): Studies on the uptake of [³H]thyrotropin-releasing hormone and its metabolites by synaptosome preparations of the rat brain. *Endocrinology,* 101:66–75.

143. Parvizi, N., and Ellendorff, F. (1975): 2-Hydroxy-oestradiol-17β as a possible link in steroid brain interaction. *Nature,* 256:59–60.

144. Parvizi, N., Elsaesser, F., Smidt, D., and Ellendorff, F. (1977): Effects of intracerebral implantation, microinjection and peripheral application of sexual steroids on plasma luteinizing hormone levels in the male miniature pig. *Endocrinology,* 101:1078–1087.

145. Pekary, A. E., Davidson, J. M., and Zondek, B. (1967): Failure to demonstrate a role of midbrain-hypothalamic afferents in reproductive processes. *Endocrinology,* 80:365–368.

146. Perkins, M. N., Demaine, C., and Whitehead, S. A. (1977): Electrophysiological and

pharmacological studies of amygdalo-hypothalamic connections in the rat. *Neuroendocrinology,* 23:200–211.

147. Perkins, M. N., and Whitehead, S. A. (1978): Responses and pharmacological properties of preoptic/anterior hypothalamic neurones following medial forebrain bundle stimulation. *J. Physiol. (Lond),* 279:347–360.

148. Pfaff, D., and Keiner, M. (1973): Atlas of estradiol-concentrating cells in the central nervous system of the female rat. *J. Comp. Neurol.,* 151:121–158.

149. Pfaff, D. W., Silva, M. T. A., and Weiss, J. M. (1971): Telemetered recording of hormone effects on hippocampal neurons. *Science,* 172:394–395.

150. Phillips, M. I., and Dafny, N. (1971): Effect of cortisol on unit activity in freely moving rats. *Brain Res.,* 25:651–655.

151. Pickford, M. (1969): Neurohypophysis-antidiuretic (vasopressor) and oxytocic hormones. In: *The Hypothalamus,* edited by W. Haymaker, E. Anderson, and W. J. H. Nauta, pp. 250–274. Thomas, Springfield, Ill.

152. Piva, F., Kalra, P. S., and Martini, L. (1973): Participation of the amygdala and of the cerebellum in the feedback effects of progesterone. *Neuroendocrinology,* 11:229–239.

153. Plapinger, L., and McEwen, B. S. (1973): Ontogeny of estradiol-binding sites in rat brain. I. Appearance of presumptive adult receptors in cytosol and nuclei. *Endocrinology,* 93:1119–1128.

154. Plapinger, L., McEwen, B. S., and Clemens, L. E. (1973): Ontogeny of estradiol-binding sites in rat brain. II. Characteristics of a neonatal binding macromolecule. *Endocrinology,* 93:1129–1139.

155. Poletti, C. E., Kinnard, M. A., and MacLean, P. D. (1973): Hippocampal influence on unit activity of hypothalamus preoptic region and basal forebrain in awake sitting squirrel monkeys. *J. Neurophysiol.,* 36:308–324.

156. Poulain, D. A., Wakerley, J. B., and Dyball, R. E. J. (1977): Electrophysiological differentiation of oxytocin- and vasopressin-secreting neurones. *Proc. R. Soc. Lond. [Biol],* 196:367–384.

157. Poulain, P. (1977): Septal afferents to the arcuate-median eminence region in the guinea pig: Correlative electrophysiological and horseradish peroxidase studies. *Brain Res.,* 137:150–153.

158. Raisman, G., Cowan, W. M., and Powell, T. P. S. (1965): The extrinsic afferent, commissural and association fibres of the hippocampus. *Brain,* 88:963–996.

159. Raisman, G., Cowan, W. M., and Powell, T. P. S. (1966): An experimental analysis of the efferent projection of the hippocampus. *Brain,* 89:83–108.

160. Raisman, G., and Field, P. M. (1971): Sexual dimorphism in the preoptic area of the rat. *Science,* 173:731–733.

161. Ranson, S. W., and Magoun, H. W. (1939): The hypothalamus. *Ergeb. Physiol.,* 41:56–163.

162. Redgate, E. S. (1970): ACTH release evoked by electrical stimulation of brain stem and limbic system sites in the cat: The absence of ACTH release upon infundibular area stimulation. *Endocrinology,* 86:806–823.

163. Redgate, E. S., and Fahringer, E. E. (1973): A comparison of the pituitary adrenal activity elicited by electrical stimulation of preoptic, amygdaloid and hypothalamic sites in the rat brain. *Neuroendocrinology,* 12:334–343.

164. Relkin, R. (1971): Relative efficacy of pinealectomy, hypothalamic and amygdaloid lesions in advancing puberty. *Endocrinology,* 88:415–418.

165. Relkin, R. (1971): Absence of alteration in puberal onset in male rats following amygdaloid lesioning. *Endocrinology,* 88:1272–1274.

166. Renaud, L. P. (1976): Influence of amygdala stimulation on the activity of identified tuberoinfundibular neurones in the rat hypothalamus. *J. Physiol. (Lond),* 260:237–252.

167. Renaud, L. P. (1976): Tuberoinfundibular neurons in the basomedial hypothalamus of the rat: Electrophysiological evidence for axon collaterals to hypothalamic and extrahypothalamic areas. *Brain Res.,* 105:59–72.

168. Renaud, L. P., and Hopkins, D. A. (1977): Amygdala afferents from the mediobasal hypothalamus: An electrophysiological and neuroanatomical study in the rat. *Brain Res.,* 121:201–213.

169. Renaud, L. P., and Martin, J. B. (1975): Microiontophoresis of thyrotropin-releasing hormone (TRH): effects on the activity of central neurons. In: *Anatomical Neuroendocrinology,* edited by W. E. Stumpf and L. D. Grant, pp. 354–356. Karger, Basel.

170. Renaud, L. P., and Martin, J. B. (1975): Thyrotropin releasing hormone (TRH): Depressant action on central neuronal activity. *Brain Res.,* 86:150–154.

171. Renaud, L. P., Martin, J. B., and Brazeau, P. (1975): Depressant action of TRH, LH-RH and somatostatin on activity of central neurones. *Nature*, 255:233–235.

172. Rezek, M., Havlicek, V., Hughes, K. R., and Friesen, H. (1976): Central site of action of somatostatin (SRIF): Role of hippocampus. *Neuropharmacology*, 15:499–504.

173. Rezek, M., Havlicek, V., Hughes, K. R., and Friesen, H. (1977): Behavioural and motor excitation and inhibition induced by the administration of small and large doses of somatostatin into the amygdala. *Neuropharmacology*, 16:157–162.

174. Rice, R. W., and Critchlow, V. (1976): Extrahypothalamic control of stress-induced inhibition of growth hormone secretion in the rat. *Endocrinology*, 99:970–976.

175. Richard, P. (1972): The reticulo-hypothalamic pathway controlling the release of oxytocin in the ewe. *J. Endocrinol.*, 53:71–83.

176. Rose, J. C., and Ganong, W. F. (1976): Neurotransmitter regulation of pituitary gland secretion. In: *Psychopharmacology*, edited by I. Essman and I. Valzelli, pp. 87–123. Spectrum, New York.

177. Rose, J. C., Goldsmith, P. C., Holland, F. J., Kaplan, S. L., and Ganong, W. F. (1976): Effect of electrical stimulation of the canine brain stem on the secretion of ACTH and growth hormone (GH). *Neuroendocrinology*, 22:352–362.

178. Rose, J. D., and Michael, R. P. (1978): Facilitation by estradiol of midbrain and pontine unit responses to vaginal and somatosensory stimulation in the squirrel monkey. *Exp. Neurol.*, 58:46–58.

179. Sawyer, C. H. (1972): Functions of the amygdala related to the feedback actions of gonadal steroid hormones. In: *The Neurobiology of the Amygdala*, edited by B. E. Eleftheriou, pp. 745–762. Plenum Press, New York.

180. Scanlon, M. F., Smith, B. R., and Hall, R. (1978): Thyroid-stimulating hormone: Neuroregulation and clinical applications. *Clin. Sci. Mol. Med.*, 55:1–10.

181. Scanlon, M. F., Smith, B. R., and Hall, R. (1978): Thyroid-stimulating hormone: Neuroregulation and clinical applications. *Clin. Sci. Mol. Med.*, 55:129–138.

182. Schalch, D. S., and Reichlin, S. (1966): Plasma growth hormone concentration in the rat determined by radioimmunoassay: Influence of sex, pregnancy, lactation, anesthesia, hypophysectomy and extrasellar pituitary transplants. *Endocrinology*, 79:275–280.

183. Segal, M. (1976): Interactions of ACTH and norepinephrine on the activity of rat hippocampal cells. *Neuropharmacology*, 15:329–333.

184. Selmanoff, M. K., Brodkin, L. D., Weiner, R. I., and Siiteri, P. K. (1977): Aromatization and 5α-reduction of androgens in discrete hypothalamic and limbic regions of the male and female rat. *Endocrinology*, 101:841–848.

185. Sherwood, N. M. (1977): Estrous cycles after electrical stimulation of the brain in conscious rats: Effect of current strength, estradiol benzoate and progesterone. *Endocrinology*, 100:18–29.

186. Simon, M. L., and George, R. (1975): Diurnal variations in plasma corticosterone and growth hormone as correlated with regional variations in norepinephrine, dopamine and serotonin content of rat brain. *Neuroendocrinology*, 17:125–138.

187. Simon, M., George, R., and Garcia, J. (1975): Chronic morphine effects on regional brain amines, growth hormone and corticosterone. *Eur. J. Pharmacol.*, 34:27–38.

188. Slusher, M. A. (1966): Effects of cortisol implants in the brain stem and neural hippocampus on diurnal corticosteroid levels. *Exp. Brain Res.*, 1:184–194.

189. Smith, G. P., and Root, A. W. (1971): Dissociation of changes in growth hormone and adrenocortical hormone levels during brain stimulation of monkeys. *Neuroendocrinology*, 8:235–244.

190. Sofroniew, M. V., and Weindl, A. (1978): Extrahypothalamic neurophysin-containing perikarya, fiber pathways and fiber clusters in the rat brain. *Endocrinology*, 102:334–337.

191. Spies, H. G., Norman, R. L., Clifton, D. K., Ochsner, A. J., Jensen, J. N. and Phoenix, C. H. (1976): Effects of bilateral amygdaloid lesions on gonadal and pituitary hormones in serum and on sexual behavior in female rhesus monkeys. *Physiol. Behav.*, 17:985–992.

192. Steiner, F. A., Ruf, K., and Akert, K. (1969): Steroid-sensitive neurones in rat brain: Anatomical localization and responses to neurohumours and ACTH. *Brain Res.*, 12:74–85.

193. Stumpf, W. E. (1970): Estrogen-neurons and estrogen-neuron systems in the periventricular brain. *Am. J. Anat.*, 129:207–218.

194. Stumpf, W. E. (1971): Autoradiographic techniques and the localization of estrogen, androgen and glucocorticoid in the pituitary and brain. *Am. Zool.*, 11:725–739.

195. Stumpf, W. E., and Sar, M. (1974): Anatomical distribution of corticosterone-concentrating neurons in rat brain. In: *Anatomical Neuroendocrinology,* edited by W. E. Stumpf and L. D. Grant, pp. 254–261. Karger, Basel.

196. Stumpf, W. E., and Sar, M. (1976): Steroid hormone target sites in the brain: The differential distribution of estrogen, progestin, androgen and glucocorticosteroid. *J. Steroid Biochem.,* 7:1163–1170.

197. Swanson, L. W., and Cowan, W. M. (1977): An autoradiographic study of the organisation of the efferent connections of the hippocampal formation in the rat. *J. Comp. Neurol.,* 172:49–84.

198. Taleisnik, S., and Carrer, H. F. (1973): Facilitatory and inhibitory mesencephalic influence on gonadotropin release. In: *Hormones and Brain Function,* edited by K. Lissák, pp. 335–345. Plenum Press, New York.

199. Taylor, A. N., and Branch, B. J. (1971) Inhibition of ACTH release by a central inhibitory mechanism in the basal forebrain. *Exp. Neurol.,* 31:391.

200. Taylor, A. N., Lindsley, D. F., and Casady, R. L. (1973): Electrical correlates of adrenal regulation. In: *Endocrinology,* edited by R. O. Scow, pp. 80–86. Excerpta Medica, Amsterdam.

201. Taylor, A. N., Lorenz, R. J., Turner, B. B., Ronnekleiv, O. K., Casady, R. L., and Branch, B. J. (1976): Factors influencing pituitary-adrenal rhythmicity, its ontogeny and circadian variations in stress responsiveness. *Psychoneuroendocrinology,* 1:291–301.

202. Taylor, A. N., Matheson, G. K., and Dafny, N. (1972): Modification of the responsiveness of components of the limbic-midbrain circuit by corticosteroids and ACTH. In: *Steroid Hormones and Brain Function,* edited by C. H. Sawyer and R. A. Gorski, pp. 67–78. University of California Press, Los Angeles.

203. Telegdy, G., and Vermes, I. (1975): Effect of adrenocortical hormones on activity of the serotoninergic system in limbic structures in rats. *Neuroendocrinology,* 18:16–26.

204. Terasawa, E., and Timiras, P. S. (1968): Electrical activity during the estrous cycle of the rat: Cyclic changes in limbic structures. *Endocrinology,* 83:207–216.

205. Terasawa, E., and Timiras, P. S. (1968): Electrophysiological study of the limbic system in the rat at onset of puberty. *Am. J. Physiol.,* 215:1462–1467.

206. Tindal, J. S., and Knaggs, G. S. (1975): Further studies on the afferent path of the milk-ejection reflex in the brain stem of the rabbit. *J. Endocrinol.,* 66:107–113.

207. Tindal, J. S., Knaggs, G. S., and Turvey, A. (1969): The afferent path of the milk-ejection reflex in the brain of the rabbit. *J. Endocrinol.,* 43:663–671.

208. Tomas, T. (1975): ADH release from cut pituitary stalk and intact pituitary gland during amygdala stimulation at various frequencies in rats. *Neuroendocrinology,* 17:139–146.

209. Tomas, T., Traczyk, W. Z., and Guzek, J. W. (1973): ADH release from cut pituitary stalk and intact pituitary gland during hippocampal stimulation of various frequencies in rats. *Neuroendocrinology,* 11:257–267.

210. Torand-Allerand, C. D. (1976): Sex steroids and the development of the newborn mouse hypothalamus and preoptic area in vitro: Implications for sexual differentiation. *Brain Res.,* 106:407–412.

211. Urban, I., Moss, R. L., and Cross, B. A. (1971): Problems in electrical stimulation of afferent pathways for oxytocin release. *J. Endocrinol.,* 51:347–358.

212. Van der Schoot, P. (1974): An evaluation of the acute effects of electrochemical stimulation of limbic structures on ovulation in cyclic female rats. *Prog. Brain Res.,* 41:363–370.

213. Van Hartesveldt, C. (1975): The hippocampus and regulation of the hypothalamic-hypophyseal-adrenal cortical axis. In: *The Hippocampus, Vol. 1: Structure and Development,* edited by R. L. Isaacson and K. H. Pribram, pp. 375–391. Plenum Press, New York.

214. Velasco, M. E., and Taleisnik, S. (1969): Release of gonadotropins induced by amygdaloid stimulation in the rat. *Endocrinology,* 84:132–139.

215. Velasco, M. E., and Taleisnik, S. (1969): Effect of hippocampal stimulation on the release of gonadotropin. *Endocrinology,* 85:1154–1159.

216. Velasco, M. E., and Taleisnik, S. (1971): Effects of the interruption of amygdaloid and hippocampal afferents to the medial hypothalamus on gonadotrophin release. *J. Endocrinol.,* 51:41–55.

217. Voloschin, L. M., and Dottaviano, E. J. (1976): The channeling of natural stimuli that evoke the ejection of milk in the rat: Effect of transections in the midbrain and hypothalamus. *Endocrinology,* 99:49–58.

218. Ward, D. G., Grizzle, W. E., and Gann, D. S. (1976): Inhibitory and facilitatory areas of the rostral pons mediating ACTH release in the cat. *Endocrinology,* 99:1220–1228.
219. Warembourg, M. (1975): Radioautographic study of the rat brain and pituitary after injection of ³H dexamethasone. *Cell Tissue Res.,* 161:183–191.
220. Warembourg, M. (1975): Radioautographic study of the rat brain after injection of [1,2-³H]corticosterone. *Brain Res.,* 89:61–70.
221. Weindl, A., and Sofroniew, M. V. (1976): Demonstration of extrahypothalamic peptide secreting neurons: A morphologic contribution to the investigation of psychotropic effects of neurohormones. *Pharmakopsychiatr. Neuropsychopharmacol.,* 9:226–234.
222. Weisz, J., and Gibbs, C. (1974): Conversion of testosterone and androstenedione to estrogens in vitro by the brain of female rats. *Endocrinology,* 94:616–622.
223. Whalen, R. E., and Luttge, G. (1971): Role of the adrenal in the preferential accumulation of progestin by mesencephalic structures. *Steroids,* 18:141–146.
224. Winokur, A., and Beckman, A. L. (1978): Effects of thyrotropin releasing hormone, norepinephrine and acetylcholine on the activity of neurons in the hypothalamus, septum and cerebral cortex of the rat. *Brain Res.,* 150:205–209.
225. Winokur, A., Kreider, M. S., Dugan, J., and Utiger, R. D. (1978): The effects of 6-hydroxydopamine on thyrotropin-releasing hormone in rat brain. *Brain Res.,* 152:203–208.
226. Winokur, A., and Utiger, R. D. (1974): Thyrotropin releasing hormone: Regional distribution in rat brain. *Science,* 185:265–267.
227. Woods, W. H., Holland, R. C., and Powell, E. (1968): Connections of cerebral structures functioning in neurohypophysial hormone release. *Brain Res.,* 12:26–46.
228. Yamada, T., and Greer, M. A. (1960): The effect of bilateral ablation of the amygdala on endocrine function in the rat. *Endocrinology,* 66:565–574.
229. Youngblood, W. W., Lipton, M. A., and Kizer, J. S. (1978): TRH-like immunoreactivity in urine, serum and extrahypothalamic brain: Non-identity with synthetic pyroglu-hist-pro-NH₂ (TRH). *Brain Res.,* 151:99–116.
230. Záborszky, L., Léránth, C., Makara, G. B., and Palkovits, M. (1975): Quantitative studies on the supraoptic nucleus in the rat. II. Afferent fiber connections. *Exp. Brain Res.,* 22:525–540.
231. Zigmond, R. E., and McEwen, B. S. (1970): Selective retention of oestradiol by cell nuclei in specific brain regions of the ovariectomized rat. *J. Neurochem.,* 17:889–899.
232. Zolovick, A. J. (1972): Effects of lesions and electrical stimulation of the amygdala on hypothalamic-hypophyseal-regulation. In: *The Neurobiology of the Amygdala,* edited by B. E. Eleftheriou, pp. 643–684. Plenum Press, New York.

The Endocrine Functions of the Brain,
edited by Marcella Motta.
Raven Press, New York, © 1980

15

Mammalian Pineal Gland:
Basic and Clinical Aspects

Steven M. Reppert and David C. Klein

Section on Neuroendocrinology, Laboratory of Developmental Neurobiology, National Institute of Child Health and Human Development, National Institutes of Health, Bethesda, Maryland 20205

Within the last 20 years a cohesive concept of the function of the mammalian pineal gland has begun to emerge. This modern concept of the pineal gland has a biochemical and physiological basis.

Biochemically, the pineal gland is unique in the capacity to synthesize melatonin (Fig. 1, below) in a rhythmic manner. The rhythm has a 24-hr period and a large amplitude (Fig. 2, below), and interestingly appears to be driven by another area of the brain, the suprachiasmatic nucleus, which is located in the hypothalamus. Environmental lighting is the only exogenous physiological factor known to significantly influence this rhythm. One effect of lighting that is of fundamental importance is to coordinate the rhythm to the 24-hr day.

Physiologically, the pineal gland has the remarkable role of mediating reproductive changes induced by photoperiod in various seasonally reproductive mammals. Thus the view has developed that the pineal gland transmits information about day length to the reproductive systems of these animals.

Although not clearly established, there is growing evidence that pineal melatonin production and the effects of the pineal gland on reproductive function are intimately related. The conceptual convergence of these two functions is largely a result of recent experiments which demonstrate that precisely timed injections of melatonin can cause the same changes in reproduction that are normally induced by changes in photoperiod (191,192,195).

BASIC ASPECTS

Indoleamine Biochemistry

The modern history of pineal indoleamine biochemistry started in 1959 when Lerner and associates (90) described the chemical structure of melatonin, a potent amphibian skin-lightening principle of the mammalian pineal gland. The skin-lightening property of the mammalian pineal gland was originally described in 1917 by McCord and Allen (108). In 1960 Axelrod and Weissbach (6) showed that the enzymes necessary for the synthesis of melatonin from serotonin were present in this tissue (6). At about the same time, Fiske and co-workers (38) demonstrated that light affected the rat pineal gland: Pineal glands of animals chronically exposed to constant light weighed significantly less than those of animals exposed to diurnal lighting and constant darkness. Three years after this finding, independent studies by Quay (141) and Wurtman and associates (216) firmly established the relationship between environmental lighting and pineal indoleamine metabolism.

Since that time, studies of one of the enzymes necessary for the biosynthesis of melatonin from serotonin, N-acetyltransferase, have provided the basis for our understanding of the circadian function of the mammalian pineal gland. This enzyme exhibits a very large daily rhythm in activity and controls the large daily changes in melatonin production (18,82,83). The extensive studies of the regulation of N-acetyltransferase activity contributed greatly to our understanding of the neural, chemical, and molecular events involved in the generation and regulation of the pineal melatonin rhythm.

With the advent of sensitive techniques for measuring melatonin in biological fluids over the past decade, considerable information has accumulated about the regulation of melatonin rhythm in a variety of mammals, including man. In general, these studies showed that regulation of the melatonin rhythm in other mammals parallels that of the N-acetyltransferase rhythm in the rat.

Synthesis of Melatonin

The biosynthetic pathway involved in the synthesis of melatonin from tryptophan can be conveniently divided into two parts (Fig. 1). The first part, synthesis of serotonin, is dependent on the availability of the essential amino acid tryptophan. The uptake of circulating tryptophan into the pinealocyte is followed by conversion to serotonin by two enzymes, tryptophan hydroxylase and aromatic amino acid decarboxylase (9,28,33,93–95). The high levels of the former enzyme and of its cofactor biotin in the pineal are responsible for the high levels of serotonin (0.5 mM) found within the gland—higher than in any other body tissue (93,168,172). Recent studies showed that tryptophan hydroxylase may be under neural control (176,177).

The second part, conversion of serotonin to melatonin (Fig. 2), is under the control of a neural mechanism which has received considerable attention over the past 10 years; this is the major regulatory system with which this chapter is concerned. Serotonin is converted to N-acetylserotonin by N-acetyltransferase (19,20,204). N-Acetylserotonin is then converted to melatonin by hydroxyindole-O-methyltransferase (4,6,76).

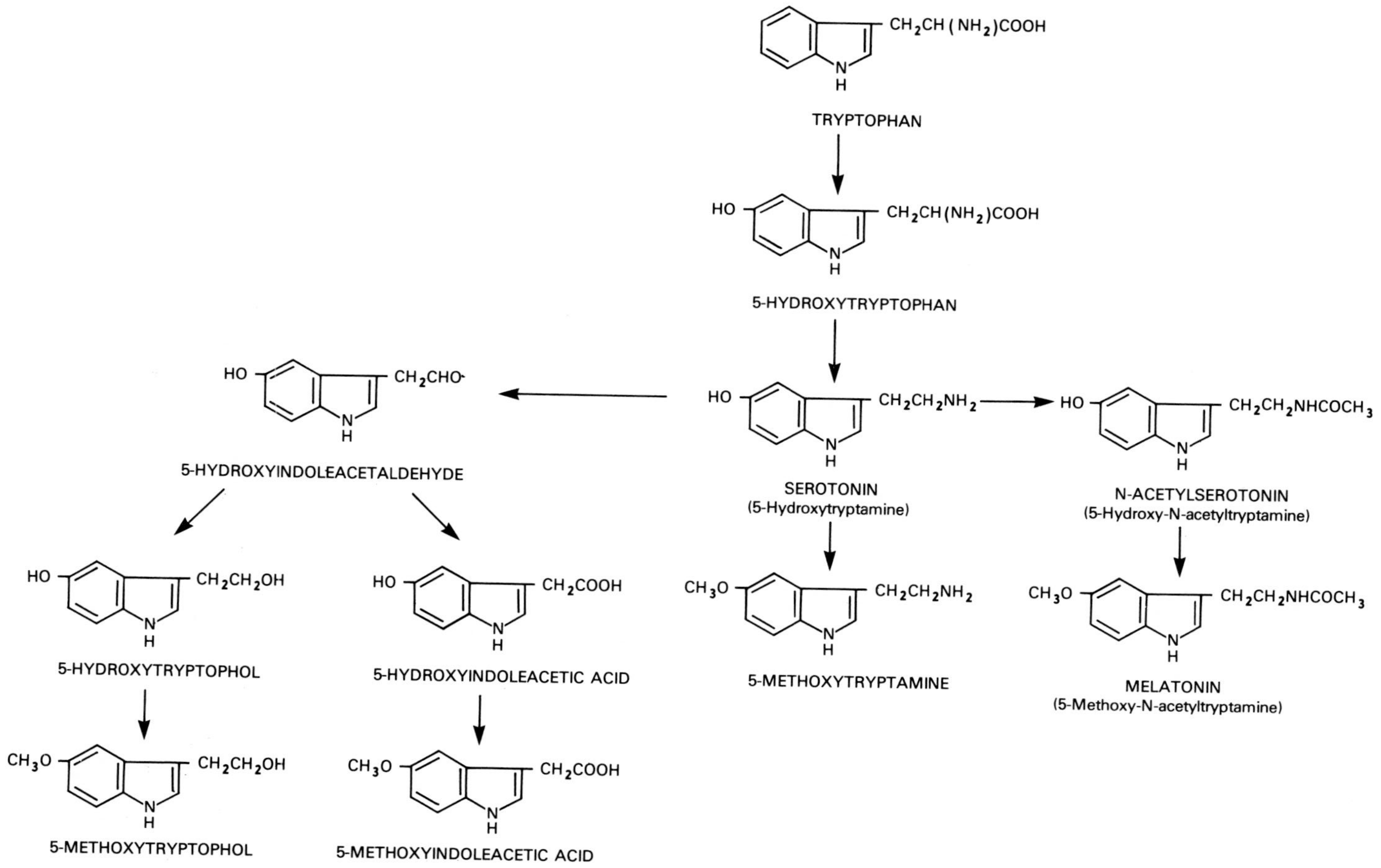

FIG. 1. Indole metabolism in the pineal gland. (From ref. 70.)

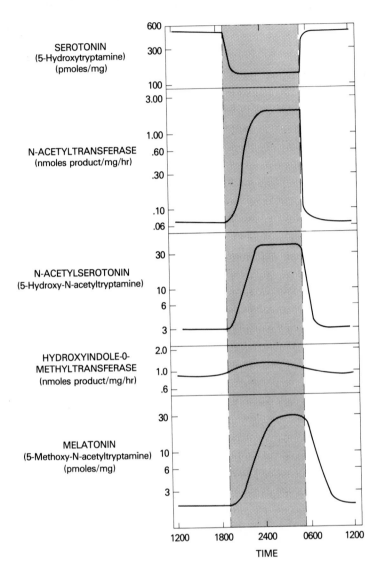

FIG. 2. Rhythms in indole metabolism in the rat pineal gland. The metabolic pathway from 5-hydroxytryptamine to melatonin is on the left. The daily variations in the concentrations of metabolites and activities of enzymes are on the right. The shaded portion indicates the dark period of the lighting cycle. The data were abstracted from reports in the literature. (AcCoA) acetyl coenzyme A. (CoA) coenzyme A. (S AdM) S-adenosyl methionine. (S AdH) S-adenosyl homocysterine. (5-HT) 5-hydroxytryptamine, serotonin. (NAcT) N-acetyltransferase. (HIOMT) hydroxyindole-0-methyltransferase. (NAc 5-MT) N-acetyl-5-methoxytryptamine, melatonin. (From ref. 69.)

Biological Fate of Melatonin

Melatonin has a short biological half-life. Studies using radiolabeled melatonin indicate that it disappears rapidly from the circulation (88,89,158) because of metabolism. It should be added that no metabolite of melatonin has been reported to be more biologically active than melatonin, or to be equally active. This indicates that melatonin is not activated by metabolism via the routes outlined below.

Metabolism by 6-Hydroxylation

The major metabolic fate (>80%) of circulating melatonin is 6-hydroxylation by liver microsomes, followed by conjugation of sulfate and, to a substantially lesser extent, glucuronic acid (88,89). Interestingly, there appears to be no change during development in the metabolic fate of melatonin (154). In the neonatal and the adult rat the primary product is the sulfate conjugate of 6-hydroxymelatonin (Fig. 3).

By altering the rate of 6-hydroxylation, the rate of disappearance of melatonin from the circulation can also be altered (212). Chlorpromazine, which blocks 6-hydroxylation, increases circulating melatonin levels in rats and humans (129,179). Alternatively, drugs which induce microsomes (e.g., barbiturates) increase melatonin metabolism *in vitro* and could thus conceivably decrease circulating melatonin levels (212).

Metabolism to N-Acetyl-5-Methoxykynurenamine

Recently Hirata and colleagues (48) identified a new metabolite of melatonin, N-acetyl-5-methoxykynurenamine. They showed that this compound was formed from melatonin *in vitro* by brain tissue via a two-step enzymatic reaction which, first, cleaves the indole ring and, second, removes the carbon adjacent to the ring nitrogen (Fig. 3). They also found that this new metabolite was the only radioactive melatonin derivative found in whole brain after radioactive melatonin was injected intracisternally. N-Acetyl-5-methoxykynurenamine appears to be the unidentified melatonin metabolite found in rat urine following intravenous injections of radiolabeled melatonin (88,89), and these investigators suggest melatonin may be normally metabolized by mammalian brain via this metabolic pathway. However, further work is needed to substantiate this interesting possibility. It is of interest to point out that the analogous metabolite of serotonin, 5-methoxykynurenamine, is a potent serotonin antagonist (196).

Potential Metabolites of Melatonin with Central Nervous System Effects

The possibility that melatonin is metabolized to a compound that has psychotropic effects has been pursued by investigators who reported unidentified, chromatographically distinct radioactive peaks in urine following administration of

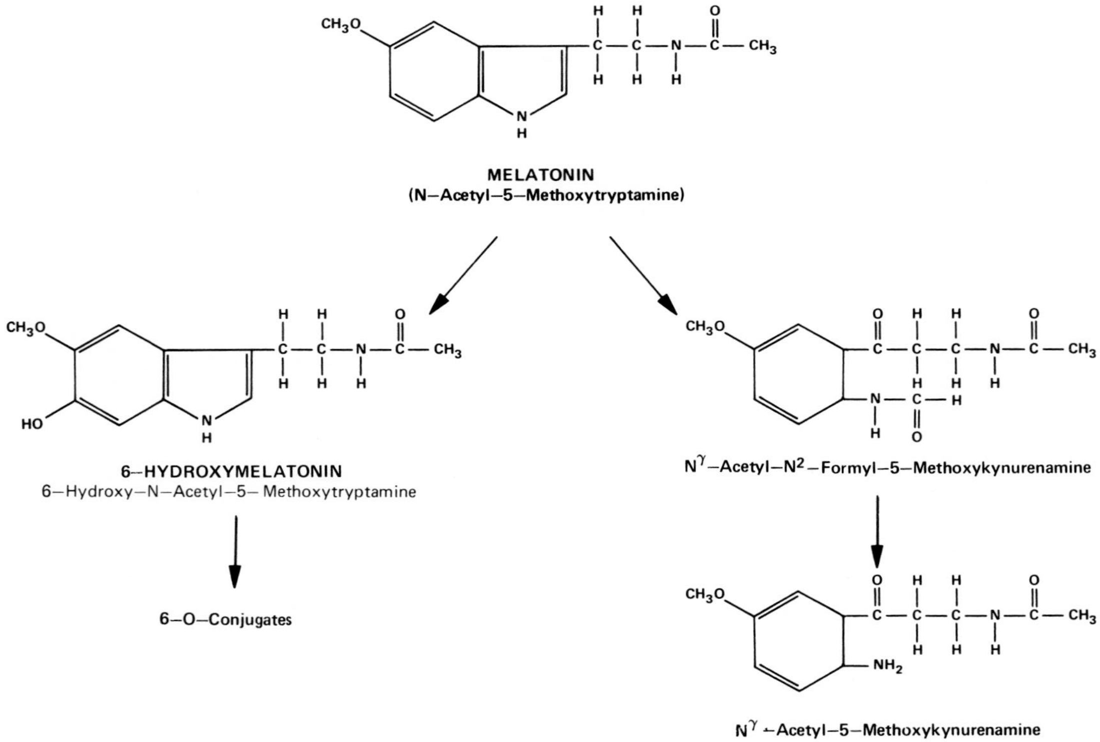

FIG. 3. Metabolism of melatonin.

radiolabeled melatonin (89). Kveder and McIsaac (89) attempted without clear success to identify one of these compounds as a β-carboline; on a chemical basis this compound is a reasonably probable derivative. β-Carbolines are of pharmacological interest because of the known hallucinogenic effects of members of this family, including the harmalan alkaloids (109).

Recently Rogawski and co-workers (161) showed that melatonin can be deacetylated *in vitro* to 5-methoxytryptamine, a potent psychoactive compound, by aryl acylamidase. This is consistent with earlier reports of the detection of a small quantity of radiolabeled 5-methoxyindoleacetic acid, a potential 5-methoxytryptamine metabolite, in rat urine following the administration of radiolabeled melatonin (88,89). The formation of 5-methoxytryptamine was demonstrated for the liver enzyme but not for the brain enzyme. Thus trace amounts of 5-methoxytryptamine could be produced from melatonin in the periphery. However, since 5-methoxytryptamine does not readily enter the brain (200), the possibility that peripheral formation of this compound affects brain function seems unlikely.

Measurement of Melatonin

A major advance in the investigation of the regulation of melatonin production and its physiological function in mammals has been the development of techniques of measuring melatonin. Four major analytical approaches have been investigated: spectrophoto fluorometry, bioassay, radioimmunoassay (RIA), and gas chromatography–mass spectrometry.

Fluorescence Microscopy

Direct detection of melatonin by fluorescence microscopy, which provided the first indication of a rhythm in pineal melatonin, has received little attention (142,143). Similarly, detection of fluorescent melatonin condensation products has been described but has not proved popular (104).

Bioassay

A melatonin rhythm in the bird, rodent, and human was first unequivocally demonstrated using a bioassay (96,137) based on the ability of melatonin to blanch amphibian skin by causing aggregation of melanin granules around the nuclei of dermal melanophores (108,148). This procedure, which is somewhat elaborate, is sensitive to about 100 pg/assay (99,219). Accordingly, relatively large volumes of bodily fluids must be concentrated prior to analysis.

Radioimmunoassay

Several practical melatonin RIA procedures have been developed within the last 5 years. At present, seven antisera are characterized in the literature (1,2,

41,64,91,163,220). Conjugation of melatonin to large antigenic proteins (e.g., bovine serum albumin) is required to generate these antibodies. The radioligands used in melatonin RIAs are either [³H]melatonin or [¹²⁵I]melatonin analogs. The RIAs using tritiated melatonin as a radioligand are sensitive to about 20 pg/assay. Higher sensitivity is achieved using the [¹²⁵I]melatonin analog [¹²⁵I]-N-3-(4-hydroxyphenyl)-propionyl-5-methoxytryptamine, which was developed by Rollag and Niswender (163). They used N-succinyl-5-methoxytryptamine conjugated to bovine serum albumin to raise antisera. Using this assay it is possible to detect about 1 pg melatonin per assay.

The RIA techniques require at least one organic extraction step to separate melatonin from interfering substances in biological samples; the extent to which samples must be processed prior to analysis appears to vary with the nature of the samples (158). In spite of this routine use of organic extraction procedures, there still appear to be problems in these assays with either specificity or contamination. For example, even though standard validation procedures [parallelism, chromatographic identity of the immunoreactive substance(s) with melatonin in several solvent systems, and testing of cross reactivity with structurally related compounds] have been used for the majority of RIAs, there is a large discrepancy in the reported concentration of melatonin detected in human plasma (92). In addition, there is a discrepancy between the RIAs and a negative ionization gas chromatography–mass spectrometry technique; the RIAs tend to give higher values (92).

Putting these absolute differences aside, however, it must be emphasized that all the RIAs confirm the existence of the melatonin rhythm under normal lighting conditions in a variety of animals including man. In all cases these assays find that melatonin values are high during the nighttime hours.

Gas Chromatography–Mass Spectrometry

Theoretically, the most accurate technique for measuring melatonin is gas chromatography–mass spectrometry (GC-MS). However, discrepancies also exist between the reported GC-MS techniques, as they do among the various RIAs. One technique, based on electron ion impact (211), provides day and night plasma melatonin values in humans which are several-fold higher than those provided by a technique based on negative chemical ionization (92). The reasons for these discrepancies are not readily apparent.

The apparent discrepancies in the values of melatonin in bodily fluids provided by bioassay, RIA, and GC-MS indicate that the values given by any one technique must be interpreted with caution. There seems to be little doubt that RIA is the most attractive routine means of detecting melatonin. However, it currently appears that it will be necessary to use alternative analytical techniques (e.g., bioassay or GC-MS) to establish the accuracy of the individual RIA techniques used for each animal species and each biological fluid of interest; this has been accomplished for only a few of the reported RIA techniques (64,99,158,194).

Also the development and use of highly specific techniques (e.g., high-pressure liquid chromatography) to effectively separate melatonin from interfering compounds may be useful as a preparatory step prior to analysis.

Locus of Melatonin Secretion

Two possible routes for pineal melatonin secretion in mammals exist (for reviews see refs. 152,155). First, since the pineal gland is an intracranial organ, melatonin could be directly secreted into cerebrospinal fluid (CSF). In all mammals this could occur by secretion into CSF in the subarachnoid space surrounding the pineal gland. In some mammals, including primates, the pineal gland forms part of the roof of the third ventricle, and thus pineal melatonin could be directly secreted into ventricular CSF. The second possible route of pineal melatonin secretion in all mammals is directly into the circulation.

The relative contribution of either direct secretion of pineal melatonin into CSF or into the circulation has been examined in sheep using a mathematical model (162). These studies indicate that the majority (greater than 99%) of pineal melatonin is secreted into the circulation before entering CSF.

However, it should be pointed out that attempts to develop mathematical models for the relationship of pineal melatonin secretion to melatonin levels in various biological fluids, including CSF, are hampered because it appears that melatonin may be produced by extrapineal sources. Reports in the literature indicate that melatonin is detectable in blood and urine after pinealectomy in the sheep and the rat (64,128). Possible sources of extrapineal melatonin include the retina, harderian gland, and enterochromaffin cells of the intestine (21, 130,146).

Melatonin in CSF

Melatonin is present in the CSF of a variety of mammals (for review see ref. 155). The reported concentrations of CSF melatonin, however, vary substantially among and within species. This variation may be due to true species differences but may also arise from differences in sampling, the age or condition of the animal and subject, or the precise location from which CSF is withdrawn. Another important variable is the assay technique used to measure melatonin.

Rapid entry of melatonin from the circulation to CSF has been demonstrated in the rhesus monkey and sheep (158,162). This is not suprising in view of the non-ionized, lipophylic nature of the molecule. Also, rapid entry of melatonin from CSF into the circulation has been shown in the sheep (162). These findings suggest that melatonin concentrations in blood and CSF are similar. However, the quantitative relationship of blood and CSF melatonin values is quite variable among and within animal species. In spite of this, a consistent dynamic relationship does exist; similar daily rhythms occur in blood and CSF melatonin (44,158) (Fig. 4).

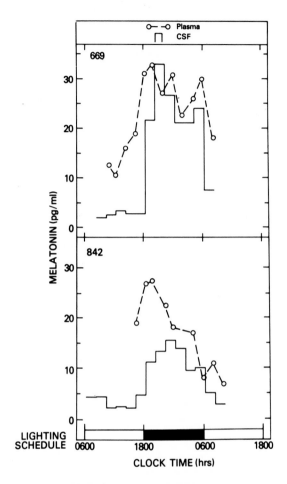

FIG. 4. Diurnal pattern of melatonin in plasma and CSF for rhesus monkeys. Plasma and CSF were collected over the same 24-hr period for each animal. The CSF was collected as 120-min fractions. Melatonin was measured by RIA. (From ref. 158.)

CSF melatonin levels are reported to be lower than corresponding circulating levels in adult humans, rhesus monkeys, and sheep (2,158,162,198,205,211). Only part of total melatonin in blood is free to cross into CSF because melatonin binds to albumin (22). Thus one factor which could influence the relative amounts of melatonin in blood and CSF is the degree of binding of melatonin to blood proteins. Lower CSF values in some mammals may be a reflection of increased binding of melatonin to serum proteins.

CSF melatonin levels that are higher than corresponding circulating values have been reported early in the development in cattle and humans (44,180). These higher melatonin concentrations in CSF may be a function of age. Perhaps there is a closer anatomical relationship of the pineal gland to ventricular CSF early in development, or there may be more melatonin-binding protein in CSF early in development. However, an additional factor to consider in the human study is that the children were undergoing therapy for acute lymphocytic leukemia. High melatonin levels in these patients may be associated with either leukemia or antileukemic therapy.

The physiological significance of melatonin in CSF is not known. It is possible that CSF is an important vehicle for the transfer of melatonin to specific areas of the brain, e.g., the hypothalamus. Interestingly, this brain area is thought to be an important site of melatonin action (112).

Rhythm in Indoleamine Metabolism

Rhythm in Melatonin Production

The rate at which serotonin is converted to melatonin exhibits a daily rhythm. The relationship of this rhythm to a diurnal lighting schedule is depicted in Fig. 2, which is based on observations made in the rat. During the day serotonin levels are high and N-acetyltransferase activity is low (80,141,144,170). After the lights are turned off at night, there is a gradual, large (50- to 100-fold) increase in N-acetyltransferase activity, causing a decrease in serotonin and an increase in N-acetylserotonin production (82,184). The increase in N-acetylserotonin results in an increase in melatonin synthesis through a mass action effect (82,96); hydroxyindole-O-methyltransferase exhibits a minimal increase in activity at night (100,145,151,169). When the lights are turned on in the morning, N-acetyltransferase activity decreases, serotonin returns to high daytime values, and pineal melatonin levels decrease to low daytime levels.

This regulatory mechanism is also present in chickens (13,16), sheep (A. Namboodiri and D. C. Klein, *unpublished results*), and, as discussed later, to a somewhat limited extent in humans (181).

In the Syrian hamster, however, large daily changes in pineal melatonin content are not paralleled by large daily changes in pineal N-acetyltransferase activity (194). This is paradoxical because the regulation of pineal melatonin content in the hamster parallels that of N-acetyltransferase activity in the rat. This discrepancy may be explained by technical problems with measuring the enzyme in the hamster. Alternatively, there may be a different regulatory scheme for pineal melatonin production in the hamster.

As indicated earlier, a day–night variation in melatonin concentrations has been detected in the pineal gland, blood, urine, or CSF of all mammals studied (1, 2, 44, 64, 92, 96, 99, 102, 129, 131, 137, 158, 163, 164, 181, 194, 197, 199, 202, 205, 208, 210, 211) including the rat, Syrian hamster (Fig. 5), sheep, cow, camel, pig, rhesus monkey (Fig. 6), and human. It is especially remarkable that high values always occur at night because some animals are active during the night and others during the day. This is in contrast to other daily rhythms where the phase relationship of the rhythm to the photoperiod varies with the innate

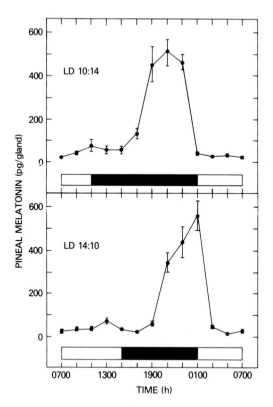

FIG. 5. Amount of melatonin in the pineal glands of Syrian hamsters maintained in LD 10:14 or LD 14:10. Melatonin was measured by RIA. Data are presented as the mean ± SE of seven determinations. (From ref. 194.)

activity pattern of the animals. For example, the daily rhythm in core body temperature is characterized by high values at night for night-active animals and high values during the day for day-active animals.

Photic Regulation of Melatonin Rhythm

The daily light–dark cycle functions to coordinate the daily rhythm in melatonin production and in melatonin levels to the 24-hr day. No other daily time cues, including feeding (29,122), are known to influence the daily N-acetyltransferase rhythm. It should be pointed out that this point has been examined so far only in the rat and hence might vary with species.

Endogenous Nature of Melatonin Rhythm

Although the daily light–dark cycle coordinates the melatonin rhythm with environmental lighting, it does not drive the daily rhythm. Rather, several inter-

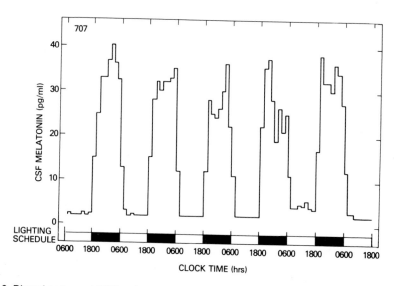

FIG. 6. Diurnal pattern of CSF melatonin for a rhesus monkey studied for 6 consecutive days. CSF was collected as 90-min fractions, and melatonin was measured by RIA. (From ref. 158.)

esting lines of evidence indicate that the daily melatonin rhythm in all mammals is generated by an endogenous oscillator.

Based on studies using rats, sheep, and monkeys, it appears that when animals are housed in constant darkness or blinded, depriving them of photic input, the daily rhythms in pineal melatonin, N-acetyltransferase activity, or serotonin persist (27,78,80,119,139,140,147,157,163,184,193). The period length of these rhythms is close to 24 hr (Fig. 7).

When an animal is maintained for longer periods (e.g., several weeks) in a constant-darkness condition, the daily melatonin rhythm is no longer coordinated with environmental lighting and becomes desynchronized from solar time; i.e., it "free runs." This, along with the fact that the period length of the free-running rhythm is slightly different for each animal, makes the interpretation of data from a population of animals difficult. Thus no melatonin rhythm may be apparent for the population when data are plotted relative to solar time. For these reasons, investigators of the rhythm in rodents monitored another circadian function—wheel-running activity—for each animal and then plotted the data for a population relative to that activity. Using this experimental technique, a clear circadian rhythm in pineal melatonin production, phase-locked to running activity, has been demonstrated for the rat, chicken, and hamster (140,147,193).

The circadian nature of the melatonin rhythm is further substantiated by studies with rats and rhesus monkeys, where it has been shown that the N-acetyltransferase rhythm (14) and CSF melatonin rhythm (S. M. Reppert, M. J. Perlow, and D. C. Klein, *unpublished results*) do not immediately re-

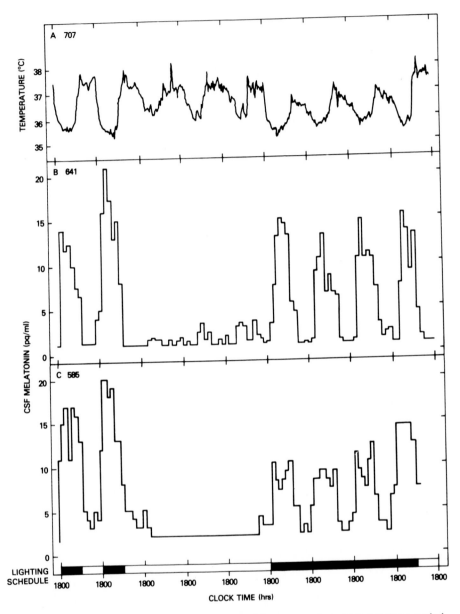

FIG. 7. Pattern of CSF melatonin concentration and brain temperature studied during a period of diurnal lighting and extended periods of constant light and constant darkness. **A:** Brain temperature was measured every 30 min. **B:** and **C:** CSF was collected in 120-min fractions. Each value represents a single determination by RIA. (From ref. 139.)

entrain to phase shifts in the daily lighting schedule but require many days for re-entrainment; the amount of time required for re-entrainment is a function of the magnitude and direction of the phase shift.

Additional evidence that the melatonin rhythm is endogenously generated is that exposure to darkness given during the light period of diurnal lighting cycle does not result in an increase in rat N-acetyltransferase activity (14) or melatonin levels in the hamster or the monkey (194; S. M. Reppert, M. J. Perlow, and D. C. Klein, *unpublished results*). Presumably this is because at that time of day the endogenous clock is not in the proper phase to stimulate the pineal gland.

Suppressive Effect of Light

Light is an active inhibitory influence causing acute suppression of N-acetyltransferase activity and melatonin production. Based on studies in the rat, sheep, rhesus monkey, and Syrian hamster (55,81,111,139,157,159,163,194), it appears that when animals are exposed to light during the dark period, at a time when N-acetyltransferase activity and melatonin levels are normally high, there is a rapid decrease in N-acetyltransferase activity to low daytime levels, resulting in a rapid decrease in pineal and circulating melatonin. Suppression persists during the period of light exposure; continued exposure to light for several days results in a continued absence of these rhythms (Fig. 7). Under these conditions, another circadian rhythm, wheel-running activity, persists. This rhythm appears to be driven by the same endogenous oscillator that drives the pineal rhythms (223), which suggests that in constant light the endogenous clock which generates the melatonin rhythm continues to function, but that pineal rhythms are selectively inhibited.

This interpretation is further substantiated by studies with the rhesus monkey (139). In these animals the daily rhythm in brain temperature persists in constant light whereas the CSF melatonin rhythm is suppressed (Fig. 7). Also, when lights are turned off at the end of several days of constant light, CSF melatonin is not increased immediately, but increases only at the time corresponding to the predicted night had the animals not been exposed to constant light.

Comparison of Melatonin Rhythm in Mammals

An interesting theory of mammalian pineal function is that the melatonin rhythm provides a daily measure of the length of the photoperiod (69,70). Elevated levels occur only during the dark period of the day. Thus the elevated levels of melatonin at night could provide a daily biochemical measure of the duration of the dark period. A gradual increase in the duration of the dark period would be reflected as a corresponding increase in the duration of elevated melatonin levels. This idea developed from studies in the rat, in which it appears that the duration of melatonin production is proportional to the duration of the dark period (69,70). The application of this hypothesis to other species can now be tested by comparing the characteristics of the rhythm in the rat to that of other mammals.

In the rat, pineal melatonin does not increase until 3 to 4 hr after lights are turned off at night (210). This lag is also found in the Syrian hamster (194), in which there is a 4- to 6-hr period after the start of the dark period before an increase in pineal melatonin (Fig. 5). In contrast, the lag period appears to be shorter in the rhesus monkey (Fig. 6). The nocturnal increase in CSF melatonin occurs within 2 hr after lights-off at night. Similarly, in sheep (163, 164), where plasma melatonin concentrations were measured, and in Geurnsey calves (44), where CSF and plasma melatonin concentrations were measured, melatonin levels also increase within 2 hr after lights-off at night. From these observations it appears that there is substantial species variation in the lag period that precedes an increase in melatonin.

There is also some variation in the relationship of when melatonin production ends and when the dark period ends. In the monkey [light–dark (LD) 12:12], calf (LD 14:10), and sheep (LD 16:8 or 8:16), the high nighttime levels of melatonin decrease rapidly when lights are turned on in the morning (44,158, 163,164). Thus in these animals it appears that light controls the duration of the increased melatonin levels at night, turning it off in the morning. In the Syrian hamster, however, the situation appears to be quite different (194). On "long" days (LD 14:10), the increased levels of pineal melatonin decrease immediately after lights-on in the morning. On the other hand, on short days (LD 10:14), high levels of pineal melatonin decrease 2 hr prior to the time lights are turned on in the morning. Indeed, the duration that pineal melatonin levels are elevated and the amplitude of the rhythm in these two photoperiods appear to be the same (Fig. 5). The only difference between these two photoperiods seems to be a 2-hr phase shift in the melatonin rhythm relative to time of day.

These findings clearly indicate that, whereas melatonin production is always elevated at night, the pattern of melatonin production exhibits significant species variation. At one end of the spectrum, sheep appear to produce melatonin essentially throughout the night, even during very long nights (164); in this case the duration of melatonin production is a proportional measure of the night period. However, at the other end of the spectrum, the hamster appears to produce melatonin only during a 4- to 6-hr period that is not substantially altered by the length of the night (194), except that it is absent during very short nights (LD 20:4) (L. Tamarkin, S. M. Reppert, D. C. Klein, and B. Goldman, *unpublished results*). The significance of these differences is not clear. However, it seems reasonable to suspect that there is some physiological importance in (a) the amount of melatonin made, and (b) the precise time it is made, and that different patterns of melatonin production have evolved to best adapt species to survive in a specific photic environment.

Regulation of Circadian Rhythms in Pineal Indoleamine Metabolism

The neural structures and the transsynaptic and molecular events involved in the generation and regulation of pineal melatonin production (Fig. 8) were elucidated primarily in studies on the rat; limited studies in other mammals have also been performed.

Neural Structures

Neural signals which appear to originate in the suprachiasmatic nuclei are transmitted to the pineal gland by way of central and peripheral neural structures. This is an unusual neural pathway, in that neural signals originating in one neural structure in the brain, the suprachiasmatic nuclei, leave it to pass through the brain to the peripheral sympathetic nervous system and then return back to another brain structure, the pineal gland.

Suprachiasmatic Nuclei

The suprachiasmatic nuclei, small paired structures in the anterior hypothalamus located close to the optic chiasm, have been proposed to function as a self-sustaining oscillator or biological "clock" (110,223). They are thought to play a major role in the organization and generation of the rhythm in rat pineal melatonin production. Evidence to support this comes from several experimental approaches. First, the metabolic activity of the suprachiasmatic nuclei in the rat, as measured by 2-deoxyglucose utilization, fluctuates in an apparent circadian manner, in contrast to other areas of the brain which do not exhibit such variation (175). Second, electrolytic lesions of the suprachiasmatic nuclei result in the loss of the rhythm in pineal N-acetyltransferase activity and presumably melatonin production (75,119). This was observed to occur for rats maintained in either diurnal lighting or constant darkness. Enzyme activity remained at low daytime levels in these animals. In addition, other circadian rhythms in rodents (rats and Syrian hamsters) are disrupted by ablation of suprachiasmatic nuclei (39,51,116,171,185,186; for reviews see refs. 110,223). These include locomotor activity, drinking, eating, core temperature, adrenocorticosteroids, and estrus. Thus the suprachiasmatic nuclei of the rodent appears to be intimately involved not only in the circadian organization of pineal function but also in the control of other circadian functions. However, it is not known whether the suprachiasmatic nuclei acts as a driving oscillator generating these rhythms or organizes rhythmic output from other oscillators, each of which controls a specific function, into a single circadian pattern.

Recent studies with the rhesus monkey also suggest that the suprachiasmatic nuclei play a key role in the generation of the CSF melatonin rhythm (156) similar to the role it plays in controlling melatonin synthesis in the rat. Destruc-

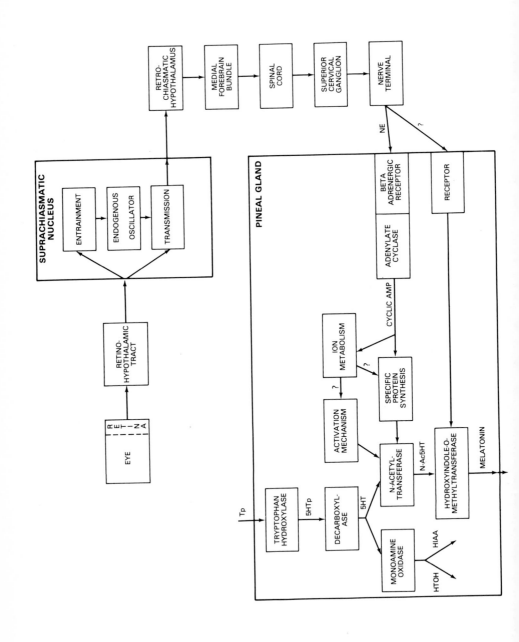

tion of the suprachiasmatic nuclei area in the monkey markedly alters the daily CSF melatonin rhythm and the regulation of this rhythm by environmental lighting. Following surgical destruction of the suprachiasmatic nuclei area, the daily CSF melatonin rhythm is either absent or abnormal in diurnal lighting. Also, CSF melatonin levels are not consistently suppressed by constant light.

Photic Input to the Suprachiasmatic Nuclei

The effects of environmental lighting on the rat pineal N-acetyltransferase rhythm are mediated by the retina through action on a rhodopsin-like photopigment (21,111). Signals from the eye to the suprachiasmatic nucleus are transmitted via retinohypothalamic projections (45,115,120). This tract, which was clearly identified by autoradiographic tracing studies, is distinct from the primary optic and the accessory optic tracts. In contrast to earlier findings (117,118), which indicated that the inferior accessory optic tracts carry photic signals which control the pineal gland, it now appears that photic regulation of the pineal enzymes N-acetyltransferase and hydroxyindole-O-methyltransferase may involve only the retinohypothalamic projections (75). These projections were recently identified in every mammal examined, including nonhuman primates (114). The presence of this tract in humans, however, has not been established.

Neural Connections from Suprachiasmatic Nuclei to the Pineal Gland

In the rat, efferents from the suprachiasmatic nuclei project caudally into the retrochiasmatic hypothalamus (174,189,190). Although the precise central neural pathway responsible for transmitting information from the suprachiasmatic nuclei to the pineal gland is unknown, it appears to pass through the median forebrain bundle and midbrain reticular formation to the intermediolateral cell column (115). This latter structure provides preganglionic input to the superior cervical ganglion, which in turn sends projections into the pineal gland. Within the pineal gland these projections form a dense plexus characterized by swollen processes called varicosities, which are located in the perivascular space (42,61,62,115). These varicosities contain the neurotransmitter substance which controls the daily fluctuations in pineal indoleamine metabolism. Neural signals, originating in the suprachiasmatic nucleus, stimulate the release of neurotransmitter.

Based on anatomical examination, postganglionic fibers from the superior cervical ganglion appear to be the sole source of innervation to the rodent

FIG. 8. Neural control of the pineal gland. (NE) norepinephrine. (cyclic AMP) adenosine 3′,5′-cyclic monophosphate. (TP) tryptophan. (OHTp) 5-hydroxytryptophan. (5-HT) 5-hydroxytryptamine, serotonin. (HIAA) 5-hydroxyindoleacetic acid. (HTOH) 5-hydroxytryptophol. (N-Ac5HT) N-acetylserotonin. The question marks indicate unproved hypotheses. (A modification of a scheme presented in ref. 75.)

pineal gland (61,62). This is supported by studies in adult rats showing that bilateral removal of this ganglion blocks the daily rhythm in pineal serotonin content (37), and ganglionectomy (surgical and chemical) and decentralization of the ganglion abolishes the daily rhythm in N-acetyltransferase activity (84). Also, superior cervical ganglionectomy abolishes the daily rhythmicity of pineal melatonin content in the Syrian hamster, with pineal melatonin levels remaining at low daytime levels (131).

Neural Regulation of Pineal Hydroxyindole-O-Methyltransferase Activity

In view of the marked differences in the dynamics of hydroxyindole-O-methyltransferase and N-acetyltransferase activities, it is surprising that the same central and peripheral neural structures outlined above regulate both enzymes. Hydroxyindole-O-methyltransferase activity responds tonically to alterations in the lighting schedule; it gradually increases during several weeks' exposure to constant darkness and decreases gradually during several weeks' exposure to constant light (7,121,130).

The following discussion of the transsynaptic and intracellular events involved in regulating N-acetyltransferase activity in the rat, however, do not apply to hydroxyindole-O-methyltransferase activity. The transsynaptic and intracellular events involved in the regulation of the latter enzyme have not been established.

Transsynaptic Events

Large daily changes in pineal N-acetyltransferase activity and consequently melatonin production are due to daily changes in the release of neurotransmitter from the sympathetic nerves in the rat pineal gland. The potential transmitter substances identified in pineal nerve endings are norepinephrine, serotonin, and octopamine (57,58,138). It is generally accepted that norepinephrine is the primary neurotransmitter responsible for the increase in N-acetyltransferase activity normally resulting from sympathetic stimulation at night (5,12,18,30,31,57,201). This is supported not only by the location of norepinephrine in nerve terminals but by the fact that norepinephrine, not serotonin, treatment mimics *in vitro* all the effects of sympathetic stimulation at night on the pineal gland. However, it should be pointed out that several lines of evidence suggest that octopamine could also function as a neurotransmitter regulating melatonin production (57,58).

There is a release of norepinephrine from nerve processes at night, in the dark (17). Extraneuronal norepinephrine interacts with a β-adrenergic receptor on the pineal cell membrane, leading to activation of a series of intracellular events discussed below, required for an increase in N-acetyltransferase activity. The pineal β-adrenoreceptors are in a dynamic state, constantly changing in number in response to the daily variation in the release of norepinephrine from the sympathetic nerves (30,32,63,165,167). Thus during the day, after receptors have been unoccupied, there is an increasing sensitivity (supersensitivity) to norepinephrine. Conversely, during the night, after receptors have been occupied, a decreasing sensitivity develops (subsensitivity). In effect, the neurotransmitter participates in regulating responsiveness to itself at the receptor level.

Intracellular Events

In vitro studies demonstrated that interaction of neurotransmitter with the pineal β-adrenoreceptor rapidly results in an adenyl-cyclase-mediated accumulation of intracellular cyclic AMP (26,73,187,188,203). The increase in this cyclic nucleotide is required for all the known effects of adrenergic stimulation of the pineal gland (11,71,72,83,85,86). These include hyperpolarization, an increase in N-acetyltransferase activity, a decrease in pineal serotonin, and an increase in N-acetylserotonin and melatonin production.

Although the cyclic AMP-mediated effects on N-acetyltransferase activity are complex and not fully understood, several distinct effects are known. First is hyperpolarization of the pinealocyte, which is required for the N-acetyltransferase activity to increase (135,173). Next, cyclic AMP initiates production of the mRNA required for N-acetyltransferase activity to increase (123,124,166). If sufficient mRNA is already available, however, this may not be required (71,166). A further effect is to stimulate a protein-synthesis-dependent increase in N-aceyltransferase activity (31,72,83,166). The nature of the protein produced by this effect is unknown. However, it is likely that it is N-acetyltransferase. Finally, cyclic AMP stabilizes N-acetyltransferase molecules in an active form (73).

Spontaneous inactivation of N-acetyltransferase is blocked by acetyl coenzyme A (15). In view of this, it is possible that the stabilizing effect of cyclic AMP may involve acetylation of N-acetyltransferase to an active form. Thus inactivation may in part involve deacetylation of the enzyme. The involvement of cyclic AMP in the rapid inactivation of N-acetyltransferase, which results from displacement or removal of norepinephrine from the adrenoreceptor, is supported by the finding that a rapid decrease in intracellular cyclic AMP precedes the drop in N-acetyltransferase activity (73,126).

Factors which Alter Pineal Indoleamine Metabolism

Light

As previously mentioned, light has an acute suppressive effect on the normally high nighttime activity of N-acetyltransferase and thus causes a parallel decrease in pineal melatonin production. From the foregoing discussion, the sequence of events involved in this effect can now be pictured as follows: Light interacts with a rhodopsin-like photopigment in the retina which results in the transmission of impulses from the retina to the suprachiasmatic nuclei via the retinohypothalamic projections. This results in a specific transsynaptic effect on neurons in the suprachiasmatic nuclei, which in turn terminates stimulation of the sympathetic nerves in the superior cervical ganglion.

At the level of the suprachiasmatic nuclei, the effects of light on pineal N-acetyltransferase activity, as mediated by the retinohypothalamic projections, may involve a cholinergic neurotransmitter. Zatz and Brownstein (222) reported that intraventricular infusions of carbacol around the area of the suprachiasmatic nuclei could mimic the acute suppressive effect of light on pineal N-acetyltransferase activity as well as the entraining effect of light. This is quite interesting since it raises the possibility that both effects of light may be mediated via the same neurotransmitter.

At the level of the pineal gland, the light-induced termination of sympathetic stimulation results in a decrease in norepinephrine release; the neurotransmitter is removed from the extraneuronal space by uptake into pineal nerve endings, and intracellular cyclic AMP decreases. This directs a rapid inactivation of N-acetyltransferase ($t_{1/2}$ = 3 to 4 min) followed by an increase in serotonin (52) and a decrease in N-acetylserotonin and melatonin production.

The rapid decrease in melatonin production is paralleled by a rapid decrease in circulating melatonin levels (55), which is due not only to decreased production and release of melatonin but also a rapid peripheral metabolism of melatonin, as described above.

Resistance to Stress

Stress could conceivably function to cause an increase in melatonin production because the associated increase in circulating catecholamines of adrenal and sympathetic origin could result in β-adrenergic stimulation of the pineal gland. This notion is supported by the fact that other sympathetically innervated systems respond to a stress-induced increase in circulating catecholamines. However, under physiological conditions this does not appear to be the case for the pineal gland.

The rich sympathetic innervation to the pineal gland, which has an efficient mechanism of reuptake of catecholamines by the pineal nerve endings, provides the gland with protection from the influence of circulating catecholamines. Only a minimal increase in N-acetyltransferase activity occurs in animals exposed to a number of forms of stress (54,77,132). However, severe stress, induced by exposing rats to 48 hr of constant light and 12 hr of starvation prior to insulin-induced hypoglycemic stress, results in an increase in N-acetyltransferase activity and pineal melatonin content (97).

The importance of the mechanism of reuptake of catecholamines by pineal nerve endings in preventing stress-induced stimulation of N-acetyltransferase activity became obvious from two experimental findings. First, it was discovered that sympathectomized animals respond to a stress-induced increase in catecholamines by a marked increase in N-acetyltransferase activity (103,132). Second, when intact animals were treated with a drug which blocks reuptake and were then stressed, there was a large increase in pineal N-acetyltransferase activity (132). These considerations point out an additional important mechanism which makes elevations of circulating melatonin a reliable indicator of the dark period of the day.

Drugs

As one would expect, there are a number of compounds which can alter pineal indoleamine metabolism at the level of the pineal gland. These agents can be broadly grouped into those which act through adrenergic mechanisms, and those which act through nonadrenergic mechanisms.

Agents acting through the adrenergic mechanism can be divided into two functional groups. First, are the β-adrenergic agonists. They mimic the effects of sympathetic stimulation, causing reversal of the normal daytime pattern of indoleamine metabolism to a nighttime pattern. These compounds can stimulate and increase N-acetyltransferase activity and melatonin production, and decrease serotonin levels. One strong β-adrenergic agonist is isoproterenol. It consistently stimulates melatonin synthesis *in vitro* and *in vivo* (31,53,194). The potency of this drug is enhanced because it is not taken up by the pineal gland nerve endings. Taurine, a sulfonate-containing amino acid found in the pineal gland, can also stimulate melatonin synthesis by interacting with the β-adrenoreceptor (209) but is far less potent than isoproterenol.

Drugs which act presynaptically to block reuptake of extraneuronal catecholamines (e.g., desmethylimipramine, cocaine, and tyramine) cause a net release of catecholamines, leading to an increase in melatonin production (5,50,125,133). Compounds such as the catecholamine precursor L-DOPA can increase net synthesis of catecholamines and thereby cause an increase in melatonin production (30,101).

The second functional category of adrenergic drugs comprises β-adrenergic antagonists. They block the effects of sympathetic stimulation, causing an acute reversal of the normal nighttime pattern of indoleamine metabolism to a daytime pattern. These compounds (e.g., propranolol) act at the pineal β-adrenoreceptor by displacing the neurotransmitter (26,134).

Compounds acting via nonadrenergic mechanisms that can alter melatonin production act through a number of processes. These include tryptophan, which increases pineal serotonin (9,147), and monoamine oxidase inhibitors, which decrease destruction of serotonin within the pineal gland (53,184). The latter agents can also stimulate N-acetyltransferase by blocking metabolism of extraneuronal catecholamines (5,31,53,79).

Another compound which alters pineal serotonin is parachlorophenylalanine, an inhibitor of tryptophan hydroxylase activity (9,11,33). By lowering pineal serotonin content, it can decrease melatonin synthesis. Ouabain is known to block the adrenergic and cyclic-AMP-stimulated increase in pineal N-acetyltransferase activity apparently through a depolarizing action (135). Inhibitors of mRNA or protein synthesis (e.g., actinomycin D and cycloheximide) can also block the nighttime increase in melatonin production (19,166).

Developmental Aspects of the Melatonin Rhythm

Development of the pineal melatonin rhythm naturally depends on the development of each of the components necessary to generate this circadian rhythm. In the rat the last element to develop appears to be hydroxyindole-O-methyltransferase (74,168). This enzyme is not detectable by available methods until the end of the second week of life. In contrast, the sheep (66) and the rhesus monkey (153) have easily detectable levels of this enzyme during late fetal life. However, whether the latter two mammals can synthesize melatonin on a circadian basis during fetal life is not known.

Prior to the development of hydroxyindole-O-methyltransferase in the rat, a rhythm in pineal N-acetyltransferase is detectable (34,56). The N-acetyltransferase rhythm is first seen during the middle of the first week of life, when the pineal gland becomes innervated. Apparently the pineal gland is capable of responding to adrenergic stimulation even earlier, 2 days prior to birth (221). By the fourth day of life, the entire neural circuitry necessary to generate an N-acetyltransferase rhythm, including the retinohypothalamic projections, suprachiasmatic nuclei, and sympathetic nervous system, is functional (115a).

The absence of the capacity of the fetus and neonate to synthesize melatonin, however, does not preclude the presence of melatonin. Evidence is now available which indicates that the mother is a source of melatonin for the developing fetus and the neonatal animal.

Placental Transfer

Placental transfer of melatonin has been demonstrated in three animal species studied: rat, sheep, and rhesus monkey (65,68,153). In the monkey this transfer is rapid and could result in transfer of a maternally generated daily melatonin rhythm to the fetus. Placental transfer of a simulated melatonin rhythm from mother to fetus is shown in Fig. 9.

This route of delivery of melatonin could provide the fetus with a circadian melatonin rhythm at the earliest stages of development. This circadian time cue may provide the fetus with a 24-hr chemical periodicity and entrain certain fetal functions with the mother and the prevailing environmental lighting time cues. Other small circulating hormones could also be transferred in a similar manner such that the fetus is exposed to a precise temporal pattern of circadian time cues similar to those in the mother. The placental transfer of melatonin leads to the exciting possibility that maternal melatonin may influence various aspects of development at any time during fetal development.

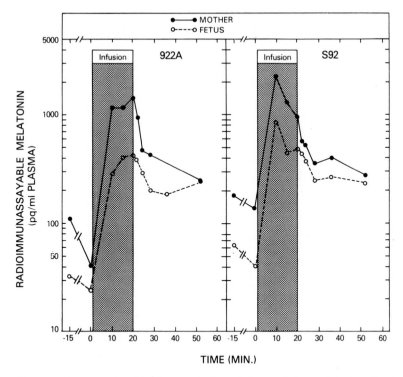

FIG. 9. Melatonin in maternal and fetal plasma before, during, and after an infusion of authentic melatonin to the mother. (From ref. 153.)

Milk Transfer

The mother may also be a source of melatonin for the neonate. It appears that melatonin can be transmitted to the neonate via milk (154). Radiolabeled melatonin injected into the circulation of lactating mothers is recovered from the stomachs of suckling pups. Similarly, when radiolabeled melatonin is instilled into the neonatal stomach, melatonin is recovered from all tissues examined including brain. The precise amount of maternal melatonin transferred by milk remains to be established.

Melatonin and Reproduction

The history of the association between the mammalian pineal gland and reproductive function starts in 1898 when Heubner (46) described the relationship of precocious puberty in man with tumors of the pineal gland. Fifty-six years later, Kitay (67) reviewed several hundred cases of pineal tumor and observed that nonparenchymal tumors were often associated with precocious puberty. This led him to speculate that the pineal gland normally produces a substance which inhibits reproductive function, and thus tumors which destroy the pineal gland (and this substance) could lead to premature sexual development. In 1963 melatonin was implicated as this inhibitory pineal substance when Wurtman and co-workers (214) reported that it could inhibit reproductive function in the rat. However, it should be noted that this effect has been difficult to reproduce and that the role of the pineal gland in reproductive function of the rat is not known.

One of the problems which most *in vitro* and *in vivo* melatonin studies share is that large amounts of the compound are required for effects to be detected (112). An exception are studies by Martin and colleagues (105,106), who showed *in vitro* that physiologic concentrations of melatonin (10^{-8} M) can inhibit luteinizing hormone releasing hormone (LHRH)-stimulated release of LH from the neonatal rat pituitary gland. This inhibition is dose-related and specific. Interestingly, this inhibitory effect of melatonin disappeared by the second postnatal week and was not found in the adult pituitary gland (105,106).

Role of Melatonin in Photoperiodic Control of Reproduction in the Hamster

An ideal mammalian model for studying the effects of the pineal gland on reproductive function was identified by Hoffman and Reiter in 1965 (49). They showed that the pineal gland was necessary for the photoperiodically induced gonadal quiescence which occurs in the Syrian hamster, an animal reproductively active only during the spring and summer. Since that time, a large number of studies of the antigonadotropic effects of the pineal gland have been directed at this rodent.

When hamsters are maintained in short days (less than 12.5 hr of light per day), gonadal quiescence is seen within about 8 weeks. This is manifested by testicular regression in males and anovulation in the female. Pinealectomy prevents this response to a short photoperiod (49). However, there has been considerable debate over which pineal product or "antigonadotropic" hormone is responsible for these pineal-dependent photoperiodically induced changes in reproductive function (149).

Tamarkin and co-workers (195) were the first to show that chronic daily injections of melatonin consistently suppressed reproductive function of hamsters maintained in long days (LD 14:10). The key element in their experimental design was careful control of the time of day the animals were injected with melatonin (Fig. 10). Single daily injections given chronically either just prior to lights-on in the morning, or from 3 hr before to the time of lights-off at night, produced reproductive collapse after several weeks (192,195); injections given at the latter time had the greatest effect.

In contrast, melatonin injections given during the midlight or middark period were not effective (192,195). Based on this, it seemed that the reason some injection paradigms were effective was that the injections extended the duration of elevated melatonin levels at night, not that they simply increased the total amount of melatonin in the animal (192). This line of thought was based on the assumption that the hamster exhibited a daily melatonin rhythm similar to that observed in other mammals. Thus, the injections, by mimicking the nocturnal melatonin pattern of a short day, induced the response.

This was further substantiated when it was found that carefully timed daily injections of melatonin to pinealectomized and superior cervical ganglionectomized animals, as well as intact animals kept in constant light, caused gonadal quiescence (39,191). The injection schedule that was most effective was three daily injections given 2 hr apart.

Parenthetically, it should be pointed out that the hormonal alterations that accompany the photoperiodically induced quiescent state (e.g., a decrease in circulating LH, FSH, prolactin, and testosterone in the male) are mimicked in the melatonin-injection-induced quiescent state (191,195). Thus the melatonin injections appear to function physiologically in the same manner as a short photoperiod.

Recently the daily pattern of pineal melatonin content in the Syrian hamster was examined by RIA as discussed above (194). Surprisingly, the pattern of the daily melatonin rhythm was different from that in the rat. The duration of elevated levels and the amplitude of the nocturnal elevation of melatonin were the same in short-day- and long-day-maintained animals. The only difference was a 2-hr phase shift in the rhythm relative to time of day (Fig. 6). Thus it appears that the duration that melatonin levels are elevated at night is not the important factor inducing reproductive collapse.

It should be pointed out that the daily activity of the Syrian hamster is precisely timed (223). Thus the 2-hr phase shift of the melatonin rhythm may be sufficient to account for the marked changes in reproductive physiology associated with long and short photoperiods. This 2-hr phase shift may be a significant alteration in the phase relationship of the melatonin rhythm and processes which may exhibit a circadian rhythm in their sensitivity to melatonin.

Extending this line of reasoning to the injection data, it is possible that in the intact animal the timed daily melatonin injections supplemented endogenous melatonin production, resulting in a modified rhythm in circulating melatonin with a new phase relationship to another circadian rhythm. This is consistent with the finding that the end of the light period was the most effective time of day for melatonin injections to induce gonadal regression in intact animals maintained in a long photoperiod. This injection schedule would extend the duration of high melatonin levels at night in the same direction as the 2-hr phase shift in the melatonin rhythm of animals maintained in short days. In the pinealectomized animals, the thrice-daily injections possibly function as an exogenous cue for other circadian rhythms and in this way establish a critical phase relationship necessary for gonadal quiescence.

Alternatively, the melatonin rhythm may not be important, but the daily

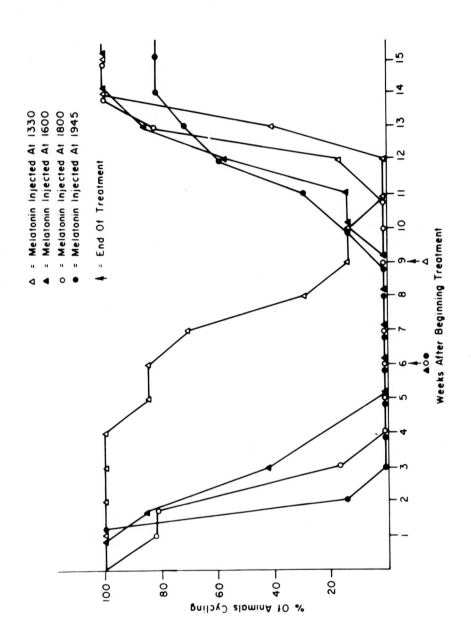

receptivity of the target tissue may vary with the photoperiod. Perhaps melatonin plays a passive permissive role, and a phase shift in tissue receptivity is important. Thus in short days serum melatonin would be elevated at a critical time when the target tissue was sensitive. However, this interpretation is not supported by the results of experiments in which pinealectomized and superior cervical ganglionectomized animals and animals maintained in constant light received thrice-daily injections (39). Indeed injection-induced regression was not dependent on the photoperiod in these animals, although the extent of regression in pinealectomized animals was influenced by photoperiod.

It should be apparent from the above discussion that further research is required to clarify the role of melatonin in the pineal-mediated seasonal reproductive events of these animals. Although there is no question that the thrice-daily injections of melatonin can cause gonadal regression in pinealectomized animals, the important question of whether these effects are pharmacologic or physiologic reflections of the effects of melatonin remains unanswered.

Pineal Peptides

An area of pineal physiology that may develop into an important one in regard to reproductive physiology is pineal peptides. Of particular interest is the peptide arginine vasotocin, which is a reputed pineal hormone with potent antigonadal properties. However, a substantial effort is needed to examine the synthesis and function of this as well as other peptides in the pineal gland. A thorough discussion of pineal peptides is not within the scope of this chapter. For an analysis of this potentially important subject, the reader is referred to several recent review articles (10,136,150).

Melatonin Receptors

There is little doubt that hormones exert their physiological effects at the target tissue by first interacting with a high-affinity receptor protein. In order to study physiologically significant hormone receptors, it follows that one must first identify the target tissue. Second, the hormone–receptor interaction must be correlated with a biological response. Unfortunately, neither has been possible for melatonin. However, recent progress in this area which has led to the identification of specific melatonin binding sites in several mammalian tissues indicates

FIG. 10. Precent of females still showing estrous cycles at the end of each weekly interval during daily administration of 10 µg melatonin. Each group contained seven animals housed in LD 14:10 with the lights on from 0600 to 2000 hr (6:00 a.m. to 8:00 p.m.). Melatonin treatment was terminated at the times indicated by the arrows for each group, and observations for the estrous vaginal discharge were continued. At each of the four injection times, a control group of oil-injected females (*N* = 6) was included (not shown here). All the oil-treated females continued to cycle regularly throughout the experiment. (From ref. 195.)

that physiologically important melatonin receptors may be clearly identified in the near future.

There is evidence for a cytoplasmic melatonin binding protein (25). High-affinity binding sites in ovarian tissue from the rat, hamster, and human appear to exist. Binding sites were also detected in the testis, uterus, liver, and eye of the rodent. No binding sites were found in several other rodent tissues including brain. However, Cohen et al. (25) point out that the possibility that binding sites in pituitary, pineal, and hypothalamus could not be ruled out. The tissue specificity and cytoplasmic location of binding sites in this study correlates well with earlier studies which identified similar tissues that concentrate radiolabeled melatonin and found a cytosol location of the binding (217).

The presence of high-affinity binding of melatonin to membrane fractions of bovine mediobasal hypothalami was recently demonstrated by Cardinali and associates (23). However, a considerable amount of additional experimental evidence is needed to verify the existence, specificity, and localization of this receptor in the hypothalamus, a suspected melatonin target (149).

In terms of binding characteristics, no major discrepancies exist between the receptors described in these two reports, although the cellular location of the receptors in the studies are distinctly different. This does not place the results of these reports in opposition. In fact, it is conceivable that melatonin could have different cellular sites of action depending on the tissue studied, and that the same receptor protein is located differently.

Hopefully these reports will stimulate further research on mammalian melatonin receptors. It may prove helpful at this point in the development of knowledge of melatonin receptors to examine the binding characteristics of melatonin to the neonatal rat pituitary gland and to amphibian skin, where clear rapid biological responses are evident (47,105,106). This in turn may provide important information about the nature of the mammalian melatonin receptor protein(s).

CLINICAL ASPECTS

A surprisingly common view is that the human pineal gland is inactive because it, like the pineal gland of some other mammalian species, undergoes varying degrees of calcification (corpora arenacea) with advancing age. However, this view is a misconception. Evidence disproving this was presented in 1963 by Wurtman and co-workers (213), who demonstrated that one aspect of human pineal function, the enzymatic capability to synthesize melatonin, persisted throughout life (age 3 to 70 years) and that this characteristic was not correlated with age or degree of pineal calcification. At about the same time, Barchas and Lerner (8) identified melatonin in adult human sciatic nerves and urine. Since that time, melatonin has been measured in the pineal gland and in various bodily fluids (blood, urine, CSF, and amniotic fluid) by bioassay (59,98,99, 102,137,149), radioimmunoassay (1,2,35,43,64,87,98,107,113,179,180,181,187, 198,202,205–208), and gas chromatography–mass spectrometry (40,92,178, 211).

Daily Rhythm in Melatonin

There is a daily melatonin rhythm in blood (1,2,35,64,107,137,178,181, 197,199,202,205,211), urine (59,87,98,99,102,208), and the pineal gland (40) of humans, with high values at night. The daily rhythm is found in the young (age 12 years) (35) and the elderly (age 65 years) (199); it persists unaltered throughout pregnancy (107) and has been demonstrated in various populations throughout the world (Japanese, Northern European, and Scandinavian) (1, 2,208), including a genetically homogenous population of African Bushmen (99). In addition to this daily pattern of secretion, secretory episodes have been observed to occur during the day and night (202).

Even though the daily melatonin rhythm in blood and urine exhibits a constant dynamic relationship to the 24-hr day, there is considerable variation in the reported daytime and nighttime concentrations of melatonin in blood. This variation may in part be due to the technique used to measure melatonin, as previously discussed. However, even when the same assay technique is used, it appears that there is considerable quantitative and qualitative variation in the daily pattern of circulating melatonin (202) and in the daily pattern of melatonin excretion among individuals (99). On the other hand, the day-to-day pattern of melatonin excretion has been reported to be remarkably similar and characteristic for an individual (99). This is consistent with observations made on a group of adult male rhesus monkeys (158).

The daily rhythm in circulating melatonin in the human, as is the case for the rat, has been found to be synchronous with the activity of pineal N-acetyltransferase activity and hydroxyindole-O-methyltransferase activity, as judged by postmortem analysis (181).

Several lines of evidence suggest that the daily melatonin rhythm in humans may indeed be circadian. First, the melatonin rhythm persists in constant environmental conditions such as constant light with sleep deprivation (59,205). Next, the rhythm does not re-entrain immediately in the majority of subjects to a phase shift in daily time cues (98,99,205). Finally, a limited study on four blind subjects (99) showed that a daily melatonin rhythm occurred in two of the four, but the high values appeared at odd times of the day. However, it should be pointed out that there was no detectable daily melatonin rhythm in the other two subjects. Long-term studies of the melatonin rhythm in humans placed in a time-cue-free environment are needed to fully investigate the circadian nature of this rhythm.

Photic Regulation of the Daily Melatonin Rhythm

In humans, in contrast to most mammals, the 24-hr light–dark cycle may not be the only entraining stimulus for the melatonin rhythm. Other cyclic daily time cues, including sleep–wake cycles and activity, may be equally important for entraining the human melatonin rhythm to the 24-hr day.

Several recent studies examined the time course of re-entrainment of the melatonin rhythm to concomitant phase shifts of the light–dark and sleep–wake cycles. These studies show that, for the most part, 5 to 7 days are required for re-entrainment of the rhythm to a 9- to 12-hr phase shift in the daily schedule (98,205). However, in another study it was found that two individuals who were accustomed to sleeping odd hours could immediately shift their melatonin rhythm, with elevated levels occurring whenever they went to sleep, even during the day (99).

The difficulty with interpreting the results of these studies is that it is difficult to separate the entraining effects of the light–dark cycle, sleep–wake cycle, and various other daily time cues on the daily melatonin rhythm. This issue will not be resolved until rigidly maintained environmental conditions with controlled variation of each cyclic cue is undertaken in humans regarding the melatonin rhythm.

Another striking difference between humans and other mammals, including a nonhuman primate, is that the circulating and urinary melatonin rhythm in humans persists in constant light (59,98,199,205). Also, acute exposure to light at night does not cause a marked decrease in circulating melatonin levels (205).

These observations indicate that the human melatonin rhythm, in contrast to that in lower mammals, is independent of environmental lighting. Such independence of human circadian rhythms from environmental lighting has been speculated as an evolutionary adaptation unique to man, freeing him from the restraints imposed by environmental lighting (160).

The nature of the difference between man and other mammals is not known. Perhaps it involves differences in the transmission of the effects of light by the retinohypothalamic projections (the presence of this tract has not been established in humans), or it may involve a change in the endogenous oscillator generating the melatonin rhythm in humans.

Neural Regulation of the Melatonin Rhythm

Although studies of the neural pathway involved in the regulation of melatonin rhythm in humans are difficult, some progress in understanding has been made. Kneisley and co-workers (87) recently showed that the sympathetic nervous system may be involved in regulation of the daily melatonin rhythm in humans. They studied melatonin excretion in six adult males with clinical evidence of cervical cord transsection. None showed a day–night variation in melatonin excretion, although they did exhibit daily rhythms in serum cortisol, aldosterone, and growth hormone. On the other hand, in normal males and in a patient with a lesion of the lumbar cord, a clear day–night variation in melatonin excretion was demonstrated. Thus these investigators suggest that the lesions of the cervical cord interrupt descending sympathetic nerves and in this way decentralize the human pineal gland. This strongly supports a role of the sympathetic nervous system in the regulation of human pineal function, similar to the role it plays in pineal function of other mammals.

Relationship of Daily Melatonin Rhythm to Other Hormonal Rhythms

Although no studies in adults have shown a causal relationship of the melatonin rhythm and other hormone rhythms (e.g., LH, prolactin, adrenocorticotropin, and growth hormone), a temporal relationship has been demonstrated (147,205). Fevre and colleagues (35) recently studied the daily pattern of plasma melatonin and LH in four pubertal males. The characteristic nocturnal sleep-related increase in LH levels in these subjects was correlated with the nighttime increase in circulating melatonin. Whether this relationship is important during human reproductive development awaits further study.

Menstrual Cycle Variation of Melatonin

Based on limited observations by Wetterburg and co-workers (206), it appears that daily 0800 hr (8:00 A.M.) serum melatonin levels vary during the menstrual cycle. Peak levels appear to occur during the premenstrual and menstrual phases and low values during the ovulatory stage, when LH concentrations peak. The authors postulate that low melatonin levels midcycle may be a permissive factor for the LH surge and subsequent ovulation. This study demonstrates that the stage of the menstrual cycle needs to be taken into consideration when studying endogenous melatonin levels in female subjects.

Annual Variation of Melatonin

There is growing evidence of an annual variation in circulating melatonin levels in humans (199). Studies by Arendt and co-workers (3), who obtained 0800 hr (8 A.M.) blood samples at monthly intervals from a group of adult volunteers in Switzerland, suggest a bimodal annual melatonin rhythm; high values appear to occur in January and July, and nadirs in April and October. It is important to determine if there is a similar annual variation in the melatonin rhythm.

Metabolism of Melatonin

Jones and associates (60) administered [14C]melatonin to schizophrenic and nonschizophrenic patients and analyzed the pattern of urinary radioactivity. They reported a pattern of radiolabeled melatonin metabolites in these subjects that was similar to the pattern reported in the rat. A rather interesting finding was that in the urine of the schizophrenic patients, compared to the nonschizophrenic patients, a higher percentage of the total radioactivity recovered from urine was an unidentified acidic melatonin metabolite. However, these results must be interpreted with caution since the number of individuals examined was small and the nonschizophrenic "controls" had major neurological diseases.

Effect of Drugs on Endogenous Melatonin

Interest in the pharmacological manipulation of melatonin production and secretion in humans has centered around the development of a "pineal function test" (219). Drugs which increase melatonin production in the rat (e.g., isoproterenol and L-DOPA) have been examined on a limited basis in humans (199,205). Neither agent consistently increased circulating melatonin levels. In the case of isoproterenol, amounts of the compound were infused which caused marked cardiovascular responses but did not consistently increase circulating melatonin levels. As pointed out by Vaughan and associates (199), species differences in tolerance and pineal response may explain the lack of effect of isoproterenol in humans compared to the rat.

Even though it appears that drugs acting through a β-adrenergic mechanism do not increase melatonin production in humans, the β-adrenergic blocking agent propranolol has been shown to consistently block the nocturnal increase in circulating melatonin (43,205). This is the second line of evidence which suggests that the sympathetic nervous system influences human melatonin production.

Effects of Stress on Endogenous Melatonin

Various forms of stress, including anesthetic stress, stress associated with lumbar puncture, and stress associated with electroconvulsive therapy, do not appear to elevate normally low daytime levels of circulating melatonin (198,205). Perhaps agents which block reuptake of catecholamines in pineal nerves and thus stimulate melatonin synthesis in the rat [e.g., imipramine (133)] may render the human pineal gland susceptible to the effects of stress. This approach may provide the basis of a useful test of pineal function in humans.

Administration of Melatonin: Effects on Psychiatric and Endocrine Parameters

Pharmacological amounts of melatonin have been administered orally and intravenously to normal humans and individuals with various psychological, neurological, and endocrinological diseases. The psychological effects of melatonin administration studies from 1960 to 1974 were recently reviewed by Carmen and colleagues (24). In general, studies involving normal subjects and patients with Parkinson's disease report mild sedation as the most frequently observed psychological effect. Also, various electroencephalographic alterations have been reported.

On the other hand, in limited studies melatonin was reported to have marked adverse effects in various psychiatric illnesses. First, two schizophrenic patients given intravenous melatonin exhibited an acute exacerbation of psychotic symptoms including hallucinations (24). Second, in a double-blind crossover study of melatonin administration to a small number of patients with primary depressive illness and Huntington's chorea, melatonin increased symptoms of dysphoria

(24). Interestingly, in three of four subjects examined in this study, melatonin caused an increase in 5-hydroxyindoleacetic acid and calcium concentrations in the CSF coincident with dysphoria. Thus altered serotonin and calcium metabolism may have been related to the dysphoria resulting form melatonin, although this association is far from conclusive. As pointed out by these investigators (24), the administration of large daily doses of melatonin to psychiatric patients may eliminate the endogenous melatonin rhythm and possibly alter abnormal circadian function. Further carefully controlled clinical studies of melatonin administration to psychiatric patients, with particular attention to dosage schedule, are clearly warranted.

Nordlund and Lerner (127) administered large daily doses of melatonin for several weeks to individuals with various hyperpigmented skin conditions. Pigmentation was altered in only one subject (with adrenogenital syndrome), in whom the skin was lightened; the authors postulate a possible suppressive effect of melatonin on pituitary MSH as a reason for this effect. It is important to point out that long-term administration of melatonin to these subjects appeared to be without toxic effects.

In this same study several endocrine parameters were monitored during melatonin administration. Melatonin appeared to decrease urinary 17-ketosteroid excretion but did not affect thyroid function (serum thyroxine or ^{131}I uptake). Also, they reported that melatonin appeared to suppress serum LH, a finding that is in contrast to those of another study (36) in which smaller doses of melatonin did not affect basal or LHRH-stimulated LH and FSH levels in men or postmenopausal women. Possibly the effects of dosage or route of administration (intramuscular versus oral) explain the differences between these studies.

The most consistent effect of melatonin administration on human endocrine function is the apparent suppressive effect on blood growth hormone (90,182, 183). This effect of melatonin has been postulated to involve blockage or interaction with serotoninergic receptors. Whether this suppression is evident physiologically has not been demonstrated.

Melatonin and Human Disease

Limited studies have shown that alterations of melatonin metabolism in many cases may be associated with various disease states (205). However, further studies are needed before a firm relationship can be established between melatonin and any human disease. Only one report in the literature describes melatonin levels in patients with pinealoma (205). In this report a single patient, who was not studied previously, was found to have no diurnal melatonin rhythm following irradiation of the tumor.

Future Direction of Human Pineal Research

One obvious area of future studies of melatonin is in patients with pinealomas. Since tumors of the parenchymal type have the enzymatic capability to synthesize melatonin (218), the measurement of melatonin in these individuals may prove useful in terms of diagnosis and effectiveness of treatment.

Two other areas of human pineal research deserve further comment. First, psychiatric diseases which display cyclic variations in symptoms may be based on altered circadian systems. Possibly the melatonin rhythm provides a marker for such abnormalities and may even be involved in pathogenesis. Second, melatonin may be involved in various physiological and pathological alterations of human reproductive function.

More knowledge of the daily melatonin rhythm in normal subjects is required before any meaningful information can be gained from studies of this rhythm in disease states. In addition, it seems appropriate now to place emphasis on describing the relationship of the melatonin rhythm to other endocrine rhythms, and to determine if the normal multicomponent circadian pattern of hormone secretion is disorganized in psychiatric, endocrine, or other disease states.

REFERENCES

1. Arendt, J., Paunier, L., and Sizonenko, P. D. (1975): Melatonin radioimmunoassay. *J. Clin. Endocrinol. Metab.*, 40:347–350.
2. Arendt, J., Wetterburg, L., Heyden, T., Sizonenko, P. C., and Paunier, L. (1977): Radioimmunoassay of melatonin: Human serum and cerebrospinal fluid. *Horm. Res.*, 8:65–75.
3. Arendt, J., Wirtz-Justice, A., and Bradtke, J. (1977): Annual rhythm of serum melatonin in man. *Neurosci. Lett.*, 7:327–330.
4. Axelrod, J., MacLean, R. D., Albers, R. W., and Weissbach, H. (1961): Regional distribution of methyl transferase enzymes in the nervous system and glandular tissues. In: *Regional Neurochemistry*, edited by S. S. Kety and J. Eikes, pp. 307–311. Pergamon Press, Oxford.
5. Axelrod, J., Shein, H. M., and Wurtman, R. J. (1969): Stimulation of C^{14}-melatonin synthesis from C^{14}-tryptophan by noradrenaline in rat pineal in organ culture. *Proc. Natl. Acad. Sci. USA*, 62:554–559.
6. Axelrod, J., and Weissbach, H. (1960): Enzymatic O-methylation of N-acetylserotonin to melatonin. *Science*, 131:1312–1313.
7. Axelrod, J., Wurtman, R. J., and Snyder, S. (1965): Control of hydroxyindole-O-methyltransferase activity in the rat pineal gland by environmental lighting. *J. Biol. Chem.*, 240:949–954.
8. Barchas, J. D., and Lerner, A. B. (1964): Localization of melatonin in the nervous system. *J. Neurochem.*, 11:489–491.
9. Bensinger, R. E., Klein, D. C., Weller, J. L., and Lovenberg, W. M. (1974): Radiometric assay of total tryptophan hydroxylation by intact cultured pineal glands. *J. Neurochem.*, 23:111–117.
10. Benson, B. (1977): Current status of pineal peptides. *Life Sci.*, 24:241–258.
11. Berg, G. T., and Klein, D. C. (1971): Pineal gland in organ culture. II. Role of adenosine 3',5'-monophosphate in the regulation of radiolabelled melatonin production. *Endocrinology*, 89:453–461.
12. Berg, G. R., and Klein, D. C. (1972): Norepinephrine stimulates ^{32}P incorporation into a specific phospholipid fraction of postsynaptic pineal membranes. *J. Neurochem.*, 19:2519–2532.
13. Binkley, S., and Geller, E. B. (1975): Pineal enzymes in chickens: Development of daily rhythmicity. *Gen. Comp. Endocrinol.*, 27:424–429.
14. Binkley, S., Klein, D. C., and Weller, J. (1974): Dark induced increase in pineal serotonin N-acetyltransferase activity: A refractory period. *Experientia*, 29:1339–1340.
15. Binkley, S., Klein, D. C., and Weller, J. L. (1976): Pineal serotonin N-acetyltransferase activity: Protection of stimulated activity by acetyl CoA and related compounds. *J. Neurochem.*, 26:51–55.

16. Binkley, S. A., MacBride, S., Klein, D. C., and Ralph, C. (1973): Pineal enzymes: Regulation of avian melatonin synthesis. *Science*, 181:273–275.

17. Brownstein, M., and Axelrod, J. (1974): Pineal gland: 24-Hour rhythm in norepinephrine turnover. *Science*, 184:163–165.

18. Brownstein, M., Saavedra, J. M., and Axelrod, J. (1973): Control of pineal N-acetyl-serotonin by a beta-adrenergic receptor. *Mol. Pharmacol.*, 9:605–611.

19. Buda, M., and Klein, D. C. (1975): Function and regulation of pineal N'-acetyltransferase activity. In: *Biochemistry and Function of Amine Enzymes*, edited by E. Usdin and N. Weiner, pp. 545–555. Pergamon Press, Elmsford, N.Y.

20. Buda, M. J., and Klein, D. C. (1978): N-Acetylation of biogenic amines. In: *Biochemistry and Function of Amine Enzymes*, edited by E. Usdin and N. Weiner, pp. 527–544. Pergamon Press, Elmsford, N.Y.

21. Cardinali, D. P., Larin, F., and Wurtman, R. J. (1971): Action spectra for effects of light on hydroxyindole-O-methyltransferases in rat pineal, retina, and harderian gland. *Endocrinology*, 91:877–886.

22. Cardinali, D. P., Lynch, H. J., and Wurtman, R. J. (1972): Binding of melatonin to human and rat plasma proteins, *Endocrinology*, 91:1213–1218.

23. Cardinali, D. P., Vacas, M. I., and Boyer, E. E. (1979): Specific binding of melatonin in bovine brain. *Endocrinology*, 105:437–441.

24. Carmen, J. S., Post, R. M., Buswell, R., and Goodwin, F. K. (1976): Negative effects of melatonin on depression. *Am. J. Psychiatry*, 133:1181–1186.

25. Cohen, M., Roselle, D., Chabner, B., Schmidt, T. J., and Lippman, M. (1978): Evidence for a cytoplasmic melatonin receptor. *Nature*, 274:894–895.

26. Deguchi, T. (1973): Role of the beta adrenergic receptor in the elevation of adenosine cyclic 3'5'-monophosphate and induction of serotonin N-acetyltransferase in rat pineal glands. *Mol. Pharmacol.*, 9:184–190.

27. Deguchi, T. (1977): Circadian rhythms of enzyme and running activity under ultradian lighting schedule. *Am. J. Physiol.*, 232:375–381.

28. Deguchi, T. (1977): Tryptophan hydroxylase in pineal gland of rat: Postsynaptic localization and absence of circadian change. *J. Neurochem.*, 28:667–668.

29. Deguchi, T. (1978): Ontogenesis of circadian rhythm of melatonin synthesis in pineal gland of rat. *J. Neural Transm. (Suppl)*, 13:115–128.

30. Deguchi, T., and Axelrod, J. (1972): Induction and superinduction of serotonin N-acetyltransferase by adrenergic drugs and denervation in the rat pineal. *Proc. Natl. Acad. Sci. USA*, 69:2547–2550.

31. Deguchi, T., and Axelrod, J. (1972): Control of circadian change in serotonin N-acetyltransferase activity in the pineal organ by the β-adrenergic receptor. *Proc. Natl. Acad. Sci. USA*, 69:2547–2550.

32. Deguchi, T., and Axelrod, J. (1973): Superinduction of serotonin N-acetyltransferase and supersensitivity of adenyl cyclase to catecholamines in denervated pineal glands. *Mol. Pharmacol.*, 9:612–619.

33. Deguchi, T., and Barchas, J. (1973): Comparative studies on the effect of parachlorophenylalanine on hydroxylation of tryptophan in pineal and brain of rat. In: *Serotonin and Behavior*, edited by J. Barchas and E. Usdin, pp. 33–47. Academic Press, New York.

34. Ellison, N., Weller, J. L., and Klein, D. C. (1972): Development of a circadian rhythm in pineal N-acetyltransferase. *J. Neurochem.*, 19:1335–1341.

35. Fevre, M., Segel, T., Marks, J. F., and Boyar, R. M. (1978): LH and melatonin secretion patterns in pubertal boys. *J. Clin. Endocrinol. Metab.*, 47:1383–1386.

36. Fideleff, H., Aparico, N. J., Guitelman, A., Debeljuk, L., Mancini, A., and Cramer, C. (1976): Effects of melatonin on the basal and stimulated gonadotropin levels in normal men and postmenopausal women. *J. Clin. Endocrinol. Metab.*, 42:1014–1017.

37. Fiske, V. M. (1964): Serotonin rhythm in the pineal organ: Control by the sympathetic nervous system. *Science*, 146:253–254.

38. Fiske, V. M., Bryant, K., and Putman, J. (1960): Effects of light on the weight of the pineal in rats. *Endocrinology*, 66:489–491.

39. Goldman, B., Hollister, C., Roychoudhury, P., Tamarkin, L., and Westrom, W. (1979): Effects of melatonin on the reproductive system in intact and pinealectomized male hamsters maintained under various photoperiods. *Endocrinology*, 104:82–88.

40. Greiner, A. E., and Chan, S. C. (1978): Melatonin content of the human pineal gland. *Science,* 199:83–84.
41. Grotta, L. J., and Brown, G. M. (1974): Antibodies to indolealkylamines: Serotonin and melatonin. *Can. J. Biochem.,* 52:196–202.
42. Hakanson, R., Lombard Des Gouttes, M. N., and Owman, C. (1967): Activities of tryptophan hydroxylase, DOPA decarboxylase and monoamine oxidase as correlated with the appearance of monoamines in the developing rat pineal. *Life Sci.,* 6:2577–2583.
43. Hanssen, T., Heyden, T., Sundberg, I., and Wetterberg, L. (1977): Effect of propranolol on serum melatonin. *Lancet,* 2:309.
44. Hedlund, L., Lischko, M., Rollag, M. D., and Niswender, G. D. (1977): Melatonin: Daily cycle in plasma and cerebrospinal fluid of calves. *Science,* 195:686–687.
45. Hendrickson, A. E., Wagoner, N., and Cowan, W. M. (1972): An autoradiographic and electron microscopic study of retino-hypothalamic connections. *Z. Zellforsch.,* 135:1–26.
46. Heubner, O. (1898): Tumor der glandula pinealis. *Dtsch. Med. Wochenschr.,* 24:214–215.
47. Heward, C. B., and Hadley, M. E. (1975): Structure-activity relationships of melatonin and related indoleamines. *Life Sci.,* 17:1167–1178.
48. Hirata, F., Hayaishi, O., Tokuyama, T., and Serioh, S. (1974): In vitro and in vivo formation of two new metabolites of melatonin. *J. Biol. Chem.,* 249:1611–1616.
49. Hoffman, R. A., and Reiter, R. J. (1965): Pineal gland: Influence on gonads of male hamsters. *Science,* 148:1609–1611.
50. Holtz, R. W., Deguchi, T., and Axelrod, J. (1974): Stimulation of serotonin N-acetyltransferase in pineal organ culture by drugs. *J. Neurochem.,* 22:205–209.
51. Ibuka, N., and Kawamura, H. (1975): Loss of circadian rhythm in sleep-wakefulness cycle in the rat by suprachiasmatic nucleus lesions. *Brain Res.,* 96:76–81.
52. Illnerova, H. (1971): Effect of light on the serotonin content of the pineal gland. *Life Sci.,* 10:955–961.
53. Illnerova, H. (1974): The effect of darkness and pargyline on the activity of serotonin N-acetyltransferase in the rat epiphysis. *Neuroendocrinology,* 16:202–211.
54. Illnerova, H. (1975): The effects of immobilization of the activity of serotonin N-act in the rat epiphysis. In: *Catecholamines and Stress,* edited by E. Usdin, R. Kvetnansky, and I. Kopin, pp. 129–131. Pergamon Press, New York.
55. Illnerova, H., Backström, M., Saaf, J., Wetterberg, L., and Yangbo, B. (1978): Melatonin in rat pineal gland and serum; rapid parallel decline after light exposure at night. *Neurosci. Lett.,* 9:189–193.
56. Illnerova, H., and Skopou, A. J. (1976): Regulation of the diurnal rhythm in rat pineal serotonin-N-acetyltransferase activity and serotonin content during ontogenesis. *J. Neurochem.,* 26:1051–1052.
57. Jaim-Etcheverry, G., and Zieher, L. M. (1974): Localizing serotonin in central and peripheral nerves. In: *Neurosciences,* edited by F. O. Schmidt, pp. 917–923. MIT Press, Cambridge, Mass.
58. Jaim-Etcheverry, G., and Zieher, L. M. (1975): Octopamine probably coexists with noradenaline and serotonin in vesicles of pineal adrenergic nerves. *J. Neurochem.,* 25:915–918.
59. Jimerson, D. C., Lynch, H. J., Post, R. M., Wurtman, R. J., and Bunney, W. E. (1977): Urinary melatonin rhythms during sleep deprivation in depressed patients and normals. *Life Sci.,* 20:1501–1508.
60. Jones, R. J., McGreer, P. L., and Greiner, A. C. (1969): Metabolism of exogenous melatonin in schizophrenic and non-schizophrenic volunteers. *Clin. Chim. Acta,* 26:281–285.
61. Kappers, J. A. (1960): The development, topographical relations and innervation of the epiphysis cerebri in the albino rat. *Z. Zellforsch.,* 52:163–215.
62. Kappers, J. A. (1965): Survey of the innervation of the epiphysis cerebri and the accessory pineal organs of vertebrates. *Prog. Brain Res.,* 10:87–153.
63. Kebabian, J. W., Zatz, M., Romero, J. A., and Axelrod, J. (1975): Rapid changes in rat pineal beta-adrenergic receptor: Alterations in L-(^{3}H)alprenolol binding and adenylate cyclase. *Proc. Natl. Acad. Sci. USA,* 72:3735–3739.
64. Kennaway, D. J., Frith, R. G., Phillipou, G., Matthews, C. D., and Seamark, R. F. (1977): A specific radioimmunoassay for melatonin in biological tissue and fluids and its validation by gas chromatography mass spectrometry. *Endocrinology,* 101:119–127.
65. Kennaway, D. J., Mathews, C. D., Seamark, R. P., and Phillipou, G. (1977): On the presence of melatonin in pineal glands and plasma of foetal sheep. *J. Steroid Biochem.,* 8:559–563.

66. Kennaway, D. J., and Seamark, R. P. (1975): The occurrence of hydroxyindole-O-methyltransferase activity in fetal sheep pineal tissue and its relationship to preparturient endocrine changes. *J. Reprod. Fertil.,* 45:529–534.

67. Kitay, J. I. (1954): Pineal lesions and precocious puberty. *J. Clin. Endocrinol. Metabol.,* 14:622–625.

68. Klein, D. C. (1972): Evidence for the placental transfer of ^{3}H-acetylmelatonin. *Nature,* 237:118–119.

69. Klein, D. C. (1974): Circadian rhythms in indole metabolism in the rat pineal gland. In: *Neurosciences,* edited by F. O. Schmidt, pp. 509–515. MIT Press, Cambridge, Mass.

70. Klein, D. C. (1978): Circadian rhythms in the pineal gland. In: *Endocrine Rhythms,* edited by D. T. Krieger, pp. 203–223. Raven Press, New York.

71. Klein, D. C., and Berg, G. R. (1970): Pineal gland: Stimulation of melatonin production by norepinephrine involves cyclic AMP-mediated stimulation of N-acetyltransferase. *Adv. Biochem. Pyschopharmacol.,* 3:241–263.

72. Klein, D. C., Berg, G. R., and Weller, J. (1970): Melatonin synthesis: Adenosine 3',5'-monophosphate and norepinephrine stimulate N-acetyltransferase. *Science,* 168:979–980.

73. Klein, D. C., Buda, M., Kappor, C. L., and Krishma, G. (1978): Pineal serotonin N-acetyltransferase activity: An abrupt disease in cyclic AMP may be the signal for "turn off." *Science,* 199:309–311.

74. Klein, D. C., and Lines, S. V. (1969): Pineal hydroxyindole-O-methyltransferase activity in the growing rat. *Endocrinology,* 89:1523–1525.

75. Klein, D. C., and Moore, R. Y. (1979): Pineal N-acetyltransferase and hydroxyindole-O-methyltransferase: Control by the retina hypothalamic tract and the suprachiasmatic nucleus. *Brain Res.,* 174:245–262.

76. Klein, D. C., and Notides, A. (1969): Thin-layer chromatographic separation of pineal gland derivatives of serotonin-^{14}C. *Anal. Biochem.,* 31:480–483.

77. Klein, D. C., and Parfitt, A. (1976): A protective role of nerve endings in stress-stimulated increase in pineal N-acetyltransferase activity. In: *Catecholamines and Stress,* edited by R. Kvetnansky and E. Usdin, pp. 119–128. Pergamon Press, New York.

78. Klein, D. C., Reiter, R. J., and Weller, J. L. (1971): Pineal N-acetyltransferase activity in blinded and anosmic rats. *Endocrinology,* 89:1020–1023.

79. Klein, D. C., and Rowe, J. (1970): Pineal gland in organ culture. I. Inhibition by harmine of serotonin-^{14}C oxidation, accompanied by stimulation of melatonin-^{14}C production. *Mol. Pharmacol.,* 6:164–171.

80. Klein, D. C., and Weller, J. L. (1970): Indole metabolism in the pineal gland: A circadian rhythm in N-acetyltransferase. *Science,* 169:1093–1095.

81. Klein, D. C., and Weller, J. L. (1972): A rapid light-induced decrease in pineal serotonin N-acetyltransferase activity. *Science,* 177:532–533.

82. Klein, D. C., and Weller, J. L. (1972): The role of N-acetylserotonin in the regulation of melatonin production. In: *Program 4th Intern. Congr. Endocrinology,* p. 52.

83. Klein, D. C., and Weller, J. L. (1973): Adrenergic-adenosine 3',5'-monophosphate regulation of serotonin N-acetyltransferase activity and the temporal relationship of serotonin N-acetyltransferase activity to synthesis of ^{3}H-N-acetylserotonin and ^{3}H-melatonin in the cultured rat pineal gland. *J. Pharmacol. Exp. Ther.,* 186:516–527.

84. Klein, D. C., Weller, J. L., and Moore, R. Y. (1971): Melatonin metabolism: Neural regulation of pineal serotonin N-acetyltransferase activity. *Proc. Natl. Acad. Sci. USA,* 68:3107–3110.

85. Klein, D. C., and Yuwiler, A. (1973): Beta-adrenergic regulation of indole metabolism in the pineal gland. In: *Frontiers in Catecholamines Research,* edited by E. Usdin and S. Snyder, p. 321–325. Pergamon Press, London.

86. Klein, D. C., Yuwiler, A., Weller, J. L., and Plotkin, S. (1973): Postsynaptic adrenergic-cyclic AMP control of the serotonin content of cultured rat pineal glands. *J. Neurochem.,* 21:1261–1272.

87. Kneisley, L. W., Moskowitz, M. A., and Lynch, H. J. (1978): Cervical spinal cord lesions disrupt the rhythm in human melatonin secretion. *J. Neural Transm. (Suppl),* 13:311–323.

88. Kopin, J. I., Pare, C. M. B., Axelrod, J., and Weissbach, H. (1961): The fate of melatonin in animals. *J. Biol. Chem.,* 236:3072–3075.

89. Kveder, S., and McIsaac, W. M. (1961): The metabolism of melatonin (N-acetyl-5-methoxytryptamine) and 5-methoxytryptamine. *J. Biol. Chem.,* 236:3214–3220.

90. Lerner, A. B., Case, J. D., and Heinzelman, R. V. (1959): Structure of melatonin. *J. Am. Chem. Soc.,* 81:6084–6085.
91. Levine, L., and Riceberg, L. J. (1975): Radioimmunoassay for melatonin. *Res. Commun. Chem. Pathol. Pharmacol.,* 10:693–702.
92. Lewy, A. J., and Markey, S. P. (1978): Analysis of melatonin in human plasma by gas chromatography negative chemical ionization mass spectrometry. *Science,* 201:741–743.
93. Lovenberg, W., Jequier, E., and Sjoerdsma, A. (1967): Tryptophan hydroxylation: Measurements in pineal gland, brain stem, and carcinoid tumor. *Science,* 155:217–218.
94. Lovenberg, W., Jequier, E., and Sjoerdsma, A. (1968): Tryptophan hydroxylation in mammalian systems. *Adv. Pharmacol.,* 6A:21–29.
95. Lovenberg, W., Weissbach, H., and Udenfriend, S. (1962): Aromatic L-amino acid decarboxylase. *J. Biol. Chem.,* 237:89–92.
96. Lynch, W. J. (1971): Diurnal oscillations in pineal melatonin content. *Life Sci.,* 10:791–795.
97. Lynch, H. J., Eng, J. P., and Wurtman, R. J. (1973): Control of pineal indole biosynthesis by changes in sympathetic tone caused by factors other than environmental lighting. *Proc. Natl. Acad. Sci. USA,* 70:1704–1708.
98. Lynch, H. J., Jimmerson, D. C., Ozaki, Y., Post, R. M., Bunney, W. E., and Wurtman, R. J. (1978): Entrainment of rhythmic melatonin secretion in man to a 12-hour phase shift in the light/dark cycle. *Life Sci.,* 23:1557–1564.
99. Lynch, H. J., Ozaki, Y., Shakl, D., and Wurtman, R. J. (1975): Melatonin excretion of man and rats: Effect of time of day, sleep, pinealectomy and food consumption. *Int. J. Biometeorol.,* 19:267–279.
100. Lynch, H. J., and Ralph, C. L. (1970): Diurnal variation in pineal melatonin and its nonrelationship to HIOMT activity. *Am. Zool.,* 10:300.
101. Lynch, H. J., Wang, P., and Wurtman, R. J. (1973): Increase in rat pineal melatonin content following L-DOPA administration. *Life Sci.,* 12:145–151.
102. Lynch, H. J., Wurtman, R. J., Moskowitz, M. A., Archer, M. C., and Ho, M. H. (1975): Daily rhythm in human urinary melatonin. *Science,* 187:169–170.
103. Machado, C. R. S., Wragg, L. E., and Machado, A. B. M. (1968): A histochemical study of sympathetic innervation and 5-hydroxytryptamine in the developing pineal body of the rat. *Brain Res.,* 8:310–318.
104. Maickel, R. P., and Miller, F. P. (1966): Fluorescent products formed by reaction of indole derivatives and O-phthalaldehyde. *Anal. Chem.,* 38:1937–1938.
105. Martin, J. E., Engle, J. N., and Klein, D. C. (1977): Inhibition of the in vitro pituitary response to lutenizing hormone-releasing hormone by melatonin, serotonin, and 5-methoxytryptamine. *Endocrinology,* 100:675–680.
106. Martin, J. E., and Klein, D. C. (1976): Melatonin inhibition of the neonatal pituitary response to luteinizing hormone-releasing factor. *Science,* 191:301–302.
107. Mathews, G. D., Kennaway, D. J., Phillipou, G., Firth, B., LeCornu, A., Schilthuis, M., and Seamark, R. F. (1977): Melatonin and pineal gland function during the fetal life of the sheep and during human pregnancy. *Br. J. Obstet. Gynaecol.,* 84:235.
108. McCord, C. P., and Allen, F. P. (1917): Evidence associating the pineal gland function with alterations in pigmentation. *J. Exp. Zool.,* 23:207–224.
109. McIsaac, W. H., Khacrallah, P. A., and Page, I. M. (1961): 10-Methoxyharmalan, a potent serotonin antagonist which affects conditioned behavior. *Science,* 134:674–675.
110. Menaker, M., Takahashi, J. S., and Eskin, A. (1978): The physiology of circadian pacemakers. *Annu. Rev. Physiol.,* 40:501–526.
111. Minneman, R. P., Lynch, H., and Wurtman, R. J. (1974): Relationship between environmental light intensity and retina-mediated suppression of rat pineal serotonin N-acetyltransferase. *Life Sci.,* 15:1791–1796.
112. Minneman, K. P., and Wurtman, R. J. (1976): The pharmacology of the pineal gland. *Annu. Rev. Pharmacol. Toxicol.,* 16:33–51.
113. Mitchell, M. D., Sayers, L., Keirse, M. J. N. C., Anderson, A. B. M., and Turnbull, A. C. (1978): Melatonin in amniotic fluid during human parturition. *Br. J. Obstet. Gynaecol.,* 85:684–686.
114. Moore, R. Y. (1973): Retinohypothalamic projection in mammals: A comparative study. *Brain Res.,* 49:403–409.
115. Moore, R. Y. (1978): The innervation of the mammalian pineal gland. In: *The Pineal and Reproduction,* edited by R. J. Reiter, pp. 1–29. Karger, Basel.

115a. Moore, R. Y. (1979): The anatomy of central neural mechanisms regulating endocrine rhythms. In: *Endocrine Rhythms,* edited by D. T. Krieger, pp. 63–87. Raven Press, New York.

116. Moore, R. Y., and Eichler, V. B. (1972): Loss of circadian adrenal corticosterone rhythm following suprachiasmatic lesions in the rat. *Brain Res.,* 42:201–206.

117. Moore, R. Y., Heller, A., Bhatnagar, R. K., Wurtman, R. J., and Axelrod, J. (1968): Central control of the pineal gland: Visual pathways. *Arch. Neurol.,* 18:208–218.

118. Moore, R. Y., Heller, A., Wurtman, R. J., and Axelrod, J. (1967): Visual pathways mediating pineal response to environmental light. *Science,* 155:220–223.

119. Moore, R. Y., and Klein, D. C. (1974): Visual pathways and the central neural control of a circadian rhythm in pineal serotonin N-acetyltransferase activity. *Brain Res.,* 71:17–33.

120. Moore, R. Y., and Lenn, N. J. (1972): A retinohypothalamic projection in the rat. *J. Comp. Neurol.,* 146:1–14.

121. Moore, R. Y., and Rapport, R. L. (1970): Pineal and gonadal function in the rat following cervical sympathectomy. *Neuroendocrinology,* 7:361–374.

122. Moore, R. Y., and Traynor, M. E. (1976): Diurnal rhythms in pineal N-acetyltransferase and hippocampal norepinephrine: Effects of water deprivation, blinding and hypothalamic lesions. *Neuroendocrinology,* 20:250–259.

123. Morrissey, J. J., and Lovenberg, W. (1978): Synthesis of RNA in the pineal gland during N-acetyltransferase induction. *Biochem. Pharmacol.,* 27:551–555.

124. Morrissey, J. J., and Lovenberg, W. (1978): Synthesis of RNA in the pineal gland during N-acetyltransferase induction: The effects of actinomycin D, alpha-amanitin, and cordycepin. *Biochem. Pharmacol.,* 27:557–562.

125. Muscholl, E. (1966): Indirectly acting sympathomimetic amines. *Pharmacol. Rev.,* 18:551–559.

126. Neff, N. H., and Oleshansky, M. A. (1975): Rat pineal adenosine cyclic 3′,5′-monophosphate phosphodiesterase activity: Modulation in vivo by a beta adrenergic receptor. *Mol. Pharmacol.,* 11:552–557.

127. Nordlund, J. J., and Lerner, A. B. (1977): The effect of oral melatonin on skin color and on the release of pituitary hormones. *J. Clin. Endocrinol. Metab.,* 45:768–774.

128. Ozaki, Y., and Lynch, H. J. (1976): Presence of melatonin in plasma and urine of pinealectomized rats. *Endocrinology,* 99:641–644.

129. Ozaki, Y., Lynch, H. J., and Wurtman, R. J. (1976): Melatonin in rat pineal, plasma, and urine: 24-Hour rhythmicity and effect of chlorpromazine. *Endocrinology,* 98:1418–1424.

130. Pang, S. F., Brown, G. M., Grota, L. J., Chambers, J. W., and Rodman, R. L. (1977): Determination of N-acetylserotonin and melatonin activities in the pineal gland, retina, harderian gland, brain and serum of rats and chickens. *Neuroendocrinology,* 23:1–13.

131. Pank, E. S., Rollag, M. D., and Reiter, R. J. (1979): Pineal melatonin concentrations in the Syrian hamster. *Endocrinology,* 104:194–197.

132. Parfitt, A. G., and Klein, D. C. (1976): Sympathetic nerve endings protect against acute stress-induced increase in N-acetyltransferase (E.C. 2.3.1.5) activity. *Endocrinology,* 99:840–854.

133. Parfitt, A., and Klein, D. C. (1977): Desmethylimipramine causes an increase in the production of [³H]melatonin by isolated pineal glands. *Biochem. Pharmacol.,* 26:906–907.

134. Parfitt, A., Weller, J. L., and Klein, D. C. (1976): Beta adrenergic blockers decrease adrenergically stimulated N-acetyltransferase activity in pineal glands in organ culture. *Neuropharmacology,* 15:353–358.

135. Parfitt, A., Weller, J. L., Sakai, K. K., Marks, B. H., and Klein, D. C. (1975): Blockade by ouabain or elevated potassium ion concentrations of the adrenergic and adenosine cyclic 3′,5′-monophosphate-induced stimulation of pineal serotonin N-acetyltransferase activity. *Mol. Pharmacol.,* 11:241–255.

136. Pavel, S. (1978): Arginine vasotocin as a pineal hormone. *J. Neural Transm. (Suppl),* 13:135–155.

137. Pelham, R. W., Vaughan, G. M., Sandock, K. L., and Vaughan, M. K. (1973): Twenty-four hour cycle of a melatonin-like substance in the plasma of human males. *J. Clin. Endocrinol. Metab.,* 37:341–344.

138. Pellegrino de Iraldi, A., and Zieher, L. M. (1966): Noradrenaline and dopamine content of normal decentralized, and denervated pineal glands of the rat. *Life Sci.,* 5:149–154.

139. Perlow, M. J., Reppert, S. M., Tamarkin, L., Wyatt, R. J., and Klein, D. C. (1979): Photic regulation of the melatonin rhythm: Monkey and man are not the same. *Brain Res. (in press).*

140. Pohl, C. R., and Gibbs, F. P. (1978): Circadian rhythms in blinded rats: Correlation between pineal and activity cycles. *Am. J. Physiol.*, 234:110–114.
141. Quay, W. B. (1963): Circadian rhythm in rat pineal serotonin and its modification by estrous cycle and photoperiod. *Gen. Comp. Endocrinol.*, 3:473–479.
142. Quay, W. B. (1963): Differential extractions for the spectrophoto fluorometric measurement of diverse 5-hydroxy- and 5-methoxy indoles. *Anal. Biochem.*, 5:51–59.
143. Quay, W. B. (1964): Circadian and estrous rhythms in pineal melatonin and 5-hydroxyindole-3-acetic acid. *Proc. Soc. Exp. Biol. Med.*, 115:710–712.
144. Quay, W. B. (1966): Twenty-four hour rhythms in pineal 5-hydroxytryptamine and hydroxyindole-0-methyl transferase activity in the macaque. *Proc. Soc. Exp. Biol. Med.*, 121:946.
145. Quay, W. B. (1967): Lack of rhythm and effect of darkness in rat pineal content of N-acetylserotonin-0-methyltransferase. *Physiologist*, 10:286.
146. Raikhlin, N. T., Kvetnoy, I. M., and Tolkachev, V. N. (1975): Melatonin may be synthesised in enterochromaffin cells. *Nature*, 255:344–345.
147. Ralph, C. L., Hull, D., Lynch, H. J., and Hedlund, L. (1971): A melatonin rhythm persists in rat pineals in darkness. *Endocrinology*, 89:1361–1366.
148. Ralph, C. L., and Lynch, H. J. (1970): A quantitative melatonin bioassay. *Gen. Comp. Endocrinol.*, 15:334–338.
149. Reiter, R. J. (1973): Comparative physiology: Pineal gland. *Annu. Rev. Physiol.*, 35:305–328.
150. Reiter, R. J. (1977): *The Pineal—1977*. Eden Press, Montreal.
151. Reiter, R. J., and Klein, D. C. (1971): Observations on the pineal glands, the harderian glands, the retinas, and the reproductive organs of adult female rats exposed to continuous light. *J. Endocrinol.*, 51:117–125.
152. Reiter, R. J., Vaughan, M. K., and Blask, D. E. (1975): Possible role of cerebrospinal fluid in the transport of pineal hormones in mammals. In: *Brain Endocrine Interaction—II*, edited by K. M. Knigge, D. E. Scott, H. Kobayashi, and J. Ishii, pp. 337–354. Karger, Basel.
153. Reppert, S. M., Chez, R. A., Anderson, A., and Klein, D. C. (1978): Maternal-fetal transfer of melatonin in the nonhuman primate. *Pediatr. Res.*, 13:788–791.
154. Reppert, S. M., and Klein, D. C. (1978): Transport of maternal [^{3}H]melatonin to suckling rats and the fate of [^{3}H]melatonin in the neonatal rat. *Endocrinology*, 102:582.
155. Reppert, S. M., Perlow, J. J., Klein, D. C. (1980): CSF melatonin. In: *Neurobiology of Cerebrospinal Fluid*, edited by J. H. Wood. Plenum Press, New York *(in press)*.
156. Reppert, S. M., Perlow, M. J., Mishkin, M., Tamarkin, L., and Klein, D. C. (1979): Effects of damage to the suprachiasmatic area of the anterior hypothalamus on the daily melatonin rhythm in the rhesus monkey. In: *Program 61st Meet. Endocrine Soc.*, p. 76.
157. Reppert, S. M., Perlow, M. D., Tamarkin, L., and Klein, D. C. (1978): Primate CSF melatonin: photic regulation of a diurnal rhythm. In: *Program 60th Meet. Endocrine Soc.*, p. 137.
158. Reppert, S. M., Perlow, M. J., Tamarkin, L., and Klein, D. C. (1979): A diurnal rhythm in primate cerebrospinal fluid. *Endocrinology*, 104: 295–301.
159. Reppert, S. M., Perlow, M. J., Tamarkin, L., and Klein, D. C. (1979): Photic regulation of the melatonin rhythm: A distinct difference between man and monkey. *Pediatr. Res.*, 13:362.
160. Richter, C. P. (1966): A hitherto unrecognized difference between man and other primates. *Science*, 154:427.
161. Rogawski, M. A., Roth, R. H., and Aghajanian, G. K. (1979): Melatonin: Deacetylation to 5-methoxytryptamine by liver but not brain aryl acylamidase. *J. Neurochem.*, 32:1219–1226.
162. Rollag, M. D., Morgan, R. J., and Niswender, G. D. (1978): Route of melatonin secretion in sheep. *Endocrinology*, 102:1–8.
163. Rollag, M. D., and Niswender, G. D. (1976): Radioimmunoassay of serum concentrations of melatonin in sheep exposed to different lighting regimens. *Endocrinology*, 98:482–488.
164. Rollag, M. D., O'Callaghan, P. L., and Niswender, G. D. (1978): Serum melatonin concentrations during different stages of the annual reproductive cycle in ewes. *Biol. Reprod.*, 18:279–285.
165. Romero, J. A., and Axelrod, J. (1974): Pineal β-adrenergic receptor: Diurnal variation in sensitivity. *Science*, 184:1091–1092.
166. Romero, J. A., Zatz, M., and Axelrod, J. (1975): Beta-adrenergic stimulation of pineal N-acetyltransferase: Adenosine 3′,5′-cyclic monophosphate stimulates both RNA and protein synthesis. *Proc. Natl. Acad. Sci. USA*, 72:2107–2111.
167. Romero, J. A., Zatz, M., Kebabian, J. W., and Axelrod, J. (1975): Circadian cycles in binding of ^{3}H-alprenolol to beta-adrenergic receptor sites in the rat pineal. *Nature*, 258:435–436.

168. Roth, W. D. (1965): Metabolic and morphologic studies on the rat pineal organ during puberty. *Prog. Brain Res.,* 10:552–563.

169. Rowe, J. W., Richert, J. R., Klein, D. C., and Reichlin, S. (1970): Relation of the pineal gland and environmental lighting to thyroid function in the rat. *Neuroendocrinology,* 6:247–254.

170. Rudeen, P. K., Reeler, R. S., and Vaughan, M. K. (1975): Pineal serotonin N-acetyltransferase activity in four mammalian species. *Neurosci. Lett.,* 1:225–229.

171. Rusak, B. (1977): The role of the suprachiasmatic nuclei in the generation of circadian rhythm in the golden hamster, Mesocricetus auratus. *J. Comp. Physiol.,* 118:145–164.

172. Saavedra, J. M., Brownstein, M., and Axelrod, J. (1973): A specific and sensitive enzymatic-isotopic microassay for serotonin in tissues. *J. Pharmacol. Exp. Ther.,* 186:508–515.

173. Sakai, K. K., and Marks, B. H. (1972): Adrenergic effects on pineal cell membrane potential. *Life Sci.,* 11:285–291.

174. Saper, C. B., Loewy, A. D., Swanson, L. W., and Cowan, W. M. (1976): Direct hypothalamoautonomic connections. *Brain Res.,* 117:305–312.

175. Schwartz, W. J., and Gainer, H. (1977): Suprachiasmatic nucleus: Use of ^{14}C-labeled deoxyglucose uptake as a functional marker. *Science,* 197:1089–1091.

176. Shibuya, H., Toru, M., and Watanabe, S. (1978): A circadian rhythm of tryptophan hydroxylase in rat pineals. *Brain Res.,* 138:364–368.

177. Sitaram, B. R., and Lees, G. J. (1978): Diurnal rhythm and turnover of tryptophan hydroxylase in the pineal gland of the rat. *J. Neurochem.,* 31:1021–1026.

178. Smith, I., Mullen, P. E., Silman, R. E., Snedden, W., and Wilson, B. W. (1976): Absolute identification of melatonin in human plasma and cerebrospinal fluid. *Nature,* 260:718–719.

179. Smith, J. A., Mee, T. J. X., and Barnes, J. D. (1978): Increased serum melatonin levels in chlorpromazine-treated psychiatric patients. *J. Neural Transm. (Suppl),* 19:397.

180. Smith, J. A., Mee, T. J. X., Barnes, N. D., Thorburn, R. J., and Barnes, J. L. C. (1976): Melatonin in serum and cerebrospinal fluid. *Lancet,* 2:425.

181. Smith, J. A., Padmick, D., Mee, T. X., Minneman, K. P., and Bird, E. D. (1977): Synchronous nyctohemeral rhythms in human blood melatonin and in human post-mortem pineal enzyme. *Clin. Endocrinol.,* 6:219–225.

182. Smythe, G. A., and Lazarus, L. (1974): Growth hormone response to melatonin in man. *Science,* 184:1373–1374.

183. Smythe, G. A., and Lazarus, L. (1974): Suppression of human growth hormone secretion by melatonin and cyproheptadine. *J. Clin. Invest.,* 54:116–121.

184. Snyder, S. H., Zweig, M., Axelrod, J., and Fischer, J. E. (1965): Control of the circadian rhythm in serotonin content of the rat pineal gland. *Proc. Natl. Acad. Sci. USA,* 53:301–303.

185. Stephan, F. K., and Zucker, I. (1972): Circadian rhythms in drinking behavior and locomotor activity of rats are eliminated by hypothalamic lesions. *Proc. Natl. Acad. Sci. USA,* 69:1583–1586.

186. Stephan, F. K., and Zucker, I. (1972): Rat drinking rhythms: Central visual pathways and endocrine factors mediating responsiveness to environmental illumination. *Physiol. Behav.,* 8:315–326.

187. Strada, S., Klein, D. C., Weller, J., and Weiss, B. (1972): Norepinephrine stimulation of cyclic adenosine monophosphate in cultured pineal glands. *Endocrinology,* 90:1470–1476.

188. Strada, S. J., and Weiss, B. (1974): Increased response to catecholamines of the cyclic AMP system of rat pineal gland induced by decreased sympathetic activity. *Arch. Biochem. Biophys.,* 160:197–204.

189. Swanson, L. W., and Cowan, W. M. (1975): The efferent connections of the suprachiasmatic nucleus of the hypothalamus. *J. Comp. Neurol.,* 160:1–12.

190. Szentagothai, J., Flerko, B., Mess, B., and Halasz, B. (1960): *Hypothalamic Control of the Anterior Pituitary.* Akademia Kiado, Budapest.

191. Tamarkin, L., Hollister, C. W., Lefebvre, N. G., and Goldman, B. D. (1977): Melatonin induction of gonadal quiescence in pinealectomized Syrian hamsters. *Science,* 198:953–955.

192. Tamarkin, L., Lefebvre, N. G., Hollister, C. W., and Goldman, B. D. (1977): Effect of melatonin administered during the night on reproductive function in the Syrian hamster. *Endocrinology,* 101:631–634.

193. Tamarkin, L., Reppert, S., Anderson, A., Pratt, B., Goldman, B. D., and Klein, D. C. (1978): Regulation of pineal melatonin in the Syrian hamster. *Pharmacologist,* 20:151.

194. Tamarkin, L., Reppert, S. M., and Klein, D. C. (1979): Regulation of pineal melatonin in the Syrian hamster. *Endocrinology,* 104:385–389.
195. Tamarkin, L., Westrom, W. K., Hamill, A. I., and Goldman, G. C. (1976): Effect of melatonin on the reproductive systems of male and female Syrian hamsters: A diurnal rhythm in sensitivity to melatonin. *Endocrinology,* 99:1534–1541.
196. Toda, N., Tokuyama, T., Senoh, S., Hirata, F., and Hayaishi (1974): Effects of 5-hydroxykynure-namine, a new serotonin metabolite, on isolated dog basal arteries. *Proc. Natl. Acad. Sci. USA,* 71:122–124.
197. Vaughan, G. M., Allen, J. P., Tullis, W., Siler-Khodr, T. M., de la Pēna, A., and Sackman, J. W. (1978): Overnight plasma profiles of melatonin and certain adenohypophyseal hormones in men. *J. Clin. Endocrinol. Metab.,* 47:566–571.
198. Vaughan, G. M., McDonald, S. A., Jordon, R. M., Allen, J. P., Bohmfalk, G. L., Abou-Samra, M., and Story, J. L. (1978): Melatonin concentration in human blood and cerebrospinal fluid: Relationship to stress. *J. Clin. Endocrinol. Metab.,* 47:220–223.
199. Vaughan, G. M., Pelham, R. W., Pand, S. F., Loughlin, L. L., Wilson, K. M., Sandock, K. L., Vaughan, M. K., Koslow, S. H., and Reiter, R. J. (1976): Nocturnal elevation of plasma melatonin and 5-hydroxyindoleacetic acid in young men: Attempts at modification by brief changes in environmental lighting and sleep and by autonomic drugs. *J. Clin. Endocrinol. Metab.,* 42:752–764.
200. Vogel, W. H. (1969): Physiological disposition of 5-methoxytryptamine and rope climbing performance of rats. *Psychopharmacologia,* 15:88–95.
201. Volkman, P. H., and Heller, A. (1971): Pineal N-acetyltranferase: Effect of sympathetic stimulation. *Science,* 173:839–840.
202. Weinberg, U., D'Eletto, R., Weitzman, E. D., Erlich, S., and Hollander, C. S. (1979): Circulating melatonin in man: Episodic secretion throughout the light-dark cycle. *J. Clin. Endocrinol. Metab.,* 48:114–118.
203. Weiss, B., and Costa, E. (1968): Selective stimulation of adenyl cyclase of rat pineal gland by pharmacologically active catecholamines. *J. Pharmacol. Exp. Ther.,* 161:310–319.
204. Weissbach, H., Redfield, B. G., and Axelrod, J. (1961): The enzymatic acetylation of serotonin and other naturally occurring amines. *Biochim. Biophys. Acta,* 54:190–192.
205. Wetterberg, L. (1978): Melatonin in human physiological and clinical studies. *J. Neural Transm. (Suppl),* 13:289–310.
206. Wetterberg, L., Arendt, J., Paunier, L., Sizonenko, P. C., van Donselaar, W., and Heyden, T. (1976): Human serum melatonin changes during the menstrual cycle. *J. Clin. Endocrinol. Metab.,* 42:185–188.
207. Wetterberg, L., Eriksson, O., Friberg, Y., and Vangbo, B. (1978): A simplified radioimmunoassay for melatonin and its application to biological fluids: Preliminary observations on the half-life of plasma melatonin in man. *Clin. Chim. Acta,* 86:169–177.
208. Wetterberg, L., Halberg, F., Tarquini, B., Cagnoni, M., Haus, E., Griffith, K., Kawasaki, T., Wallach, L. A., Ueno, M., Uezo, K., Matsuoka, M., Kuzel, M., Halberg, E., and Omae, T. (1979): Circadian variation in urinary melatonin in clinically healthy women in Japan and the United States of America. *Experientia,* 35:415–418.
209. Wheler, G. H. T., Weller, J. L., and Klein, D. C. (1979): Taurine: Stimulation of pineal N-acetyltransferase activity and melatonin production via a beta-adrenergic mechanism. *Brain Res.,* 166:65–74.
210. Wilkinson, M., Arendt, J., and de Ziegler, D. (1977): Determination of a dark-induced increase in pineal N-acetyltransferase activity and simultaneous radioimmunoassay of melatonin in pineal, serum, and pituitary tissue of the male rat. *J. Endocrinol.,* 72:243–244.
211. Wilson, B. W., Snedden, W., Silman, R. E., Smith, I., and Mullen, P. (1977): A gas chromatography-mass spectrometry method for the quantitative analysis of melatonin in plasma and cerebrospinal fluid. *Anal. Biochem.,* 81:283–291.
212. Wurtman, R. J., Axelrod, J., and Anton-Tay, F. (1968): Inhibition of the metabolism of ^{3}H-melatonin by phenothiazines. *J. Pharmacol. Exp. Ther.,* 161:367–372.
213. Wurtman, R. J., Axelrod, J., and Barchas, J. D. (1964): Age and enzyme activity in the human pineal. *J. Clin. Endocrinol. Metab.,* 24:299–301.
214. Wurtman, R. J., Axelrod, J., and Chu, E. W. (1963): Melatonin, a pineal substance: Effect on the rat ovary. *Science,* 141:277–278.
215. Wurtman, R. J., Axelrod, J., and Kelley, D. E. (1968): *The Pineal.* Academic Press, New York.

216. Wurtman, R. J., Axelrod, J., and Phillips, L. S. (1963): Melatonin synthesis in the pineal gland: Control by light. *Science,* 142:1071–1073.
217. Wurtman, R. J., Axelrod, J., and Potter, L. T. (1964): The uptake of H³-melatonin in endocrine tissues and the effects of constant light exposure. *J. Pharmacol. Exp. Ther.,* 143:314–318.
218. Wurtman, R. J., and Krammer, H. (1966): Melatonin synthesis by an ectopic pinealoma. *N. Engl. J. Med.,* 274:1233–1236.
219. Wurtman, R. J., and Moskowitz, M. A. (1977): The pineal organ. *N. Engl. J. Med.,* 296:1383–1386.
220. Wurzburger, R. J., Kawashima, K., Miller, R. L., and Spector, S. (1976): Determination of rat pineal gland melatonin content by radioimmunoassay. *Life Sci.,* 18:867–878.
221. Yuwiler, A., Klein, D. C., Buda, M., and Weller, J. L. (1977): Pineal N-acetyltransferase activity: Development aspects. *Am. J. Physiol.,* 233:141–146.
222. Zatz, M., and Brownstein, M. J. (1979): Intraventricular carbachol mimics the effects of light on the circadian rhythm in the rat pineal gland. *Science,* 203:358–360.
223. Zucker, I., Rusak, B., King, R. C. (1976): Neural basis for circadian rhythms in rodent behavior. *Adv. Psychobiol.,* pp. 35–74.

The Endocrine Functions of the Brain,
edited by Marcella Motta.
Raven Press, New York, © 1980

16

The Isorenin and Tonin Systems

Roger Boucher and Jacques Genest

Clinical Research Institute of Montreal, Montreal, Quebec H2W 1R7, Canada

Although the physiological role of angiotensin in the central nervous system (CNS) is at present uncertain, it is now clear that angiotensin II (AII) has a number of central actions in addition to its peripheral vasoconstrictor effect and its stimulating action of aldosterone biosynthesis. Microinjections of AII directly into the brain ventricles stimulate drinking behavior in animals of various species (2,21,24,30,50,51,57) more easily and reliably than does intravenous administration (33,54,69,81), although both routes are effective. In 1961, it was demonstrated that AII exerts a pressor effect by acting directly on the brain (5). Subsequent investigations have shown clearly that doses of AII yielding blood levels well within the physiological range for AII induce a centrally mediated pressor response in many species (38,93). Other reported effects of AII in the brain are the increased secretion of vasopressin (46,54,66,80) and adrenocorticotropic hormone (ACTH) (28,32,59,66). In addition, there is evidence that angiotensin may inhibit norepinephrine uptake by central adrenergic neurons (63) and increase the release of acetylcholine at central cholinergic nerve terminals (3,20).

It seemed unlikely that, except for effects on limited areas of the circumventricular organs, these responses to AII represent physiological effects of circulating AII. In some areas of the brain in which receptors for at least some of the central effects of angiotensin are located, the blood–brain barrier is weak or absent; these would therefore be accessible to circulating angiotensin. They include the area postrema (pressor effect) (22,53,78), the subfornical organ (1) and the organum vasculosum of the lamina terminalis (dipsogenic action) (83), the median eminence (ACTH secretion) (27), and the pituitary (ACTH and vasopressin secretions) (26,58). Thus, plasma-borne AII may be able to reach a limited number of brain sites.

Several investigators have demonstrated cerebral penetration in areas in which the blood–brain barrier breaks down in arterial hypertension (18,49); likewise, in the presence of acute hypertension, anesthesia is associated with protein transport across the blood–brain barrier (25). Under normal conditions, however, evidence that systemic angiotensin reaches the same sites as central angiotensin remains inconclusive, mostly because peripheral saralasin [Sar^1,Ala^8]-AII (P113) at levels that do not cause increased blood pressure is not antagonistic to central AII, whereas saralasin (intraventricular) (87,89) blocks the increase in blood pressure induced by intraventricular administration of AII.

Other studies showed that radioactivity can be detected in the cerebrospinal fluid (CSF) after labelled AII has been injected systematically (49,77,91). However, electrophoresis studies (32,66,77) revealed that no intact AII had crossed into the CSF and suggested a rapid degradation of AII by angiotensinases in plasma as well as in tissues (40). Furthermore, the doses employed in the studies were extremely high (66) and may have disrupted the blood–brain barrier. Horseradish peroxidase could be detected in periventricular tissue 5 min after the simultaneous i.v. injection of 2 μg AII and enzyme, while at lower doses of AII, no horseradish peroxidase crossed from the blood to the brain (64).

The effects produced by circulating AII appear to be different from those of CSF-borne angiotensin, and there appear to be different receptors for AII within the blood–brain barrier. These receptors may be activated by administration of AII directly into the cerebral ventricles or by iontophoretic applications (60), but not by injection of AII into the blood supply to the brain. Examples of receptor areas include the subnucleus medialis (pressor effect) (17,39) and the supraoptic nucleus (vasopressin secretion) (60,75). This is substantiated by the pressor response of AII. Blood pressure increases are obtained by injection via both routes, but the responses are different (70). The pressor response to angiotensin rises more slowly to a peak and is more prolonged after intraventricular than after intravenous injection. Intraventricular AII consistently produces a release of vasopressin (46,54,66,80). Whether intravenous AII releases vasopressin, on the other hand, is still a matter of controversy (66,82). Thus, although plasma-borne AII could reach brain sites, the eventual effects appear to be somewhat different from those of CSF-borne AII. Such differences in vasopressin release and pressor responses argue against a simple diffusion of AII in the CSF to receptor sites outside the brain and vice versa.

The fact that the area postrema is stimulated by circulating plasma AII whereas the injection of AII onto the area postrema surface does not stimulate a pressor response (22,38,66) suggests that there is not only a blood–brain barrier to AII, but also a CSF–brain barrier which prevents brain stimulation from the CSF side (10,22,38,53,78,80).

Another important finding is that there is saturable, high-affinity binding of AII by brain tissue—binding which is inhibited by unlabelled AII and AII antagonists. This strongly suggests that AII receptors are present in the brain (4,52,65,75,84,86). Adrenal glands and brain bind AII more than any other organs studied. Receptors in the brain seem to be confined to the area occupied by the organum vasculosum of the laminae terminalis, which is very sensitive to AII. Other areas may also be sensitive, but appear to be reached by peripheral AII and not by intraventricular AII.

The mechanism by which AII can be produced locally remains to be determined. One popular suggestion is that AII is synthesized within the CNS and is, therefore, available to interact with brain AII receptors. A pathway for the local formation of AII was first suggested in 1971 by Ganten et al. (35) and Fischer-Ferraro et al. (23), who observed that isorenin, renin substrate, and AI converting enzyme are present within the brain. These observations have been confirmed (15,33,44), and it is now generally assumed that there is a functional brain renin–angiotensin system. Indeed, it has been proposed that such a system participates in the control of water intake, blood pressure, vasopressin secretion, and a variety of other physiological functions.

A second possibility is that AII is produced through a new enzymatic system reported recently, namely the tonin–angiotensin II system (7–9). Tonin may lead to the formation of AII without the intermediate formation of angiotensin I and play a major role in controlling water balance and blood pressure. Moreover, large concentrations of this enzyme have recently been demonstrated in the brain (13). The pathways of AII formation are summarized in Fig. 1. For a complete discussion on the renin and tonin angiotensin system, the reader is referred to earlier reviews (37,61). The purpose of this chapter is to summarize the current knowledge concerning the formation of angiotensin II in the brain and to evaluate the evidence that the systems for such formation could be involved in physiological regulation.

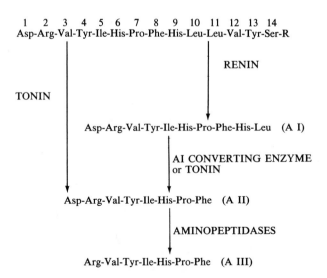

FIG. 1. Pathways for angiotensin formation. R = α-globulin. AI, AII, and AIII are readily fragmented by a group of peptidases called angiotensinases.

THE BRAIN ISORENIN–ANGIOTENSIN I–ANGIOTENSIN II SYSTEM

Isorenin

The renin–angiotensin I–angiotensin II system was originally associated with the kidney and with mechanisms of renal hypertension and sodium and blood volume regulation (37,61). High concentrations of isorenin can also be present in uterus, salivary glands, tumors, and various other tissues (6,30–32,61).

Isorenin activity has been demonstrated in the brain of nephrectomized dogs (23,35), man (15), and rats (44,47). Although some aspects of the subject are controversial (71,72), there is considerable evidence that the brain contains its own isorenin–angiotensin system. Isorenin that forms AI from the natural substrate has been measured in brain tissues of different species (15,23,28,32,44, 55,79). This type of isorenin is similar to kidney renin in having a molecular weight of 40,000 to 60,000. It hydrolyzes renin substrates (angiotensinogens), it does not destroy AI, and its activity can be inhibited by antirenin. Until a few years ago, brain isorenin had not been obtained in pure form, and its existence in the brain has been debated (42,43,71,72).

Another point which has given rise to controversy (73) is that brain isorenin has a pH optimum of 4.0 to 6.5, depending on the species, whereas that for kidney renin is 5.0 to 7.0.

Because a wide variety of neutral and acid proteases has also been observed in brain extracts, it has been suggested that the activity observed in brain extracts could merely be that of the lysosomal acid protease cathepsin D (42,43,62,71,72). Separation of renin from cathepsins is difficult, and most of the renin preparations available have been found to be contaminated by cathepsin-like acid protease activity.

More recently, brain isorenin has been separated from cathepsin (48,62) and has been claimed to satisfy all criteria of specificity *in vitro* and *in vivo*. Various renin substrates injected into the brain ventricles of nephrectomized rats produce drinking behavior, which indicates that the substrates are hydrolyzed by an endogenous enzyme active at the CSF pH. Synthetic renin tetradecapeptide substrate produced the greatest amount of drinking. One must remember that AI converting enzyme catalyzes the formation of AII from this substrate, which is not the case with the natural protein substrate.

Angiotensinogen

Angiotensinogen was first demonstrated in brain tissue in dogs (34), and was later confirmed in brain tissue of rabbits and sheep (69) and the CSF of various species (29). Drinking and pressor responses increased when renin was injected directly into the ventricles (74). The responses observed after intraventricular injection of angiotensinogen are not clearly defined, and conflicting results are reported (70).

Experimentally induced changes in plasma angiotensinogen do not parallel changes in CSF angiotensinogen (28,72). Furthermore, a protein with molecular weight 40,000 to 60,000 would not be expected to cross the blood–brain barrier, and this is another argument in favor of local synthesis of brain angiotensinogen. Additional investigation is required to determine the source of angiotensinogen in the central nervous system.

Angiotensin I Converting Enzyme

AI converting enzyme, which converts AI into AII by cleaving leucyl-histidine from the carboxyl end of the decapeptide, is present in high concentrations in brain tissue (29,68,92). A blockade of dipsogenesis is observed if an inhibitor of AI converting enzyme, the nonapeptide SQ 20881, is injected into the brain ventricles together with renin or substrate. This strongly suggests that AII, not AI, is the biologically active peptide. Thus, all the components of a brain renin–angiotensin system are present.

Brain Angiotensins

AI and AII have been extracted from brain tissue (14,23,28,85). The physico-chemical characteristics are similar to those of synthetic angiotensins. Measurements of the concentrations of these peptides have been attempted (14,23,28,85), but results must be interpreted with caution, as the high proteolytic activities present in brain tissue (29,40) may falsify results. The presence of AII in CSF has been reported (76,81), and its concentration seems to be higher in spontaneously hypertensive rats (32). Although antagonists to AII have been reported to decrease blood pressure in spontaneously hypertensive rats (31,32,66,67), the picture is not as clear as one would wish. Conflicting results have been obtained (19,57,88,90), and the effects of central administration of angiotensin antagonist in spontaneously hypertensive rats must still be clarified. The presence of angiotensin III has also been reported.

THE TONIN–ANGIOTENSIN II SYSTEM

Among the proteases presently known, tonin is unique in its ability to hydrolyze AI, the renin–tetradecapeptide renin substrate, and angiotensinogen to form AII rapidly and directly. In the circulation as well as in most tissues, its enzymatic activity is inhibited by a protein (7,8). Tonin has been purified to a state of homogeneity from rat submaxillary glands (16) and crystallized (45). Studies in brain carried out to date strongly suggest the local formation of AII. This alters our present concept from one based exclusively on the classical renin–angiotensin system to one involving a different pathway.

Intraventricular administration of tonin consistently stimulated water drinking (Fig. 2) and increased blood pressure (Fig. 3) in rats. These responses were

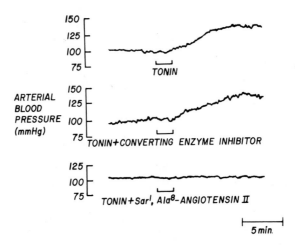

FIG. 2. Effect of intraventricular administration of tonin (10 μg), tonin (10 μg) + AI converting enzyme inhibitor (SQ 20881) (15 μg), and tonin (10 μg) + [Sar[1]-Ala[8]]-AII (12 μg) on the mean blood pressure of anesthetized rats.

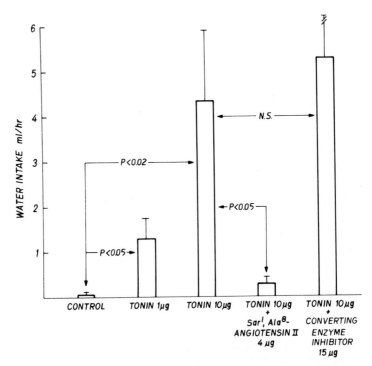

FIG. 3. Effect of intraventricular administration of tonin on water drinking. [Sar[1]-Ala[8]]-AII and AI converting enzyme inhibitor (SQ 20881) were administered simultaneously with tonin. Water intake during the hour after injection was recorded. Seven rats were examined in each group. Values represent the mean ± SEM; significance by Student's unpaired t-test.

abolished by the simultaneous administration of [Sar[1]-Ala[8]]-AII, but were unaffected by the AI converting enzyme inhibitor SQ 20881 (36). Intravenous administration of the same amount of tonin had no effect on blood pressure because of the presence of a strong protein inhibitor of tonin in plasma.

Preliminary studies using both radioimmunoassay of tonin (41) and the fluorimetric detection of His-Leu derived from the cleavage of AI to AII (7,9) showed that tonin is present in large amounts in rat brain and pituitary extracts (13). These results confirm the presence of angiotensinogen in brain tissue and strongly suggest that the effects of intraventricular tonin are mediated mainly by the local generation of AII.

CONCLUSIONS

When injected into the brain, AII produces drinking behavior, blood pressure increase, vasopressin release, and other effects. These effects differ in certain respects from the responses obtained when AII is administered intravenously. Whether intravenous AII acts on the same receptor sites as intraventricular AII remains unsettled. It seems that at least under normal situations and at low doses of angiotensin, the intravenous and the intraventricular routes produce different effects.

The brain isorenin–angiotensin system is still not universally accepted, mainly because of the difficulty of separating cathepsin D from brain isorenin. Although this problem appears to have been solved, the purity and physicochemical properties of isorenin isolated from brain must still be confirmed. Nevertheless, the evidence reviewed here supports the existence of a brain isorenin system.

Early experiments were not convincing because of the large, unphysiological doses of AII used. Subsequent investigations, however, have clearly shown that much smaller doses of peptide and physiological levels of AII induce a centrally mediated pressor and dipsogenic response. The dose levels of AII, AII antagonists, and anesthetic agents (11,12) and the depth of anesthesia are extremely important; under certain experimental conditions they could be misleading.

The contribution of the renin–angiotensin system to thirst has also been questioned (56). Administration of SQ 20881—the enzyme inhibitor that blocks the conversion of AI to AII—did not abolish thirst in rats during hypovolemia, caval ligation, and water intake caused by isoproterenol, whereas it sharply reduced drinking evoked by exogenous renin.

Intraventricular injection of saralasin has also been reported (88,90) to lower blood pressure in rats with renal hypertension. However, central administration of pepstatin or SQ 20881 failed to lower blood pressure. Such findings are consistent with the properties of tonin, which forms AII directly and is not inhibited by pepstatin or AI converting enzyme inhibitors.

Central administration of AII antagonists and AI converting enzyme inhibitors have, in general, failed to provide evidence for the existence of a functional brain isorenin system. These agents, when injected intraventricularly, do not decrease water intake, vasopressin secretion, or arterial blood pressure. It must be admitted that stimulation of water intake, vasopressin secretion, or blood pressure by locally formed AII under physiological conditions has not been proved, neither has the ultimate mechanism whereby it might be elucidated.

The pathways for the formation of AII remain to be determined. No conclusion is possible at present except that the central nervous system and the isorenin and/or tonin–angiotensin systems are particularly exciting areas for research.

ACKNOWLEDGMENTS

The authors wish to thank Mrs. Vivianne Lacombe for her skillful secretarial assistance in preparing this manuscript.

This work was supported by an M.R.C. Group Grant to the Multidisciplinary Research Group on Hypertension at the Clinical Research Institute of Montreal. (Other members of the group are Drs. W. Nowaczynski and O. Kuchel.)

REFERENCES

1. Abdelaal, A. E., Assaf, S. Y., Kucharczyk, J., and Morgenson, G. J. (1974): Effect of ablation of the S.F.O. on water intake elicited by systematically administered AII. *Can. J. Physiol. Pharmacol.*, 52:362–363.
2. Abraham, S. F., Baker, R. M., Blaine, E. H., Denten, D. A., and McKinely, M. J. (1975): Water drinking induced in sheep by angiotensin—a physiological or pharmacological effect? *J. Comp. Physiol. Psychol.*, 88:503–518.
3. Barker, J. L. (1976): Peptides: Role in neuronal excitability. *Physiol. Rev.*, 56:435–452.
4. Bennett, J. B., and Snyder, S. H. (1976): Angiotensin II binding to mammalian brain membranes. *J. Biol. Chem.*, 251:7423–7430.
5. Bickerton, R. K., and Buckley, J. P. (1961): Evidence for a central mechanism in angiotensin induced hypertension. *Proc. Soc. Exp. Biol. Med.*, 106:834–836.
6. Bing, J., and Poulsen, K., (1971): The renin system in mice. Effects of removal of kidneys or (and) submaxillary glands in different strains. *Acta Pathol. Microbiol. Scand.* [*A*], 79:134–138.
7. Boucher, R., Asselin, J., and Genest, J. (1974): A new enzyme leading to the direct formation of angiotensin II. *Circ. Res.*, 34–35 (Suppl. I):203–212.
8. Boucher, R., Demassieux, S., Garcia, R., and Genest, J. (1977): Tonin, angiotensin II system: A review. *Circ. Res.*, 41 (Suppl. II):26–29.
9. Boucher, R., Saidi, M., and Genest, J., (1972): A new "angiotensin I converting enzyme" system. In: *Hypertension 1972*, edited by J. Genest and E. Koiw, pp. 512–523. Springer, Berlin.
10. Brightman, M. W. (1968): The intracerebral movement of proteins injected into blood and cerebrospinal fluid of mice. *Prog. Brain Res.* 29:19–40.
11. Brody, M. J., Fink, G. D., Buggy, J., Haywood, J. R., Gordon, F. J., and Johnson, A. K. (1978): The role of the anteroventral third ventricle (AV3V) region in experimental hypertension. *Circ. Res.*, 43 (Suppl. I):2–13.
12. Buggy, J., Fink, G. D., Johnson, A. K., and Brody, M. J. (1977): Prevention of the development of renal hypertension by anteroventral third ventricular tissue lesions. *Circ. Res.*, 40 (Suppl. I):110–117.
13. Chan, J. S. D., Seidah, N. G., Chrétien, M., Gutkowska, J., Boucher, R., and Genest, J. (1979): *J. Biol. Chem. (in press)*.
14. Changaris, D. G., Demers, L. M., Keil, L. C., and Severs, W. B. (1977): Immunopharmacology of angiotensin I in brain. In: *Central Actions of Angiotensin and Related Hormones*, edited by J. P. Buckley and C. M. Ferrario, pp. 233–243. Pergamon Press, New York.
15. Daul, C. B., Heath, R. M., and Garey, R. E. (1975): Angiotensin-forming enzyme in human brain. *Neuropharmacology*, 14:75–80.

16. Demassieux, S., Boucher, R., Grisé, C., and Genest, J. (1976): Purification and characterization of tonin. *Can. J. Biochem.*, 54:788–795.
17. Deuben, R. R., and Buckley, J. P. (1970): Identification of a central site of action of angiotensin II. *J. Pharmacol. Exp. Ther.*, 175:139–146.
18. Dinsdale, H. B., Robertson, D. M., and Hass, R. A. (1974): Cerebral blood flow in acute hypertension. *Arch. Neurol.*, 31:80–87.
19. Elghozi, J. L., Altman, J., Devynck, M. A., Liard, J. F., Grunfeld, J. P., and Meyer, P. (1977): Lack of hypotensive effect of central infection of angiotensin inhibitors in spontaneously hypertensive and normotensive rats. In: *Central Actions of Angiotensin and Related Hormones*, edited by J. P. Buckley and C. M. Ferrario, pp. 514–519. Pergamon Press, New York.
20. Elie, R., and Panisset, J. C. (1970): Effect of angiotensin and atropine on the spontaneous release of acetylcholine from cat cerebral cortex. *Brain Res.*, 17:297–305.
21. Epstein, A. N. (1978): The neuroendocrinology of thirst and salt appetite. In: *Frontiers of Neuroendocrinology, Vol. 5*, edited by W. F. Ganong and L. Martini, pp. 101–134. Raven Press, New York.
22. Ferrario, C. M., Gildenberg, P. L., and McCubbin, J. W. (1972): Brief reviews: Cardiovascular effects of angiotensin mediated by the central nervous system. *Circ. Res.*, 30:257–262.
23. Fischer-Ferraro, C., Nahmad, V. E., Goldstein, D. J., and Finkielman, S. (1971): Angiotensin and renin in rat and dog brain. *J. Exp. Med.*, 133:353–361.
24. Fitzsimons, J. T., (1972): Thirst. *Physiol. Rev.*, 52:468–561.
25. Forster, A., Van Horn, K., Marshall, F., and Shapiro, H. M. (1978): Anesthetic effects on blood–brain barrier function during acute arterial hypertension. *Anesthesiology*, 49:26–30.
26. Gagnon, D. J., Cousineau, D., and Boucher, P. J. (1973): Release of vasopressin by angiotensin II and prostaglandin E_2 from the rat neurohypophysis in vitro. *Life Sci.*, 12:487–497.
27. Gann, D. S. (1969): Parameters of the stimulus initiating the adrenocortical response to hemorrhage. *Ann. N.Y. Acad. Sci. U.S.A.*, 156:740–755.
28. Ganten, D., Fuxe, K., Phillips, M. I., Mann, J. F. E., and Ganten, U. (1978): The brain isorenin–angiotensin system: Biochemistry, localization, and possible role in drinking and blood pressure regulation. In *Frontiers in Neuroendocrinology, Vol. 5*, edited by W. F. Ganong and L. Martini, pp. 61–69. Raven Press, New York.
29. Ganten, D., Ganten, U., Schelling, P., Boucher, R., and Genest, J. (1975): The renin and iso-renin–angiotensin systems in rats with experimental pituitary tumors. *Proc. Soc. Exp. Biol. Med.*, 148:568–572.
30. Ganten, D., Hutchinson, J. S., Haebara, H., Schelling, P., Fischer, H., and Ganten, U. (1976): Tissue isorenins. *Clin. Sci. Mol. Med.*, 51:117–120.
31. Ganten, D., Hutchinson, J. S., and Schelling, P. (1975): The intrinsic brain isorenin–angiotensin system in the rat: Its possible role in central mechanism of blood pressure regulation. *Clin. Sci. Mol. Med.*, 48:265–268.
32. Ganten, D., Hutchinson, J. S., Schelling, P., Ganten, U., and Fischer, H. (1976): The iso-renin angiotensin systems in extrarenal tissue. *Clin. Exp. Pharmacol. Physiol.*, 3:103–126.
33. Ganten, D., Kusumoto, M., Constantopoulos, G., Ganten, U., Boucher, R., and Genest, J. (1973): Iso-renin, electrolytes and catecholamines in dog brain: Possible interrelationship. *Life Sci.*, 12:1–8.
34. Ganten, D., Marquez-Julio, A., Granger, P., Hayduk, K., Karsunky, K. P., Boucher, R., and Genest, J. (1971): Renin in dog brain. *Am. J. Physiol.*, 221:1733–1737.
35. Ganten, D., Minnich, J. L., Granger, P., Hayduk, K., Brecht, H. M., Barbeau, A., Boucher, R., and Genest, J. (1971): Angiotensin-forming enzyme in the brain tissue. *Science*, 173:64–65.
36. Garcia, R., Boucher, R., Kondo, K., Schiffrin, E. L., Gutkowska, J., and Genest, J. (1979): The role of tonin in experimental hypertension. *Clin. Sci. Mol. Med. (in press)*.
37. Genest, J., Koiw, E., and Kuchel, O., editors (1977): *Hypertension*. McGraw Hill, New York.
38. Gildenberg, P. L., and Ferrario, C. M. (1977): A technique for determining the site of action of angiotensin and other hormones in the brain stem. In: *Central Actions of Angiotensin and Related Hormones*, edited by J. P. Buckley and C. M. Ferrario, pp. 157–164. Pergamon Press, New York.
39. Gildenberg, P. L., Ferrario, C. M., and McCubbin, J. W. (1973): Two sites of cardiovascular action of angiotensin II in the brain of the dog. *Clin. Sci.*, 44:417–420.
40. Goldstein, D. J., Diaz, A., Finkielman, S., Nahmad, V. E., and Fischer-Ferraro, C. (1972): Angiotensinase activity in rat and dog brain. *J. Neurochem.*, 19:2451–2452.

41. Gutkowska, Y., Boucher, R., Demassieux, S., Garcia, R., and Genest, J. (1978): A direct radioimmunoassay for tonin. *Can. J. Biochem.,* 56:769–773.
42. Hackenthal, E., Hackenthal, R., and Hilgenfeldt, U., (1978): Iso-renin, pseudo-renin, cathepsin D and renin. A comparative enzymatic study of angiotensin-forming enzymes. *Biochim. Biophys. Acta,* 522:574–588.
43. Hackenthal, E., Hackenthal, P., and Hilgenfeldt, U. (1978): Purification and partial characterization of rat brain acid proteinase (iso-renin). *Biochim. Biophys. Acta,* 522:561–573.
44. Haulica, I., Branistaenu, D. D., Rosca, V., Stratone, A., Berbeleu, V., Balan, G., and Ionescu, L. (1975): A renin-like activity in pineal gland and hypophysis. *Endocrinology,* 96:508–510.
45. Hayakawa, K., Kelly, J. A., and James, M. N. G. (1978): Crystal data for tonin, an enzyme involved in the formation of angiotensin II. *J. Mol. Biol.,* 123:107–111.
46. Hoffman, W. E., and Phillips, M. I. (1977): The role of ADH in the pressor response to intraventricular angiotensin II. In: *Central Actions of Angiotensin and Related Hormones,* edited by J. P. Buckley and C. M. Ferrario, pp. 307–314. Pergamon Press, New York.
47. Hoffman, W. E., Schelling, P., Phillips, M. I., and Ganten, D. (1976): Evidence for local angiotensin formation in brain of nephrectomized rats. *Neuroscience,* 3:299–303.
48. Inagami, T., and Murakami, K., (1977): Pure renin: Isolation from hog kidney and characterization. *J. Biol. Chem.,* 252:2978–2983.
49. Johanson, B., (1974): Blood–brain barrier dysfunction in acute arterial hypertension after papaverine-induced vasodilation. *Acta Neurol. Scand.,* 50:573–580.
50. Johnson, A. K. (1975): The role of the cerebral ventricular system in angiotensin-induced thirst. In: *Control Mechanisms of Drinking,* edited by G. Peters, J. T. Fitzsimons, and L. Peters-Maefeli, pp. 117–122. Springer, Berlin.
51. Johnson, A. K., and Buggy, J., (1977): A critical analysis of the site of action for the dipsogenic effect of angiotensin II. In: *Central Actions of Angiotensin and Related Hormones,* edited by J. P. Buckley and C. M. Ferrario, pp. 357–386. Pergamon Press, New York.
52. Johnson, A. K., and Schwob, J. E. (1975): Cephalic angiotensin receptors mediating drinking to systemic angiotensin II. *Pharmacol. Biochem. Behav.,* 3:1076–1084.
53. Joy, M., (1977): The regulation of vasomotor centre activity by angiotensin. In: *Central Actions of Angiotensin and Related Hormones,* edited by J. P. Buckley, and C. M. Ferrario, pp. 165–168. Pergamon Press, New York.
54. Keil, L. C., Summy-Long, J., and Severs, W. B. (1975): Release of vasopressin by angiotensin II. *Endocrinology,* 96:1063–1065.
55. Lee, M. R. (1969): *Renin and Hypertension.* Lloyd-Luke, London.
56. Lehr, D., Goldman, H. W., and Casner, P., (1973): Renin–angiotensin role in thirst: Paradoxical enhancement of drinking by angiotensin converting enzyme inhibitor. *Science,* 182:1031–1034.
57. Mann, J. F. E., Phillips, M. I., Dietz, R., Haebara, H., and Ganten, D., (1978): Effects of central and peripheral angiotensin blockage in hypertensive rats. *Am. J. Physiol.,* 89:234–235.
58. Maran, J. W., and Yates, F. E., (1974): Locus of ACTH-releasing action of angiotensin II. *Program 56th Meeting Endocrine Soc.,* p. 118.
59. Morgan, J. M., and Routtenberg, A. (1977): Angiotensin injected into the neostriatum after learning disrupts retention performance. *Science,* 196:87–89.
60. Nicoll, R. A., and Barker, J. L. (1971): Excitation of supraoptic neurosecretory cells by angiotensin II. *Nature,* 233:172–174.
61. Oparil, S., (1977): *Renin 1976.* Eden Press, Montreal.
62. Osman, M. Y., Sen, S., and Smeby, R. R. (1978): Separation of renin activity from acid protease activity in brain extracts. *Fed. Proc.,* 37:354.
63. Palaic, D., and Khairallah, P. A. (1967): Effect of angiotensin on uptake and release of norepinephrine by brain. *Biochem. Pharmacol.,* 16:2291–2298.
64. Phillipps, M. I. (1978): Angiotensin in the brain. *Neuroendocrinology,* 25:354–377.
65. Phillips, M. I., and Felix, D., (1976): Specific angiotensin II receptive neurons in the cat subfornical organ. *Brain Res.,* 109:531–540.
66. Phillips, M. I., Felix, S., Hoffman, W. E., and Ganten, D. (1977): Angiotensin-sensitive sites in the brain ventricular system. In: *Approaches to the Cell Biology of Neurons,* edited by W. M. Cowan, and J. A. Ferrendelli, pp. 308–339. Neuroscience Society, Bethesda, Maryland.
67. Phillips, M. I., Phipps, J., Hoffman, W., and Leavitt, M. (1975): Reduction of blood pressure by intracranial injection of angiotensin blocker (P113) in spontaneously hypertensive rats. *Physiologist,* 18:350.

68. Poth, M. M., Heath, R. G., and Ward, M. (1975): Angiotensin-converting enzyme in human brain. *J. Neurochem.,* 25:83–85.
69. Printz, M. P., and Lewicki, J. A. (1977): Renin substrate in the CNS: Potential significance to central regulatory mechanisms. In: *Central Actions of Angiotensin and Related Hormones,* edited by J. P. Buckley and C. M. Ferrario, pp. 57–64. Pergamon Press, New York.
70. Reid, I. A., (1976): The brain renin–angiotensin system; New observations. In: *Regulation of Blood Pressure by the Central Nervous System,* edited by G. Onesti, M. Fernandes, and E. Kim, pp. 161–173. Grune & Stratton, New York.
71. Reid, I. A. (1977): Is there a brain renin–angiotensin system? *Circ. Res.,* 41:147–153.
72. Reid, I. A., and Day, R. P. (1977): Interactions and properties of some components of the renin–angiotensin system in brain. In: *Central Actions of Angiotensin and Related Hormones,* edited by J. P. Buckley and C. M. Ferrario, pp. 267–282. Pergamon Press, New York.
73. Reid, I. A., and Moffat, B. (1978): Angiotensin II concentration in cerebrospinal fluid after intraventricular injection of angiotensinogen or renin. *Endocrinology,* 103:1494–1498.
74. Reid, I. A., and Ramsay, D. J. (1975): The effects of intracerebroventricular administration of renin on drinking and blood pressure. *Endocrinology,* 97:536–542.
75. Sakai, K. K., Marks, B. H., George, J., and Koestner, A., (1974): Specific angiotensin II receptors in organ-cultured canine supra-optic nucleus cells. *Life Sci.,* 14:1337–1344.
76. Schelling, P., Ganten, D., Heckl, R., Hayduk, K., Hutchinson, J. S., Sponer, G., and Ganten, U. (1977): On the origin of angiotensin-like peptides in cerebrospinal fluid. In: *Central Actions of Angiotensin and Related Hormones,* edited by J. P. Buckley and C. M. Ferrario, pp. 519–526. Pergamon Press, New York.
77. Schelling, P., Hutchinson, J. S., Ganten, U., Sponer, G., and Ganten, D. (1976): Impermeability of the blood-cerebrospinal fluid barrier for angiotensin II in rats. *Clin. Sci. Mol. Med.,* 51:399–402.
78. Scroop, G. C., Katic, F. P., Brown, M. J., Cain, M. D., and Zeegers, P. J. (1975): Evidence for a significant contribution from central effects of angiotensin in the development of acute renal hypertension in the greyhound. *Clin. Sci. Mol. Med.,* 48:115–119.
79. Sen. S., Ferrario, C. M., and Bumpus, F. M. (1974): Alteration in the feedback control of renin release by an angiotensin antagonist. *Acta Physiol. Lat. Am.,* 24:529–532.
80. Severs, W. B., and Daniel-Severs, A. E. (1973): Effects of angiotensin on the central nervous system. *Pharmacol. Rev.,* 25:415–449.
81. Severs, W. B., Changaris, D. G., Kapsha, J. M., Keil, L. C., Petro, D. J., Reid, I. A., and Summy-Long, J. Y. (1977): Presence and significance of angiotensin in cerebrospinal fluid. In: *Central Actions of Angiotensin and Related Hormones,* edited by J. P. Buckley and C. M. Ferrario, pp. 225–232. Pergamon Press, New York.
82. Shade, R. E., and Share, L., (1975): Vasopressin release during nonhypotensive hemorrhage and angiotensin II infusion. *Am. J. Physiol.,* 228:149–154.
83. Simpson, J. B., and Routtenberg, A. (1973): Subfornical organ: Site of drinking elicitation by angiotensin II. *Science,* 181:1172–1175.
84. Sirett, N. E., McLean, A. M., Bray, J. J., and Hubbard, J. I., (1977): Distribution of angiotensin II receptors in rat brain. *Brain Res.,* 122:299–312.
85. Slaven, B., (1975): Influence of salt and volume on changes in rat brain angiotensin. *J. Pharm. Pharmacol.,* 27:782–783.
86. Snyder, S. H., (1978): Peptide neurotransmitter candidates in the brain: focus on enkephalin, angiotensin II, and neurotensin. In: *The Hypothalamus,* edited by S. Reichlin, R. J. Baldessarini, and J. B. Martin, pp. 233–243. Raven Press, New York.
87. Solomon, T. A., and Buckley, J. P., (1974): Inhibitory effects of central hypertensive activity of angiotensin I and II by 1-Sar-8-Ala-angiotensin II (saralasin acetate). *J. Pharm. Sci.,* 63:1109–1113.
88. Sweet. C. S., Columbo, J. M., and Gaul, S. L., (1977): Inhibitors of the renin–angiotensin system in the malignant hypertensive rat: comparative antihypertensive effects of central vs. peripheral administration. In: *Central Actions of Angiotensin and Related Hormones,* edited by J. P. Buckley and C. M. Ferrario, pp. 271–280. Pergamon Press, New York.
89. Sweet. C. S., Ferrario, C. M., Khosla, M. C., and Bumpus, F. M. (1973): Antagonism of peripheral and central effects of angiotension II by (1-sarcosine,8-isoleucine) angiotensin II. *J. Pharmacol. Exp. Ther.,* 185:35–41.
90. Vogel, H. G., Jung, W., and Schoelkens, B. A. (1976): Hypotensive action of central injection

of angiotensin II antagonist in conscious rats with experimental hypertension. In: *Program 5th Intern. Congr. Endocrinology,* p. 117.
91. Volicer, L., and Loew, C. G. (1971): Penetration of angiotensin II into the brain. *Neuropharmacology,* 10:631–636.
92. Yang, H.-Y., and Neff, N. H. (1973): Differential distribution of angiotensin converting enzyme in the anterior and posterior lobe of the rat pituitary. *J. Neurochem.,* 21:1035–1036.
93. Yu, R., and Dickinson, C. J., (1965): Neurogenic effects of angiotensin. *Lancet,* 2:1276–1277.

The Endocrine Functions of the Brain,
edited by Marcella Motta.
Raven Press, New York © 1980

17

Posterior Pituitary Hormones and Neurophysins

Guy Valiquette

Department of Endocrinology, University of Milan, Milan, Italy

The posterior pituitary has long been the main organ of interest for the study of the endocrine functions of the brain. Our knowledge of the posterior pituitary has increased in parallel with the technical means at our disposal, but recently a second neuroendocrine organ of major importance, the median eminence, has come to light. Other intracranial structures, such as the circumventricular organs (51,280) (see also Chapter 1) and the pineal (44) (see also Chapter 15), are also now being recognized as neuroendocrine transducers. Nevertheless, the neurohypophysial system has kept precedence, as the expression "classical" neurosecretion tacitly recognizes, as the neuroendocrine unit "par excellence."

PHYLOGENESIS OF THE NEUROHORMONES

In most vertebrates, the neurohypophysis has three secretory products, of which two are neurohormones. In mammals, including man, these are vasopressin (or antidiuretic hormone, VP) and oxytocin (OT); the third secretory product of the posterior pituitary is made up of the carrier proteins of the neurohormones, the neurophysins. Neurohypophysial hormones can be divided into two groups, based on their action in mammals: vasopressor peptides, and OT-like, or neutral, peptides (Table 1). Of all known naturally occurring neurohypophysial hormones, vasotocin stands out in more than one respect. It is the most ubiquitous peptide in the evolutionary tree (Table 1) and is the vasopressor peptide of all submammalian vertebrate species so far examined. It is also the only peptide to combine in its molecule both vasopressor and oxytocic activities to a relevant extent.

It therefore seems quite clear that arginine-vasotocin is the "primitive" neurohypophysial hormone, ancestral to all the other octapeptides. Also of great phyletic interest is the fact that the lampreys, probably the most primitive living vertebrates, unlike all other vertebrates, have only one neurohypophysial hormone, arginine-vasotocin (210,211). It would seem that the gene for vasotocin duplicated early in the evolution of vertebrates, which eventually allowed for the evolution of two different hormones. In all other vertebrates, the vasopressor peptide is concerned with the control of blood pressure and/or salt and water metabolism, while the OT-like peptide is involved in reproduction (15,150).

TABLE 1. *Naturally occurring neurohypophysial peptides*

Octapeptides[a]	Amino acid in position			Vertebrates where present
	3	4	8	
Vasopressor peptides:				
Arginine-vasotocin (AVT)	Ile	Gln	Arg	All vertebrates except some Suina[b]
Arginine-vasopressin (AVP)	Phe	Gln	Arg	All mammals except some Suina[b]
Lysine-vasotocin (LVT)	Ile	Gln	Lys	Suina[b]
Lysine-vasopressin (LVP)	Phe	Gln	Lys	Suina[b]
Oxytocin-like peptides:				
Oxytocin (OT)	Ile	Gln	Leu	Mammals, holocephali (chimeras) (birds, reptiles, amphibians [disputed[c]])
Mesotocin (MT)	Ile	Gln	Ile	Sarcopterygii (lungfishes), amphibians, reptiles, birds[c]
Isotocin (IT)	Ile	Ser	Ile	Actinopterygii (bony fishes)
Glumitocin (GT)	Ile	Ser	Glu	Some Elasmobranchii (skates)
Asparatonin (AT)	Ile	Asn	Leu	Some Elasmobranchii (sharks)[d]
Valitocin (VT)	Ile	Gln	Val	Some Elasmobranchii (sharks)[d]

Common structure: Cys-Tyr- - -Asn-Cys-Pro- -Gly(NH$_2$)
              1   2   3   4   5   6   7   8   9

[a] Although the neurohypophysial hormones are in fact nonapeptides, they are conventionally called octapeptides for historical reasons, counting one cystine instead of two cysteines.

[b] See text.

[c] The presence of OT has been challenged in amphibians, reptiles, and birds. OT-MT polymorphism may exist in amphibians, reptiles, and birds.

[d] VT-AT polymorphism seems to exist in sharks.

However, this straightforward, mind-pleasing scheme does not explain all the known facts. It would seem that mammals did not replace vasotocin with VP, but added VP as a third peptide. Vasotocin has recently been found to be produced by the fetal neurohypophysis of mammals (170,237,270) and by the pineal gland of both fetal and adult mammals (159,179,180), although it has not yet been identified in the circulation or in the cerebrospinal fluid (CSF). More surprisingly, the genes for VP and vasotocin seem to be somehow linked together: pigs, along with a few other members of the suborder Suina, produce lysine-VP instead of arginine-VP, as do all the other mammals, but would also produce lysine-vasotocin instead of arginine-vasotocin (177). That two different, independent genes would both mutate in an analogous manner simultaneously is highly improbable, and this piece of evidence is, as yet, completely unexplainable. However, this linkage between these two genes in mammals is not absolute, since the Brattleboro rat, which is genetically incapable of producing arginine-VP, does nevertheless produce arginine-vasotocin in its pineal gland (41). Many evolutionary schemes have been proposed to account for the distribution of the neurohypophysial peptides across the species, but none is entirely satisfactory and, to date, relatively few species have been examined.

The hypothalamo-neurohypophysial system is functionally quite similar in most vertebrates, despite a considerable degree of anatomical variability, particularly of the degree of contact between the posterior pituitary and the intermediate and anterior lobes (for an excellent review on the anatomy of the hypophysis in mammals, see reference 97). This is not surprising when one considers that its role is to deliver the octapeptides to the general circulation and, to a certain extent, to the adenohypophysis. In most mammals, including the rat, the primates, and man, the neurohypophysis intermingles with the intermediate lobe, whereas in very few species, such as the whale and the elephant, it is cleanly separated by an avascular fibrous septum; unfortunately, these species are not readily adaptable to laboratory experimentation. But even these differences in the degree of anatomical intimacy between the posterior and the intermediate/anterior pituitaries are functionally of little importance when the median eminence, the neurohypophysis, and the adenohypophysis are considered in a more holistic context.

NEUROPHYSINS AND THE BIOSYNTHESIS OF NEUROHYPOPHYSIAL HORMONES

The neurophysins are the third secretory product of the neurohypophysis. To date, these proteins have no known biological activity. Many authors in the past have claimed for the neurophysins lipolytic (80), hypocalcemic (79), positive chronotropic (126), natriuretic (201), and anabolic (259) activities. Later studies demonstrated that these activities were caused by the use of impure preparations of neurophysins (136,201); for example, the observed natriuretic activity might be due to VP, 1-13 ACTH, and α-MSH contaminations (42).

Despite the fact that they do not have any intrinsic biological activity, the neurophysins remain of great interest for their close association with the neurohypophysial hormones as binding proteins, both before and after neurosecretion. The neurophysins and the octapeptides are found loosely bound together in the neurosecretory granules (46,88) and are usually, if not always, secreted together (109,133) by exocytosis. Once secreted into the circulation, the neurophysin-hormone complex dissociates, since the affinity constant of the neurophysins is too low for them to function as binding proteins at the circulating concentrations of the hormones.

A model that explains this association satisfactorily has been proposed by Sachs and coworkers (213): in the perikaria of the magnocellular neurons of the supraoptic and paraventricular nuclei, a precursor protein, common to both the neurophysin and the octapeptide, would be synthesized on ribosomes and packaged by the Golgi into the neurosecretory granules. While the granule travels down the axon toward the neurohypophysis, a proteolytic enzyme, called "maturase," would split both the neurohormone and the neurophysin from this precursor, leaving them loosely but noncovalently bound together. This model has received further support from the demonstration of the existence of a 20,000-dalton protein (161), synthesized in the supraoptic nucleus and showing common antigenic determinants with both the neurophysin and the neurohormone (84). This precursor is slowly transformed into neurophysin (MW approximately 10,000 dalton) during axonal transport. There would be one such prohormone for each neurohormone.

All mammalian species studied to date, with one exception (the guinea pig), show two different "major" neurophysins, known in some species, and presumed in the others, to be specifically associated with VP and OT, and one or more "minor" neurophysins. Pickering and coworkers (185) have proposed, with good indirect evidence in the case of the rat, that the "maturase" enzyme, after having split OT and its associated neurophysin from their precursor, would then further manifest its proteolytic activity by slowly metabolizing the OT-neurophysin into the "minor" neurophysins. More recently, other data supporting this theory have been published (172,288).

Since, in the hypothalamo-hypophysial system, the neurophysins are coupled to the neurohormones in their synthesis and in their secretion, one may wonder whether these concepts hold true for all tissues and organs that secrete any of the octapeptides. It would seem reasonable to think so. Neurophysins have been identified in the pineal gland of mammals (138,190), where secretion of vasotocin is known to occur from the ependymal cells (180). They have also been found in the CSF (202), into which they presumably have been secreted by one or more of the circumventricular organs, whereas vasotocin has been found in the subcommissural organ (206), one of the circumventricular organs specializing in the secretion of peptides and other substances into the CSF. However, it has not been established to date that there is a specific vasotocin-neurophysin, as has been demonstrated for the pituitary octapeptides, or that it is produced from a precursor common both to the neurophysin and the octapeptide. Whenever looked for, neurophysins were also found in association with the octapeptides in lower vertebrates, including birds (181) and fishes (184,218), thus lending further support to the "maturase" model.

The one exception mentioned above is the guinea pig (278) and another, possibly, is the hedgehog (64), in which only one apparently homogenous neurophysin has been found. Although this may seem to challenge the "maturase" model since, as there are two neurohormones, these should be two prohormones and two neurophysins, it has been argued (185) that the two neurophysins liberated by the "maturase" would be so similar as to be indistinguishable by the analytical methods available.

Interestingly, immunoreactive and peptide-binding neurophysin-like substances have been identified in the octapeptide target tissues: renal cortex, mammary gland, and uterus (89,90,139). Although, particularly in the case of the kidney, these substances could be metabolic products of the neurohypophysial neurophysins, it has been shown that the uterine neurophysin-like protein is produced *in situ* by the endometrium, and that on gel chromatography and on analytical disk-gel electrophoresis it is indistinguishable from the neurohypophysial neurophysin believed to be associated with oxytocin (198). The significance of these neurophysin-like proteins in the target organs of the neurohypophysial hormones is completely unknown.

The Neurophysins As Tools

Since neurophysins accompany the neurohypophysial hormones through all stages of synthesis, transport, storage, and secretion, and since they seem to be specifically associated with one or the other hormone, they quite naturally came to be used as tracers for these. The neurohypophysial hormones are in fact particularly difficult to work with; they are small peptides, nine amino acids long, and are therefore generally nonantigenic and must be coupled to carrier proteins for immunization (238). They circulate at very low concentrations and, before radioimmunoassay, must be extracted from plasma to eliminate nonspecific activity and to concentrate them. In addition, they tend to leach out of tissue during immunohistochemical preparatory procedures and may give rise to false-negative results (235). Neurophysins were therefore welcomed and used to localize and assay the neurohormones indirectly and to provide corroborative evidence.

Of paramount importance to these uses are obtaining specific antibodies and identifying the neurophysin (or neurophysins, when the minor components are considered) associated with each hormone. This second requisite has actually been more challenging than might be anticipated. All neurophysins will bind both neurohormones indiscriminately; OT and VP will actually compete for the binding site (24). The conclusions reported in Table 2, where the nomenclature and the hormonal specificity of the main neurophysins are summarized, were obtained by demonstrating the association of one hormone with one neurophysin in intact granules, or by demonstrating simultaneous secretion of one neurophysin with one hormone, or by showing secretion of one neurophysin in response to stimuli known or believed to be specific to one hormone.

TABLE 2. *Nomenclature of the main neurophysins and their association with the neurohypophysial hormones*

		Neurophysin associated with	
Main investigator	Species	VP	OT
Robinson (109,197,200)	Human	NSN[a] (II)	ESN[b] (I)
Legros (133,137)	Human	I	II
Robinson (203)	Bovine	II	I
Legros (140,141)	Bovine	II	I
Dean (46)	Bovine	II	I
Dax (45)	Porcine	I	II
Pickering (28,157)	Rat	A	B
Sokol (252)	Rat	I	II

[a] NSN = nicotine-stimulated neurophysin.
[b] ESN = estrogen-stimulated neurophysin.

The neurophysins are usually identified according to their electrophoretic mobility, the more anodal migrating neurophysin being called neurophysin I (or A), etc. The results obtained from this use of the neurophysins as tools will be mentioned later as relevant to the individual hormones.

VASOPRESSIN

The antidiuretic hormone of most mammals is arginine-VP. Its existence was first recognized by its vasopressor effects (173), and the presence of a functional linkage between the pituitary gland and water excretion was recognized 14 years later (217). We owe our knowledge of the control of VP, and thereby of water excretion, by plasma osmolarity to the classical series of experiments done by Verney in the second quarter of this century (267). In the meantime, arginine-VP was being purified; its structure was determined and it was synthesized in 1954 by du Vigneaud (59,60).

Arginine-VP, as stated above, is the antidiuretic hormone of all mammals examined so far, except the members of the suborder Suina and one strain of mice. In domestic pigs, lysine-VP has replaced arginine-VP, and the latter hormone seems to be completely lacking in this species. In the other members of the Suina, including, for example, the European wild boar, the pecaries, the warthog, the bushpig, and the hippopotamus, one can find arginine-VP exclusively, or lysine-VP exclusively, or both VPs in any given animal (68,69). When enough animals of one species could be examined to deduce the gene frequency, the results were compatible with the existence of a single allelic gene pair determining the structure of the VP; furthermore, no evidence of any selective pressure toward one hormone or the other could be found (67). It is not clear why the domestic pig has lost the arginine-VP gene, but it may be relevant to point out that only races of West-European descent have been examined so far. That this might be important is illustrated by a South American strain of mice that has also been reported to produce lysine-VP instead of arginine-VP (251).

The VP released at the neurohypophysis is synthesized in the supraoptic and paraventricular nuclei of the hypothalamus. As discussed above, its synthesis is coupled to that of the corresponding neurophysin and VP itself would actually be liberated from a prohormone within the neurosecretory granule as it travels down the axon. In the neurohypophysis, two pools of VP can be identified: a "readily releasable" pool of hormone, accounting for up to 10% of the total content of the gland, and a larger "storage" pool (185). The newly-synthesized hormone would first enter the readily releasable pool before equilibrating with the storage pool.

It was generally believed that the supraoptic and paraventricular nuclei were specifically dedicated to the production of VP and OT, respectively. Although there is a specialization in that direction, it is quite clear now that both nuclei secrete both hormones (254). In most species, VP-containing neurons seem to be concentrated in the more central part of the supraoptic nucleus and in the more medial part of the paraventricular nucleus (291). Virtually all neurons of the supraoptic nucleus contain neurophysins, but some (up to 25%) magnocellular neurons in the paraventricular nucleus seem not to contain any neurophysin. These neurons probably represent enkephalin-containing neurons, which have been found in the paraventricular nucleus and also in the supraoptic nucleus, and which project their axons to the posterior pituitary (207). Furthermore, it would seem that both VP and OT may be produced by the same cell (293) (For a detailed discussion of the distribution of the neuropeptides, see chapters 7 and 8).

In rats and mice, but not in monkeys or in man, VP and its neurophysin, but not OT, have been identified in the suprachiasmatic nucleus (266,293). This finding may be relevant to VP's function as a corticotropin-releasing hormone *(see below)*. The electrophysiological aspects of VP secretion are discussed in Chapter 2.

Stimuli to Vasopressin Secretion and Their Neural Mediation

Osmolar Control of Vasopressin

The main physiological function of VP is to control the renal excretion of water, and its secretion is constantly regulated by many factors, of which two are of major importance: plasma osmolarity and blood volume.

Plasma osmolarity is maintained within very narrow limits; in normal human subjects given a water load and then a hypertonic saline infusion, maximal water diuresis is seen at a plasma osmolarity of approximately 282 mOsm/kg, and the onset of antidiuresis at a plasma osmolarity of 287 mOsm/kg (166). Maximal antidiuresis is attained when plasma osmolarity rises to approximately 293 mOsm/kg (195). Experimental animals also show a similarly tight control of plasma osmolarity. To account for this remarkably sensitive control of plasma osmolarity, Verney (268) proposed that "osmoreceptors" are present in the forebrain, that they are sensitive to the osmolar concentration of body fluids, and that they control the release of antidiuretic hormone.

Much work has been done to find out where these osmoreceptors are located and which stimulus or stimuli they react to. Verney (268) had already established, by selective arterial infusion of hypertonic saline, that they were in the vascular territory of the internal carotid artery, although this has been challenged recently (17). Hypothalamic "islands," produced by total deafferentation, were used to demonstrate that the region immediately surrounding the supraoptic nucleus does contain osmoreceptors and can provide for apparently normal secretion of VP in response to hyperosmolarity (253,286). Hypothalamo-hypophysial explants in organ culture also maintain normal responsiveness to the osmolarity of the medium (248). These results, however, do not exclude that osmoreceptors may also be present in more remote locations.

That the osmoreceptors are not the VP-secreting magnocellular neurons has been shown, using electrophysiological recording techniques, by Hayward and Vincent (105). By electrophysiological (269) and intracranial injection techniques (182), osmoreceptor cells have been identified not only in the immediate paranuclear zone of the supraoptic nucleus but also elsewhere in the anterior hypothalamus. Furthermore, the latter (182) and another study (158) have provided evidence suggesting that the osmoreceptors for thirst and for VP secretion might be different and distinct.

However, one aspect remains controversial. The concept of the osmoreceptors, as proposed by Verney (267) and later elaborated on, implies that solute concentration, whatever the nature of the solute, is sensed by the intracellular dehydration that is induced in the osmoreceptors. Their molar efficiency should therefore depend on only two factors: their ease of diffusion across the bloodbrain barrier (to gain access to the osmoreceptors), and their lack of access to the intracellular space (to cause "cell shrinkage" by osmotically induced water shifts). Andersson and Olsson (4,5) have challenged this model. They have presented evidence suggesting that the osmoreceptors are in fact sodium receptors, monitoring the sodium concentration of the CSF and that this sodium receptor would depend on its $Na^+K^+ATPase$ activity (142,174). However, the two models are not necessarily mutually exclusive, and a dual sensing system may be involved (154).

Since the magnocellular neurons are not the osmoreceptors, they must receive their control information from the osmoreceptors by synaptic transmission. Among the classical neurotransmitters, acetylcholine activates the magnocellular neurons (56,57,167) and stimulates VP release (247); VP is also released by nicotine (103,109), while norepinephrine inhibits the magnocellular neurons *in vitro* (167), but may stimulate VP secretion *in vivo* (25,128). Finally, dopamine may stimulate VP secretion (25), although this has been challenged (118), at least in man. However, this tells us little about the nature of the neurotransmitters implicated in the transmission of information from the osmoreceptors to the magnocellular neurons. Very few well-designed studies are available wherein a physiological or physiological-like osmotic stimulus has been applied to animals pretreated with neurotransmitter antagonists in reasonable doses. Furthermore, the systemic administration of these antagonists usually leads to side effects (e.g., hypotension) and unrelated stimulations and inhibitions that render the interpretation of the results difficult if at all possible.

These problems can be partially circumvented by studying the hypothalamoneurohypophysial system in organ culture, since, as seen above, this preparation maintains normal responses to osmotic stimulation. In these conditions, VP release in response to osmotic and acetylcholine stimulation is blocked by hexamethonium but not by atropine (246). Furthermore, saralasin, a specific inhibitor of angiotensin II, blocks the osmotic stimulation of VP, but not the cholinergic or the nicotinic stimulations, whereas hexamethonium does not block the angiotensin II-stimulated response of VP (245,246). Angiotensin II has also been shown to excite neurosecretory cells of the cat and dog supraoptic nucleus (170,215), and has long been known to stimulate VP secretion, although it was usually thought to be implicated only in the hypovolemic stimulation of VP *(see below)*. These results imply that at least one interneuron and two neurotransmitters (acetylcholine and angiotensin II) are necessary to link the osmoreceptors to the VP-secreting neuron (Fig. 1).

One other point of interest in the osmolar control of VP is how the VP secretion is related to the osmolarity. The most generally accepted model proposes that above a certain "osmotic threshold," more and more osmoreceptors are activated as the osmolarity increases, and therefore, proportionally more and more VP is secreted (9,104,192). This model requires a population of osmoreceptors with randomly distributed levels of activation (above the osmotic threshold), and predicts a linear relationship between the plasma osmolarity and the VP secretion rate. However, the available data are equally well accounted for by a model based on an exponential relationship between the plasma osmolarity and plasma VP levels (205), and the controversy, although the minimal practical relevance, remains unsettled.

There also is some evidence for the existence of osmoreceptors in the splanchnic circulation (1), although there seems to be considerable species variation (219); furthermore, it is not clear whether or not the hepatic osmoreceptors are true osmoreceptors or sodium receptors (7,171). Preliminary data indicate

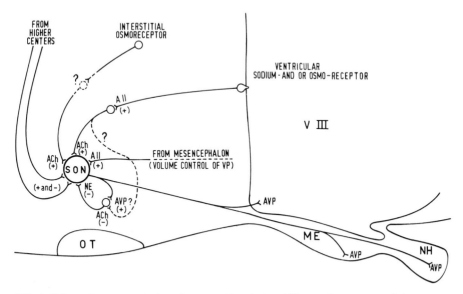

FIG. 1. Schematic representation of neuronal inputs to a VP-secreting magnocellular neuron in the supraoptic nucleus. The neurotransmitter and its action [excitatory (+) or inhibitory (−)] are indicated at each synapse. Question marks indicate postulated but not demonstrated neuronal connections or neurotransmitters. VP neurons in the paraventricular nucleus are presumed to have similar inputs. Abbreviations used: V III, third ventricle; ME, median eminence; NH, neurohypophysis; OT, optic tract; SON, supraoptic nucleus; A II, angiotensin II; ACh, acetylcholine; NE, norepinephrine; AVP, arginine-vasopressin.

that a splanchnic sodium intake monitoring mechanism would exist in man (30), although its relevance to VP secretion has not been studied.

Finally, it may be interesting to point out that VP, like many other hormones, may be secreted episodically in response to hyperosmolarity, particularly at high levels of stimulation (281).

Volume Control of Vasopressin

Although the minute-to-minute control of VP secretion is osmolar in nature, there is also a second control mechanism of major importance, dependent on the circulating or "effective" blood volume. Various receptors monitor the circulatory status of the organism and feed this information to the hypothalamus.

That hemorrhage could stimulate the secretion of VP was established as long ago as 1938 by Ryden and Verney (212), and much work has been done since then to identify the receptors involved and the parameters monitored. Unfortunately, much of this is difficult to interpret, since there seem to be considerable interspecies differences in the sensitivity and threshold of these receptors, and since many of the data have been obtained from anesthetized animals, with the obviously profound hemodynamic perturbations that this entails.

The first hemodynamic parameter to be influenced by a small to moderate hemorrhage is left atrial pressure. It has been shown that in both conscious and anesthetized dogs, a modest hemorrhage without any concurrent hypotension stimulates VP secretion, and that the plasma VP levels correlate well with central venous pressure (36,107,223). Atrial stretch receptors monitor left atrial pressure and increase their firing rate in proportion to the blood volume (94); this signal, sent via the vagi, would tonically inhibit VP secretion (225). Comparable results have been obtained in sheep (113) and in rats (58), but not in men (91), for whom normotensive hypovolemia seems to be very poor stimulus for VP (194).

Arterial baroreceptors also participate in the control of VP secretion. Receptors in the aortic arch (19,227) and, probably more importantly, in the carotid bodies (35,227,262,289) inhibit VP secretion on sensing hypertension and stimulate it on hypotension. The carotid bodies would sense a reduction of the pulse pressure rather than of the mean arterial pressure (229). The chemoreceptors of the carotid bodies will also stimulate VP secretion on hypoxemia (228,289), and this reflex may be relevant in cases of severe hemorrhage.

The pathways involved in the transmission of these signals to the hypothalamus are still ill-defined. Most data have been obtained from electrical stimulation techniques, providing valuable information on the central structures involved in the control of VP secretion but little on the origin of the physiological inputs to these structures. Stimulation of the vagal nuclei will release VP (27,125). The reticular formation, and more particularly the tractus solitarius, may also stimulate VP release (160,208); this has recently been corroborated by the finding of a neurophysin-containing pathway from the paraventricular nucleus to the nucleus solitarius (285), suggesting a negative feedback. Further rostrally, stimulation experiments have shown, for example, that the release of VP can be stimulated from nearly all the mesencephalon (111,125,208,287), but it has been impossible so far to identify one or more pathways as specifically carrying signals from the cardiovascular receptors to the hypothalamus, or even less so, to the magnocellular neurons.

Closely related to the volume control of VP is its possible stimulation by angiotensin II. It is well established that angiotensin plays an important role in the physiological control of thirst (for review, see reference 65); however, its function in the control of VP secretion is still controversial. This originates from the observation that centrally administered angiotensin II induces VP secretion and VP-dependent hypertension (20,110,116,221). However, peripherally administered angiotensin does not reliably stimulate VP if given in physiological doses (176,223,234). Nevertheless, it is quite clear that angiotensin may modulate the response to other, and particularly osmolar, stimuli of VP secretion (234), and that VP itself can inhibit the release of renin (222).

The osmolar and hemodynamic control mechanisms for VP secretion are generally described and studied separately. Osmolar stimuli undoubtedly provide most of the minute-to-minute control of VP, whereas hemodynamic stimuli may be seen as an emergency mechanism, capable of rapidly stimulating VP to levels far beyond those necessary for maximal urinary concentration into a range where it may have a relevant vasoconstrictor effect *(see below)*. That the hemodynamic control mechanism is insufficient in itself to adequately regulate VP secretion is dramatically demonstrated by the rare clinical cases of osmoreceptor dysfunction (52,96).

However, moderate hemodynamic perturbations without hypotension also modulate the osmotic stimulation of VP; for example, a hypovolemia of little or no consequence in itself to plasma VP levels will amplify the VP response to hyperosmolarity. Although in most conscious animals and in man, a hemorrhage of 10% to 20% of the blood volume is necessary to stimulate VP in the absence of an osmotic stimulus, the physiological significance of these modulatory influences should not be underestimated, since they come into play for such everyday occurrences as assuming the upright posture (194), as well as in more exotic circumstances, such as orbital flight (279). These interactions have been studied in detail in rats (58) and in men (165) and have recently been reviewed by Moses and Miller (164).

Other Stimuli to Vasopressin Secretion

Pain and stress have long been seen as stimuli to VP secretion (212). However, their exact role and significance are not clearly demonstrated. In rats, hypoglycemia (both insulin- and 2-deoxy-D-glucose-induced) markedly stimulate VP (11,12), but exposure to ether vapor, immersion in water, and intraperitoneal injection of normal saline—all procedures that markedly stimulate plasma corticosterone—fail to stimulate VP (23); ether and centrifugation stresses even reduce osmotically stimulated VP secretion (115).

Surgical procedures have been repeatedly demonstrated to increase plasma VP levels (162,236,261); however, it is obviously very difficult to distinguish, in the total response, the effects of blood loss, anesthetics and other drugs, and the surgical stress itself. This issue therefore remains controversial, although it has recently been suggested that painful conditions, in man, are associated with higher VP levels (117).

Emesis has been associated with considerable elevations of plasma VP levels (193). It is not clear whether or not this stimulus should be considered as nonspecific stress, although nausea, even when severe, is not sufficient to stimulate VP.

The influence of glucocorticoids on the secretion of VP has also been a controversial subject for more than 20 years. The well known impairment of water load excretion in adrenal insufficiency and its correction by glucocorticoids has led to the proposal of two theories. Some authors maintain that glucocorticoids inhibit VP secretion at the hypothalamic level (9), and others have proposed that the phenomenon could be explained by a direct renal effect (120).

The requirement, at the renal level, of glucocorticoids for a normal water diuresis has been clearly established by Green and coworkers (92) in Brattleboro rats; these animals with a hereditary VP deficiency are unable to excrete a water load normally if adrenalectomized. Also, VP levels are elevated in adrenalectomized dogs without replacement therapy, mostly in response to volume depletion and hypotension (230,231). However, in some circumstances, cortisol may be necessary to bring VP levels back to normal (257), either by modulating the hypothalamic control mechanisms or by attenuating the emotional response to stressful situations. Furthermore, recent data tend to demonstrate that VP hypersecretion may be a significant factor in the impaired water diuresis of adrenalectomized rats (220).

Recently, it has been suggested that VP secretion may be influenced by other hormones. Plasma VP levels and urinary excretion rates are elevated in hypothyroid patients and in thyroidectomized sheep (239,240,277), and thyrotropin-releasing hormone inhibits VP secretion *in vitro* (242) and *in vivo* (249). Other neuroactive peptides may also affect VP release, although most of the data are preliminary. For example, enkephalins, substance P, and neurotensin can stimulate VP after intraventricular injection, but probably via the induced systemic hypotension (241). Similarly, β-endorphin stimulates VP secretion *in vivo* but not *in vitro* from the neural lobe (282), and luteinizing hormone-releasing hormone and somatostatin stimulate VP release *in vitro* from the neural lobe (242). Sex steroids have also been shown to influence circulating VP levels (243,244,263). It is still too early to determine the relevance of these modulatory influences on the physiological (or pathophysiological) control of VP, but they may, with further research, completely change our present understanding of

VP control, entirely based on responses to plasma osmolarity, effective blood volume, and stress.

VP secretion is increased at night (for which we should be grateful), but without any clear relationship to electroencephalographic sleep stage (85,209). VP levels are also elevated in the human fetus during labor (34); whether this is in response to stress, or hypoxia, or hemodynamic modifications, or a combination of these and other factor(s) is not clear.

Effects of Vasopressin

Antidiuresis and Electrolyte Transport

Antidiuresis is certainly the best known and probably the most important effect of VP. The whole of the renal concentrating and diluting capability is controlled by VP in a relatively narrow range of plasma levels, from approximately 0.5 to 5 pg/ml, when the kidneys reach maximal urinary concentration. The importance of this effect for homeostasis is obvious, and for a discussion of its mechanism, the reader is referred to several excellent reviews (cellular basis of antidiuretic hormone action in mammalian kidney: reference 6; physiology of the mammalian antidiuretic response: references 16,216; effects of VP on electrolyte transport: reference 131; effects of neurohypophysial hormones on nonmammalian vertebrates: references 15,150).

Cardiovascular Effects of Vasopressin

VP is generally recognized as being a vasopressor peptide; it also indirectly reduces heart rate and aortic blood flow. However, it can also cause vasodilation, and its cardiovascular effects cannot be summarized in a few words. It is most important to point out that most of these effects are seen at physiological concentrations and that arginine-VP may have an important physiological function in vascular control in mammals. For further discussion, the reader is referred to recent reviews on this subject (3,168).

Vasopressin as a Corticotropin-Releasing Factor

Hypothalamic regulation of hypophysial hormone secretion was postulated more than 30 years ago (93); the hormones of the neurohypophysis were among the first to be examined as putative releasing factors. As early as 1952, it was suggested that VP might be involved in the release of ACTH (152).

VP can stimulate the release of ACTH from the anterior pituitary (214) and is present at high concentrations in the hypophysial portal blood (292). VP- and neurophysin-containing axon terminals are present in the zona externa of the median eminence (291) and there are indications that individual hypothalamic neurons innervate both the median eminence and the neurohypophysis (149,186).

That VP is not the only corticotropin-releasing factor (CRF) (53,189) is also clearly illustrated by the various studies of the Brattleboro rat. The ACTH response of these VP-deficient animals has been found to be normal (8) or impaired (153) but present, and they have CRF in their mediobasal hypothalamus, albeit in reduced quantities (127). It has also been suggested that VP, although not acting as a CRF in the strict sense of the word, would nevertheless be important in the control of ACTH secretion by acting as a potentiator of CRF (290). VP is also known to potentiate the adrenal response to ACTH (284).

This question is not yet resolved, particularly regarding the origin of the VP secreted at the median eminence [it has been suggested that it could be produced in the suprachiasmatic nucleus as well as, or instead of, in the magnocellular nuclei (235,265)] and the independence of the secretion of VP at the median eminence from that at the neurohypophysis. However, the concept of VP as a physiologically important CRF potentiator is gaining wide acceptance (29) and it has even been proposed that VP could be not an adjuvant but the basis of the CRF activity modulated and potentiated by other factors (87).

Other Effects of Vasopressin

VP, and possibly also other peptides, has a physiological role in memory processes and may also control some aspects of behavior. This function of vasopressin has been reviewed recently (50).

It has lately been proposed that centrally released VP may control brain capillary water permeability and thereby brain volume (188). VP injected in the CSF, but not systemically, increases brain water permeability, and the VP-containing axons projecting into the third ventricle (291) may be involved in this function.

Metabolism of Vasopressin

This subject has been extensively reviewed recently (132) and only a very brief outline will be given here.

The state of circulating VP is of great importance to its metabolism. This has been investigated with a great variety of techniques and, partly for this reason and partly because major differences seem to exist between various species, the results have often been contradictory (132). In normal human subjects, VP is not bound to plasma proteins and its distribution space is approximately equal to the extracellular fluid volume (10).

VP seems to be quite stable in whole blood and in plasma, although it is significantly degraded by serum and hemolyzed blood (260). The half-life of VP in plasma is variably estimated to be from 3 to 25 min. VP seems to be cleared from plasma not according to a single but to at least two exponential curves; determinations made at supraphysiological plasma levels may therefore be misleading. Most authors working at near-physiological levels in man agree to a half-life between 5 and 10 min (13,14,163,195). Although the results are not unanimous, the circulating half-life of VP does not seem to be affected by the state of hydration nor to be different in patients with diabetes insipidus.

The kidneys and the liver seem to be the two main organs responsible for the clearance of circulating VP. Their relative importance is unclear but each could account for 20% to 50% of the total clearance. Again, the results are widely divergent according to the blood levels used in the experiment. A fraction of the VP cleared by the kidney appears intact in the urine, and this fraction would be higher in patients with nephrogenic diabetes insipidus, raising interesting questions concerning the metabolism of VP in these and in normal subjects.

The plasma of pregnant women and primates (but not subprimate mammals) contains an enzyme capable of destroying VP and OT (260). This pregnancy oxytocinase appears soon after conception (as early as 2 weeks) and rises during the pregnancy, disappearing gradually after delivery. It is higher in twin and triplet pregnancies. This enzyme is not very active, even at term, when it reaches its highest levels, and the circulating half-lives of VP and OT are similar in pregnant women and in men. Its function, if it has any, is unknown. It is a rather nonspecific enzyme, capable of attacking other small peptides, such as angiotensin, and its role may not be related to OT or to VP. So far, its only known importance is as a hindrance in the assay of the neurohypophysial hormones from pregnant primates.

Assay of Vasopressin

Before discussing the assay methods for VP, one fact must be underlined. VP circulates at molar concentrations much lower than those of most hormones. For example, while insulin, in normal fasting subjects, is present in plasma at a concentration of approximately 1×10^{-10}M, and prolactin at approximately 5×10^{-10}M, a plasma level of 5 pg/ml of VP (a level sufficient to induce maximum urinary concentration) represents a molar concentration of only 4.6×10^{-12}M.

Bioassays of VP are based on essentially two methods, the so-called antidiuretic and vasopressor assays. The vasopressor assay, introduced by Dekansky (49), is no longer in current use, since it is quite insensitive (detection limit: approximately 1 mU or 2 ng); it is mentioned only because it is still the official standardization method of posterior pituitary extracts.

The antidiuretic assay remains the bioassay method of choice. It is based on the antidiuretic response of ethanol-anesthetized rats and was introduced by Jeffers and coworkers (112). It has since been modified and in good hands can reach a sensitivity of 1 μU (2 pg) or less, although an extraction procedure is usually necessary; details of the assay method have been reviewed (72,76,226).

Radioimmunoassays for VP were developed in the early 1970s. It was originally hoped that they would eliminate the problems of the bioassays; unfortunately, these hopes have not been completely fulfilled. The limit of sensitivity of most radioimmunoassays is comparable to, or only slightly lower than, that of the rat antidiuretic assay and an extraction is still necessary to assay from plasma. The radioimmunoassay has advantages in specificity, reproducibility, and convenience, but cannot be considered a "routine" radioimmunoassay, and the results obtained must always be examined with care. (For detailed reviews on the subject, see references 32, 193, 196, and 199.)

OXYTOCIN

Oxytocin is the second hormone of the neurohypophysis. It is chemically very similar to VP, differing by two out of nine amino acids (Table 1). Its existence, or rather, the existence of an oxytocic (43) and of a galactokinetic (175) substance in the posterior pituitary was recognized at the beginning of the century, and in 1953 it was the first polypeptide hormone to by synthesized (59,61,62).

The phylogenesis and chemistry of OT were discussed at the beginning of this chapter. The biosynthesis of the neurohypophysial hormones and their secretory processes have been studied mostly in relation to VP, but seem to be identical for the two neurohypophysial hormones (see the corresponding sections on VP).

One distinctive characteristic of OT-secreting neurons is their electrical pattern. VP and OT cells can be distinguished by their firing patterns after physiological stimulation, VP neurons being characterized by a phasic, or bursting, type of activity, and OT neurons by a brief, high-frequency discharge type of activity (26,55,100,187,275,276) (see also chapter 2).

Stimuli to Oxytocin Secretion and Their Neural Mediation

Before considering the various stimuli to OT secretion, it must be pointed out that OT is secreted in response to many stimuli classically considered to be specific to VP secretion. For example, homozygous Battleboro rats, which have a genetic deficiency of VP, have a reduced OT pituitary content, presumably due to hypersecretion, and they return to normal after a chronic VP treatment (264). OT is also secreted in response to dehydration, hypertonic saline infusion, and hemorrhage (54,283); this has also been corroborated by electrophysiological data showing that both OT- and VP-secreting magnocellular neurons are responsive to plasma osmolarity (26).

Suckling and the Milk-Ejection Reflex

Suckling is probably the only stimulus that will specifically release OT, normally without VP. This has been quite well established in rats (274), rabbits (18), and cows (140), but less so in humans. In response to suckling, to milking, or to other stimuli associated with suckling or milking, OT is secreted in one or more short bursts (37,39,75), and completes the efferent arc of the milk-ejection reflex. The milk-ejection reflex is essential if the young are to obtain milk on suckling in most mammals, including humans, cows, sows, cats, dogs, and rats, but not goats and sheep (256).

The pathways involved in the afferent arc have been studied for quite some time. Sensory nerves in the mammary gland are essential, as shown by experiments on transplanted mammary glands (147,148). Although in the human, milk ejection can be obtained despite local anesthesia of the nipple (255), conditioned reflexes may circumvent the lack of sensory input from the breast (70). From the dorsal roots, the afferent pathway runs ipsilaterally in the deep part of the lateral funiculus of the cord (63). In the midbrain and in the hypothalamus, the afferent pathway is diffuse and requires extensive lesions for its interruption (272). Both the supraoptic and paraventricular nuclei are involved in OT secretion (146), but lesions in the vicinity of the supraoptic nucleus will abolish it, since neurosecretory fibers from the paraventricular nucleus will also be interrupted.

As was mentioned above, OT is secreted in bursts or spurts, each lasting less than a minute. Although the mechanism of this periodicity is unknown, it seems to depend on a "neural trigger function," partially modulated by afferent inputs (mammary gland congestion and intensity of suckling) (145); in the rat it has been shown not to be dependent on a negative feedback of OT on itself (144).

There is, however, some evidence that α-adrenergic synapses are involved in this "neural trigger mechanism"; in the rat, α-adrenergic antagonists markedly inhibit the milk-ejection reflex and increase the interval between two successive milk-ejections (258). On the other hand, β-adrenergic receptors might mediate the stress-induced "central inhibition" of milk ejection (258).

Parturition

Oxytocin is extensively used in obstetric practice to induce and stimulate labor in parturient women; despite this, its role in physiological labor and delivery is unclear. In animals, plasma OT levels are low or undetectable during pregnancy and the first stage of labor, and are elevated only during the expulsive phase (2,33,81,95,121,156). VP may or may not be released simultaneously with OT, and this seems to be variable from individual to individual, as well as from one species to another (2,82,156).

In humans, OT levels are also low or undetectable during pregnancy; during labor, the pattern of OT release would also seem to be in spurts, just as in the response to suckling (33,86). The plasma OT levels reported in human during labor are considerably lower than in experimental animals, but these results are difficult to interpret, since many animal studies have been done using jugular vein blood samples.

The indirect data obtained in humans from the assay of neurophysins are in conflict with those obtained by direct assay of OT. Oxytocin-associated neurophysin plasma levels are elevated in pregnancy, as they are with estrogen administration, whereas OT itself is not, and show no further elevation at delivery (200), whereas the VP-associated neurophysin levels rise at delivery. This discrepancy may in part be accounted for by plasma pregnancy oxytocinase and by the short burst mode of OT secretion, but it remains disturbing.

Similarly, urinary OT excretion is not increased during labor (21), possibly because the spurt release of OT contributes little to the overall secretion. Furthermore, labor is more or less normal in women with diabetes insipidus, despite the presence of a confirmed deficit in OT (38,106).

OT and VP are also elevated in fetal blood at delivery, and are higher in umbilical artery than in umbilical vein plasma (33,34,130,135). This indicates that OT, and also VP, are secreted by the fetus and metabolized by the placenta or transferred to the mother.

The role of OT in physiological parturition is uncertain. Its use in obstetric practice shows beyond doubt that it is an efficient oxytocic, and yet it generally is undetectable in maternal plasma at the onset of labor. Conversely, alcohol is known to inhibit neurohypophysial hormone secretion (40,83,273) and is widely used in clinical practice, but its efficacy cannot be automatically ascribed to its hypothalamic effect, since it is also known to act at the uterine level and to inhibit prostaglandin-induced uterine contractions (114). There is little doubt that OT secretion by the mother is of great value in reducing the duration of the second phase of labor, and therefore of the period of anoxia for the fetus, but maternal OT would not seem to be involved in the onset of labor.

Oxytocin secreted by the fetus might be more important; OT can cross the placenta and stimulate the myometrium when administered from the fetal side (169). It is therefore not unreasonable to propose that fetal OT, accumulating in the amniotic fluid and/or secreted in ever greater quantities by the fetal neurohypophysis, could trigger parturition by acting directly on the myometrium, without appearing in significant amounts in the maternal circulation. Similarly, the VP secreted before and during labor may be an important trigger. As seen above, VP is an important CRF and it has been proposed that labor is triggered by increased cortisol secretion by the fetus (143). It might therefore be that the primordial trigger to parturition is neurohypophysial hormone secretion by the fetus. However, studies of OT and VP in the fetus before delivery are necessary to evaluate this hypothesis.

Other Stimuli to Oxytocin Secretion

Genital stimuli other than parturition will stimulate OT secretion in female mammals. Vaginal distension stimulates OT secretion; this neuroendocrine reflex, also known as Ferguson's reflex, was first described scientifically in 1938 (101), but has been known and used in dairy husbandry for untold centuries (74).

This reflex was examined and most convincingly ascribed to OT secretion by Debackere and Peeters (47,48). Ferguson's reflex is probably at the origin of OT secretion by the mother at parturition; it can be modified and even abolished by hormonal manipulations (48,191).

Oxytocin is also released during coitus; milk ejection has been reported during coitus in mares, cows, and humans (99,102) and antidiuresis (indicating vasopressin release) in women and rats (66,78). In the goat, OT levels have been measured in jugular vein plasma and have been found to be elevated during mating, but are not associated specifically with any phase of the mating process (155). In human females, also, OT has been shown to be elevated in peripheral plasma during coitus (77).

Coitus may also be a stimulus to OT and VP secretion in the male. Antidiuresis has been observed during mating in men and in rams (78,183) and OT secretion during genital manipulation in rams (48) and in bulls (232), but not in men during coitus (77).

Functions of Oxytocin

The only well established functions of OT are its milk-ejecting action in lactation and its oxytocic action in parturition. These two functions, discussed above, are undoubtedly of great importance for survival, since they are essential for the young to obtain milk and for the reduction of the period of anoxia at delivery. However, the fact that OT performs a known, useful function for only a few hours in a lifetime and in only one-half of the species (the female half) has led investigators to search for other roles for the peptide.

It has been proposed that OT may assist sperm transport in the female genital tract (98). Despite the fact that OT is released at coitus in the female mammal *(see above),* there is no clear evidence for any functional role of the hormone. Sperm transport has been found to be normal in female rats with diabetes insipidus induced by hypophysectomy (151); however, OT secretion was not measured in these animals and it is known to recuperate quite rapidly after hypophysectomy (54).

Oxytocin has been shown to increase ovarian contractility *in vitro* (250) and intraovarian pressure *in vivo* (204) in the rat, with a greater response on the day of proestrus in both cases. It was suggested that OT plays a role in follicular rupture, but this needs further confirmation.

In male mammals, OT has been reported to increase semen volume and sperm concentration and/or total number per ejaculate (73,119,123,124,271) as well as sexual drive (73). OT also stimulates contractions of the male genital ducts (122) and seminiferous tubules (108). However, to the author's knowledge, only one study has shown that the inhibition of OT adversely effects fertility (reduced number of spermatozoa per ejaculate) (233).

It has also been suggested that OT might act as a releasing factor for prolactin. This hypothesis has been infirmed and indeed, supraphysiological doses of OT inhibit the prolactin response to suckling in the rat (129).

At the renal level, OT has been found to be diuretic, antidiuretic, or natiuretic, according to the dosage and the experimental conditions (31); however, no physiologically significant effect could be demonstrated. Recently, it has been suggested that OT, with VP and other small peptides, may play a physiological role in memory processes and behavioral control (50).

The functions of OT and its analogs in submammalian vertebrates has been reviewed recently by Maetz and Lahlou (150) and by Bentley (15).

Metabolism of Oxytocin

The metabolism of OT is quite comparable to that of VP. OT at physiological concentrations seems to circulate free in plasma, although it could be bound to plasma proteins to some extent at supraphysiological concentrations in some species. The peptide, like VP, is stable in the plasma of nonpregnant mammals, but is inactivated by the plasma pregnancy oxytocinase of primates. The role of this enzyme, which increases the clearance of both neurohypophysial peptides by approximately 20%, is entirely obscure (see also the discussion of the metabolism of VP).

In all mammals studied (excluding pregnant primates), the half-life of OT in circulation is approximately 2 min; in one study in the rat, a second component with a half-life of approximately 15 min was demonstrated. Again, as in the case of VP, the liver and the kidney seem to be the main organs responsible for the clearance of OT, although the lactating mammary gland has a non-negligible importance. A very small portion of the cleared OT appears intact in the urine and, interestingly, the amount of OT excreted is proportional to the urine flow rate (22), so that the urinary concentration, and not the urinary content, of OT reflects the mean plasma concentration. For references and for further details on the metabolism of OT, the reader is referred to two excellent and exhaustive reviews (132,260).

Assay of Oxytocin

Oxytocin, like VP, circulates at very low concentrations and indeed, no method developed to date is capable of measuring basal unstimulated levels.

The bioassay of OT is usually based on the response of the uterus or the mammary gland of small mammals (for increased sensitivity), usually the rat or the guinea pig. The isolated rat uterus method, of which many variants have been described (72), can reach a minimum sensitivity of approximately 10 μU (20 pg) for the perfused everted organ method, and is usually preferred for its relative convenience and reliability. The assays based on the response of the mammary gland *in vivo* (measuring the milk-ejection pressure) are generally considered more specific for OT but less sensitive; using mammary gland strips *in vitro*, a very sensitive (approximately 1 μU-2 pg) but less specific assay can be obtained (71). The isolated pulmonary vein of the duck has also been used *in vitro* as the basis of an assay that is claimed to be more sensitive and more specific than the rat uterus method (71). All methods require a preliminary extraction procedure to obtain a satisfactory sensitivity and specificity.

Although the radioimmunoassay of oxytocin has provided an increase in specificity and convenience over the bioassay, it has not pushed the limit of sensitivity much below that of the best of the bioassays. The details of the assay are quite similar to those of VP and it also requires, in most cases, prior extraction. Most of the antibodies used for the radioimmunoassay of OT also seem to measure, to a variable extent, biologically inactive fragments, particularly in urine, thus leading to a dissociation of biological and immunological activities (32). VP radioimmunoassays seem to be more immune to this artifact.

ACKNOWLEDGMENTS

This review was written during the tenure of a research fellowship of the Medical Research Council of Canada; this support is gratefully acknowledged.

The author also wishes to thank Ms. Elena De Vincenzo and Ms. Matilde Daniotti for their expert secretarial help.

REFERENCES

1. Adachi, A., Niijima, A., and Jacobs, H. L. (1976): A hepatic osmoreceptor mechanism in the rat: Electrophysiological and behavioral studies. *Am. J. Physiol.,* 231:1043–1049.
2. Allen, W. E., Chard, T., and Forsling, M. L. (1973): Peripheral plasma levels of oxytocin and vasopressin in the mare during parturition. *J. Endocrinol.,* 57:175–176.
3. Altura, B. M., and Altura B. T. (1977): Vascular smooth muscle and neurohypophysial hormones. *Fed. Proc.,* 36:1853–1860.
4. Andersson, B. (1977): Regulation of body fluids. *Annu. Rev. Physiol.,* 39:185–200.
5. Andersson, B., and Olsson, K. (1977): Evidence for periventricular sodium-sensitive receptors of importance in the regulation of ADH secretion. In: *Neurohypophysis,* edited by A. M. Moses and L. Share, pp. 118–127. Karger, Basel.
6. Andreoli, T. E., and Schafer, J. A. (1977). Some considerations on the role of antidiuretic hormone in water homeostasis. *Recent Prog. Horm. Res.,* 33:387–434.
7. Andrews, W. H. H., and Orbach, J. (1974): Sodium receptors activating some nerves of perfused rabbit livers. *Am. J. Physiol.,* 227:1273–1275.
8. Arimura, A., Saito, T., Bowers, C. Y., and Schally, A. V. (1967): Pituitary-adrenal activation in rats with hereditary hypothalamic diabetes insipidus. *Acta Endocrinol. (kbh.),* 54:155–165.
9. Aubry, R. H., Nankin, H. R., Moses, A. M., and Streeten, D. H. (1965): Measurement of the osmotic threshold for vasopressin release in human subjects, and its modification by cortisol. *J. Clin. Endocrinol. Metab.,* 25:1481–1492.
10. Baumann, G., and Dingman, J. F. (1976): Distribution, blood transport, and degradation of antidiuretic hormone in man. *J. Clin. Invest.,* 57:1109–1116.
11. Baylis, P. H., Cunningham, M., and Robertson, G. L. (1978): Effect of 2-deoxy-D-glucose on plasma vasopressin in rats. *Program 60th Annu. Meeting Endocrine Soc.,* p. 189.
12. Baylis, P. H., and Heath, D. A. (1977): Plasma arginine vasopressin response to insulin induced hypoglycemia. *Lancet,* 2:428–430.
13. Beardwell, C. G. (1971): Radioimmunoassay of arginine vasopressin in human plasma. *J. Clin. Endocrinol. Metab.,* 33:254–260.
14. Beardwell, C. G., Geelan, G., Palmer, H. M., Roberts, D., and Salamonson, L. (1975): Radioimmunoassay of plasma vasopressin in physiological and pathological states in man. *J. Endocrinol.,* 67:189–202.

15. Bentley, P. J. (1974): Actions of neurohypophysial peptides in amphibians, reptiles, and birds. In: *Handbook of Physiology,* Section 7: Endocrinology; Volume 4: The Pituitary Gland and its Neuroendocrine control, Part 1, edited by E. Knobil and W. H. Sawyer, pp. 545–563. American Physiological Society, Washington, D.C.

16. Berliner, R. W. (1976): The concentrating mechanism in the renal medulla. *Kidney Int.,* 9:214–222.

17. Bie, P. (1977): Sustained water diuresis in anesthetized dogs: Antidiuresis in response to intravenous and bilateral intracarotid infusion of hyper-osmolar solutions of sodium chloride. *Acta Physiol. Scand.,* 101:446–457.

18. Bisset, G. W., Clark, B. J., and Haldar, J. (1970): Blood levels of oxytocin and vasopressin during suckling in the rabbit and the problem of their independent release. *J. Physiol. (Lond.),* 206:711–722.

19. Bond, G. C., and Frank, J. W. (1970): Effect of bilateral aortic nerve section on plasma ADH titer. *Physiologist,* 13:152.

20. Bonjour, J. P., and Malvin, R. L. (1970): Stimulation of ADH release by the renin-angiotensin system. *Am. J. Physiol.,* 218:1555–1559.

21. Boyd, N. R. H., and Chard, T. (1973): Human urine oxytocin levels during pregnancy and labor. *Am. J. Obstet. Gynecol.,* 115:827–829.

22. Boyd, N. R. H., Jackson, D. B., Hollingsworth, S., Forsling, M. L., and Chard, T. (1972): The development of a radioimmunoassay for oxytocin: The extraction of oxytocin from urine and determination of the excretion rate for exogenous and endogenous oxytocin in human urine. *J. Endocrinol.,* 52:59–67.

23. Brennan, T. C., Shelton, R. L., and Robertson, G. L. (1975): Effect of stress on plasma vasopressin and corticosterone in rats. *Clin. Res.,* 23:234A.

24. Breslow, E. (1975): On the mechanism of binding of neurohypophysial hormones and analogs to neurophysins. *Ann. N. Y. Acad. Sci.,* 248:423–441.

25. Bridges, T. E., Hillhouse, E. W., and Jones, M. T. (1976): The effect of dopamine on neurohypophysial hormone release *in vivo* and from the rat neural lobe and hypothalamus *in vitro. J. Physiol. (Lond.),* 260:647–666.

26. Brimble, M. J., and Dyball, R. E. J. (1977): Characterization of the responses of oxytocin and vasopressin-secreting neurones in the supraoptic nucleus to osmotic stimulation. *J. Physiol. (Lond.),* 271:253–271.

27. Brooks, C. M., Ushiyama, J., and Lange, G. (1962): Reactions of neurons in or near the supraoptic nuclei. *Am. J. Physiol.,* 202:487–490.

28. Burford, G. D., Jones, C. W., and Pickering, B. T. (1971): Tentative identification of a vasopressin-neurophysin and an oxytocin-neurophysin in the rat. *Biochem. J.,* 124:809–813.

29. Burlet, A., Chateau, M., and Czernichow, P. (1979): Infundibular localization of vasopressin, oxytocin and neurophysins in the rat; its relationships with corticotrope function. *Brain Res.,* 168:275–286.

30. Carey, R. M. (1977): Evidence for a splanchnic sodium input monitor regulating renal sodium excretion in man. *Program 59th Annu. Meeting Endocrine Soc.,* p. 119.

31. Chard, T. (1971): Recent trends in the physiology of the posterior pituitary. In: *Current Topics in Experimental Endocrinology, Vol 1,* edited by L. Martini and V. H. T. James, pp. 81–120. Academic Press, New York.

32. Chard, T. (1973): The radioimmunoassay of oxytocin and vasopressin. *J. Endocrinol.,* 58:143–160.

33. Chard, T., Boyd, N. R. H., Forsling, M. L., McNeilly, A. S., and Landon, J. (1970): The development of a radioimmunoassay for oxytocin: The extraction of oxytocin from plasma, and its measurement during parturition in human and goat blood. *J. Endocrinol.,* 48:223–234.

34. Chard, T., Hudson, C. N., Edwards, C. R. W., and Boyd, N. R. H. (1971): The release of oxytocin and vasopressin by the human foetus during labour. *Nature,* 234:352–354.

35. Chien, S., Peric, B., and Usami, S. (1962): The reflex nature of release of antidiuretic hormone upon common carotid occlusion in vagotomized dogs. *Proc. Soc. Exp. Biol. Med.,* 111:193–196.

36. Claybaugh, J. R., and Share, L. (1973): Vasopressin, renin, and cardiovascular responses to continuous slow hemorrhage. *Am. J. Physiol.,* 224:519–523.

37. Cleverley, J. D., and Folley, S. J. (1970): The blood levels of oxytocin during machine milking in cows with some observations on its half-life in the circulation. *J. Endocrinol.,* 46:347–361.

38. Cobo, E., de Bernal, M. M., and Gaitan, E. (1972): Low oxytocin secretion in diabetes insipidus associated with normal labor. *Am. J. Obstet. Gynecol.,* 114:861–866.
39. Cobo, E., de Bernal, M. M., Gaitan, E., and Quintero, C. A. (1967): Neurohypophysial hormone release in the human. II. Experimental study during lactation. *Am. J. Obstet. Gynecol.,* 97:519–529.
40. Cobo, E., and Quintero, C. A. (1969): Milk-ejecting and antidiuretic activities under neurohypophysial inhibition with alcohol and water overload. *Am. J. Obstet. Gynecol.,* 105:877–887.
41. Coculescu, M., Matulevičius, V., Goldstien, R., and Pavel, S. (1978): Presence and synthesis of vasotocin in the pineal gland of Brattleboro rats. *J. Endocrinol.,* 77:145–146.
42. Cort, J. H., Sedláková, E., Kluk, I., and Mulder, J. L. (1975): Neurophysin binding and natriuretic peptides from the posterior pituitary. *Ann. N.Y. Acad. Sci.,* 248:336–344.
43. Dale, H. H. (1906): On some physiological actions of ergot. *J. Physiol.,* 34:163–206.
44. David, G. F. X., Umberkoman, B., Kumar, K., and Kumar, T. C. A. (1975): Neuroendocrine significance of the pineal. In: *Brain-Endocrine Interaction II. The ventricular system,* edited by K. M. Knigge, D. E. Scott, M. H. Kobayashi, and S. Ishii, pp. 365–375. Karger, Basel.
45. Dax, E. M., Cumming, I. A., Lawson, R. A. S., and Johnston, C. I. (1977): The physiological release of specific individual neurophysins into the circulation of pigs. *Endocrinology,* 100:635–641.
46. Dean, C. R., Hope, D. B., and Kazic, T. (1968): Evidence for a storage of oxytocin with neurophysin-I and of vasopressin with neurophysin-II in separate neurosecretory granules. *Br. J. Pharmacol.,* 34:192P–193P.
47. Debackere, M., and Peeters, G. (1960): The influence of vaginal distention on milk ejection and diuresis in the lactating cow. *Arch. Int. Pharmacodyn. Ther.,* 123:462–471.
48. Debackere, M. Peeters, G., and Tuyttens, N. (1961): Reflex release of an oxytocic hormone by stimulation of genital organs in male and female sheep studied by a cross-circulation technique. *J. Endocrinol.,* 22:321–334.
49. Dekansky, J. (1952): The quantitative assay of vasopressin. *Br. J. Pharmacol.,* 7:567–572.
50. De Kloet, R., and De Wied, D. (1980): The brain as target tissue for hormones of pituitary origin: behavioral and biochemical studies. In: *Frontiers in Neuroendocrinology, Vol. 6,* edited by L. Martini and W. F. Ganong, pp. 203–218. Raven Press, New York.
51. Dellmann, H. D., and Simpson, J. B. (1975): Comparative ultrastructure and function of the subfornical organ. In: *Brain-Endocrine Interaction II. The Ventricular System,* edited by K. M. Knigge, D. E. Scott, M. H. Kobayashi, and S. Ishii, pp. 166–189. Karger, Basel.
52. De Rubertis, F. R., Michelis, M. J., Beck, N., Field, J. B., and Davis, B. B. (1971): Essential hypernatremia due to ineffective osmotic and intact volume regulation of vasopressin secretion. *J. Clin. Invest.,* 50:97–111.
53. Dhariwal, A. P. S., Antunes-Rodrigues, J., Reeser, F., Chowers, I., and McCann, S. M. (1966): Purification of hypothalamic corticotrophin-releasing factor (CRF) of ovine origin. *Proc. Soc. Exp. Biol. Med.,* 121:8–12.
54. Dogterom, J., Van Wimersma Greidanus, Tj. B., and Swaab, D. F. (1977): Evidence for the release of vasopressin and oxytocin into cerebrospinal fluid: Measurements in plasma and CSF of intact and hypophysectomized rats. *Neuroendocrinology,* 24:108–118.
55. Dreifuss, J. J., Harris, M. C., and Tribollet, E. (1976): Excitation of phasically firing hypothalamic supraoptic neurones by carotid occlusion in rats. *J. Physiol. (Lond.),* 257:337–354.
56. Dreifuss, J. J., and Kelly, J. S. (1970): Excitation of identified supraoptic neurones by iontophoretic application of acetylcholine. *J. Physiol. (Lond.),* 210:170P–172P.
57. Dreifuss, J. J., and Kelly, J. S. (1972): The activity of identified supraoptic neurones and their response to acetylcholine applied by iontophoresis. *J. Physiol. (Lond.),* 220:105–118.
58. Dunn, D. L., Brennan, T. J., Nelson, A. E., and Robertson, G. L. (1973): The role of blood osmolality and volume in regulating vasopressin secretion in the rat. *J. Clin. Invest.,* 52:3212–3219.
59. du Vigneaud, V. (1956): Hormones of the posterior pituitary gland: oxytocin and vasopressin. *Harvey Lect., 1954–1955:* 1–26.
60. du Vigneaud, V., Gish, D. T., and Kalsoyannis, P. G. (1954): A synthetic preparation possessing biological properties associated with arginine-vasopressin. *J. Am. Chem. Soc.,* 76:4751–4752.
61. du Vigneaud, V., Ressler, C., Swan, J. M., Roberts, C. W., and Katsoyannis, P. G. (1954): The synthesis of oxytocin. *J. Am. Chem. Soc.,* 76:3115–3121.
62. du Vigneaud, V., Ressler, C., Swan, J. M., Roberts, C. W., Katsoyannis, P. G., and Gordon, S. (1953): The synthesis of an octapeptide amide with the hormonal activity of oxytocin. *J. Am. Chem. Soc.,* 75:4879–4880.

63. Eayrs, J. T., and Baddeley, R. M. (1956): Neural pathways in lactation. *J. Anat.,* 90:161–171.

64. Ellis, H. K., Watkins, W. B., and Evans, J. J. (1972): Distribution of soluble proteins in the mammalian neurohypophysis and their cross-species reactivity with anti-neurophysin. *J. Endocrinol.,* 55:565–575.

65. Epstein, A. N. (1978): The neuroendocrinology of thirst and salt-appetite. In: *Frontiers in Neuroendocrinology, Vol. 5,* edited by W. F. Ganong and L. Martini, pp. 101–134.

66. Eränkö, O., Friberg, O., and Karnoven, M. J. (1953): The effect of the act of copulation on water diuresis in the rat. *Acta Endocrinol. (kbh.),* 12:197–200.

67. Ferguson, D. R. (1969): The genetic distribution of vasopressins in the peccary (Tayassu angulatus) and warthog (Phacochoerus aethiopicus). *Gen. Comp. Endocrinol.,* 12:609–613.

68. Ferguson, D. R., and Heller, H. (1965): Distribution of neurohypophysial hormones in mammals. *J. Physiol. (Lond.),* 180:846–863.

69. Ferguson, D. R., and Pickering, B. T. (1969): Arginine and lysine vasopressins in the hippopotamus neurohypophysis. *Gen. Comp. Endocrinol.,* 13:425–429.

70. Findlay, A. L. R. (1968): The effect of teat anasthesia on the milk-ejection reflex in the rabbit. *J. Endocrinol.,* 40:127–128.

71. Fitzpatrick, R. J. (1973): Oxytocin-measurement-bioassay. *In: Methods in Investigative and Diagnostic Endocrinology, Vol. 2A: Peptide Hormones,* edited by S. A. Berson and R. S. Yalow, pp. 694–704. North-Holland, Amsterdam.

72. Fitzpatrick, R. J., and Bentley, P. J. (1968): The assay of neurohypophysial hormones in blood and other body fluids. In: *Handbook of Experimental Pharmacology, Vol. XXIII: Neurohypophysial Hormones and Similar Polypeptides,* edited by B. Berde, pp. 190–285. Springer, Berlin.

73. Fjellstrom, D., Kihlstrom, J. E., and Melin, P. (1968): The effect of synthetic oxytocin upon seminal characteristics and sexual behavior in male rabbits. *J. Reprod. Fertil.,* 17:207–209.

74. Folley, S. J. (1969): The milk-ejection reflex: A neuroendocrine theme in biology, myth and art. *J. Endocrinol.,* 44:X–XX.

75. Folley, S. J., and Knaggs, G. S. (1966): Milk-ejection activity (oxytocin) in the external jugular vein blood of the cow, goat and sow, in relation to the stimulus of milking or suckling. *J. Endocrinol.,* 34:197–214.

76. Forsling, M. L., Jones, J. J., and Lee, J. (1968): Factors influencing the sensitivity of the rat to vasopressin. *J. Physiol. (Lond.),* 196:495–505.

77. Fox, C. A., and Knaggs, G. S. (1969): Milk-ejection activity (oxytocin) in peripheral venous blood in man during lactation and in association with coitus. *J. Endocrinol.,* 45:145–146.

78. Friberg, O. (1953): The antidiuretic effect of coitus in human subjects. *Acta Endocrinol. (Kbh.),* 12:193–196.

79. Friesen, H. (1964): Hypocalcemic effect of pituitary polypeptides in rabbits. *Endocrinology,* 75:692–697.

80. Friesen, H. (1964): Pituitary peptides and fat mobilization. *Metabolism,* 13:1214–1229.

81. Fuchs, A. R., and Dawood, M. Y. (1978): Oxytocin levels and uterine activity during parturition and lactation in rabbits. *Program 60th Annu. Meeting, Endocrine Soc.,* p. 188.

82. Fuchs, A. R., and Saito, S. (1971): Pituitary oxytocin and vasopressin content of pregnant rats before, during, and after parturition. *Endocrinology,* 88:574–578.

83. Fuchs, A. R., and Wagner, G. (1963): Effect of alcohol on release of oxytocin. *Nature,* 198:92–96.

84. Gainer, H., Sarne, Y., and Brownstein, M. J. (1977): Neurophysin biosynthesis: Conversion of a putative precursor during axonal transport. *Science,* 195:1354–1356.

85. George, C. P. L., Messerli, F. H., Genest, J., Nowaczynski, W., Boucher, R., Kuchel, O., and Rojo-Ortega, M. (1975): Diurnal variation of plasma vasopressin in man. *J. Clin. Endocrinol. Metab.,* 41:332–338.

86. Gibbens, D., Boyd, N. R. H., and Chard, T. (1972): Spurt release of oxytocin during human labour. *J. Endocrinol.,* 53:LIV–LV.

87. Gillies, G., and Lawry, P. (1979): Corticotrophin releasing factor may be modulated vasopressin. *Nature,* 278:463–466.

88. Ginsburg, M., and Ireland, M. (1966): The role of neurophysin in the transport and release of neurohypophysial hormones. *J. Endocrinol.,* 35:289–298.

89. Ginsburg, M., and Jayasena, K. (1968): The distribution of proteins that bind neurohypophysial hormones. *J. Physiol. (Lond.),* 197:65–76.

90. Ginsburg, M., and Jayasena, K. (1968): The occurrence of antigen reacting with antibody to porcine neurophysin. *J. Physiol. (Lond.),* 197:53–63.
91. Goetz, K. L., Bond, G. C., and Smith, W. E. (1974): Effect of moderate hemorrhage in humans on plasma ADH and renin. *Proc. Soc. Exp. Biol. Med.,* 145:277–280.
92. Green, H. H., Harrington, A. R., and Valtin, H. (1970): On the role of antidiuretic hormone in the inhibition of acute water diuresis in adrenal insufficiency and the effects of gluco- and mineralocorticoids in reversing the inhibition. *J. Clin. Invest.,* 49:1724–1736.
93. Green, J. D., and Harris, G. W. (1947): The neurovascular link between the neurohypophysis and adenohypophysis. *J. Endocrinol.,* 5:136–146.
94. Gupta, P. D., Henry, J. P., Sinclair, R., and von Baumgarten, R. (1966): Responses of atrial and aortic baroreceptors to non-hypotensive hemorrhage and to transfusion. *Am. J. Physiol.,* 211:1429–1437.
95. Haldar, J. (1970): Independent release of oxytocin and vasopressin during parturition in the rabbit. *J. Physiol. (Lond.),* 206:723–730.
96. Halter, J. B., Goldberg, A. P., Robertson, G. L., and Porte, D., Jr. (1977): Selective osmoreceptor dysfunction in the syndrome of chronic hypernatremia. *J. Clin. Endocrinol. Metab.,* 44:609–616.
97. Hanström, B. (1966): Gross anatomy of the hypophysis in mammals. In: *The Pituitary Gland, Vol. 1,* edited by G. W. Harris and B. T. Donovan, pp. 1–57. Butterworths, London.
98. Harris, G. W. (1947): The innervation and action of the neurohypophysis; an investigation using the method of remote control stimulation. *Trans. R. Soc. Lond. (Biol.),* 232:385–441.
99. Harris, G. W., and Pickles, V. R. (1953): Reflex stimulation of the neurohypophysis (posterior pituitary gland) and the nature of the posterior pituitary hormone(s). *Nature,* 172:1049.
100. Harris, M. C., Dreifuss, J. J., and Legros, J. J. (1975): Excitation of phasically firing supraoptic neurones during vasopressin release. *Nature,* 258:80–82.
101. Haterius, H. O., and Ferguson, J. K. W. (1938): Evidence for the hormonal nature of the oxytocic principle of the hypophysis. *Am. J. Physiol.,* 124:314–321.
102. Hays, R. L., and Van Demark, N. L. (1953): Effect of stimulation of the reproductive organs of the cow on the release of an oxytocin-like substance. *Endocrinology,* 52:634–637.
103. Hayward, J. N., and Pavasuthipaisit, K. (1976): Vasopressin released by nicotine in the monkey, *Neuroendocrinology,* 21:120–129.
104. Hayward, J. N., Pavasuthipaisit, K., Perez-Lopez, F. R., and Sofroniew, M. V. (1976): Radioimmunoassay of arginine vasopressin in rhesus monkey plasma. *Endocrinology,* 98:975–981.
105. Hayward, J. N., and Vincent, J. D. (1970): Osmosensitive single neurones in the hypothalamus of unanaesthetized monkeys. *J. Physiol. (Lond.),* 210:947–972.
106. Hendricks, C. H. (1954): The neurohypophysis in pregnancy. *Obstet. Gynecol. Surv.,* 9:323–341.
107. Henry, J. P., Gupta, P. D., Meekan, J. P., Sinclair, R., and Share, L. (1968): The role of afferents from the low-pressure system in the release of antidiuretic hormone during nonhypotensive hemorrhage. *Can. J. Physiol. Pharmacol.,* 46:287–295.
108. Hib, J. (1974): The contractility of the cauda epididymidis of the mouse, its spontaneous activity in vitro and the effect of oxytocin. *J. Reprod. Fertil.,* 36:191–193.
109. Husain, M. K., Frantz, A. G., Ciarochi, F., and Robinson, A. G. (1975): Nicotine-stimulated release of neurophysin and vasopressin in humans. *J. Clin. Endocrinol. Metab.,* 41:1113–1117.
110. Hutchinson, J. S., Schelling, P., Möhring, J., and Ganten, D. (1976): Pressor action of centrally perfused angiotensin II in rats with hereditary hypothalamic diabetes insipidus. *Endocrinology,* 99:819–823.
111. Ishikawa, T., Koizumi, K., and Brooks, C. M. (1966): Activity of supraoptic nucleus neurones of the hypothalamus. *Neurology,* 16:101–106.
112. Jeffers, W. A., Livezey, M. M., and Austin, J. H. (1942): A method for demonstrating an antidiuretic action of minute amounts of pitressin; statistical analysis of results. *Proc. Soc. Exp. Biol. Med.,* 50:184–188.
113. Johnson, J. A., Zehr, J. E., and Moore, W. W. (1970): Effects of separate and concurrent osmotic and volume stimuli on plasma ADH in sheep. *Am. J. Physiol.,* 218:1273–1280.
114. Karim, S. M. M., and Sharma, S. D. (1971): The effect of ethyl alcohol on prostaglandins E_2 and F_2 induced uterine activity in pregnant women. *J. Obstet. Gynecol. Br. Commonw.,* 78:251–256.
115. Keil, L. C., and Severs, W. B. (1977): Reduction in plasma vasopressin levels of dehydrated rats following ether stress. *Endocrinology,* 100:30–38.

116. Keil, L. C., Summy-Long, J., and Severs, W. B. (1975): Release of vasopressin by angiotensin II. *Endocrinology,* 96:1063–1068.
117. Kendler, K. S., Weitzman, R. E., and Fisher, D. A. (1978): The effect of pain on plasma arginine vasopressin concentrations in man. *Clin. Endocrinol. (Oxf.),* 8:89–94.
118. Kendler, K. S., Weitzman, R. E., and Rubin, R. T. (1978): Lack of arginine vasopressin response to central dopamine blockade in normal adults. *J. Clin. Endocrinol. Metab.,* 47:204–207.
119. Kihlström, J. E., and Melin, P. (1963): The effect of oxytocin upon some seminal characteristics in the rabbit. *Acta Physiol. Scand.,* 59:363–369.
120. Kleeman, C. R., Czaczkes, J. W., and Cutler, R. (1964): Mechansim of impaired water excretion in adrenal and pituitary insufficiency IV. Antidiuretic hormone in primary and secondary adrenal insufficiency. *J. Clin. Invest.,* 43:1641–1668.
121. Knaggs, G. S. (1963): Blood oxytocin levels in the cow during milking and in the parturient goat. *J. Endocrinol.,* 26:XXIV–XXV.
122. Knight, T. W. (1972): *In vivo* effects of oxytocin on the contractile activity of the cannulated epididymis and vas deferens in rams. *J. Reprod. Fertil.,* 28:141.
123. Knight, T. W. (1974): The effect of oxytocin and adrenalin on semen output of rams. *J. Reprod. Fertil.,* 39:329–336.
124. Knight, T. W., and Lindsay, D. R. (1970): Short- and long-term effects of oxytocin on quality and quantity of semen from rams. *J. Reprod. Fertil.,* 21:523–529.
125. Kogel, J. E., and Rothballer, A. B. (1962): Brainstem localization of a neurohypophysial activating system in the rat. *Fed. Proc.,* 21:353.
126. Krayer, O., Astwood, F. B., Wand, D. R., and Alper, M. H. (1961): Rate-increasing action of corticotropin and of α-intermedin in the isolated mammalian heart. *Proc. Natl. Acad. Sci. USA,* 47:1227–1236.
127. Krieger, D. T., Liotta, A., and Browstein, M. J. (1977): Corticotropin releasing factor distribution in normal and Brattleboro rat strain, and effect of deafferentation, hypophysectomy and steroid treatment in normal animals. *Endocrinology,* 100:227–237.
128. Kühn, E. R. (1974): Cholinergic and adrenergic release mechanism for vasopressin in the male rat: A study with injections of neurotransmitters and blocking agents into the third ventricle. *Neuroendocrinology,* 16:255–264.
129. Kühn, E. R., Krulich, L., and McCann, S. M. (1973): Influence of exogenously administered oxytocin on prolactin release in the lactating rat. *Neuroendocrinology,* 11:11–21.
130. Kumaren, P., Anandarangam, P. B., Dianzon, W., and Vasicka, A. (1974): Plasma oxytocin levels during human pregnancy and labor as determined by radioimmunoassay. *Am. J. Obstet. Gynecol.,* 119:215–223.
131. Kurtzman, N. A., Boonjarern, S. (1975): Physiology of antidiuretic hormone and the interrelationship between the hormone and the kidney. *Nephron,* 15:167–185.
132. Lauson, H. D. (1974): Metabolism of the neurohypophysial hormones. In: *Handbook of Physiology, Section 7: Endocrinology; Vol. 4: The Pituitary Gland and Its Neuroendocrine Control,* edited by E. Knobil and W. H. Sawyer, pp. 287–393. American Physiological Society, Washington, D.C.
133. Legros, J. J., Conte-Devolx, B., Rougon-Rapuzzi, G., Millette, Y., and Franchimont, P. (1977): Libération simultanée de vasopressin (A.D.H.) et de neurophysines lors de la perfusion de nicotine chez l'homme. *C.R. Soc. Biol. (Paris),* 171:478–483.
134. Legros, J. J., and Crabbè, J. (1978): Serum neurophysins in familial central diabetes insipidus. *J. Clin. Endocrinol. Metab.,* 47:1065–1072.
135. Legros, J. J., and Franchimont, P. (1972): Human neurophysin blood levels under normal, experimental, and pathological conditions. *Clin. Endocrinol.,* 1:99–113.
136. Legros, J. J., and Lefebvre, P. (1974): Lack of effect of human neurophysin I on the metabolism of rat adipose tissue. *Horm. Metab. Res.,* 6:83.
137. Legros, J. J., and Louis, F. (1973–4): Identification of a vasopressin-neurophysin and of an oxytocin-neurophysin in man. *Neuroendocrinology,* 13:371–375.
138. Legros, J. J., Louis, F., Demoulin, A., and Franchimont, P. (1976): Immunoreactive neurophysins and vasotocin in human foetal pineal glands. *J. Endocrinol.,* 69:289–290.
139. Legros, J. J., Louis, F., Grötschel-Stewart, U., and Franchimont, P. (1975): Presence of immunoreactive neurophysin-like material in human target organs and pineal gland: physiological meaning. *Ann. N.Y. Acad. Sci.,* 248:157–171.

140. Legros, J. J., Reynaert, R., and Peeters, G. (1974): Specific release of bovine neurophysin I during milking and suckling in the cow. *J. Endocrinol.,* 60:327–332.
141. Legros, J. J., Reynaert, R., and Peeters, G. (1975): Specific release of bovine neurophysin II during arterial or venous haemorrhage in the cow. *J. Endocrinol.,* 67:297–302.
142. Leksell, L. G., Lishajko, F., and Rundgren, M. (1976): Negative water balance induced by intracerebroventricular infusion of deuterium. *Acta Physiol. Scand.,* 97:142–166.
143. Liggins, G. C., Fairclough, R. J., Grieves, S. A., Kendall, J. Z., and Knox, B. S. (1973): The mechanism of initiation of parturition in the ewe. *Recent Prog. Horm. Res.,* 29:111–159.
144. Lincoln, D. W. (1974): Does a mechanism of negative feedback determine the intermittent release of oxytocin during suckling? *J. Endocrinol.,* 60:193–196.
145. Lincoln, D. W., Hill, A., and Wakerley, J. B. (1973): The milk-ejection reflex of the rat: An intermittent function not abolished by surgical levels of anesthesia. *J. Endocrinol.,* 57:459–476.
146. Lincoln, D. W., and Wakerley, J. B. (1974): Electrophysiological evidence for the activation of supraoptic neurones during the release of oxytocin. *J. Physiol. (Lond.),* 242:533–554.
147. Linzell, J. L. (1960): Transplantation of mammary glands. *Nature,* 188:596–598.
148. Linzell, J. L. (1963): Some effects of denervating and transplanting mammary glands. *Q. J. Exp. Physiol.,* 48:34–60.
149. LuQui, I. J., and Fox, C. A. (1976): The supraoptic nucleus and the supraoptico-hypophysial tract in the monkey (Macaca mulatta). *J. Comp. Neurol.,* 168:7–40.
150. Maetz, J., and Lahlou, B. (1974): Actions of neurohypophysial hormones in fishes. In: *Handbook of Physiology, Section 7: Endocrinology; Vol. 4: The Pituitary Gland and Its Neuroendocrine Control,* edited by E. Knobil and W. H. Sawyer, pp. 521–544. American Physiological Society, Washington, D.C.
151. Manabe, Y. (1969): Sperm migration in rats with experimental diabetes insipidus. *J. Reprod. Fertil.,* 18:371–373.
152. Martini, L. (1966): Neurohypophysis and anterior pituitary activity. In: *The Pituitary Gland, Vol. 3,* edited by G. W. Harris and B. T. Donovan, pp. 535–577. Butterworths, London.
153. McCann, S. M., Antunes-Rodrigues, J., Naller, R., and Valtin, H. (1966): Pituitary-adrenal function in the absence of vasopressin. *Endocrinology,* 79:1058–1066.
154. McKinley, M. J., Denton, D. A., and Weisinger, R. S. (1978): Sensors for antidiuresis and thirst-osmoreceptors or CSF sodium detectors? *Brain Res.,* 141:89–103.
155. McNeilly, A. S., and Ducker, H. A. (1972): Blood levels of oxytocin in the female goat during coitus and in response to stimuli associated with mating. *J. Endocrinol.,* 54:399–406.
156. McNeilly, A. S., Martin, M. J., Chard, T., and Hart, I. C. (1972): Simultaneous release of oxytocin and neurophysin during parturition in the goat. *J. Endocrinol.,* 52:213–216.
157. McPherson, M. A., and Pickering, B. T. (1978): Preparation of antisera to three individual rat neurophysins and their use for radioimmunoassays. *J. Endocrinol.,* 76:461–471.
158. Mendelsohn, J., Feinberg, L. E., and Berman, J. (1971): Dissociation of diencephalic mchanisms controlling water intake and water retention in the rat. *Am. J. Physiol.,* 220:1768–1776.
159. Milcu, S. M., Pavel, S., and Neascu, C. (1963): Biological and chromatographic characterization of a polypeptide with pressor and oxytocic activities isolated from bovine pineal gland. *Endocrinology,* 72:563–566.
160. Mills, E., and Wang, S. C. (1964): Liberation of antidiuretic hormone: Location of ascending pathways. *Am. J. Physiol.,* 207:1399–1404.
161. Moore, G. J., Swann, R. W., Fisher, A. W. F., and Lederis, K. (1978): A high molecular-weight substance in the supraoptic region of the rat hypothalamus which cross-reacts with a specific antiserum against arginine-vasopressin. *J. Endocrinol.,* 79:23P–24P.
162. Moran, W. H., Mittenberger, F. W., Shuyab, W. A., and Zimmerman, B. (1964): The relationship of antidiuretic hormone secretion to surgical stress. *Surgery,* 56:99–108.
163. Morton, J. J., Padfield, P. L., and Forsling, M. L. (1975): A radioimmunoassay for plasma arginine-vasopressin in man and dog: Application to physiological and pathological states. *J. Endocrinol.,* 65:411–424.
164. Moses, A. M., and Miller, M. (1974): Osmotic influences on the release of vasopressin. In: *Handbook of Physiology, Section 7: Endocrinology; Vol. 4: The Pituitary Gland and Its Neuroendocrine Control,* edited by E. Knobil and W. H. Sawyer, pp. 225–242. American Physiological Society, Washington, D.C.

165. Moses, A. M., Miller, M., and Streeten, D. H. P. (1967): Quantitative influence of blood volume expansion on the osmotic threshold for vasopressin release. *J. Clin. Endocrinol. Metab.,* 27:655–662.

166. Moses, A. M., and Streeten, S. H. P. (1967): Differentiation of polyuric states by measurement of responses to changes in plasma osmolarity induced by hypertonic saline infusions. *Am. J. Med.,* 42:368–377.

167. Moss, R. L., Dyball, R. E. J., and Cross, B. A. (1971): Responses of antidromically identified supraoptic and paraventricular units to acetylcholine, noradrenaline and glutamate applied iontophoretically. *Brain Res.,* 35:573–575.

168. Nakano, J. (1974): Cardiovascular responses to neurohypophysial hormones. In: *Handbook of Physiology, Section 7: Endocrinology; Vol. 4: The Pituitary Gland and Its Neuroendocrine Control,* edited by E. Knobil and W. H. Sawyer, pp. –442. American Physiological Society, Washington, D.C.

169. Nathanielsz, P. W., Comline, R. S., and Silver, M. (1973): Uterine activity following intravenous administration of oxytocin to the foetal sheep. *Nature,* 243:471–472.

170. Nicoll, R. A., and Barker, J. L. (1971): Excitation of supraoptic neurosecretory cells by angiotensin II. *Nature,* 223:172–176.

171. Niijima, A. (1969): Afferent discharges from osmoreceptors in the liver of the guinea pig. *Science,* 166:1519–1520.

172. North, W. G., Valtin, H., Morris, J. F., and La Rochelle, Jr., F. T. (1977): Evidence for metabolic conversions of rat neurophysins within neurosecretory granules of the hypothalamoneurohypophysial system. *Endocrinology,* 101:110–118.

173. Oliver, G., and Schäfer, E. A. (1895): On the physiological action of extracts of pituitary body. *J. Physiol.,* 18:277.

174. Olsson, K., Fyhrquist, F., Larsson, B., and Eriksson, L. (1978): Inhibition of vasopressin release during developing hypernatremia and plasma hyperosmolarity: An effect of intracerebroventricular glycerol. *Acta Physiol. Scand.,* 102:399–409.

175. Ott, I., and Scott, J. C. (1910): The action of infundibulin upon the mammary secretion. *Proc. Soc. Exp. Biol. Med.,* 8:48–49.

176. Padfield, P. L., and Morton, J. J. (1977): Effects of angiotensin II on arginine vasopressin in physiological and pathological situations in man. *J. Endocrinol.,* 74:251–259.

177. Pavel, S. (1965): Evidence for the presence of lysine-vasotocin in the pig pineal gland. *Endocrinology,* 77:812–817.

178. Pavel, S. (1975): Vasotocin biosynthesis by neurohypophysial cells from human fetuses. Evidence for its ependymal origin. *Neuroendocrinology,* 19:150–159.

179. Pavel, S., Dorcescu, M., Petrescu-Holban, R., and Ghinea, E. (1973): Biosynthesis of a vasotocin-like peptide in cell cultures from pineal glands of human fetuses. *Science,* 181:1252–1253.

180. Pavel, S., Goldstein, R., Ghinea, E., and Calb, M. (1977): Chromatographic evidence for vasotocin biosynthesis by cultured pineal ependymal cells from rat fetuses. *Endocrinology,* 100:205–208.

181. Peck, J. C., and Walkins, W. B. (1979): Identification of neurophysin-like proteins in the posterior pituitary gland of the chicken. *Neuroendocrinology,* 28:52–63.

182. Peck, J. W., and Blass, E. M. (1975): Localization of thirst and antidiuretic osmoreceptors by intracranial injections in rats. *Am. J. Physiol.,* 228:1501–1509.

183. Peeters, G., and Debackere, M. (1963): Influence of massage of the seminal vesicles and ampullae and of coitus on water diuresis of the ram. *J. Endocrinol.,* 26:249–258.

184. Pickering, B. T. (1968): A neurophysin from cod (Gadus morrhua) pituitary glands: Isolation and properties. *J. Endocrinol.,* 42:143–152.

185. Pickering, B. T., Jones, C. W., Burford, G. D., McPherson, M., Swann, R. W., Heap, P. S., and Morris, J. F. (1975): The role of neurophysin proteins: Suggestions from the study of their transport and turnover. *Ann. N.Y. Acad. Sci.,* 248:15–35.

186. Pittman, Q. J., Blume, H. W., and Renaud, L. P. (1978): Electrophysiological indications that individual hypothalamic neurons innervate both median eminence and neurohypophysis. *Brain Res.,* 157:364–368.

187. Poulain, D. A., Wakerley, J. B., and Dyball, R. E. J. (1977): Electrophysiological differentiation of oxytocin- and vasopressin-secreting neurones. *Proc. R. Soc. Lond. (Biol.),* 196:367–384.

188. Raichle, M. E., and Grubb, R. L., Jr. (1978): Regulation of brain water permeability by centrally-released vasopressin. *Brain Res.,* 143:191–196.

189. Ramirez, V. D., and McCann, S. M. (1964): Thioglycollate-stable luteinizing hormone and corticotrophin-releasing factors. *Am. J. Physiol.,* 207:441–445.
190. Reinharz, A. C., Czernichow, P., and Vallotton, B. (1974): Neurophysin-like protein in bovine pineal gland. *J. Endocrinol.,* 62:35–44.
191. Roberts, J. S., and Share, L. (1969): Effects of progesterone and estrogen on blood levels of oxytocin during vaginal distention. *Endocrinology,* 84:1076–1081.
192. Robertson, G. L. (1974): Vasopressin in osmotic regulation in man. *Annu. Rev. Med.,* 25:315–322.
193. Robertson, G. L. (1977): Vasopressin function in health and disease. *Recent Prog. Horm. Res.,* 33:333–374.
194. Robertson, G. L., and Athar, S. (1976): The interaction of blood osmolality and blood volume in the regulation of plasma vasopressin in man. *J. Clin. Endocrinol. Metab.,* 42:613–620.
195. Robertson, G. L., Mahr, E. A., Athar, S., and Sinha, T. (1973): Development and clinical application of a new method for the radioimmunoassay of arginine vasopressin in human plasma. *J. Clin. Invest.,* 52:2340–2352.
196. Robertson, G. L., Roth, J., Beardwell, C., Klein, L. A., Petersen, M. J., and Gorden, P. (1973): Vasopressin measurement radioimmunoassay. In: *Methods in Investigative and Diagnostic Endocrinology, Vol. 2A: Peptide Hormones,* edited by S. A. Berson and R. S. Yalow, pp. 656–668. North-Holland, Amsterdam.
197. Robinson, A. G. (1975): Isolation and secretion of individual human neurophysins. *J. Clin. Invest.,* 55:360–367.
198. Robinson, A. G., Ciarochi, F. F., Markovitz, B., Sinding, C., and Zimmerman, E. A. (1977): Rat uterus neurophysin—product of local synthesis? Program *59th Annu. Meeting, Endocrine Soc.,* p. 240.
199. Robinson, A. G., and Frantz, A. G. (1973): Radioimmunoassay of posterior pituitary peptides: A review. *Metabolism,* 22:1047–1057.
200. Robinson, A. G., Haluszczak, C., Wilkins, J. A., Huellmantel, A. B., and Watson, C. G. (1977): Physiologic control of two neurophysins in humans. *J. Clin. Endocrinol. Metab.,* 44:330–339.
201. Robinson, A. G., Michelis, M. F., Warms, P. C., and Davis, B. B. (1975): Biologic activity of neurophysin: Natriuresis. *Ann. N.Y. Acad. Sci.,* 248:317–323.
202. Robinson, A. G., and Zimmerman, E. A. (1973): Cerebrospinal fluid and ependymal neurophysin. *J. Clin. Invest.,* 52:1260–1267.
203. Robinson, A. G., Zimmerman, E. A., and Franz, A. G. (1971): Physiologic investigation of the posterior pituitary binding proteins neurophysin I and neurophysin II. *Metabolism,* 20:1148–1155.
204. Roca, R. A., Garófalo, E. G., Périz, H., Martino, I., and Rieppi, G. (1977): Influence of the estrous cycle on the action of oxytocin on rat ovarian contractility *in vivo. Fertil. Steril.,* 28:205–208.
205. Rodbard, D., and Munson, P. J. (1978): Is there an osmotic threshold for vasopressin release? *Am. J. Physiol.,* 234:340–342.
206. Rosenbloom, A. A., and Fisher, D. A. (1975): Arginine vasotocin in the rabbit subcommissural organ. *Endocrinology,* 96:1038–1039.
207. Rossier, J., Battenberg, E., Pittman, Q., Bayon, A., Koda, L., Miller, R., Guillemin, R., and Bloom, F. (1979): Hypothalamic enkephalin neurones may regulate the neurohypophysis. *Nature,* 277:653–655.
208. Rothballer, A. B. (1966): Pathways of secretion and regulation of posterior pituitary factors. *Res. Publ. Assoc. Res. Nerv. Ment. Dis.,* 43:86–131.
209. Rubin, R. T., Poland, R. E., Ravessoud, F., Gouin, P. R., and Tower, B. B. (1975): Antidiuretic hormone: Episodic nocturnal secretion in adult men. *Endocrine Res. Commun.,* 2:459–469.
210. Rurak, D. W., and Perks, A. M. (1976): The neurohypophysial principles of the western brook lamprey, Lampetra richardisoni: Studies in the adult. *Gen. Comp. Endocrinol.,* 29:301–312.
211. Rurak, D. W., and Perks, A. M. (1977): The neurohypophysial principles of the western brook lamprey, Lampetra richardisoni: Studies in the ammocoete larva. *Gen. Comp. Endocrinol.,* 31:91–100.
212. Ryden, H., and Verney, E. B. (1938): The inhibition of water-diuresis by emotional stress and by muscular exercise. *Q. J. Exp. Physiol.,* 27:343–375.

213. Sachs, H., Fawcett, P., Takabatake, Y., and Portanova, R. (1969): Biosynthesis and release of vasopressin and neurophysin. *Recent Prog. Horm. Res.,* 25:447–491.

214. Saffran, M. (1974): Chemistry of hypothalamic hypophysiotropic factors. In: *Handbook of Physiology, Section 7: Endocrinology; Vol. 4: The Pituitary Gland and Its Neuroendocrine Control,* edited by E. Knobil and W. H. Sawyer, pp. 563–586. American Physiological Society, Washington, D.C.

215. Sakai, K. K., Marks, B. H., George, J., and Koestner, A. (1974): Specific angiotensin II receptors in organ-cultured canine supraoptic nucleus cells. *Life Sci.,* 14:1337–1344.

216. Sawyer, W. H. (1974): The mammalian antidiuretic response. In: *Handbook of Physiology, Section 7: Endocrinology; Vol. 4: The Pituitary Gland and Its Neuroendocrine Control,* edited by E. Knobil and W. H. Sawyer, pp. 443–468. American Physiological Society, Washington, D.C.

217. Schäfer, E. A. (1909): Cronian lecture: Functions of the pituitary body. *Proc. R. Soc. Lond. (Biol.),* 81:442–468.

218. Schlesinger, D. H., Pickering, B. T., Watkins, W. B., Peek, J. C., Moore, L. G., Audhyo, T. K., and Walter, R. (1977): A comparative study of partial neurophysin protein sequences of cod, guinea pig, rat and sheep. *FEBS Lett.,* 80:371–373.

219. Schneider, E. G., Davis, J. O., Robb, C. A., Baumber, J. S., Johnson, J. A., and Wright, F. S. (1970): Lack of evidence for a hepatic osmoreceptor mechanism in conscious dogs. *Am. J. Physiol.,* 218:42–45.

220. Seif, S. M., Robinson, A. G., Zimmerman, E. A., and Wilkins, J. (1978): Plasma neurophysin and vasopressin in the rat: Response to adrenalectomy and steroid replacement. *Endocrinology,* 103:1009–1015.

221. Severs, W. B., Summy-Long, J., Taylor, J. S., and Connors, J. D. (1970): A central effect of angiotensin: Release of pituitary pressor material. *J. Pharmacol. Exp. Ther.,* 174:27–34.

222. Shade, R. E., Davis, J. O., Johnson, J. A., Gotshall, R. W., and Spielman, W. S. (1973): Mechanism of action of angiotensin II and antidiuretic hormone on renin secretin. *Am. J. Physiol.,* 224:926–929.

223. Shade, R. E., and Share, L. (1975): Vasopressin release during non-hypotensive hemorrhage and angiotensin II infusion. *Am. J. Physiol.,* 228:149–154.

224. Shade, R. E., and Share, L. (1975): Volume control of plasma antidiuretic hormone concentration following acute blood volume expansion in the anesthetized dog. *Endocrinology,* 97:1048–1057.

225. Share, L. (1968): Control of plasma ADH titer in hemorrhage: Role of atrial and arterial receptors. *Am. J. Physiol.,* 215:1384–1389.

226. Share, L. (1973): Vasopressin-measurement-bioassay and extraction from blood. In: *Methods in Investigative and Diagnostic Endocrinology, Vol. 2A: Peptide Hormones,* edited by S. A. Berson and R. S. Yalow, pp. 652–656. North-Holland, Amsterdam.

227. Share, L., and Levy, M. N. (1962): Cardiovascular receptors and blood titer of antidiuretic hormone. *Am. J. Physiol.,* 203:425–428.

228. Share, L., and Levy, M. N. (1966): Effect of carotid chemoreceptor stimulation on plasma antidiuretic hormone titer. *Am. J. Physiol.,* 210:157–161.

229. Share, L., and Levy, M. N. (1966): Carotid sinus pulse pressure, a determinant of plasma antidiuretic hormone concentration. *Am. J. Physiol.,* 211:721–724.

230. Share, L., and Travis, R. H. (1970): Plasma vasopressin concentration in the adrenally insufficient dog. *Endocrinology,* 86:196–201.

231. Share, L., and Travis, R. H. (1971): Interrelations between the adrenal cortex and the posterior pituitary. *Fed. Proc.,* 30:1378–1382.

232. Sharma, O. P., and Hays, R. L. (1973): Release of an oxytocic substance following genital stimulation in bulls. *J. Reprod. Fertil.,* 35:359–363.

233. Sharma, O. P., and Hays, R. L. (1976): A possible role for oxytocin in sperm transport in the male rabbit. *J. Endocrinol.,* 68:43–47.

234. Shimizu, K., Share, L., and Claybaugh, J. R. (1973): Potentiation by angiotensin II of the vasopressin response to an increasing plasma osmolality. *Endocrinology,* 93:42–50.

235. Silverman, A. J., and Zimmerman, E. A. (1975): Ultrastructural immunocytochemical localization of neurophysin and vasopressin in the median eminence and posterior pituitary of the guinea pig. *Cell Tissue Res.,* 159:291–301.

236. Sinnatamby, C., Edwards, C. R. W., Kitau, M., and Irving, M. H. (1974): Antidiuretic hormone

response to high and conservative fluid regimens in patients undergoing operation. *Surg. Gynecol. Obstet.,* 139:715–719.

237. Skowsky, W. R., and Fisher, D. A. (1977): Fetal neurohypophysial arginine vasopressin and arginine vasotocin in man and sheep. *Pediatr. Res.,* 11:627–630.

238. Skowsky, W. R., and Fisher, D. A. (1972): The use of thyroglobulin to induce antigenicity to small molecules. *J. Lab. Clin. Med.,* 80:134–144.

239. Skowsky, W. R., and Fisher, D. A. (1977): Arginine vasopressin secretion in thyroidectomized sheep. *Endocrinology,* 100:1022–1026.

240. Skowsky, R., Nielsen, T., and Fisher, D. (1974): Arginine vasopressin (AVP) kinetics in the thyroidectomized sheep. *Program 56th Annu. Meeting Endocrine Soc.,* p. 164.

241. Skowsky, R., Smith, P., and Swan, L. (1978): The effects of enkephalins, substance P, and neurotensin on arginine vasopressin (AVP) release in the unanesthetized rat. *Program 60th Annu. Meeting Endocrine Soc.,* p. 523.

242. Skowsky, R., and Swan, L. (1976): Effects of hypothalamic releasing hormones on neurohypophysial arginine vasopressin (AVP) secretion. *Clin. Res.,* 24:101A.

243. Skowsky, R., and Swan, L. (1977): Effects of androgens and estrogens on arginine vasopressin (AVP) in the rat and the human. *Program 59th Annu. Meeting Endocrine Soc.,* p. 241.

244. Skowsky, W. R., Swan, L., and Smith, P. (1979): Effects of sex steroid hormones on arginine vasopressin in intact and castrated male and female rats. *Endocrinology,* 104:105–108.

245. Sladek, C. D., and Joynt, R. J. (1978): Cholinergic involvement in the osmotic control of vasopressin release by the organ cultured rat hypothalamohypophysial system. *Neurology,* 28:366.

246. Sladek, C. D., and Joynt, R. J. (1978): Role of acetylcholine and angiotensin in the osmotic control of vasopressin release by the organ cultured rat hypothalamo-neurohypophysial system. *Program 8th Annu. Meeting Am. Soc. Neurosci.,* p. 356.

247. Sladek, C. D., and Knigge, K. M. (1977): Cholinergic stimulation of vasopressin release from the rat hypothalamo-neurohypophysial system in organ culture. *Endocrinology,* 101:411–420.

248. Sladek, C. D., and Knigge, K. M. (1977): Osmotic control of vasopressin release by rat hypothalamo-neurohypophysial explants in organ culture. *Endocrinology,* 101:1834–1838.

249. Sowers, J. R., Hershman, J. M., Skowsky, R., and Carlson, H. E. (1976): Effect of TRH on serum arginine vasopressin in euthyroid and hypothyroid subjects. *Horm. Res.,* 7:232–237.

250. Sterin-Borda, L., Borda, E., Gimeno, M. F., and Gimeno, A. L. (1976): Spontaneous and prostaglandin- or oxytocin-induced motility of rat ovaries isolated during different stages of the estrous cycle: Effects of norepinephrine. *Fertil. Steril.,* 27:319–327.

251. Stewart, A. D. (1968): Genetic variation in the neurohypophysial hormones of the mouse (Mus musculus), *J. Endocrinol.,* 11:XIX–XX.

252. Sunde, D. A., and Sokol, H. W. (1975): Quantification of rat neurophysins by polyacrylamide gel electrophoresis (PAGE): Application to the rat with hereditary hypothalamic diabetes insipidus. *Ann. N.Y. Acad. Sci.,* 248:345–364.

253. Sundsten, J. W., and Sawyer, C. H. (1961): Osmotic activation of neurohypophysial hormone release in rabbits with hypothalamic islands. *Exp. Neurol.,* 4:548–561.

254. Swaab, D. F., Nijveldt, F., and Pool, C. W. (1975): Distribution of oxytocin and vasopressin in the rat supraoptic and paraventricular nucleus. *J. Endocrinol.,* 67:461–462.

255. Theobald, G. W. (1959): The separate release of oxytocin and antidiuretic hormone. *J. Physiol. (Lond.),* 149:443–461.

256. Tindal, J. S. (1974): Stimuli that cause the release of oxytocin. In: *Handbook of Physiology, Section 7: Endocrinology; Vol. 4: The Pituitary Gland and Its Neuroendocrine Control,* edited by E. Knobil and W. H. Sawyer, pp. 257–267. American Physiological Society, Washington, D.C.

257. Travis, R. H., and Share, L. (1971): Vasopressin-renin-cortisol interrelations. *Endocrinology,* 89:246–253.

258. Tribollet, E., Clarke, G., Dreifuss, J. J., and Lincoln, D. W. (1978): The role of central adrenergic receptors in the reflex release of oxytocin. *Brain Res.,* 142:69–84.

259. Trygstad, O., Foss, I., and Sletten, K. (1975): Metabolic activities of human neurophysins. *Ann. N.Y. Acad. Sci.,* 248:304–316.

260. Tuppy, H. (1968): The influence of enzymes on neurohypophysial hormones and similar peptides. In: *Handbook of Experimental Pharmacology, Vol. XXIII: Neurohypophysial Hormones and Similar Peptides,* edited by B. Berde, pp. 67–129. Springer, Berlin.

261. Ukai, M., Moran, W. H., and Zimmerman, B. (1968): The role of visceral afferent pathways

on vasopressin secretion and urinary excretory patterns during surgical stress. *Ann. Surg.,* 168:16–28.

262. Usami, S., Peric, B., and Chien, S. (1962): Release of antidiuretic hormone due to common carotid occlusion and its relation with vagus nerve. *Proc. Soc. Exp. Biol. Med.,* 111:189–193.

263. Valiquette, G., and Martini, L. (1978): The effects of castration and aging on osmoregulation in the rat. *J. Steroid Biochem.,* 9:877–878.

264. Valtin, H., Sokol, H. W., and Sunde, D. (1975): Genetic approaches to the study of the regulation and actions of vasopressin. *Recent Prog. Horm. Res.,* 31:447–486.

265. Vandesande, F., De Mey, J., and Diericks, K. (1974): Identification of neurophysin producing cells. The origin of the neurophysin-like substance-containing nerve fibers of the external region of the median eminence of the rat. *Cell Tissue Res.,* 151:187–200.

266. Vandesande, F., Diericks, K., and De Mey, J. (1975): Identification of vasopressin-neurophysin producing neurons of the rat suprachiasmatic nuclei. *Cell Tissue Res.,* 156:337–342.

267. Verney, E. B. (1946): Absorption and excretion of water: The antidiuretic hormone. *Lancet,* 2:739–744; 781–783.

268. Verney, E. B. (1947): The antidiuretic hormone and the factors which determine its release. *Proc. R. Soc. London (Biol.),* 135:25–106.

269. Vincent, J. D., Arnaud, E., and Bioulac, B. (1972): Activity of osmosensitive single cells in the hypothalamus of the behaving monkey during drinking. *Brain Res.,* 44:371–384.

270. Vizsolyi, E., and Perks, A. M. (1969): New neurohypophysial principle in foetal mammals. *Nature,* 223:1169–1171.

271. Volgmayr, J. K. (1975): Output of spermatozoa and fluid by the testis of the ram and its response to oxytocin. *J. Reprod. Fertil.,* 43:119–122.

272. Voloschin, L. M., and Dottaviano, E. J. (1976): The channeling of natural stimuli that evoke the ejection of milk in the rat. Effect of transections in the mid-brain and hypothalamus. *Endocrinology,* 99:49–58.

273. Wagner, G., and Fuchs, A. R. (1968): Effect of ethanol on uterine activity during suckling in post-partum women. *Acta Endocrinol. (Kbh.),* 58:133–141.

274. Wakerley, J. B., Dyball, R. E. J., and Lincoln, D. W. (1973): Milk ejection in the rat: The result of a selective release of oxytocin. *J. Endocrinol.,* 57:557–558.

275. Wakerley, J. B., Poulain, D. A., and Brown, D. (1978): Comparison of firing patterns in oxytocin- and vasopressin-releasing neurones during progressive dehydration. *Brain Res.,* 148:425–440.

276. Wakerley, J. B., Poulain, D. A., Dyball, R. E. J., and Cross, B. A. (1975): Activity of phasic neurosecretory cells during hemorrhage. *Nature,* 258:82–84.

277. Waters, A. K. (1978): Increased vasopressin excretion in patients with hypothyroidism. *Acta Endocrinol. (Kbh.),* 88:285–290.

278. Watkins, W. B., and Ellis, H. K. (1973): The designation of the major guinea pig neural lobe protein as a neurophysin. *J. Endocrinol.,* 59:31–41.

279. Webb, P. (1967): Weight loss in men in space. *Science,* 155:558–560.

280. Weindl, A., and Schinkl, I. (1975): Vascular and ventricular neurosecretion in the organum vasculosum of the lamina terminalis of the golden hamster. In: *Brain-Endocrine Interaction II,* edited by K. M. Knigge, D. E. Scott, M. H. Kobayashi, and S. Ishii, pp. 190–203. Karger, Basel.

281. Weitzman, R. E., Di Stefano, J. J., III, Bennett, C. M., and Fisher, D. A. (1977): Episodic release of arginine vasopressin to osmotic stimulation. *Am. J. Physiol.,* 233:32–36.

282. Weitzman, R. E., Fisher, D. A., Minick, G., Ling, N., and Guillemin, R. (1977): β-Endorphin stimulates secretion of arginine vasopressin *in vivo. Endocrinology,* 101:1643–1646.

283. Weitzman, R. E., Glatz, T. H., and Fisher, D. A. (1978): The effect of hemorrhage and hypertonic saline upon plasma oxytocin and arginine vasopressin in conscious dogs. *Endocrinology,* 103:2154–2160.

284. Wiley, M. K., Pearlmutter, A. F., and Miller, R. E. (1974): Decreased adrenal sensitivity to ACTH in the vasopressin-deficient (Brattleboro) rat. *Neuroendocrinology,* 14:257–270.

285. Wilkins, J. Michaels, J., Nilaver, G., and Zimmerman, E. A. (1978): Hypothalamic pathways to the lower brainstem containing neurophysins, oxytocin and vasopressin in rat. *Program 60th Annu. Meeting, Endocrine Soc.,* p. 269.

286. Woods, J. W., Bard, P., and Bleir, R. (1966): Functional capacity of the deafferented hypothalamus: Water balance and responses to osmotic stimuli in decerebrate cat and rat. *J. Neurophysiol.,* 29:751–767.

287. Woods, W. H., Holland, R. C., and Powell, E. W. (1969): Connections of cerebral structures functioning in neurohypophysial hormone release. *Brain Res.,* 12:26–46.
288. Wuu, T. C., and Crumm, S. E. (1976): Characterization of porcine neurophysin III. Its resemblance and possible relationship to porcine neurophysin I. *J. Biol. Chem.,* 251:2735–2739.
289. Yamashita, H. (1977): Effect of baro- and chemoreceptor activation on supraoptic nuclei neurons in the hypothalamus. *Brain Res.,* 126:551–556.
290. Yates, F. E., Russel, S. M., Dallman, M. F., Hedge, G. A., McCann, S. M., and Dhariwal, A. P. S. (1971): Potentiation by vasopressin of corticotropin release induced by corticotropin-releasing factor. *Endocrinology,* 88:3–15.
291. Zimmerman, E. A. (1976): Localization of hypothalamic hormones by immunocytochemical techniques. In: Frontiers in Neuroendocrinology, Vol. 4, edited by L. Martini and W. F. Ganong, pp. 25–62. Raven Press, New York.
292. Zimmerman, E. A., Carmel, P. W., Husain, M. K., Ferin, M., Tannenbaum, M., Frantz, A. G., and Robinson, A. G. (1973): Vasopressin and neurophysin: High concentrations in monkey hypophysial portal blood. *Science,* 182:925–927.
293. Zimmerman, E. A., and Defendini, R. (1975): The distribution of neurophysin-secreting pathways in the mammalian brain: Light microscopic studies using the immunoperoxidase technique. *Ann. N.Y. Acad. Sci.,* 248:92–111.

The Endocrine Functions of the Brain,
edited by Marcella Motta.
Raven Press, New York © 1980

18

Clinical Aspects of Hypothalamic Disease

Lawrence A. Frohman

Division of Endocrinology and Metabolism, Michael Reese Medical Center and Department of Medicine, University of Chicago, Chicago, Illinois 60616

The earliest recognition of the role of the hypothalamus in the pathogenesis of endocrine-metabolic disorders was by Fröhlich (26), who described a teenage boy with obesity and hypogonadism attributed to a tumor in the region of the sella turcica that was compressing the anterior hypothalamus. Although the tumor was subsequently shown to be a chromophobe adenoma and the etiology of the gonadotropin deficiency was probably due to primary pituitary failure, the concept that central nervous system (CNS) disorders could produce alterations in endocrine function and in metabolic homeostasis antedated the development of neuroendocrinology as a discipline by at least three decades.

While other reports of patients with similar clinical manifestations appeared in the literature in a sporadic manner, it was not until 1959 that a work concerning series of endocrine disorders related to hypothalamic disease was published. In a now classic review, Bauer (6) described 60 cases of severe (and ultimately fatal) CNS disease with endocrine dysfunction, of which the most common disorders were diabetes insipidus and gonadal dysfunction, including hypogonadism and precocious puberty. Thyroid dysfunction was uncommon and disturbances of adrenocorticoid function or of growth were rare. It must be recognized, however, that the selection of patients was limited to those in whom pathology was demonstrated at autopsy, thereby excluding patients with nonlethal hypothalamic disorders whose endocrine disturbances were less severe. Since much of the current knowledge concerning hypothalamic-pituitary physiology was unknown at that time and assays for pituitary (and hypothalamic) hormones were virtually nonexistent, many of the reports were insufficiently documented to exclude the presence of pituitary disease, using current criteria. However, in some patients it was quite evident, as is now well recognized, that hypothalamic disease, in the absence of any demonstrable pituitary pathology, was responsible for the disturbances in endocrine function. Today, more than 20 years later, it is well accepted that disorders of anterior and pituitary function can occur on the basis of CNS disease. However, the distinction of hypothalamic (or other CNS) from pituitary disorders cannot always be made with certainty on either a clinical or a laboratory basis and endocrine therapy is frequently directed not at the primary hypothalamic disorder but at pituitary or target glands.

This chapter will review the pathophysiologic mechanisms and the clinical and laboratory features of endocrine disorders secondary to hypothalamic and other CNS diseases from both anatomic and hormonal considerations.

HYPOTHALAMIC DISEASES

The anatomic structure of the hypothalamus, like that of many other brain regions, exhibits a reticular organization. Some hypothalamic functions can be localized to a precise anatomic area (i.e., vasopressin synthesis is restricted to the magnocellular neurons of the supraoptic and paraventricular nuclei) (see Chapters 2, 9, and 17) whereas others are more widely distributed (i.e., temperature-sensitive neurons are found throughout large regions of the preoptic anterior hypothalamus as are neurons that regulate anterior pituitary function). Furthermore, neurons residing in a single region may subserve different hypothalamic functions (within the ventromedial nucleus there are neuronal populations that regulate both sympathetic pathways mediating pancreatic islet hormone secretion and hepatic glucose output as well as the stimulatory control of growth hormone secretion). Consequently, the location rather than the size of a hypothalamic region usually determines the extent of endocrine or metabolic disturbances.

Certain generalizations concerning hypothalamic disease can be made. Slowly growing lesions of the hypothalamus often will not produce symptoms until they reach considerable size (although exceptions do occur) whereas rapidly enlarging lesions, depending on their location, can produce dramatic clinical manifestations even when they are quite small. Acute destruction of the hypothalamus is responsible for most disturbances of consciousness, for sustained hyperthermia, and for severe disturbances of cardiovascular, gastrointestinal, or pulmonary function that can be related to hypothalamic disease. In contrast, chronic hypothalamic damage is generally manifested by alterations in cognition and complex homeostatic behavior involving neurometabolic regulation. Neuroendocrine control is altered primarily by chronic hypothalamic disturbances, but also by acute lesions that destroy a final common pathway (i.e., trauma to the median eminence or pituitary stalk). The complexity of the functions mentioned requires integration of the hypothalamus with various other neural regions and results in effector mechanisms involving neuroendocrine or autonomic nervous system-mediated pathways. In many instances the component parts of these symptoms can be shown to operate in the absence of an intact hypothalamus. However, the loss of the integrated functions of the hypothalamus resulting from chronic disturbances tends to cause alterations in normal regulatory tone or impaired responses to exteroceptive stimuli rather than in acute or severe fluctuations in consciousness, temperature, or autonomic discharge.

With the exception of sympathetic efferent pathways, hypothalamic neuronal projections in humans are not lateralized. Consequently, unilateral hypothalamic damage seldom causes significant or prolonged endocrine symptoms. Thus, disturbances of hypothalamic function are seen most commonly with infiltrative or inflammatory diseases that affect the region diffusely, with tumors that originate in the midline and expand bilaterally to affect predominately those structures adjacent to the third ventricle (paraventricular region) and in relation to diseases of the median eminence.

A summary of the causes of hypothalamic disease is provided in Table 1. The frequency of hypothalamic dysfunction due to each disease within specific age groups is listed in descending order. The anterior pituitary regulatory function of the hypothalamus is still immature at birth and as a consequence, some types of hypothalamic damage may not be clinically apparent in the newborn. In addition, numerous patients will exhibit disturbed neuroendocrine function unassociated with anatomic evidence of CNS disease. Many of these abnormalities have been attributed to disturbances of neurotransmitter function though proof that the abnormality involves the hypothalamus is lacking, as is, in most instances, the nature of the specific neurochemical defect.

Inflammatory Diseases

Sarcoidosis

Involvement of the CNS in sarcoidosis, although relatively uncommon, may appear at any time during the illness and exhibit either a self-limited or a progressive course. Infiltrative granulomatous nodules may be present in the pituitary, the stalk, or the hypothalamus. Manifestations of hypothalamic-pituitary dysfunction include polyuria and polydipsia associated with diabetes insipidus, galactorrhea due to hyperprolactinemia, and varying degrees of anterior pituitary insufficiency. Other evidence of hypothalamic involvement includes somnolence or hyperphagia, and hypopituitarism has been reported in a patient with a preserved anterior and posterior pituitary but with extensive hypothalamic involvement (69). Systemic manifestations of sarcoidosis usually facilitate the diagnosis and CSF abnormalities include elevated protein, pleocytosis, and decreased glucose levels. Steroid therapy has been reported to ameliorate the diabetes insipidus on occasion (70) but it is usually ineffective in reversing diabetes insipidus, galactorrhea, or anterior pituitary insufficiency, if present. Substitution hormone therapy is generally required.

Infiltrative Diseases

Histiocytosis X

This term is applied to a family of granulomatous diseases of unknown etiology. There are three clinical patterns observed: Hand-Schüller-Christian disease, the

TABLE 1. *Etiology of hypothalamic disease*

Neonatal period:
  Intraventricular hemorrhage
  Meningitis: bacterial
  Tumors: glioma, hemangioma
  Trauma
  Hydrocephalus, hydranencephaly, kernicterus

1 month–2 years:
  Tumors: glioma, especially optic glioma
    histiocytosis X
    hemangiomas
  Hydrocephalus, meningitis
  "Familial" disorders: Laurence-Moon: Bardet-Biedl; Prader-Labhart-Willi; etc.

2–10 years:
  Tumors: craniopharyngioma
    glioma, dysgerminoma, hamartoma, histiocytosis X, leukemia
    ganglioneuroma, ependymoma, medulloblastoma
  Meningitis: bacterial
    tuberculous
  Encephalitis: viral and demyelinating
    various viral encephalitides and exanthematous demyelinating
    encephalitides
    disseminated encephalomyelitis
  "Familial" disorders: diabetes insipidus, etc.
  Damage from nasopharyngial radiation therapy

10–25 years:
  Tumors: craniopharyngioma, pituitary tumors
    glioma, hamartoma, dysgerminoma
    histiocytosis X, leukemia
    dermoid, lipoma, neuroblastoma
  Trauma
  Subarachnoid hemorrhage, vascular aneurysm, arteriovenous malformation
  Inflammatory diseases: meningitis, encephalitis, sarcoid, tuberculosis
  Associated with midline brain defects: agenesis of corpus callosum
  Chronic hydrocephalus or increased intracranial pressure

25–50 years:
  Nutritional: Wernicke's disease
  Tumors: glioma, lymphoma, meningioma
    craniopharyngioma, pituitary tumors
    angioma, plasmacytoma, colloid cysts
    ependymoma, sarcoma, histiocytosis X
  Inflammatory: sarcoid
    tuberculosis, viral encephalitis
  Subarachnoid hemorrhage, vascular aneurysms, arteriovenous malformation
  Damage from pituitary radiation therapy

After 50 years:
  Nutritional: Wernicke's disease
  Tumors: sarcoma, glioblastoma, lymphoma
    meningioma, colloid cysts, ependymoma, pituitary tumors
  Vascular: infarct, subarachnoid hemorrhage
    pituitary apoplexy
  Infectious: encephalitis, sarcoid, meningitis

Modified from Plum, F. and Van Uitert, R. (1978): Nonendocrine diseases and disorders of the hypothalamus. In: *The Hypothalamus,* edited by S. Reichlin, R. J. Baldessarini, and J. B. Martin, pp. 415–473.

most common type, characterized by polyuria, exophthalmos, and skull defects; Letterer-Siwe disease, a much more rapidly progressive form; and eosinophilic granuloma, in which solitary bone lesions are found. When the CNS is involved, granulomas of the histiocytic type with eosinophilic elements occur in the tuber cinereum and in the hypothalamus and may be associated with diabetes insipidus, galactorrhea, or hypopituitarism similar to what has been described in sarcoidosis (3). Diabetes insipidus occurs in almost 50% of patients with histiocytosis X and the disease should be suspected in any child presenting with posterior pituitary insufficiency. Although 90% of patients will eventually develop skeletal lesions, most commonly in the skull, diabetes insipidus may exist as a solitary abnormality for several years. Growth failure due to growth hormone (GH) deficiency, hypogonadism, and panhypopituitarism are also seen, but less frequently and at a later stage of the disease. Hyperprolactinemia is common and some patients exhibit galactorrhea. The diagnosis is established by biopsy of a bone or an intracranial lesion. The course of the disease is generally good through the overall mortality is about 15%. Local disease is usally treated with curettage and radiotheraphy of bone lesions whereas the disseminated forms often respond to high dose glucocorticoids or chemotherapy utilizing alkylating agents. Pituitary hormone dysfunction, once established, generally does not respond to the above treatment (76).

Vascular Diseases

Ischemic and hemorrhagic lesions of the hypothalamus have been observed as a result of rupture of aneurysms of the anterior or posterior communicating arteries. Microhemorrhages in the supraoptic and paraventricular nuclei have also been noted (16). Impaired metyrapone responsiveness and a loss of diurnal rhythm of cortisol secretion has been reported in patients after subarachnoid hemorrhage, though there have been no studies of vasopressin secretion in such patients (39).

Internal Hydrocephalus

Patients with internal hydrocephalus can exhibit a variety of alterations in endocrine function including primary amenorrhea, oligomenorrhea, diminished dexamethasone suppressiveness, absent insulin hypoglycemia responsiveness, and panhypopituitarism (23,42). In some patients, correction of the hydrocephalus has been associated with disappearance of symptoms and reversion of the abnormal responses.

Tumors

The most common types of hypothalamic tumors originate from cell rests or developmental abnormalities and tend to be located in the region of the third ventricle. Craniopharyngiomas constitute the most frequent cell type, followed by astrocytomas and dysgerminomas. Most tumors occur in patients under 25 years of age though they have been observed as late as the seventh decade (4). The disturbances produced by these tumors are dependent on their location. Alterations in endocrine function are most commonly produced by tumors in the inferior portion of the third ventricle or the anterior mediobasal hypothalamus. Both anterior and posterior pituitary function can be altered though the increased frequency of diabetes insipidus in primary hypothalamic tumors helps in distinguishing them from pituitary tumors that extend into the suprasellar region and compress hypothalamic structures.

Nonendocrine aspects of hypothalamic tumors vary with the location of the tumor. Olfactory and visual disturbances are common with tumors in the anterior and ventromedial portion of the hypothalamus whereas internal hydrocephalus (caused by blockage of the foramina of Munro), dementia (due to interference with dorsomedial thalamic-frontal lobe pathways), and symptoms of increased intracranial pressure (papilledema, headache, nausea, and vomiting) are seen in association with tumors in the anterior and superior portion of the third ventricle. Tumors in the epithalamic or pineal region of the third ventricle cause disturbances of extraocular and pupillary muscle movements along with brainstem signs, whereas hydrocephalus, ocular nerve palsies, and cerebellar and pyramidal tract signs are seen with tumors located more posteriorly.

Craniopharyngiomas are benign tumors of congenital origin, frequently cystic, and histologically consisting of bands of interwoven epithelium, often similar to tumors of the enamel organ. The cysts frequently contain a brownish fluid with a high cholesterol content and calcifications develop in more than 15%. Tumor appearance may vary and the distinction between ependymomas and epidermoid cysts is often difficult. The tumors grow at a variable rate and may cease to grow entirely. Most originate in the midline at the upper end of the pituitary stalk though some are derived from lower portions of the stalk and about 15% are intrasellar in origin. Upward pressure of the pituitary stalk can displace the hypothalamus and third ventricle whereas downward pressure tends to compress both anterior and posterior lobes of the pituitary. A previous belief that craniopharyngiomas originated from remnants of Rathke's pouch has recently been questioned because of the infrequency of a primary intrasellar site and the rarity of the tumor along the embryonic migration tract through the sphenoid bone.

The production of endocrine disturbances by hypothalamic tumors is generally caused by destruction of those neural elements required for hypothalamic hormone secretion, resulting (with the exception of prolactin) in decreased pituitary function. On occasion, however, hypothalamic tumors have been associated with precocious puberty. One type of tumor, the hamartoma, appears to produce this effect not by destruction of neural tissue but a stimulatory effect. Hamartomas are masses of redundant partially disoriented glial and ganglion cells or a collection of normal nerve tissue lodged in an abnormal location. Those tumors associated with precocious puberty consist of encapsulated nodules attached to the posterior hypothalamus between the anterior portion of the mammillary body and the posterior region of the tuber cinereum. The neurons resemble those within the hypothalamus and contain membrane-bound secretory granules similar in size and character to synaptosomal granules in the median eminence. The vascular supply is usually from the posterior communicating artery and tumor vessels have the characteristic fenestrations of those in the median eminence that allow transport of neurosecretory products directly into the blood stream, with potential access to the pituitary portal system being provided by the vessels of the tuber cinereum. Although the mechanism whereby early sexual maturation is induced remains uncertain, it has been suggested that some neurons within the tumor could stimulate the hypothalamus or serve as accessory hypophysiotropic neurons with specific connections to the median eminence. Luteinizing hormone-releasing-hormone (LHRH) has been found in both cerebrospinal fluid and in the tumor itself (7,40).

Hypothalamic tumors are diagnosed by standard neuroradiologic and neuroophthalmologic procedures. Arteriography and pneumoencephalography are, with increasing frequency, being replaced by computerized tomography but may be necessary if surgical intervention is planned. The presence of atypical visual field defects (i.e., inferior rather than superior field loss) and normal sellar tomography in patients with pituitary insuffiency, particularly when diabetes insipidus is present, along with intact responses to hypothalamic releasing hormones, suggests a primary hypothalamic disease.

The treatment of hypothalamic tumors must be considered only partially successful at present. The location of the tumor frequently precludes its removal without sacrificing intact tissues critical for maintenance of normal homeostatic mechanisms. Since developmental tumors, particularly those that are cystic, tend to grow very slowly and may even undergo a spontaneous growth arrest, aspiration of cyst fluid will frequently relieve pressure symptoms for long periods of time. Marsupialization of the cyst into the CSF has also been effective in some patients. Radiotherapy of craniopharyngiomas appears to be a useful technique (45), particularly in adults, where surgical excision is less successful (4) than in children (57). Endocrine function, once lost, is rarely regained and permanent hormonal replacement therapy is required. An exception to this statement, however, is the "catch-up growth" occasionally observed in GH-deficient children after successful removal of a craniopharyngioma and that occurs without a return of normal GH secretion.

Trauma

Diabetes insipidus and panhypopituitarism occur in association with basal skull fractures secondary to transsection of the pituitary stalk. Impairment of the hypothalamic-pituitary-thyroid and gonadal axes has been reported in comatose patients with skull fractures with or without demonstrable subdural hematomas (41). Gonadal and thyroid function returned to normal with improvement of coma, though the use of high dose dexamethasone during the period of coma has made the etiology of these findings open to quesiton.

Growth deficiency is also beginning to be recognized in children who are victims of child abuse. It remains to be determined whether the GH deficiency observed is the permanent result of hypothalamic injury or is recoverable, as seen in psychosocial dwarfism (discussed later in this chapter).

Radiation-Induced Disorders

The use of radiation therapy for the treatment of intracranial neoplasms (pituitary tumors, gliomas, ependymomas, medulloblastomas) and for carcinomas of the nasopharynx and maxillary sinus has been followed by the development of signs and symptoms of hypopituitarism with an interval of 1 to 10 years or possibly longer. Growth failure associated with reduced GH responses, hypogonadotropic hypogonadism, and hypothyroidism have been observed and in some patients, preservation of LHRH and thyrotropin-releasing hormone (TRH) responsiveness has indicated the site of the abnormality to be the hypothalamus. The critical dose appears to be about 4,000 rads and children appear to be more susceptible than do adults (62). In addition to the endocrine dysfunction, papilledema, dementia, and localized neurologic signs provide evidence of radiation damage. A commonly used practice of prophylactic head irradiation (2,400 rads) in children with CNS leukemia has not been associated with significant neurologic dysfunction, though studies of neuroendocrine function are limited. The only available therapy involves hormonal replacement.

DISTURBANCES OF NEUROENDOCRINE FUNCTION DUE TO HYPOTHALAMIC DISEASE

Neuroendocrine dysfunction in man is manifested by quantitative or qualitative alterations in pituitary and target organ gland hormone secretion. The earliest descriptions of endocrine abnormalities associated with hypothalamic tumors (6) focused on diabetes insipidus and gonadal dysfunction. Decreased pituitary hormone secretion resulting from impaired hypothalamic hormone secretion can mimic primary hypopituitarism although the extent of impairment is generally less than with primary pituitary disease. Panhypopituitarism has, however, been reported in a patient with a histologically normal pituitary and two small areas of hemorrhagic necrosis adjacent to the third ventricle, just above the median eminence (30). Increased pituitary hormone secretion occurs primarily in relation to GH, prolactin, ACTH, and vasopressin, and differentiation from primary pituitary disorders is also not always possible.

The increased understanding of hypothalamic control of anterior pituitary hormone secretion has resulted in an appreciation that abnormalities of neuroendocrine function may be manifested by altered feedback, stress-induced release, or circadian periodicity, which are less apparent clinically, rather than by changes in basal hormone levels. Thus, abnormalities in hypothalamic-pituitary regulation can occur without overt clinical evidence of endocrine dysfunction. Alterations in plasma cortisol circadian rhythm, for example, are often seen in patients with hypothalamic or limbic system lesions but not with disorders of other areas of the CNS (46).

The differential diagnosis of hypothalamic and pituitary disorders has been greatly aided by the availability of the hypothalamic releasing hormones TRH and LHRH, which has permitted evaluation of the pituitary hormone secretory capability independent of hypothalamic input. With increasing use of these peptides, however, a previously unexpected complexity in the normal hypothalamic-pituitary control has been recognized and the ability to distinguish between hypothalamic and pituitary disorders on the basis of the responses to releasing hormones is less than complete. The following section will describe those clinically recognized disturbances in neuroendocrine regulation though, for many of the examples, evidence for a specific hypothalamic disease is lacking. The details of hypothalamic pituitary testing will be found in Chapter 19.

Adrenocorticotropic Hormone

Hypofunction

Diminished ACTH secretion secondary to hypothalamic or other CNS dysfunction is less common than that of the other anterior pituitary hormones for reasons not entirely clear. Relative adrenal insufficiency can occur in association with each of the hypothalamic disorders described above. It is also seen in the absence of any recognized disease as an isolated hormonal deficiency or in association with impaired secretion of other anterior pituitary hormones, usually in children. Because corticotropin-releasing factor (CRF) is unavailable for clinical use, differentiation between hypothalamic and pituitary disorders cannot generally be made with certainty. However, the presence of intact pituitary hormone responses to TRH and LHRH in children with idiopathic hypopituitarism implies a hypothalamic etiology for the deficiency of ACTH as well. In some patients, the preservation of ACTH (or cortisol) response to vasopressin, which has CRF-like activity together with the absence of a response to insulin hypoglycemia (which requires an intact hypothalamic-pituitary axis) can be used as evidence for a primary hypothalamic disorder.

Qualitatively Altered Function

Disturbances of circadian rhythmicity of ACTH secretion and of glucocorticoid suppressibility of ACTH are common in patients with intracranial diseases or severe behavioral disturbances and reflect early deficiencies in neuroendocrine control mechanisms. These changes are not recognized to be of major clinical significance, but subtle effects on behavior cannot be excluded.

Hyperfunction: Cushing's Disease

The association of bilateral adrenocortical hyperplasia and the clinical features of excessive cortisol secretion with pituitary adenomas was first described by Cushing (19). The small tumor size and the infrequency with which they were detected at the time patients presented with manifestations of adrenal hyperplasia resulted in attention being focused on the adrenal cortex as the cite of the primary disease. The recent results obtained at transsphenoidal surgery have indicated, however, that ACTH-secreting pituitary tumors are present in nearly all patients with Cushing's disease. The appearance of pituitary tumors after bilateral adrenalectomy in patients with Cushing's disease, first described by Nelson et al. (61), suggested that the development of an ACTH-secreting tumor could occur as a consequence of adrenalectomy. At the same time, demonstration of a variety of neuroendocrine disturbances in patients with Cushing's disease have raised the possibility of a CNS etiology.

The clinical features of ACTH-secreting tumors include those related to adrenocortical hyperplasia and excessive cortisol secretion, and those involving extraadrenal effects of ACTH and associated peptides. The major features of hypercortisolemia include centripetal obesity, hypertension, diabetes, amenorrhea, hirsutism, acne, osteoporosis and compression fractures, muscular wasting, violaceous striae, capillary fragility, impaired wound healing, decreased resistance to infection, and behavioral changes.

The increased secretion of ACTH, β-LPH, and possibly other peptides results in increased pigmentation similar to that seen in Addison's disease. Skin darkening occurs over the pressure points (knees, elbows, knuckles) and in the areoli, genitalia, mucous membranes, and at sites of new scar formation. ACTH secretion by pituitary tumors is not autonomous but is partially suppressed by hypercortisolemia. Hyperpigmentation, therefore, is not pronounced in the early stages of the disease but is prominent after adrenalectomy when ACTH levels increase markedly. Although ACTH fragments and endorphins exert pronounced CNS effects, behavioral changes that occur in patients with Cushing's disease (euphoria, decreased sleep requirement, and psychoses) can be explained by the elevated cortisol levels inasmuch as they are corrected after bilateral adrenalectomy.

Plasma ACTH values are increased in about half of patients with Cushing's disease (74) and diurnal variation is absent. Even the values in the normal range are relatively elevated in relation to the circulating levels of cortisol. Morning plasma cortisol levels are elevated in most but not all patients with Cushing's disease. Because of the absence of diurnal variation in plasma cortisol, elevated levels are more readily recognized in the late afternoon. The 24-hr urinary free cortisol level is the most useful urine measurement for distinguishing between normal and increased adrenocortical function (21).

The most reliable procedure for distinguishing between normals, Cushing's disease, and adrenal tumors relates to the alteration in the negative feedback control of the hypothalamic-pituitary-adrenal axis. The dexamethasone suppression test, either as a single overnight dose or as the standard serial 24-hr urine test, provides characteristic findings in Cushing's disease patients who exhibit impaired suppression of cortisol secretion with the low dose and at least 50% suppression with the high dose. Infrequently, patients with ACTH-secreting tumors will not suppress with the high dose (15). The cortisol response to exogenous ACTH is increased as is the adrenocortical response to interruption of the cortisol feedback with metyrapone. In contrast, the cortisol response to insulin hypoglycemia is diminished.

Tomography of the sella often provides evidence of localized bony erosion, though 40% of patients have normal findings and in patients with radiologic changes, the tumor location may not correspond to that of the abnormality (74).

ACTH-secreting pituitary tumors are present in approximately 80% of patients with hypercortisolemia. The differential diagnosis includes adrenocortical tumors, the ectopic ACTH syndrome caused by nonendocrine neoplasms that secrete ACTH of CRF, and patients with some clinical features of the disease but normal hormonal secretion. Loss of periodicity of cortisol secretion and glucocorticoid suppressibility as well as mild elevations of plasma cortisol are often seen in patients under stress, during periods of bereavement, and with depressive illnesses. It may be possible to distinguish such patients from those with classical Cushing's disease on a biochemical basis, though the clinical features of the disease are generally absent.

The etiology of Cushing's disease is still open to question. The major abnormalities seen in this disorder may be explained by functional alterations in hypothalamic control mechanisms that regulate periodicity, stress responsiveness, and the set point at which glucocorticoid suppression occurs (47). The hypothesis of a hypothalamic etiology is supported by the presence of lesions at autopsy in the paraventricular and supraoptic hypothalamic nuclei (36) and the association of Cushing's disease with CNS tumors and increased intracranial pressure in which symptoms have regressed after tumor removal. In pituitaries removed transsphenoidally for treatment of Cushing's disease, Lüdecke et al. (53) found tumors in 73% and diffuse or nodular corticotrope hyperplasia in 87%. The similarity between the loss of ACTH periodicity and glucocorticoid suppressibility in Cushing's disease and that occurring in primary CNS disorders suggests a common etiology mediated by increased CRF secretion and similar findings in CRF-producing lung tumors support this concept. Alterations in other periodic phenomena also suggest primary CNS disturbances. The loss of GH and cortisol periodicity and the decrease in slow wave sleep that occur in patients with active Cushing's disease are corrected by normalization of cortisol levels after surgery in only some patients (48,50). Finally, the responses of some patients with Cushing's disease to neuropharmacological agents such as the serotonin antagonist, cyproheptadine (49), which has been reported to alter CNS control of ACTH secretion in animals, provide additional strong support for a primary CNS abnormality.

The major argument for a pituitary origin of Cushing's disease has been based on the results of transsphenoidal surgery that, when successful, lead to an initial deficiency of ACTH secretion followed by a recovery of the hypothalamic-pituitary-adrenal axis (8,9,51,74). The impairment of ACTH secretion is presumed to be secondary to suppression of normal corticotropes by the ACTH-secreting tumor analogous to that seen after removal of an adrenocortical adenoma. In these patients the re-establishment of cortisol secretion, normal periodicity, and glucocorticoid suppressibility argues for a pituitary origin of the disease. The difficulty in reconciling the two arguments relates to the limited numbers of patients treated by the various methods and the relatively short duration of follow-up in most patients. It is possible that two varieties of Cushing's disease exist, one of pituitary origin and the other secondary to excessive hypothalamic CRF secretion.

ACTH-secreting pituitary tumors, irrespective of size, providing the clearest indication for definitive therapy of all the hyperfunctioning pituitary tumors because of the problems associated with prolonged adrenocortical hypersecretion. Although considerable success has been achieved with bilateral total adrenalectomy, the need for permanent replacement therapy with cortisone limits the enthusiasm for this procedure. The current procedure of choice is that of a transsphenoidal adenomectomy of the pituitary tumor (53,68,74). Up to 2 years may be required for recovery of the hypothalamic-pituitary-adrenal axis, during which time glucocorticoid replacement therapy may be required. Cure rates, based on postoperative reduction of cortisol hypersecretion, have in some series reached 90%. The results in patients with Nelson's syndrome, in whom large tumors are encountered, are less encouraging with reduction in hyperpigmentation and ACTH secretion reported in only 30% (74). Radiation therapy with conventional irradiation or proton beam has also been reported to reduce cortisol secretion in a comparable percentage of patients (71). In a few patients, cyproheptadine has been used with encouraging results. Reductions of plasma ACTH, plasma cortisol, and the cortisol secretory rate to normal have been observed, as has been a restoration of diurnal periodicity and dexamethasone suppressibility (2,49). Many patients with Cushing's disease, however, appear not to respond to cyproheptadine. Responses have been seen in patients with Nelson's syndrome and the drug has been used successfully as an adjunct in patients treated with irradiation to produce a more rapid response.

Luteinizing Hormone Stimulating Hormone and Follicle Stimulating Hormone

Hypothalamic hypogonadism is defined as an impairment of the pituitary-gonadal axis attributed to decreased or disordered secretion of LHRH. It may be seen in the presence or absence of hypothalamic destruction and the manifestations vary, depending on the age at which it occurs.

Pre-Pubertal Hypofunction

When hypothalamic hypogonadism occurs prior to puberty, there is failure of normal sexual maturation and, in girls, primary amenorrhea. In children other evidence of hypothalamic hypopituitarism is frequently present. Nocturnal plasma LH rises that normally occur during puberty are absent and clinically the disorder resembles pre-pubertal primary hypopituitarism. In some males, anosmia or hyposmia is also present and these findings constitute Kallman's syndrome, or olfactory-genital dysplasia, which may be associated with color blindness, nerve deafness, or other neurologic defects. It occurs primarily as a genetic disorder, though sporadic cases have been reported (56). In some patients (33), hypoplasia of the region of the anterior commissure, olfactory bulb, and/ or hypothalamus has been reported.

The gonadotropin responses to a single injection of LHRH are markedly impaired or absent in subjects with hypothalmic hypogonadism, indicating a lack of prior (endogenous) LHRH stimulation. Repeated administration of LHRH results in priming of the gonadotropes leading to a normal or supranormal response, thereby providing a means to differentiate this disorder from that of primary hypopituitarism (72). Intermittent (repeated bolus) injections of LHRH have been used successfully in these subjects to produce normal pubertal development (17).

Post-Pubertal Hypofunction

Hypothalamic hypogonadism post-pubertally is a disorder predominately of women, generally manifested by secondary amenorrhea or oligomenorrhea and occasionally by infertility associated with anovulatory cycles. The terms "functional" and "psychogenic" amenorrhea probably represent the same disorder(s). Circulating estrogen levels are decreased, plasma LH and FSH levels are inappropriately low, and the pulsatile LH fluctuations seen in normal women tend to be absent (79). A single injection of LHRH produces a rise in both LH and FSH levels and a normal response to clomiphene administration is also generally present, suggesting the existence of a functional derangement in hypothalamic release mechanisms. This disorder, in the absence of any other neuroendocrine disturbances, is usually a self-limited condition.

Similar physiologic disturbances occur in women with hyperprolactinemia, irrespective of etiology. Extensive studies have indicated that the gonadotropin responses to the negative estrogen feedback are present but those to the positive feedback are absent, suggesting a selective effect of hyperprolactinemia on the CNS (1). It is presently unclear whether the hypothalamic disturbances are due specifically to hyperprolactinemia or to alterations in neurotransmitter metabolism (primarily dopamine) that occur as a result of hyperprolactinemia. In men, hyperprolactinemia has been associated with varying degrees of hypogonadism, with diminished libido and impotence being the most frequent symptoms.

Severe alterations in weight (both marked increases and decreases) are frequently accompanied by amenorrhea. Amenorrhea is quite common in ballerinas and female athletes and occurs in virtually all patients with anorexia nervosa. Hypogonadism is also seen in other CNS disorders in which the nature of the pathology remains to be clarified. These include the Laurence-Moon, Bardet-Biedl, and Prader-Willi syndromes.

Therapeutic decisions depend on the etiology and severity of the disease and the patient's desire for fertility. In most women, no therapy is indicated unless restoration of menses and/or pregnancy is desired. In others, the effects of hypoestrogenemia (primarily dyspareunia due to decreased vaginal secretions and decreased libido) may justify replacement therapy. In men, testosterone replacement therapy is indicated if endogenous hormone levels are subnormal. Treatment of hyperprolactinemia is discussed later in this section.

Polycystic Ovary Syndrome

The polycystic ovary (Stein-Leventhal) syndrome, the clinical features of which are amenorrhea, hirsutism, and obesity, has been seen in association with a history of childhood CNS disease or "encephalitis" (5). LH levels are consistently elevated though below the level observed at the midcycle ovulatory peak in normals. The suggestion of a functional CNS disturbance is based on the experimental induction of the disorder by neonatal adrogenization in the rat, in which ovarian transplantation into a normal host corrects the abnormalities. Other evidence, however, has implicated adrenal or ovarian etiologies. The Stein-Leventhal syndrome has been seen in association with hyperprolactinemia but the significance of this association is not entirely clear.

Thyroid Stimulating Hormone

Hypofunction

Hypothalamic hypothyroidism or "tertiary" hypothyroidism is a disorder manifested by clinical features of hypothyroidism, decreased plasma thyroid hormone and TSH levels, and an exaggerated delayed TSH response to thyrotropin-releasing hormone (TRH). The peak TSH value after TRH occurs at 15 to 30 min in most normal subjects whereas in these patients it may be as late as 90 or 120 min (25). In children with this disorder, basal TSH levels may be slightly elevated but respond in a similar manner (37). Hypothalamic hypothyroidism is believed to be caused by TRH deficiency but this remains to be proven. It occurs as an isolated defect or more commonly, in children, associated with other anterior pituitary hormone deficiencies. The frequency of this disorder as a cause for hypothyroidism is probably quite low.

Another form of hypothalamic hypothyroidism has been recognized in children receiving GH therapy for GH deficiency states (see below). During the course of therapy, hypothyroidism associated with a low TSH may be observed and can most probably be explained by the stimulation of somatostatin secretion by exogenous GH which, in turn, suppresses TSH secretion.

Growth Hormone

Hypofunction

Idiopathic GH deficiency (IGHD) occurs as both a familial and a sporadic disorder, either as an isolated hormone deficiency or together with other anterior pituitary hormone deficiencies. The diagnosis is often made as early as 2 or 3 years of age and is manifested by growth retardation and, occasionally, fasting hypoglycemia. GH deficiency may be complete or partial. Although the unavailability of GH-releasing factor precludes distinguishing between hypothalamic and pituitary etiologies, the absence of neuroradiologic abnormalities of the sella and the frequent coexistence of TRH- and LHRH-responsive deficiencies of TSH, LH, and FSH provide evidence for a hypothalamic etiology. To date, no histologic studies of brain or hypothalamus are available. It has been proposed that the disorder may be secondary to a neurotransmitter abnormality rather than to a structural defect in the hypothalamus. In one series, a group of children with IGHD responded to propranolol with a stimulation of GH release, suggesting the existence of enhanced β-adrenergic inhibitory tone (38). However, this has not been confirmed in other studies.

The diagnosis is established by characteristic changes in bone age and height age, the absence of other disorders that can cause GH deficiency, and impaired responsiveness to GH stimulation (54). Treatment of IGHD requires administration of human GH during the pre-pubertal period. Therapy may be required for several years in order to achieve near normal stature, and is continued until a height of at least 1.5 to 1.6 meters is reached or until the post-pubertal fusion of the epiphyseal growing centers of the long bones.

Another form of GH deficiency, "emotional deprivation dwarfism" or "psychosocial dwarfism" is characterized by short stature, normal sellar size, and clinical findings suggestive of hypopituitarism (63). Children with this disorder have a history of a disturbed home environment. The biochemical and physiologic disturbances are rapidly reversed on removal from this environment and it has been suggested that excessive β-adrenergic inhibitory effects may be the mediators of the GH deficiency (38).

Hyperfunction: Acromegaly

GH hypersecretion is usually associated with a pituitary tumor, though in some patients there is evidence for a hypothalamic etiology. Signs and symptoms of GH hypersecretion (acromegaly) often begin in mid-life and develop slowly. The earliest recognizable findings include soft tissue swelling and hypertrophy of the extremities and the face, resulting in coarsening of features, increased glove and shoe size, and skin thickening. Generalized hirsutism and increased pigmentation can be seen; sebaceous gland hypersecretion leading to oiliness of the skin and cyst formation is common, as is increased sweating. Osseous changes that develop more slowly include osteophyte proliferation and tufting of the terminal phalanges; hypertrophic arthropathy which may lead to a crippling arthritis; prognathism; increased teeth spacing; sinus and vocal cord hypertrophy; generalized visceromegaly including salivary glands, liver, spleen, and kidneys; hyperfunction of other endocrine glands; cardiomegaly; hypertension; peripheral neuropathy due to both nerve entrapment and axonal demyelination; and impaired carbohydrate tolerance leading in some patients to diabetes. When GH hypersecretion begins during childhood prior to epiphyseal plate fusion, the increase in skeletal growth is proportional, resulting in gigantism. Mixtures of gigantisms and acromegaly are quite common.

The diagnosis of acromegaly is established by demonstrating elevated plasma GH levels that do not respond normally to stimulatory and suppressive agents. In patients with acromegaly, plasma GH levels do not suppress with glucose as occurs in normals, usually increase after TRH and occasionally LHRH, whereas these agents have no effect in normals, and decrease after L-DOPA in contrast with the increase observed in normals. The latter two effects appear to represent the development of receptors (for TRH, LHRH, and dopamine) on the neoplastic somatotrope, which are normally not present. Measurement of somatomedin C levels has been suggested as an alternate means of diagnosing acromegaly though experience with this measurement is still limited (14).

GH levels are elevated in patients with chronic renal failure, cirrhosis, starvation, anorexia nervosa, and protein calorie malnutrition, and also exhibit a stimulatory response to TRH. Patients with these diseases, however, do not present with clinical features of acromegaly. Elevated levels of GH also occur in several types of dwarfism, presumably due to biologically altered GH or to impaired GH receptors. A form of gigantism during childhood occurs in the absence of GH hypersecretion (cerebral gigantism) and is associated with accelerated bone age and mental retardation (73).

Several lines of evidence support a hypothalamic etiology of acromegaly. GH secretion is usually not autonomous but responds to stimuli mediated through the hypothalamus including glucose, insulin hypoglycemia, and arginine, implying that the somatotropes do respond to hypothalamic signals. Hypothalamic tumors, particularly in the ventromedial region, have been associated with GH hypersecretion and acromegaly, suggesting the overproduction of a GH-releasing factor. GH-releasing activity has been reported in plasma of patients with acromegaly when tested *in vitro* and acromegaly caused by GH-secreting pituitary tumors is reversible after removal of carcinoid or pancreatic pituitary tumors that contain a GH-releasing factor (28,80), indicating GH hypersecretion and even pituitary tumors can develop in response to prolonged GH-releasing factor stimulation. In addition, GH secretion is altered by neuropharmacologic agents that are believed to act within the CNS (18) and, in some patients, dynamic studies of GH secretions have remained abnormal even after successful tumor removal and return of basal levels to normal. In other patients, secretory dynamics have returned to normal after successful surgery, suggesting that there may be two subgroups of acromegaly with different etiologies.

The goals of therapy in acromegaly are to correct the metabolic disturbances, reverse as much as possible the soft tissue changes, and arrest the progression of the musculoskeletal abnormalities. In some patients, reduction of GH levels has been reported to improve existing cardiovascular disease as well. Although current therapy does not depend on whether the disease is of pituitary or hypothalamic origin, one must consider the possibility of an extra-pituitary tumor, removal of which may reverse the GH hypersecretion. Surgical removal of GH-secreting tumors is a rapid and effective treatment for acromegaly. The success rate varies in different series but has been reported as high as 92% (53), using as criterion the reduction of plasma GH to normal levels. Success is inversely related to the size of the tumor and the likelihood of normalizing GH levels is considerably lower when the initial value is greater than 100 ng/ml. Both conventional and proton beam irradiation have been used successfully for treatment of acromegaly. Although improvement is more gradual, success rates of greater than 80% have been reported. Neuropharmacologic therapy of acromegaly using bromocriptine is based on the presence of dopamine receptors on the neoplastic somatrope. Approximately 80% of patients respond to the drug with a reduction of GH levels to the normal range. The drug must be given continuously, since GH hypersecretion returns with its discontinuation. In as much as bromocriptine does not appear to affect tumor growth in GH-secreting tumors, its use is best reserved for those patients who are not surgical candidates, and in patients in whom surgery and/or radiation therapy has not restored GH levels to normal.

Prolactin

Since interference with the integrity of the hypothalamic-pituitary axis results in increased prolactin secretion, the consequence of most hypothalamic disorders is hyperprolactinemia. Idiopathic hyperprolactinemia (IH) has been defined as the presence of elevated prolactin levels unassociated with demonstrable pituitary or CNS disease or with other recognized causes of increased prolactin secretion. Prolactin levels may vary from slightly above normal to values greater than 10 times normal. The diagnosis must remain inferential, since the coexistence of a nondetectable pituitary microadenoma cannot be excluded. In fact, IH may represent the earliest stage of prolactin-secreting pituitary tumor formation.

Hyperprolactinemia is generally manifested in women by galactorrhea and amenorrhea, though neither is invariably present, and in males by decreased libido and hypogonadism. The development of galactorrhea requires the presence of both gonadal steroids as well as prolactin. Its frequent association with previous oral contraceptive use is believed due to the sudden removal of progestins in patients whose breasts have been prepared by the previous combination of estrogens, progestins, and hyperprolactinemia. In patients with IH, ultradian secretion of LH is inhibited (10), as is the positive feedback response to exogenous estrogen (1,52). In men, the effect of prolactin appears to be at the negative feedback site of testosterone on endogenous LHRH secretion.

The etiology of IH has been attributed to a neurotransmitter defect in the CNS related to dopamine metabolism. Agents that impair dopaminergic neurotransmission (most commonly the neuroleptic dopamine receptor antagonists) increase prolactin secretion. Patients with IH, in contrast with normals, or absent responses to such agents. Administration of nomifensine, a synaptosomal dopamine reuptake inhibitor, fails to suppress prolactin secretion in IH patients as it does in normals (60) and enhancement of central dopaminergic tone by a combination of L-DOPA and a peripheral decarboxylase inhibitor, carbidopa, also fails to suppress prolactin release in patients with IH and prolactin-secreting tumors, in contrast with normals (24). Stimulation of prolactin secretion by TRH and cimetidine, an H-2 histamine receptor antagonist, is also decreased in patients with IH (35,44). At present, there are no tests that can reliably differentiate patients with IH from those with prolactin-secreting tumors and long-term follow-up of all IH patients is, therefore, mandatory.

Hyperprolactinemia has also been observed in patients on chronic neuroleptic therapy, in hypothyroidism, cirrhosis, chronic renal failure, after spinal cord lesions and injuries to the chest wall, and in association with ectopic tumors.

Further evidence that prolactin-secreting tumors are of hypothalamic origin includes the presence of lactotrope hyperplasia in up to one-third of patients (58) and a report of prolacting-releasing activity in serum of patients with tumors (32). The success of pituitary microsurgery in eliminating hyperprolactinemia and restoring normal cyclic ovulatory function argues against this hypothesis, though conflicting reports on dynamic studies of prolactin secretion in the postoperative period suggest that, as in the case of the other hormone secreting tumors of the pituitary, there may be more than one etiology.

The most widely employed therapy for prolactin-secreting tumors is surgical removal. However, with the recognition that the natural history of many microadenomas is benign, a more conservative therapeutic approach is becoming increasingly popular. Bromocriptine is capable of reducing prolactin levels into the normal range in greater than 90% of patients with idiopathic hyperprolactinemia and prolactin-secreting tumors. The drug is effective in restoring ovulatory menses and fertility and its greatest use has been for this purpose. In patients not desirous of becoming pregnant, therapy may be withheld in as much as some patients with IH will show spontaneous remissions. In patients with moderate to large prolactin-secreting tumors, bromocriptine has also been used successfully in reducing tumor size (34,55). Studies are currently underway to assess the efficacy of this form of therapy as compared with surgery.

Vasopressin

Hypofunction

Decreased or absent secretion of vasopressin results in diabetes insipidus, which is characterized by an inability of the renal tubular cells to conserve water, leading to the excretion of large volumes of dilute urine (polyuria), hypertonicity of circulating fluids, and a compensatory increase in thirst and water intake (polydipsia). The causes of diabetes insipidus can vary on an anatomic basis and with respect to both etiology and the precise mechanism responsible for the deficient vasopressin secretion.

The neurohypophyseal system may fail to develop normally, as in sporadic or familial disorders and the disease may be present at birth. Alternately, destruction of the hypothalamus, stalk, or posterior pituitary can impair the ability to maintain normal vasopressin secretion. Diabetes insipidus is the most common endocrinopathy occurring in destructive lesions of the hypothalamus.

Impaired vasopressin secretion may be total or partial. When the hormone is completely absent, polyuria of up to 10 to 12 liters per day can occur, severe plasma hyperosmolality is present, particularly if the patient is unable to maintain a large fluid intake, and the diagnosis is relatively easy to establish. With milder forms of the disease, however, plasma osmolality may be maintained in the normal range (281–287 mOsm/kg) and the diagnosis will require performance of a fluid deprivation test. Normal subjects achieve maximal urine concentration (600–1400 mOsm/kg) and a maximum reduction in urine volume within 6 to 8 hr with plasma osmolality remaining in the normal range. At that time, an injection of aqueous vasopressin does not further increase urine osmolality. Patients with diabetes insipidus may show a variety of responses. Most commonly, there is only a limited increase in urinary osmolality in the period of water deprivation associated with a rise in plasma osmolality. With exogenous vasopressin administration, urine osmolality increases to the normal range. In some patients with diabetes insipidus, sufficient vasopressin may be secreted to prevent a constant diuresis, but only when plasma osmolality is elevated. If the thirst mechanism is intact, these patients exhibit polydipsia due to increasing plasma osmolality before the osmotic stimulus is sufficiently high to stimulate endogenous vasopressin release.

Hyperosmolality has been reported in patients with intracranial lesions, particularly in the presence of serious disturbances of sensorium but also in fully conscious patients (20). These patients exhibit normal renal function, adequate fluid intake, absence of thirst, failure of forced fluid intake to completely correct the hyperosmolality, effective release of vasopressin in response to osmotic stimuli, and occasionally, the presence of anterior pituitary insufficiency and obesity. These findings are best explained by an impaired hypothalamic regulation of thirst as well as of vasopressin secretion. In some patients, there is evidence that ADH release is regulated primarily by changes in effective circulating volume rather than plasma osmolality. The neural centers involved in modulating water intake and in the production and release of vasopressin are situated in close proximity in the anterior hypothalamus. Experimentally, lesions in the ventromedial hypothalamus produce a syndrome of adipsia, dehydration, hypernatremia, and obesity. Similar lesions might, therefore, be expected to produce these findings in humans. The syndrome has been described in association with histiocytosis, craniopharyngiomas, optic nerve gliomas, inflammatory disturbances of undetermined origin, ruptured aneurysms, and pineal tumors.

Proper treatment of diabetes insipidus requires establishing the extent of the quantitative and qualitative defects in the secretion of vasopressin, assessing the intactness of the thirst mechanism, and excluding other causes of polyuria and hypertonicity. In patients with partial vasopressin deficiency, chlorpropamide alone or in combination with clofibrate, both of which stimulate endogenous vasopressin release, are frequently effective. Chlorpropamide also enhances the effect of vasopressin by stimulation of renal adenylate cyclase. In severe forms of the disease, substitution therapy is required. Posterior pituitary extract (Pitressin) in oil or, when only short-term therapy is required, in an aqueous solution, remains the therapy of choice. A synthetic analog of vasopressin (DDAVP), which can be given intranasally and is devoid of nearly all side effects, represents a major therapeutic improvement, though its increased cost has limited its widespread acceptance. In patients with "essential" or "cerebral" hypernatremia, the difficulty in correcting the hyperosmolality with forced fluid intake underscores the necessity for specific treatment, if possible, of the causative lesion.

A condition frequently confused with diabetes insipidus is "psychogenic polydipsia." Patients with this disorder will exhibit polyuria and polydipsia but in contrast with patients with diabetes insipidus, plasma osmolality is decreased rather than increased. The disorder may be seen on the basis of chronic overingestion of water or by intermittent ingestion of very large quantities of water, resulting in water intoxication. Originally attributed to a psychiatric disturbance, it is now believed that some of these patients may have an alteration in the set point of the thirst regulatory center that is activated at lower plasma osmolality levels.

Hyperfunction

Hypersecretin of vasopressin results in the syndrome of inappropriate secretion of antidiuretic hormone (SIADH). In this disorder, vasopressin is released continuously and without relation to plasma osmolality. Patients are unable to excrete a dilute urine; extracellular fluid volume expands because of retention of ingested fluids and results in dilutional hyponatremia. In many patients with SIADH, blood and urine vasopressin levels are within normal limits, but are inappropriately high for the concomitant plasma osmolality (65). Patients with SIADH exhibit weight gain without edema, weakness, lethargy, mental confusion, and eventually convulsions and coma. This syndrome has been described in a variety of disease states involving both central and peripheral nervous systems including metastatic carcinoma to brain, primary brain tumors, skull fractures, intermittent cerebral dysrhythmias, cerebrovascular disorders, infection, acute intermittent porphyria, and hypothyroidism. Physical and emotional stress and pain have been implicated as etiologic factors, as have pulmonary tuberculosis, lung abscess, and carcinoma of the lung associated with ectopic production of vasopressin.

Criteria for diagnosis include hyponatremia, renal sodium loss, the presence of normal renal, pituitary, adrenal, and thyroid function, inability to excrete a dilute urine after water ingestion, resistance to correction by hypertonic saline, and reversibility after water restriction. The increased sodium excretion appears to be a consequence of expanded intracellular volume which suppresses aldosterone secretion. A variety of hypoglycemic and antineoplastic drugs have also been reported to induce SIADH. Therapy consists primarily of restricting fluid intake, though, if sufficient salt wasting has occurred, replacement may be required. The narcotic antagonists oxilorphan and butorphanol have been used successfully in reducing vasopressin secretion in patients with SIADH. Their effects are probably mediated by interference with endorphin-enkaphalin stimulation of vasopressin secretion. Although they are ineffective in patients with vasopressin-secreting lung tumors, demeclocycline, which interferes with vasopressin action on the renal tubule, has proven to be very effective (59).

OTHER HYPOTHALAMIC DISORDERS

Disturbances of Neurometabolic Regulation

The hypothalamus serves as integrated locus for those autonomic nervous system components involved in regulating carbohydrate and lipid metabolism. Its effects are mediated by direct neuronal connections to the pancreatic islets, liver, adipose tissue, gastrointestinal tract, and by adrenal medullary catecholamine release. Acute disturbances of this system are frequently seen in stress states that activate the sympathetic nervous system. Thus, in the presence of general anesthesia, trauma, sepsis, burns, and hyperthermia, patients may exhibit hyperglycemia and hyperglucagonemia and/or impairment of insulin secretion (27). These disturbances generally do not produce significant clinical problems and disappear with resolution of the stress. However, in patients with severe burns or sepsis, persistent or nonsuppressible hyperglucagonemia and gluconeogenesis have been implicated as etiologic factors in producing a life-threatening catabolic state (78).

The hypothalamus, with imput from extra hypothalamic structures, particularly the limbic system and telencephalon, is also involved in the control of caloric homeostasis, which is responsible for maintenance of body weight. A ventromedial satiety center and a ventrolateral feeding center have been well established, though the specific signals remain a subject of controversy (29,66). Destruction of the ventromedial hypothalamus leads to an obesity state whereas damage to the ventrolateral hypothalamus results in anorexia and emaciation. In only a small percentage of patients with severe obesity or inanition can the disorder be attributed to defined anatomic destruction of the hypothalamus. However, the inability to distinguish between clinical and biochemical features of obesity or inanition in patients with and without recognizable hypothalamic disease has led to the belief that "functional" disorders of caloric balance such as "essential" obesity and/or anorexia nevosa, may represent biochemical disturbances of hypothalamic function.

Hypothalamic Obesity

Destruction of the ventromedial hypothalamus, irrespective of etiology, has been associated with the development of obesity (12). Hyperphagia and weight gain continue until a new set point has been reached at which time food intake diminishes somewhat. The increase in adipose tissue mass is primarily the result of hypertrophy rather than hyperplasia, insulin resistance is quite marked, and diabetes may be present. GH secretion is invariably impaired though thyroid function is normal. Alterations in gonadal function and sexual behavior are common in obesity and range from inpaired infertility or decreased libido to true hypogonadism. In most patients these changes are reversible after successful weight reduction.

There are a number of well recognized syndromes, many of which are familial, which have been associated with obesity and are believed to be of hypothalamic origin. These include the Laurence-Moon, Bardet-Biedl, Allstrom-Hallgren, and Prader-Willi syndromes (22). Evidence of other hypothalamic disturbances includes hypogonadism, temperature tolerance, and loss of diurnal rhythms, though there are, in addition, extrahypothalamic disturbances (deafness, pigmentary retinopathy, and mental retardation).

Therapy of hypothalamic obesity is for the most part unsuccessful. With the exception of a few patients in whom the underlying disease is responsive to therapy (i.e., childhood CNS leukemia, where chemotherapy-induced remission results in loss of hyperphagia and weight reduction), the functional alterations appear irreversible. Therapeutic measures aimed at treatment of the morbidly obese patient constitute the only approach.

Anorexia Nervosa

This disorder, recognized for more than 300 years, is manifested primarily by weight loss, amenorrhea, and behavioral disturbances and occurs almost exclusively in young women of higher socioeconomic status. It has been attributed to a psychiatric disturbance, an endocrine metabolic disturbance, or a combination of the two (75). Features of the disease include age of onset less than 25 years, weight loss of at least 25% of original body weight, a distorted and implacable attitude toward eating, amenorrhea which may precede significant weight loss, and the absence of other medical and psychiatric illnesses. There is a loss of pulsatile secretion of LH, indirect evidence for decreased secretion of endogenous LHRH, normal to elevated GH levels with a paradoxic increase after glucose, and elevations in plasma cortisol levels with maintenance of responsiveness to insulin hypoglycemia. Impaired body temperature maintenance in response to environmental changes has been observed as has reduced urine concentrating ability suggestive of partial diabetes insipidus. Pituitary hormone secretion generally reverts to normal with successful therapy though persistence of amenorrhea in many patients even after restoration of weight to normal suggests that a factor other than malnutrition may be present (67). Therapy, which consists of improving nutritional intake and appropriate psychotherapeutic measures, has led to a reasonably good prognosis. Mortality is 5% or less and the vast majority of patients regain sufficient weight to return to within 10% of original body weight. Only 40%, however, will maintain this weight permanently and resume normal ovulatory menses.

Diencephalic Syndrome of Infancy

A syndrome of emaciation and hyperkinesis occasionally with large hands and feet has been described in association with invasive tumors of the optic chiasm or anterior hypothalamus in infants (13). Most infants are alert and cheerful, though they may exhibit irritability, and usually maintain a good appetite and exhibit normal linear growth. Neuroendocrine disturbances include absent circadian variations in plasma cortisol and elevated GH levels with paradoxical responses to alterations in glucose levels. Most children die within the first 2 years of life because of inanition and the accompanying complications. In those who survive, the illness frequently undergoes a dramatic transformation. Appetite continues, emaciation ceases, and extreme obesity develops (31). Irritability and rage replace the previous euphoric behavior and the prognosis for survival improves dramatically, for unexplained reasons. It is unclear why destruction of the immature hypothalamus produces symptoms different from those in the older child and adult. However, experimental data indicates that the food intake-controlling activity of the ventromedial nucleus does not exert an important role until after weaning. Thus, destruction of a nonfunctional ventromedial hypothalamus would produce few symptoms and the effects of ventrolateral destruction would predominate. With increasing maturity, the lack of ventromedial hypothalamic function would become the dominant feature, resulting in obesity.

Pseudomotor Cerebri

Pseudomotor cerebri, characterized by headache, papilledema, and raised intracranial pressure in the absence of a focal lesion or obstructive hydrocephalus, is also known as "benign intracranial hypertension." Most cases occur in obese females with an abrupt clinical onset consisting of severe headache or visual symptoms (loss or blurring of vision or diplopia). Somnolence and hyperphagia may also be present. Spontaneous recovery is seen in one-fourth of patients whereas in others recovery is coincident with repeated lumbar punctures or corticosteroid therapy (77). In a few patients, the disorder has been associated with venus sinus obstruction, vitamin A intoxication, iron deficiency anemia, steroid withdrawal, Addison's disease, pregnancy, or the use of oral contraceptives. Sellar enlargement with evidence of an empty sella has also been noted when symptoms have been of prolonged duration. With few exceptions, endocrine studies have been normal.

Pineal Diseases

Although the pineal is not a hypothalamic structure, diseases of the pineal gland have been associated with disturbances of gonadal function (see also Chapter 15). Pineal tumors and rarely pineal hypoplasia or aplasia have been associated with precocious puberty and with hypogonadism. When viewed in perspective, only a small percentage of parenchymatous pineal tumors cause sexual precocity (43,64) and it is only those tumors that extend well beyond the pineal region that have been implicated. The most likely basis for the endocrine disturbance is, therefore, a destruction of other brain regions during the pre-pubertal period that tonically inhibit LHRH secretion. Nonparenchymatous tumors are more commonly associated with precocious puberty and it has been suggested that destruction of the normal pineal by the tumor results in loss of a pineal secretory product (possibly melatonin, arginine vasotocin, or another factor) that normally inhibits initiation of sexual maturation. At least some pineal tumors exhibit endocrine function and the production of an anti-gonadotropic factor by the tumor could provide an explanation for the delayed puberty frequently encountered. By the time of diagnosis, most pineal tumors are no longer surgically resectable. If the tumor is of the germinoma type, which histologically constitutes nearly half the pineal tumors, radiotherapy can be used successfully (11).

REFERENCES

1. Aono, T., Miyaki, A., Shioji, T., Kinugasa, T., Onishi, T., and Kurachi, K. (1976): Impaired LH release following exogenous estrogen administration in patients with amenorrhea-galactorrhea syndrome. *J. Clin. Endocrinol. Metab.,* 42:696–702.
2. Aronin, N., and Kreiger, D. T. (1980): Sustained remission of Nelson's syndrome after stopping cyproheptadine treatment. *N. Engl. J. Med.,* 302:453–455.
3. Avery, M. E., McAfee, J. G., and Guild, H. G. (1957): The course and prognosis of reticuloendotheliosis (eosinophilic granuloma, Schüller-Christian disease and Letterer-Siwe disease). *Am. J. Med.,* 22:636–652.
4. Bartlett, J. R. (1971): Craniopharyngiomas—a summary of 85 cases. *J. Neurol. Neurosurg. Psychiatry,* 34:37–41.
5. Bartuska, D. G., Eskin, B. A., Smith, E. M., Dacou, C., and Dratman, M. B. (1967): Brain damage, hypertrichosis and polycystic ovaries. *Am. J. Obstet. Gynecol.,* 99:387–389.

6. Bauer, H. G. (1959): Endocrine and metabolic conditions related to pathology in the hypothalamus: A review. *J. Nerv. Ment. Dis.,* 128:323–338.

7. Bierich, J. R. (1975): Sexual precocity. In: *Clinics in Endocrinology, Vol. 4,* edited by J. R. Bierich, pp. 107–142. Saunders, Philadelphia.

8. Bigos, S. T., Robert, F., Pelletier, G., and Hardy, J. (1977): Cure of Cushing's disease by transsphenoidal removal of a microadenoma from a pituitary gland despite a radiographically normal sella turica. *J. Clin. Endocrinol. Metab.,* 45:1251–1260.

9. Bigos, S. T., Somma, M., Rasio, E., Eastman, R. C., Lanthier, A., Johnston, H. H., and Hardy, J. (1980): Cushing's disease: Management by transsphenoidal pituitary microsurgery. *J. Clin. Endocrinol. Metab.,* 50:348–354.

10. Boyar, R. M., Capen, S., Finkelstein, J. W., Perlow, M., Sassin, J. F.; Fukushima, D. K., Weitzman, E. D., and Hellman, L. (1974): Hypothalamic-pituitary function in diverse hypoprolactinemic states. *J. Clin. Invest.,* 53:1588–1598.

11. Bradfield, J. S., and Perez, C. A. (1972): Pineal tumors and ectopic pinealomas. Analysis of treatment and failures. *Radiology,* 103:399–406.

12. Bray, G. A., and Gallagher, T. F. Jr. (1975): Manifestations of hypothalamic obesity in man: A comprehensive investigation of eight patients and a review of the literature. *Medicine,* 54:301–330.

13. Burr, I. M., Slonim, A. E., Danish, R. K., Gadoth, N., and Butler, I. J. (1976): Diencephalic syndrome revisited. *J. Pediatr.,* 88:439–444.

14. Clemmons, D. R., Van Wyk, J. J., Ridgeway, E. C., Kliman, B., Kjellberg, R. N., and Underwood, L. E. (1979): Evaluation of acromegaly by radioimmunoassay of somatomedin-C. *N. Engl. J. Med.,* 301:1138–1142.

15. Crapo, L. (1979): Cushing's syndrome: A review of diagnostic tests. *Metabolism,* 28:955–977.

16. Compton, M. R. (1963): Hypothalamic lesions following the rupture of cerebral berry aneurysms. *Brain,* 86:301–314.

17. Crowley, W. F. Jr., and McArthur, J. W. (1980): Induction of puberty in hypogonadotropic males: Use of low-dose pulsatile luteinizing hormone releasing hormone (LHRH) administration. In: *Progr. Endocrine Society 62nd Annual Meeting,* Washington, Abstr. 743.

18. Cryer, P. E., and Daughaday, W. H. (1974): Adrenergic modulation of growth hormone secretion in acromegaly: Suppression during phentolamine and phentolamine-isoproterenol administration. *J. Clin. Endocrinol. Metab.,* 39:658–663.

19. Cushing, H. (1932): The basophil adenomas of the pituitary body and their clinical manifestations (pituitary basophilism). *Bull. Johns Hopkins Hosp.,* 50:137–195.

20. DeRubertis, R., Michelis, M. F., and Davis, B. B. (1974): Essential hypernatremia. *Arch. Intern. Med.,* 134:889–895.

21. Eddy, R. L., Jones, A. L., Gilliland, P. F., Ibarra, J. D. Jr., Thompson, J. Q., and McMurry J. F. Jr. (1973): Cushing's syndrome: A prospective study of diagnostic methods. *Am. J. Med.,* 55:621–630.

22. Edwards, J. A., Sethi, P. K., Scoma, A. J., Bannerman, R. M., and Frohman, L. A. (1976): A new familial syndrome characterized by pigmentary retinopathy, hypogonadism, mental retardation, nerve deafness and glucose intolerance. *Am. J. Med.,* 60:23–32.

23. Fiedler, R., and Krieger, D. T. (1975): Endocrine distrubances in patients with congenital aqueductal stenosis. *Acta Endocrinol.,* 80:1–13.

24. Fine, S. A., and Frohman, L. A. (1978): Loss of central nervous system component of dopaminergic inhibition of prolactin secretion in patients with prolactin-secreting pituitary tumors. *J. Clin. Invest.,* 61:973–980.

25. Fleischer, N., Lorente, M., Kirkland, J., Kirkland, R., Clayton, G., and Calderon, M. (1972): Synthetic thyrotropin releasing factor as a test of pituitary thyrotropin reserve. *J. Clin. Endocrinol. Metab.,* 34:617–624.

26. Frohlich, A. (1901): Ein Fall von Tumor Hypophysis cerebri ohne Akromegalie. *Wiener Klin. Radsch.,* 15:883–886.

27. Frohman, L. A. (1978): The central nervous system and metabolic regulation. In: *Advances in Modern Nutrition, Vol. 2: Diabetes, Obesity, and Vascular Disease,* edited by H. M. Katzen and R. J. Mahler, pp. 493–515. Hemisphere, Washington, D.C.

28. Frohman, L. A., Szabo, M., Berelowitz, M., and Stachura, M. E. (1980): Partial purification and characterization of a peptide with growth hormone-releasing activity from extrapituitary tumors in patients with acromegaly. *J. Clin. Invest.,* 65:43–54.

29. Frohman, L. A. (1980): Hypothalamic control of energy metabolism. In: *Handbook of the Hypothalamus,* edited by P. J. Morgane and J. Panksepp. Marcel Dekker, New York.
30. Gailani, S. D., Roque, A. L., Band, P., and Ross, C. (1970): Hypopituitarism due to localized hypothalamic lesions. *Arch. Intern. Med.,* 126:284–286.
31. Gamstorp, I., Kjellman, B., and Palmgren, B. (1967): Diencephalic syndrome of infancy. *J. Pediatr.,* 70:383–390.
32. Garthwaite, T. L., and Hagen, T. C. (1978): Plasma prolactin-releasing factor-like activity in the amenorrhea-galactorrhea syndrome. *J. Clin. Endocrinol. Metab.,* 47:885–888.
33. Gauthier, G. (1961): La Dyplasie olfacto-génitale (agénésie des lobes olfactifs avec absence de dévelopement gonadique à la puberté). *Acta Neuroveg.,* 21:345–394.
34. George, S. R., Burrow, G. N., Zinman, B., and Ezrin, C. (1979): Regression of pituitary tumors, possible effect of bromergocryptine. *Am. J. Med.,* 66:697–702.
35. Gonzalez, C., Szabo, M., and Frohman, L. A. (1979): Comparison of the stimulatory effects of cimetidine on prolactin secretion in vivo, in vitro and in patients with prolactin-secreting tumors. *Clin. Res.,* 27:448A.
36. Heinbecker, P. (1944): Pathogenesis of Cushing's syndrome. *Medicine,* 23:225–247.
37. Illig, R., Krawczynska, H., Torresani, T., and Prader A. (1975). Elevated plasma TSH and hypothyroidism in children with hypothalamic hypopituitarism. *J. Clin. Endocrinol. Metab.,* 41:722–728.
38. Imura, H., Nakai, Y., Kato, Y., Yoshimoto, Y., and Moridera, K. (1973): Effect of adrenergic agents on growth hormone and ACTH secretion. In: *Endocrinology,* edited by R. O. Scow, pp. 156–162. Excerpta Medica, Amsterdam.
39. Jenkins, J. S. (1969): Hypothalamic pituitary-adrenal function after subarachnoid hemorrhage. *Br. Med. J.,* 2:707–709.
40. Judge, D. M., Kulin, H. E., Page, R., Santen, R., and Trapukdi, S. (1977): Hypothalamic hamartoma. *N. Engl. J. Med.,* 296:7–10.
41. Kepes, J. J., and Kepes M. (1969): Predominantly cerebral forms of histiocytosis-X. A reappraisal of "Gagel's hypothalamic granuloma," "granuloma infiltrans of the hypothalamus" and "Ayala's disease" with a report of four cases. *Acta Neuropathol. (Berl.),* 14:77–98.
42. Kim, C. S., Bennett, D. R., and Roberts, T. S. (1969): Primary amenorrhea secondary to noncommunicating hydrocephalus. *Neurology (Minneap.),* 19:533–535.
43. Kitay, J. I. (1954): Pineal lesions and precocious puberty: A review. *J. Clin. Endocrinol. Metab.,* 14:622–625.
44. Kleinberg, D. L., Noel, G. L., and Frantz, A. G. (1977): Galactorrhea: A study of 235 cases, including 48 with pituitary tumors. *N. Engl. J. Med.,* 296:589–600.
45. Kramer, S., Southard, M., and Mansfield, C. M. (1968): Radiotherapy in the management of craniopharyngiomas. Further experience and late results. *Am. J. Roentgenol.,* 103:44–52.
46. Krieger, D. T., and Krieger, H. P. (1966): The circadian variation of the plasma 17-OHCS in central nervous system disease. *J. Clin. Endocrinol. Metab.,* 26:929–940.
47. Krieger, D. T. (1972): The central nervous system and Cushing's syndrome. *Mt. Sinai J. Med.,* 39:416–428.
48. Krieger, D. T., and Glick, S. M. (1974): Sleep EEG stages and plasma growth hormone concentration in states of endogenous and exogenous hypercortisolemia or ACTH elevation. *J. Clin. Endocrinol. Metab.,* 39:986–1000.
49. Krieger, D. T., Amorosa, L., and Linick, F. (1975): Cyproheptadine-induced remission of Cushing's disease. *N. Engl. J. Med.,* 293:893–896.
50. Krieger, D. T., Howanitz, P. J., and Frantz, A. G. (1976): Absence of nocturnal elevation of plasma prolactin concentrations in Cushing's disease. *J. Clin. Endocrinol. Metab.,* 42:260–272.
51. Lagerquist, L. W., Meikle, A. W., West, C. D., and Tyler, F. H. (1974): Cushing's disease with cure by resection of a pituitary adenoma. Evidence against a primary hypothalamic defect. *Am. J. Med.,* 57:830–836.
52. L'Hermite, M., Delonge-Desnoeck, J., Michaux-Duchene, A., and Robyn, C. (1978): Alteration of feedback mechanisms of estrogen on gonadotropin by sulpiride-induced hyperprolactinemia. *J. Clin. Endocrinol. Metab.,* 47:1132–1136.
53. Lüdecke, D., Kautzky, R., Saeger, W., and Schrader, D. (1976): Selective removal of hypersecreting pituitary adenomas? *Acta Neurochirurgica,* 35:27–42.
54. MacGillivray, M., and Voorhess, M. (1981): Disorders of growth and development. In: *Endocri-*

nology and Metabolism, edited by P. Felig, A. Broadus, J. Baxter, and L. Frohman. McGraw Hill, New York.

55. MacGregor, A. M., Scanlon, M. F., Hall, K., Cook, D. B., and Hall, R. (1979): Reduction in size of a pituitary tumor by bromocriptine therapy. *N. Engl. J. Med.,* 300:291–293.

56. Males, J. L., Townsend, J. L., and Schneider, R. (1973): Hypogonadotropic hypogonadism with anosmia-Kallmann's syndrome. A disorder of olfactory and hypothalamic function. *Arch. Intern. Med.,* 131:501–507.

57. Matson, D. D., and Crigler, J. F. Jr. (1969): Management of craniopharyngioma in childhood. *J. Neurosurg.,* 30:377–390.

58. McKeel, D. W. Jr., Fowler, M., and Jacobs, L. S. (1978): The high prevalence of prolactin call hyperplasia in the human adenohypophysis. In: *Progr. Endocrine Society 60th Annual Meeting,* Miami Beach. Abstr. 353.

59. Moses, A. M. (1980): Diabetes insipidus. In: *Neuroendocrinology,* edited by D. T. Krieger and J. C. Hughes, pp. 141–148. Sinauer Associates, Sunderland, Massachusetts.

60. Müller, E. E., Genazzani, A. R., and Murru, S. (1978). Nomifensine: Diagnostic test in hyperprolactinemic states. *J. Clin. Endocrinol. Metab.,* 47:1352–1357.

61. Nelson, D. H., Meakin, J. W., Dealy, J. B. Jr., Matson, D. D. Emerson, K. Jr., and Thorn, G. W. (1958): ACTH-producing tumor of the pituitary gland. *N. Engl. J. Med.,* 259:161–164.

62. Peck, F. C. Jr., and McGovern, E. R. (1966): Radiation necrosis of the brain in acromegaly. *Neurosurgery,* 25:536–542.

63. Powell, G. E., Brasel, J. A., Raiti, S., and Blizzard, R. M. (1967): Emotional deprivation and growth retardation simulating idiopathic hypopituitarism. II. Endocrinologic evaluation of the syndrome. *N. Engl. J. Med.,* 276:1279–1284.

64. Ringertz, N., Nordenstam, H., and Flyger, G. (1954): Tumors of the pineal region. *J. Neuropathol. Exp. Neurol.,* 13:540–561.

65. Robertson, G. L. (1977): The regulation of vasopressin function in health and disease. In: *Recent Progress in Hormone Research, Vol. 33,* edited by R. O. Greep, pp. 333–385. Academic, New York.

66. Russek, M. (1975): Current hypothesis on the control of feeding behavior. In: *Neural Integration of Physiological Mechanisms and Behavior,* edited by C. J. Morgenson, pp. 128–145. University of Toronto Press, Toronto.

67. Russell, G. F. (1977): General management of anorexia nervosa and difficulties in assessing the efficacy of treatment. In: *Anorexia Nervosa,* edited by R. Vigersky, pp. 277–289. Raven Press, New York.

68. Salassa, R. M., Laws, E. R. Jr., Carpenter, P. C., and Northcutt, R. C. (1978): Transsphenoidal removal of pituitary microadenoma in Cushing's disease. *Mayo Clin. Proc.,* 53:24–28.

69. Selenkow, H. A., Tyler, H. R., Matson, D. D., and Nelson, D. H. (1959): Hypopituitarism due to hypothalamic sarcoidosis. *Am. J. Med. Sci.,* 238:456–463.

70. Shealy, C. N., Kahana, L., Engel, F. L., and McPherson, H. T. (1961): Hypothalamic pituitary sarcoidosis. *Am. J. Med.,* 30:46–55.

71. Sheline, G. E. (1973): Treatment of chromophobe adenomas of the pituitary gland and acromegaly. In: *Diagnosis and Treatment of Pituitary Tumors,* edited by P. O. Kohler and G. T. Ross, pp. 201–216. Excerpta Medica, Amsterdam.

72. Snyder, P. J., Rudenstein, R. S., Gardner, D. F., and Rothman, J. G. (1979): Repetitive infusion of gonadotropin-releasing hormone distinguishes hypothalamic from pituitary hypogonadism. *J. Clin. Endocrinol. Metab.,* 48:864–868.

73. Sotos, J. F., Dodge, P. R., Muirhead, D., Crawford, J. D., and Talbot, N. B. (1964): Cerebral gigantism in childhood. *N. Engl. J. Med.,* 271:109–116.

74. Tyrrell, J. B., Brooks, R. M., Fitzgerald, P. A., Cofoid, P. B., Forsham, P. H., and Wilson, C. B. (1978): Cushing's disease: Selective trans-sphenoidal resection of pituitary microadenomas. *N. Engl. J. Med.,* 298:753–758.

75. Vigersky, R. (ed) (1977): Anorexia Nervosa, pp. 1–392. New York, Raven Press.

76. Vogel, J. M., and Vogel, P. (1972): Idiopathic histiocytosis: A discussion of eosinophilic granuloma, the Hand-Schüller-Christian syndrome and the Letterer-Siwe syndrome. *Semin. Hematol.,* 9:349–369.

77. Weisberg, L. A. (1975): Benign intracranial hypertension. *Medicine,* 54:197–207.

78. Wilmore, D. W., Lindsey, C. A., Moylan, J. A., Faloona, G. R., Pruitt, B. A., and Unger, R. H. (1974): Hyperglucagonaemia after burns. *Lancet,* 1:73–75.
79. Yen, S. S. C., Rebar, R., Vandenberg, G., and Judd, H. (1973): Hypothalamic amenorrhea and hypogonadotropism: Responses to synthetic LRH. *J. Clin. Endocrinol. Metab.,* 36:811–816.
80. Zafar, M. S., Mellinger, R. C., Fine, G., Szabo, M., and Frohman, L. A. (1979): Acromegaly associated with a bronchial carcinoid tumor: Evidence for ectopic production of growth hormone-releasing activity. *J. Clin. Endocrinol. Metab.,* 48:66–71.

The Endocrine Functions of the Brain,
edited by Marcella Motta.
Raven Press, New York, © 1980

19

Hormonal Tests in Hypothalamo-Pituitary Dysfunctions

Antonio Liuzzi, Pier Giorgio Chiodini, Renato Cozzi, Giorgio Verde, and Giuseppe Oppizzi

Endocrine Unit, Ente Ospedaliero di Niguarda, Milan, Italy

The purpose of this chapter is to evaluate the diagnostic meaning of dynamic tests employed in the hormonal assessment of endocrine disorders that depend on pathological processes primarily localized in the hypothalamo-pituitary system (HPS). The endocrine function of the HPS can be affected by neurological or psychiatric diseases, as well as by peripheral hormonal or metabolic disorders; these secondary derangements of the HPS function are discussed here when they are involved in problems of differential diagnosis.

The study of the hormonal levels under basal conditions combined with a careful clinical and neuroradiological evaluation allows one to diagnose most cases of HPS dysfunction; the aim of dynamic tests is mainly to clarify pathophysiological problems and in particular to obtain information on the hypothalamic or pituitary site of the lesion.

We do not attempt to review all the tests proposed for the study of HPS dysfunction but critically evaluate tests which may have diagnostic value. In addition, we do not discuss those tests whose meanings are well established (e.g., metyrapone or dexamethasone).

We first consider the importance of evaluating the hormonal secretion of HPS under basal conditions. Thereafter we deal with tests currently thought to affect hormone secretion either by acting at the pituitary level or by modifying the activity of brain neurotransmitters.

BASAL LEVELS OF PITUITARY HORMONES

The spontaneous secretion of pituitary hormones is characterized by the presence of circadian rhythms and/or by episodic bursts of release which differ for each hormone in frequency, amplitude, and relation to sleep phases (94). Although the mechanisms of these secretory episodes remain to be clarified, it is likely that they depend mainly on changes in the activity of brain neurotransmitters and neurohormones.

Misleading information about the basal secretion of pituitary hormones can be obtained if only a single plasma sample is collected during a secretory burst or a quiescent phase. In addition, some of the pituitary hormones (e.g., growth hormone, ACTH, and prolactin) undergo stress-related increases. For these reasons plasma samples must be collected under carefully controlled conditions. This technique must be considered as a preliminary to any further dynamic evaluation since it offers invaluable information from a diagnostic point of view. Indeed if spontaneous fluctuations of plasma levels of the hormone are seen, it suggests that the hypothalamo-pituitary axis is functioning properly. Moreover, this kind of study is of particular relevance in view of the fact that the dynamic tests performed by neuropharmacological manipulations explore the HPS activity after challenge by unphysiological stimulation or inhibition.

Growth Hormone

When evaluating patients with suspected growth hormone (GH) secretory failure, studying basal secretion of the hormone by frequent plasma sampling may be of great diagnostic value. Indeed spontaneous secretory bursts which occur during a saline infusion rule out a condition of GH secretory failure; their absence, however, does not allow any conclusion to be drawn since even in normal subjects plasma GH levels can be at very low or undetectable levels for many hours (76). The presence of the sleep-related GH increase, which is the most repeatable of the GH secretory episodes (86), appears to be a reliable index for excluding a situation of GH secretory deficiency. The wide application of this test in clinical practice is limited by the observation that the sleep-related peak may be absent even in normal subjects, mainly in women (86). In addition, the onset of the GH increase is unpredictable (42,95), and a prolonged period of sampling is required.

For the assessment of GH hypersecretory states, a careful evaluation of the unstimulated GH levels is necessary mainly in acromegaly, since in this condition GH levels may fluctuate widely (20). In this disease, multiple GH samples can fully define the GH secretory status, permitting correct evaluation of the changes in the plasma hormone values in response to dynamic tests.

Prolactin

Hyperprolactinemia is perhaps the most frequent finding in patients with HPS dysfunctions. Indeed increased prolactin (PRL) secretion can arise from pathological processes localized in the hypothalamus or the pituitary. Many tests have been proposed in an attempt to distinguish between "functional" (i.e., without evidence of hypothalamic or pituitary lesions) and tumoral hyperprolactinemia, but this problem is still unsolved. There is a general agreement

(84) that the degree of hyperprolactinemia under basal conditions is, at present, a reliable parameter for distinguishing between these two conditions, since PRL levels consistently above 100 ng/ml allow diagnosis of PRL-secreting adenoma. On the contrary, basal PRL levels are generally below this value in patients with "functional" hyperprolactinemia. However, below 100 ng/ml there is an overlapping of values between tumoral and "functional" hyperprolactinemia, since PRL levels slightly above normal are a common finding in patients with neuroradiological evidence of a pituitary or hypothalamic tumor. In a series of craniopharyngiomas (84), for example, a 66% incidence of slight hyperprolactinemia (i.e., 15 to 19 ng/ml) has been reported.

The assessment of daily fluctuations of PRL levels does not help solve the problem of the origin of the hyperprolactinemia. In most patients with a PRL-secreting adenoma, PRL levels do not show the physiological sleep-related increase (52), but this is also common in patients with nontumoral hyperprolactinemia (91) or Cushing's disease (46).

In conclusion, all patients with hyperprolactinemia must be strongly suspected of having a disease of the hypothalamo-pituitary region. In particular, very high PRL levels are indicative of a tumoral origin of the hyperprolactinemia. Lower levels are consistent with either "functional" or tumoral hyperprolactinemia. It should be stressed, however, that there are some doubts about the existence of "functional" hyperprolactinemia (unless related to pregnancy or induced by drugs), since this diagnosis is only presumptive in the majority of patients and possibly due to a technical inability to visualize intrasellar microadenomas.

Gonadotropins

In female patients with menstrual disorders or in hypogonadal men, low or normal gonadotropin levels under basal conditions point to the existence of HPS disorders. However, as with the other pituitary hormones, evaluation of the actual basal secretion of gondotropins requires a prolonged period of observation, with plasma sampling at 20-min intervals to see if there are secretory episodes (102). The failure to observe a pulsatile release of gonadotropins is strongly indicative of a dysfunction of either hypothalamic or pituitary origin. Indeed this is a frequent finding in patients with anorexia nervosa (10), hypothalamic amenorrhea (100) [whether associated with pathological hyperprolactinemia (7) or not], isolated gonadotropin deficiency, or pituitary tumors (29). On the other hand in some of these patients plasma gonadotropin levels fluctuate, and therefore pulsatile gonadotropin release does not exclude an HPS dysfunction (10).

The study of gonadotropin release during sleep is of interest in particular conditions, e.g., true precocious puberty, where the sleep-related pulsatile increase of LH characteristic of the puberal phase is present (9). A similar pattern of response has also been observed in patients with anorexia nervosa (10).

Thyroid Stimulating Hormone

Basal thyroid stimulating hormone (TSH) levels are in the normal range in most hypothyroid patients with HPS dysfunctions; however, in some of these patients they have been found to be elevated although not to the values encountered in primary hypothyroidism (24,73). TSH in these patients is immunologically identical to the hormone secreted by the normal pituitary, but it may be biologically inactive (26).

Elevated basal TSH levels can be found in the rare patient with TSH-secreting pituitary adenoma or ectopic production of TSH. In these conditions, however, a clinical picture of hyperthyroidism and elevated thyroxine values are easily demonstrable (25).

Adrenocorticotropin

Basal ACTH levels are slightly elevated or in the normal range in most patients with Cushing's disease and appear to have an episodic pattern of secretion as in normal subjects (82). Frequent plasma sampling shows, however, that in Cushing's disease the ACTH nadir is higher than normal, as is the average level of ACTH; secretory spikes are more frequent and often greater than normal in amplitude; and the circadian rhythm is lacking (44,83,94).

A lack or an abnormality of this rhythm is not specific for Cushing's disease since it may be observed in a variety of acute and chronic illnesses, including neurological diseases, pituitary tumors, and psychiatric disorders, particularly depressive states (80). The study of basal plasma ACTH levels is also important in patients with Cushing's disease treated by pituitary irradiation or microadenectomy, since the restoration of normal periodicity of ACTH concentrations indicates that the disease has been cured (89). On the contrary, the persistence of abnormal ACTH periodicity in patients with clinical remission has been taken to indicate that, because of a primitive malfunction at the central nervous system (CNS) level, the disease has not been cured (45). In patients treated by bilateral adrenalectomy, the frequent evaluation of basal ACTH levels is useful for detecting as early as possible any evolution toward Nelson's syndrome.

NEUROPHARMACOLOGICAL TESTS

During recent years many pharmacological tests have been proposed in the study of HPS dysfunctions. These tests are employed in clinical practice to evaluate the existence of a condition of excessive or deficient hormonal secretion as well as to distinguish the hypothalamic or the pituitary origin of the dysfunction. For this purpose, synthetic releasing hormones or drugs acting at the hypothalamic or pituitary level have been employed. The rationale for the use of releasing hormones in patients with suspected or proved HPS dysfunctions is that a reduced hormone response implies a primary impairment of the pituitary cells (i.e., a diagnosis of primary pituitary failure), whereas a normal or even exaggerated hormonal release suggests a lack of stimulatory influence from the hypothalamus.

However, the application of these criteria in clinical practice may be misleading. Indeed in conditions of hypothalamic impairment, a single acute dose of the exogenous neurohormone may fail to restore the secretory activity of the pituitary cells unstimulated by a chronic lack of the endogenous neurohormone, and an erroneous diagnosis of primary pituitary failure could be made.

On the other hand, in a condition of partial pituitary failure, the administration of a pharmacological dose of the neurohormone can unphysiologically stimulate maximal secretion of the reserve, leading to the incorrect conclusion that the pituitary cells are functioning normally.

A normal hormone response after the administration of drugs capable of modifying the activity of brain neurotransmitters indicates that the neural mechanisms controlling secretion of the hormone and the pituitary cells are functioning properly. On the contrary, reduced responsiveness to these agents suggests the existence of an HPS dysfunction but does not allow one to establish the site of the lesion. In some cases a combination of tests can be useful for this purpose. For example, a normal response to gonadotropin releasing hormone (GnRH) and an impaired response to clomiphene suggest hypothalamic impairment in patients with amenorrhea.

However, in most cases the hypothalamic or pituitary site of the HPS derangement cannot be localized on a hormonal basis; it requires the combination of a careful clinical, hormonal, and neuroradiological evaluation.

In the presence of a functional hypothalamic derangement, pharmacological tests have also been employed to clarify which of the neural mechanisms controlling secretion of the pituitary is impaired. An attempt has been made to solve this point by studying in normal subjects the changes induced in the hormonal responses to the dynamic tests by drugs able to modify the activity of specific brain neurotransmitters and by comparing the results with those observed in HPS dysfunctions. However, because of the lack of specificity of the majority of neuroactive drugs, and mainly because of the complex interactions among the neurotransmitter systems, definite conclusions have not been reached.

Finally, when evaluating the results obtained with the use of neuroactive drugs, it should be remembered that some of these can change the release of pituitary hormones by acting at the CNS level and directly on the pituitary cells.

Thyrotropin Releasing Hormone Test

Thyrotropin releasing hormone (TRH) was the first neurohormone to be isolated from hypothalamic tissues and shown to be effective in releasing TSH in humans (2). Further studies gave evidence that TRH is also a powerful releaser of PRL (8) and in some pathological conditions of GH and ACTH (47,78).

Most of the studies refer to the intravenous injection of TRH, given either as a single bolus, repeated pulses, or an intravenous infusion. In normal humans the maximal TSH response after a bolus injection occurs over the dose range between 100 and 800 μg (2); the most commonly used dose is 200 μg.

When evaluating TRH-induced TSH release, one must consider quantitative and qualitative parameters: According to the rationale of the TRH test, the release of TSH is expected to be low in patients with hypothyroidism secondary to pituitary failure and normal in patients with hypothyroidism due to hypothalamic failure. This pattern of response is indeed frequently observed, but in clinical practice low responses in patients with hypothalamic tumors and normal responses in patients with intrasellar pituitary lesions are also encountered (85).

It has been claimed (24) that delayed, prolonged, or exaggerated responses are pathognomonic of an impairment of the TSH-secreting mechanisms operating at the hypothalamic level. However, the occurrence of "hypothalamic" responses has also been reported in patients with clear-cut evidence of pituitary impairment (13). Thus the evaluation of TSH release after TRH injection is of value in the differential diagnosis between hypothalamic and pituitary hypothyroidism only when there is a complete lack of response. An alteration of the temporal pattern of the release of the hormone after TRH is, however, strongly indicative of HPS dysfunction.

The TRH test has also been widely employed to study the secretion of PRL in patients with HPS dysfunction owing to the frequent occurrence of hyperprolactinemia in these conditions. The results of these studies (see ref. 84 for a review) showed that, independent of neuroradiological evidence of a hypothalamic or pituitary tumor, the TRH-induced PRL release can be either normal or impaired in patients with slightly elevated basal PRL levels, and that it is almost always impaired when basal PRL levels are well above the normal range.

TRH, which does not increase GH levels in normal humans, does so in several pathological conditions. An increase of GH levels after TRH has been observed in acromegaly (78), depression (59), anorexia nervosa (60), renal failure (32), hepatic cirrhosis (71), and primary hypothyroidism (34). This anomalous response has been taken to indicate either a derangement in brain catecholamines (15) or a functional disconnection between the hypothalamus and the pituitary (68). The finding of a TRH-induced GH release is of major clinical interest in acromegaly, where it is present in about 50% of patients (56). In the responsive patients, this test has been employed to evaluate the outcome of the surgical treatment (27,79). Indeed the persistence of TRH-induced GH increase after surgery suggests incomplete removal of the adenoma even when the basal levels of the hormone are in the normal range.

A paradoxical increase of ACTH after TRH injection in patients with Cushing's disease was reported by Krieger and Luria (47). This finding has not been confirmed, so the possible usefulness of this test awaits further consideration.

Gonadotropin Releasing Hormone Test

In normal adults GnRH given as a single intravenous bolus of 25 to 500 μg causes a dose-related increase in plasma concentrations of LH and FSH. The increase of FSH is weaker than that of LH in adults, whereas the secretory pattern of the two gonadotropins is reversed during the prepuberal stage (30,40). In clinical practice the test is usually performed by giving GnRH as an intravenous bolus with doses ranging between 10 and 150 μg. In many clinical studies a dose of 100 μg was used because it allows study of the acutely releasable pool as well as the pituitary reserve (96).

This test would distinguish between hypothalamic and pituitary hypogonadism, but a single acute administration of GnRH was found to increase plasma levels of gonadotropins independent of the site of the pathological process. Patients with pituitary adenomas and with Sheehan's syndrome show a great variability in gonadotropin responsiveness to GnRH, ranging from absent or impaired to normal responses. On the other hand, in patients with hypothalamic tumors the GnRH-induced LH release may be absent (65).

In most patients who fail to release gonadotropins following a single dose of GnRH, the repeated administration of the neurohormone evokes a positive response. This phenomenon can be appreciated mainly in patients with isolated gonadotropin deficiency. These patients usually do not release gonadotropins when tested with 100 μg GnRH; however, when given repeated doses of 500 μg they almost invariably show an appreciable increase in plasma gonadotropin levels. Thus it appears that in most cases of secondary hypogonadism the pituitary can secrete gonadotropins when adequately stimulated by GnRH (77).

Exaggerated responses to GnRH are frequently observed in patients with hypothalamic hypogonadism: They are common in hyperprolactinemic amenorrhea and are also frequent in patients with anorexia nervosa or in the so-called hypothalamic amenorrhea without hyperprolactinemia (65). The reasons for this behavior can probably be found in a lack of the long loop feedback by gonadal hormones in patients with a normal pituitary reserve of gonadotropins, and resembles the exaggerated response to GnRH observed in primary hypogonadism.

In conclusion, since an appreciable release of gonadotropins after GnRH can be achieved independent of the origin of hypogonadism, this test does not discriminate between a hypothalamic or a pituitary site of the lesion. However, the finding of an impaired or exaggerated response indicates an alteration of the HPS. On the other hand, when an HPS dysfunction is suspected, a normal responsiveness to GnRH does not rule out this possibility.

Tests with Dopamine Agonist or Antagonist Drugs

The effects of dopamine agonists on the secretion of pituitary hormones are complex as these drugs can alter the release of GH, PRL, TSH, LH (51), and

ACTH acting at the hypothalamic and/or the pituitary level (6). From a diagnostic point of view, the effects of these agents have been investigated mainly with respect to the secretion of PRL and GH.

PRL is predominantly under inhibitory influence from the hypothalamus; in particular, there is evidence that dopamine inhibits the release of PRL by acting on dopaminergic receptors present on the lactotrophs (58). Thus the administration of dopamine agonists explores the sensitivity of the PRL-secreting cells to one of the possible PRL inhibiting factors. For this purpose, oral administration of L-DOPA (43) or bromocriptine (23), subcutaneous injection of apomorphine (48), and infusion of dopamine (16) have been employed. The acute administration of 2.5 mg bromocriptine is followed by a decrease in PRL levels, which is evident by about the second hour and lasts 6 to 7 hr. In normal subjects the decrease in plasma PRL concentrations is to at least 50% below baseline values. In about 25% of patients with pathological hyperprolactinemia, with or without evidence of hypothalamic or pituitary tumors, the sensitivity to the PRL-lowering effect of a single dose of bromocriptine is reduced. Moreover, even in patients unresponsive to the acute test, chronic administration of bromocriptine usually results in a consistent decrease in PRL levels (84). Thus the acute administration of dopamine receptor stimulating drugs is neither of value for the differential diagnosis between "functional" and organic hyperprolactinemic states nor predictive of the outcome of chronic therapy with these drugs. Also, the acute administration of nomifensine (200 mg p.o.), an inhibitor of dopamine reuptake, is, in our experience and contrary to the suggestion of Muller et al. (67), unsuitable for the former purpose.

Since the first demonstration by Boyd et al. (12), a large body of evidence has accumulated that dopaminergic drugs can increase GH levels in humans. The oral administration of 500 mg L-DOPA is at present the most widely used tool to investigate the GH releasing effect of pharmacological stimulation of the dopaminergic system. The use of the L-DOPA test to evoke GH release has been proposed primarily for the diagnosis of hyposomatotropic dwarfism (see also *Insulin Hypoglycemia,* below). Normal subjects, however, may fail to respond to L-DOPA; in addition, peaks of GH levels after oral L-DOPA are erratic, occurring 30 to 100 min after ingestion of the drug (41). The unresponsiveness to L-DOPA may be explained on the basis of an extensive gastrointestinal degradation of the drug (19), but more recent studies (11) indicate that the negative response to L-DOPA is due to refractoriness of the neural centers which control GH release to the drug.

Although the L-DOPA test may be useful to assess the release of GH in suspected secretory failure of the hormone, it should not be used as a specific means to investigate the influence of the dopaminergic system on GH secretion. In fact, the effects of L-DOPA are more complex than those predicted from its conversion to dopamine, which accounts for only one aspect of its action on the brain. Apomorphine is a far more specific dopamine agonist (1). However, injection of this drug is followed in most cases by marked side effects (49) so that apomorphine is unsuitable for wide clinical use especially in children.

Paradoxically dopaminergic drugs inhibit GH secretion in acromegalic patients (53); there is clear-cut evidence that this effect acts at the pituitary level on the dopaminergic receptors of tumoral GH-secreting cells (63). The acute oral administration of 2.5 mg bromocriptine is followed by a marked decrease in GH levels in about 50% of acromegalics. In the remaining patients the GH-lowering effect of the drug is weak or absent. A patient whose GH levels fall at least 50% below the basal values after the acute administration of dopamine agonists has been arbitrarily defined a "responder" (55). This finding is of great pathophysiological interest, but from a clinical point of view the usefulness of this test lies mainly in its capability to predict if a given acromegalic subject is amenable to medical treatment with dopamine agonist. Indeed, in our patients treated with either bromocriptine or lisuride, we found a significant correlation between the responsiveness to the acute test and to the chronic administration of the drug (92).

Since the dopaminergic system inhibits PRL secretion, antidopaminergic drugs have been used in clinical studies as agents capable of releasing PRL. At present, sulpiride is one of the most widely employed drugs; because of its poor ability to cross the blood–brain barrier (5), it is probable that most of its PRL-releasing effect is exerted at the pituitary level. Although doses of sulpiride as low as 1 mg i.v. can significantly increase PRL levels, the majority of the studies were performed with a dose of 100 mg i.m. After the injection of sulpiride, PRL levels increase within 5 min and peak between 15 and 30 min. Comparative studies between the PRL-releasing activities of TRH and sulpiride have shown that the latter is the more powerful stimulator of PRL release in the normal subject (88). However, when used in the study of HPS dysfunctions, the results of the two tests are generally superimposable. Indeed, as in the case of TRH, PRL release after sulpiride depends mainly on the degree of hyperprolactinemia. In the presence of high basal levels of the hormone, sulpiride fails to further increase PRL levels. When plasma PRL levels are slightly elevated, a negative response can be observed independent of the presence of a pituitary tumor. Therefore this test too does not enable us to distinguish between "functional" and tumoral hyperprolactinemia. It has been observed, however (97), that in patients with pituitary tumors and normal PRL levels TRH can increase PRL levels but not sulpiride. These results do not suggest that sulpiride can disclose pathological changes in PRL secretion more subtly than TRH.

Insulin Hypoglycemia

It is well known that insulin-induced hypoglycemia is a powerful stimulus for the release of ACTH and GH; recently it was reported that hypoglycemia can also increase PRL levels in normal subjects (17). The test is generally performed by intravenous injection of regular insulin 0.1 unit/kg, but smaller doses are used in patients suspected of having pituitary or adrenal failure and larger doses in patients with acromegaly, diabetes mellitus, or Cushing's disease, where insulin resistance is present. GH, PRL, and ACTH levels generally increase 30 to 90 min after the insulin injection. A fall in blood glucose levels to at least 50% below the baseline is required to avoid false-negative responses. Much consideration has been given to the mechanism(s) which links these hormonal responses to changes in glucose levels (17). An overall evaluation of the studies on this topic indicates that modifications of glucose levels affect hormone release by acting at the hypothalamic level (76), and the pituitary hormonal responses are mainly related to the appearance of the symptoms of stress rather than being functions of any specific glucose level.

The importance of brain monoamines in regulating the hormonal responses to hypoglycemia, first recognized by Muller et al. (69) in rats, was largely confirmed also in humans. There are data suggesting that the response to insulin hypoglycemia is modulated by adrenergic, serotoninergic, and dopaminergic pathways, but the respective roles of these neurotransmitters are still to be established (62). In consequence, it is not possible to deduce the functional activity of a given neurotransmitter from the pattern of the hormonal response.

Impaired GH responsiveness to insulin hypoglycemia, which is one of the most frequent hormonal disturbances in HPS dysfunctions, is observed not only in patients with pituitary dwarfism and tumors of the hypothalamo-pituitary region (39) but also in those with other conditions where GH neuroregulation is impaired as a consequence of hormonal, metabolic, neurological, or psychiatric alterations.

Reversible impairment of GH release after hypoglycemia can be observed in obese subjects (18) as well as in patients with primary hypothyroidism (36), diabetes (66), glucocorticoid excess (35), delayed puberty, and hypogonadism (22). In neurological and affective disease (e.g., Parkinson's disease and depression), impaired GH response to hypoglycemia has also been observed (33,50). Thus the diagnosis of true GH secretory failure requires careful clinical and endocrinological evaluation to rule out other conditions in which impaired GH responsiveness may be found.

Another problem of evaluating the results of the insulin hypoglycemia test is the wide variability of peak GH values in normal subjects. Some authors (103) report that patients with complete GH deficiency do not show a rise greater than 3 ng/ml, whereas others (72) indicate as the lowest normal limit peak values ranging from 5 to 10 ng/ml.

The many other tests proposed to evaluate the release of GH—e.g., arginine infusion (72), L-DOPA (12), sleep-related increase (57), Bovril (37), and glucagon (81)—do not provide better results than hypoglycemia. Indeed all these provocative tests have the potential disadvantage that they may fail to release GH even in normal subjects (72,74). Thus to reach a conclusive diagnosis of GH deficiency, a failure to respond to at least two of the provocative tests usually employed (e.g., arginine, insulin, or L-DOPA) is required. In acromegaly, insulin hypoglycemia, like arginine, induces a repeatable GH response in only some cases; therefore it is of limited value in establishing the status of HPS in this disease (54).

The evaluation of ACTH and cortisol increase after insulin hypoglycemia is one of the most used tests in clinical practice, as it allows study of the hypothalamo-pituitary-adrenal axis, particularly its ability to respond to stress. This test gives invaluable information for the assessment of patients with hypothalamo-pituitary tumors before and after neurosurgery and for the diagnosis of Cushing's syndrome, a condition where the insulin-induced ACTH release is low (38). Since patients with Cushing's syndrome often present psychiatric symptoms, it may be difficult to distinguish them from those with severe endogenous depression, who have high plasma and urinary cortisol levels, with loss of circadian rhythm and resistance to dexamethasone suppression (14). Insulin hypoglycemia is useful in these conditions, since a normal response has been reported in patients with depressive states without Cushing's syndrome (75).

Conflicting results have been reported on the effectiveness of hypoglycemia for releasing PRL in normal subjects, probably because of the different doses of insulin employed. When an adequate insulin dose is injected (0.1 unit/kg), PRL levels are constantly increased (98). Thus the hypoglycemic stimulus is a reliable test to assess the integrity of the HPS in regulating PRL secretion. Our study of patients with pituitary tumors demonstrated a reduced PRL response to insulin hypoglycemia even when TRH responsiveness was present (92a). The absence of PRL release after insulin hypoglycemia may thus represent a very sensitive index of a deranged control of PRL secretion in patients with hypothalamo-pituitary tumors.

Tests with Clomiphene and Estrogens

Estrogens regulate the release of gonadotropins by positive and/or negative feedback mechanisms which probably operate at different hypothalamic sites (64). Clinical evaluation of the functional integrity of the negative feedback may be obtained by determining plasma levels of gonadotropins after the administration of clomiphene. Clomiphene citrate is a weak synthetic estrogen which competes with endogenous estradiol at the receptor level (93,99). The mechanism of the clomiphene-induced gonadotropin release might thus depend on an increased release of GnRH as a consequence of a decreased inhibition by estradiol (87).

In normal female subjects of reproductive age, clomiphene, when administered during the early follicular phase at doses of 50 to 100 mg/day for 5 days, induces a progressive increase in FSH and LH during its administration. This first peak is followed by a decline of both hormones and by a rise of estradiol which triggers the midcycle peak of LH and a moderate surge of FSH (second peak) (61). Vanderberg and Yen (90) showed that the quantitative rise in LH during treatment with clomiphene is greater during the late follicular phase of the cycle, and the reverse is true for FSH. Thus it is suggested that a decrease in the negative feedback effect of estradiol exists for LH but not for FSH. In contrast, in postmenopausal women (21) clomiphene inhibits gonadotropin release as the absence of endogenous estradiol allows the weak estrogenic activity of the drug to be effective. A clomiphene dose of 100 to 200 mg/day given to men generally induces an increase in LH levels which are evident within 2 days and which have approximately doubled by 6 days (28). The clomiphene-induced gonadotropin release in men may be explained by experimental data showing that androgens exert their action at the CNS level after conversion to estrogens (70).

In conclusion, the clomiphene test allows evaluation of the ability of the hypothalamus to release GnRH. Obviously, a normal responsiveness to the drug also implies the integrity of gonadotropic cells to secrete FSH and LH as well as sufficient plasma concentration of estradiol. An impaired responsiveness alone does not allow any conclusion to be drawn as to the site of the lesion. In fact, a reduced response to clomiphene may be due to a deficit of GnRH, to a primary impairment of gonadotrophs, or to a low concentration of estradiol. For these reasons the responsiveness to clomiphene is abolished in most patients with HPS dysfunctions, mainly when gonadotropin and estrogen levels are low.

The integrity of estradiol positive feedback for gonadotropins may be evaluated employing estradiol benzoate, a depot ester with prolonged estrogen activity (101). The administration of estradiol benzoate 1 mg/day i.m. for 1 to 3 days, by raising plasma estradiol levels to values near those seen during the late follicular phase, triggers a midcycle-like peak of LH after 48 to 72 hr. The LH rise is usually unaccompanied by a concomitant increase in plasma FSH levels. LH increase is greater during the late than during the early follicular phase, suggesting that a concomitant increase in the sensitivity of the positive feedback mechanism occurs during the course of a follicular phase. This positive feedback mechanism is not simply a function of some threshold concentration of estradiol; it is also critically dependent on a time component. The release of gonadotropins is in fact demonstrable only if the increase in blood estrogen concentration is sustained for at least 24 hr. It is not yet known whether the positive feedback occurs primarily at the hypothalamus, the pituitary, or both. It has been reported, however, that estrogens modulate the sensitivity of the gonadotropic cells to the action of GnRH (4,104). Therefore a normal responsiveness of gonadotropins to estradiol, like that of clomiphene, requires not only the integrity of gonadotropic cells but also the presence of endogenous GnRH.

In clinical practice, the study of gonadotropin release after estradiol administration is useful in patients who secrete normal amounts of LH, FSH, and estradiol under basal conditions and after GnRH but yet fail to menstruate cyclically. In these conditions the absence of gonadotropin release after estradiol administration has been reported to be reduced mainly in patients with hypothalamic amenorrhea and in women with the amenorrhea–galactorrhea syndrome and a normal response to GnRH (3,31).

TABLE 1. Basic tests in the study of hypothalamo-pituitary dysfunctions

Hormone	Hypersecretory conditions		Hyposecretory conditions	
	Condition	Tests	Condition	Tests
GH	Acromegaly Gigantism	Spontaneous fluctuations TRH Glucose load Dopamine agonists	HP tumors[a] Pituitary necrosis Pituitary dwarfism	Spontaneous fluctuations Sleep Arginine Hypoglycemia L-DOPA
Prolactin	Tumoral and "functional" hyperprolactinemia	Spontaneous fluctuations Sleep TRH Hypoglycemia Dopamine antagonists Dopamine agonists	Pituitary necrosis	TRH Hypoglycemia
Gonadotropins	Gonadotropin-secreting adenomas Precocious puberty	Spontaneous fluctuations Sleep GnRH TRH (?)[b]	Isolated gonadotropin deficiency HP tumors Pituitary necrosis "Functional" hyperprolactinemia Hypothalamic amenorrhea	Spontaneous fluctuations GnRH Clomiphene Estradiol benzoate
TSH	TSH-producing adenomas	TRH Triiodothyronine	Pituitary necrosis HP tumors Isolated TSH deficiency	TRH
ACTH	Cushing's disease	Spontaneous fluctuations Circadian rhythm Metyrapone Hypoglycemia Lysin vasopressin TRH Cortisol infusion (?)	Pituitary necrosis Pituitary tumors Isolated ACTH deficiency	Hypoglycemia Metyrapone Lysine vasopressin

TABLE 1. *(Continued)*

| Hormone | Hypersecretory conditions | | Hyposecretory conditions | |
	Condition	Tests	Condition	Tests
Antidiuretic hormone	Diabetes insipidus	Dexamethasone Dopamine agonists (?) Water deprivation Exogenous vasopressin Hypertonic saline Nicotine Exercise		

[a] HP tumors = hypothalamo-pituitary tumors.
[b] (?) indicates that the test is of potential but still unproved value.

SYNOPSIS OF BASIC TESTS USED TO STUDY HYPOTHALAMO-PITUITARY DYSFUNCTIONS

We summarized in Table 1 the tests used most frequently for studying the principal HPS dysfunctions. We stress, however, that some of these tests are useful mainly in pathophysiological studies. Hyperprolactinemic patients, for example, often undergo a number of tests (e.g., TRH, sulpiride, hypoglycemia, L-DOPA) which add no information to that provided by a careful evaluation of the basal PRL levels when the practical problem is the differential diagnosis between "functional" and tumoral hyperprolactinemia. Thus when studying HPS dysfunctions, the clinician should always evaluate which tests are really useful for the diagnosis and therapy of the individual patient.

ACKNOWLEDGMENT

This study was partially supported by grant 79.00695.95 from CNR.

REFERENCES

1. Andén, N. E., Rubensson, E., Fuxe, K., and Hökfelt, T. (1967): Evidence for dopamine receptor stimulation by apomorphine. *J. Pharm. Pharmacol.*, 19:626–629.
2. Anderson, M. S., Bowers, C. U., Kastin, A. J., Schalch, D. S., Schally, A. V., Snyder, P. J., Utiger, R. D., Wilber, J. F., and Wise, A. J. (1971): Synthetic thyrotropin releasing hormone: A potent stimulator of thyrotropin secretion in man. *N. Engl. J. Med.*, 285:1279–1283.
3. Aono, T., Myake, A., Shiosi, T., Kinugasa, T., Onishi, T., and Kurachi, K. (1976): Impaired LH release following exogenous estrogen administration in patients with amenorrhea-galactorrhea syndrome. *J. Clin. Endocrinol. Metab.*, 42:696–702.
4. Ayer, M. S., and Fink, G. (1974): The role of sex steroid hormones in modulating the responsiveness of the anterior pituitary gland to luteinizing hormone releasing factor in the female rat. *J. Endocrinol.*, 62:553–572.
5. Benakis, A., and Stefan, Y. (1977): Argument in favor of the direct effect of psychotropic drugs on hypophysis prolactin and gonadotrope cells. In: *Prolactin and Human Reproduction,* edited by P. G. Crosignani and C. Robyn, pp. 125–134. Academic Press, New York.
6. Besser, G. M., Jeffcoate, W. J., and Tomlin, S. (1976): The use of metyrapone and bromocriptine in the control of Cushing's syndrome. In: *Program 5th Intern. Congr. Endocrinology,* p. 202.
7. Bohnet, H. G., and Schneider, H. P. G. (1977): Prolactin as cause of anovulation. In: *Prolactin and Human Reproduction,* edited by P. G. Crosignani and C. Robyn, pp. 153–159. Academic Press, New York.
8. Bowers, C. Y., Friesen, H., Hwang, P., Guyda, H., and Folkers, K. (1971): Prolactin and thyrotropin release in man by synthetic pyroglutamylhistidyl-prolinamide. *Biochem. Biophys. Res. Commun.*, 45:1033–1041.
9. Boyar, R. M., Finkelstein, J. W., Roffwarg, H., Kapen, S., Weitzman, E. D., and Hellman, L. (1972): Synchronization of augmented luteinizing hormone secretion with sleep during puberty. *N. Engl. J. Med.*, 287:582–586.
10. Boyar, R. M., Katz, J., Finkelstein, J. W., Kapen, S., Weiner, H., Weitzman, E. D., and Hellman, L. (1974): Anorexia nervosa: Immaturity of the 24 hour luteinizing hormone secretory pattern. *N. Engl. J. Med.*, 291:861–865.
11. Boyd, A. E., Angoff, G., Long, A., and Mager, M. (1978): L-DOPA absorption and the pituitary-hypothalamic axis. *J. Clin. Endocrinol. Metab.*, 47:1341–1347.
12. Boyd, A. E., Lebovitz, H. E., and Pfeiffer, J. B. (1970): Stimulation of human growth hormone secretion by L-DOPA. *N. Engl. J. Med.*, 283:1425–1429.
13. Burger, H. G., and Patel, Y. C. (1977): TSH and TRH: their physiological regulation and

the clinical applications of TRH. In: *Clinical Neuroendocrinology,* edited by L. Martini and G. M. Besser, pp. 67–131. Academic Press, New York.

14. Butler, P. W. B., and Besser, G. M. (1968): Pituitary-adrenal function in severe depressive illness. *Lancet,* 1:1234–1236.

15. Collu, R., Leboeuf, G., Letarte, J., and Ducharme, J. R. (1977): Increase in plasma growth hormone levels following thyrotropin-releasing hormone injection in children with primary hypothyroidism. *J. Clin. Endocrinol. Metab.,* 44:743–747.

16. Colussi, G., Cremascoli, G., Botalla, L., De Stefano, L., Oppizzi, G., Verde, G., Chiodini, P. G., and Liuzzi, A. (1976): La neuroregolazione della prolattina. In: *Atti 16th Congr. Soc. It. Endocrinol.,* p. 40.

17. Copinschi, G., L'Hermite, M., Leclercq, R., Goldstein, J., Vanhaelst, L., Virasoro, E., and Robyn, C. (1975): Effects of glucocorticoids on pituitary hormonal responses to hypoglycemia: Inhibition of prolactin release. *J. Clin. Endocrinol. Metab.,* 40:442–449.

18. Copinschi, G., Wegienka, L. C., Hore, S., and Forsham, P. H. (1967): Effect of arginine on serum levels of insulin and growth hormone in obese subjects. *Metabolism,* 16:402–412.

19. Cotler, S., Holazo, A., Boxenbaum, H., and Kaplan, S. (1976): Influence of route of administration on physiological availability of levodopa in dogs. *J. Pharm. Sci.,* 65:823–827.

20. Cryer, P. E., and Daughaday, W. H. (1969): Regulation of GH secretion in acromegaly. *J. Clin. Endocrinol. Metab.,* 29:386–393.

21. Czygan, P. J., and Schulz, K. D. (1972): Studies on the anti-oestrogen and oestrogen-like action of clomiphene citrate in women. *Gynecol. Invest.,* 3:126–134.

22. Deller, J. J., Plunket, D. C., and Forsham, P. H. (1966): Growth hormone studies in growth retardation: Therapeutic response to administration of androgens. *Calif. Med.,* 104:359–362.

23. Del Pozo, E., Brun del Re, R., Varga, R., and Friesen, H. (1972): The inhibition of prolactin secretion in man by CB 154 (2-Br-α-ergocriptine). *J. Clin. Endocrinol. Metab.,* 35:768–770.

24. Faglia, G., Beck Peccoz, P., Ferrari, C., Ambrosi, B., Spada, A., Travaglini, P., and Paracchi, A. (1973): Plasma TSH response to TRH in patients with pituitary and hypothalamic disorders. *J. Clin. Endocrinol. Metab.,* 37:595–601.

25. Faglia, G., Ferrari, C., Neri, V., Beck Peccoz, P., and Valentini, F. (1972): High plasma thyrotropin levels in two patients with pituitary tumors. *Acta Endocrinol. (Kbh),* 69:649–658.

26. Faglia, G., Ferrari, C., Paracchi, A., and Pinchera, A. (1977): Thyrotropin secretion in patients with secondary hypothyroidism. *Acta Endocrinol. [Suppl] (Kbh),* 212:170.

27. Faglia, G., Paracchi, A., Ferrari, C., and Beck Peccoz, P. (1978): Evaluation of the results of trans-sphenoidal surgery in acromegaly by assessment of the growth hormone response to thyrotropin releasing hormone. *Clin. Endocrinol.,* 8:373–380.

28. Franchimont, P. (1973): Human gonadotropin secretion in male subjects. In: *The Endocrine Function of the Human Testis,* edited by V. H. T. James, M. Serio, and L. Martini, pp. 439–458. Academic Press, New York.

29. Franks, S., Murray, M. A., Jequier, A. M., Steela, J. J., Nabarro, J. D., and Jacobs, H. S. (1975): Incidence and significance of hyperprolactinemia in women with amenorrhea. *Clin. Endocrinol.,* 4:597–607.

30. Garnier, P. E., Chaussain, J. L., Binet, E., Schlumberger, A., and Job, J. L. (1974): Effect of synthetic luteinizing hormone-releasing hormone (LHRH) on the release of gonadotrophins in children and adolescents. VI. Relations to age, sex and puberty. *Acta Endocrinol. (Kbh),* 77:422–429.

31. Glass, M. R., Shaw, R. W., Butt, W. R., Logan Edwards, R., and London, D. R. (1975): An abnormality of oestrogen feedback in amenorrhea-galactorrhea syndrome. *Br. Med. J.,* 3:274–275.

32. Gonzales-Barcena, D., Kastin, A. J., Schalch, D. S., Torres-Zamora, M., Perez-Pasten, E., Kato, A., and Schally, A. V. (1973): Response to thyrotropin releasing hormone in patients with renal failure and after infusion in normal men. *J. Clin. Endocrinol. Metab.,* 36:117–120.

33. Gruen, P. H., Sachar, E. J., Altman, N., and Sassin, J. (1975): Growth hormone response to hypoglycemia in depressed women. *Arch. Gen. Psychiatry,* 32:31–33.

34. Hamada, N., Uoi, K., Nishizawa, Y., Okamoto, T., Hasegawa, K., Morii, H., and Wada, M. (1976): Increase of serum GH concentration following TRH injection in patients with primary hypothyroidism. *Endocrinol. Jpn.,* 23:5–10.

35. Hartog, M., Gaafar, M. A., and Fraser, R. (1964): Effects of corticosteroids on serum growth hormone. *Lancet,* 2:376–378.

36. Iwatsuho, H., Kiyohiko, O., Yoshiaki, O., Fukuchi, M., Miyai, K., Hiroshi, A., and Kumahara, Y. (1967): Human growth hormone secretion in primary hypothyroidism before and after treatment. *J. Clin. Endocrinol. Metab.*, 27:1751–1754.
37. Jackson, D., Grant, D. B., and Clayton, B. E. (1968): A simple oral test of growth hormone secretion in children. *Lancet*, 2:373–375.
38. James, V. H. T., and Landon, J. (1968): Control of corticosteroid secretion: Current views and methods of assessment. In: *Recent Advances in Endocrinology*, edited by V. H. T. James, pp. 50–94. Churchill, London.
39. Jenkins, J. S., Gilbert, C. J., and Ang, V. (1976): Hypothalamic-pituitary function in patients with craniopharyngioma. *J. Clin. Endocrinol. Metab.*, 43:394–399.
40. Job, J. C., Garnier, P. E., Chaussain, J. L., and Milhaud, G. (1972): Elevation of serum gonadotropin (LH and FSH) after releasing hormone (LHRH) injection in normal children and patients with disorders of puberty. *J. Clin. Endocrinol. Metab.*, 35:473–476.
41. Kansal, P. C., Buse, J., Talbert, O. R., and Bore, M. G. (1972): The effect of L-DOPA on plasma growth hormone, insulin and thyroxine. *J. Clin. Endocrinol. Metab.*, 34:99–105.
42. Karacan, I., Rosenbloom, A. L., Williams, R. L., Finley, W. H., and Husch, C. J. (1971): Slow wave deprivation in relation to plasma growth hormone concentration. *Behav. Neuropsychiatry*, 2:11–24.
43. Kleinberg, D. L., Noel, G. L., and Frantz, A. G. (1971): Chlorpromazine stimulation and L-DOPA suppression of plasma prolactin in man. *J. Clin. Endocrinol. Metab.*, 33:873–876.
44. Krieger, D. T., and Allen, W. (1975): Relationship of bioassayable and immunoassayable plasma ACTH and cortisol concentrations in normal subjects and in patients with Cushing's disease. *J. Clin. Endocrinol. Metab.*, 40:675–687.
45. Krieger, D. T., and Glick, S. M. (1972): Growth hormone and cortisol responsiveness in Cushing's syndrome: Relation to a possible central nervous system etiology. *Am. J. Med.*, 52:25–40.
46. Krieger, D. T., Howanitz, P. J., and Frantz, A. G. (1976): Absence of nocturnal elevation of plasma prolactin concentrations in Cushing's disease. *J. Clin. Endocrinol. Metab.*, 42:260–272.
47. Krieger, D. T., and Luria, M. (1977): Plasma ACTH and cortisol responses to TRF, vasopressin or hypoglycemia in Cushing's disease and Nelson's syndrome. *J. Clin. Endocrinol. Metab.*, 44:361–368.
48. Lal, S., De La Vega, C. E., Sourkes, J. L., and Friesen, H. G. (1973): Effect of apomorphine on growth hormone, prolactin, luteinizing hormone and follicle stimulating hormone levels in human serum. *J. Clin. Endocrinol. Metab.*, 37:719–724.
49. Lal, S., Martin, J. B., De La Vega, C. E., and Friesen, H. (1975): Comparison of the effect of apomorphine and L-DOPA on serum growth hormone levels in normal men. *Clin. Endocrinol.*, 4:277–285.
50. Lebovitz, H. E., Skyler, J. S., and Boyd, A. E. (1974): L-DOPA and growth hormone secretion in man. *Adv. Neurol.*, 5:461–469.
51. Leebaw, W. F., Lee, L., and Woolf, P. (1978): Dopamine affects on basal and augmented pituitary hormone secretion. *J. Clin. Endocrinol. Metab.*, 47:480–487.
52. L'Hermite, M., Caufriez, A., and Robyn, C. (1977): Pathophysiology of human prolactin secretion with special reference to prolactin-secreting pituitary adenomas and isolated galactorrhea. In: *Prolactin and Human Reproduction*, edited by P. G. Crosignani and C. Robyn, pp. 179–202. Academic Press, New York.
53. Liuzzi, A., Chiodini, P. G., Botalla, L., Cremascoli, G., and Silvestrini, F. (1972): Inhibitory effect of L-DOPA on GH release in acromegalic patients. *J. Clin. Endocrinol. Metab.*, 35:941–943.
54. Liuzzi, A., Chiodini, P. G., Botalla, L., Cremascoli, G., and Tosi, M. (1973): Indagini sul controllo ipotalamico della increzione somatotropica nell'acromegalia. *Folia Endocrinol. (Roma)*, 26:503–510.
55. Liuzzi, A., Chiodini, P. G., Botalla, L., Cremascoli, G., Muller, E. E., and Silvestrini, F. (1974): Decreased plasma growth hormone levels in acromegalics following CB 154 administration. *J. Clin. Endocrinol. Metab.*, 38:910–912.
56. Liuzzi, A., Chiodini, P. G., Botalla, L., Silvestrini, F., and Muller, E. E. (1974): Growth hormone-releasing activity of TRH and GH-lowering effect of dopaminergic drugs in acromegaly: Homogeneity of the two responses. *J. Clin. Endocrinol. Metab.*, 39:871–876.
57. Mace, J. W., Gotlin, R. W., Sassin, J. F., Parker, D. C., and Rossman, L. G. (1970): Usefulness

of post-sleep human growth hormone release as a test of physiological growth hormone secretion. *J. Clin. Endocrinol. Metab.*, 31:225–226.

58. MacLeod, R. M., and Lehmeyer, J. E. (1974): Studies on the mechanism of the dopamine mediated inhibition of PRL secretion. *Endocrinology,* 94:1077–1085.

59. Maeda, K., Kato, Y., Ohgo, S., Chihara, K., Yoshimoto, Y., Yamaguchi, N., Kuromaru, S., and Imura, K. (1975): Growth hormone and prolactin release after injection of thyrotropin-releasing hormone in patients with depression. *J. Clin. Endocrinol. Metab.,* 40:501–505.

60. Maeda, K., Kato, Y., Yamaguchi, N., Chihara, K., Ohgo, S., Iwasaki, Y., Yoshimoto, Y., Moridera, K., Kuromaru, S., and Imura, H. (1976): Growth hormone release following thyrotropin-releasing hormone injection into patients with anorexia nervosa. *Acta Endocrinol. (Kbh),* 81:1–8.

61. Marshall, J. C., Morris, R., Count, J., and Butt, N. R. (1975): Absent positive feed-back of estrogens: A cause of amenorrhea. *J. Endocrinol.,* 59:xxiv.

62. Martin, J. B. (1976): Brain regulation of growth hormone secretion. In: *Frontiers in Neuroendocrinology,* Vol. 4, edited by L. Martini and W. F. Ganong, pp. 129–168. Raven Press, New York.

63. Mashiter, K., Adams, E., Beard, M., and Halley, A. (1977): Bromocriptine inhibits prolactin and growth hormone release by human pituitary tumours in culture. *Lancet,* 2:197–202.

64. McCann, S. M., Krulich, L., Cooper, K. J., Kalra, P. S., Kalra, S. P., Libertun, C., Negro-Vilar, A., Orias, R., Ronnekleiv, K., and Fawcett, C. P. (1973): Hypothalamic control of gonadotropin and prolactin secretion. *J. Reprod. Fertil. (Suppl),* 20:43–59.

65. Mortimer, C. H. (1977): Gonadotropin-releasing hormone. In: *Clinical Neuroendocrinology,* edited by L. Martini and G. M. Besser, pp. 213–236. Academic Press, New York.

66. Muggeo, M., Tiengo, A., Fedele, D., Nosadini, R., Molinari, M., and Crepaldi, G. (1975): Insulina e ormoni cotroinsulari nel prediabete e nel diabete clinico. In: *Atti Giornate Endocrinologiche Senesi,* edited by E. E. Muller and S. Piazzi, pp. 139–149. Sclavo, Siena.

67. Muller, E. E., Genazzani, A. R., and Murru, S. (1978): Nomifensine: Diagnostic test in hyperprolactinemic states. *J. Clin. Endocrinol. Metab.,* 47:1352–1357.

68. Muller, E. E., Panerai, A. E., Cocchi, D., Gil-Ad, I., Rossi, G. L., and Olgiati, V. R. (1976): Nonspecific release of GH by hypothalamic neurohormones following experimental interruption of central nervous system-anterior pituitary connections. In: *Program 58th Meet. Endocrine Soc.,* p. 120.

69. Muller, E. E., Saito, T., Arimura, A., and Schally, A. V. (1967): Hypoglycemia, stress and growth hormone release: Blockade of growth hormone release by drugs acting on the central nervous system. *Endocrinology,* 80:109–117.

70. Naftolin, F., Ryan, K. J., Davies, I. J., Reddy, V. V., Flores, F., Petro, Z., Kuhn, M., White, R. J., Takaoka, Y., and Wolin, L. (1975): The formation of estrogens by central neuroendocrine tissues. *Recent Prog. Horm. Res.,* 31:295–315.

71. Panerai, A. E., Salerno, F., Manneschi, M., Cocchi, D., and Muller, E. E. (1977): Growth hormone and prolactin responses to thyrotropin releasing hormone in patients with severe liver disease. *J. Clin. Endocrinol. Metab.,* 45:134–140.

72. Parker, M. L., Hammond, J. M., and Daughaday, W. H. (1967): The arginine provocative test: An aid in the diagnosis of hyposomatotropinism. *J. Clin. Endocrinol. Metab.,* 27:1129–1136.

73. Patel, Y. C., and Burger, H. G. (1973): Serum thyrotropin in pituitary and/or hypothalamic hypothyroidism: Normal or elevated basal levels and paradoxical responses to thyrotropin-releasing hormone. *J. Clin. Endocrinol. Metab.,* 37:190–196.

74. Raiti, S., Davis, W. T., and Blizzard, R. M. (1976): A comparison of the effect of insulin hypoglycemia and arginine infusion on release of human growth hormone. *Lancet,* 2:1182–1183.

75. Rees, L. H. (1977): Human adrenocorticotropin and lipotropin. In: *Clinical Neuroendocrinology,* edited by L. Martini and G. M. Besser, pp. 401–441. Academic Press, New York.

76. Reichlin, S. (1974): Regulation of somatotrophic hormone secretion. In: *Handbook of Physiology—Endocrinology,* Vol. IV, part 2, edited by E. Knobil and W. H. Sawyer, pp. 405–447. American Physiological Society, Washington.

77. Reitano, J. F., Caminos-Torres, R., and Snyder, P. J. (1975): Serum LH and FSH responses to the repetitive administration of gonadotropin-releasing hormone in patients with idiopathic hypogonadotropic hypogonadism. *J. Clin. Endocrinol. Metab.,* 41:1035–1042.

78. Saito, S., Abe, K., Yoshida, H., Kaneko, T., Nakamura, E., Shiruzu, N., and Yanainara, N.

(1971): Effects of synthetic thyrotropin releasing hormone on plasma thyrotropin, growth hormone and insulin levels in man. *Endocrinol. Jpn.,* 17:101–108.

79. Samaan, S. A., Leavens, M. E., and Jesse, R. H. (1974): Serum GH and PRL response to TRH in patients with acromegaly before and after surgery. *J. Clin. Endocrinol. Metab.,* 38:957–963.

80. Sawin, C. T., and Clark, T. (1968): Measurement of plasma cortisol in the diagnosis of Cushing's syndrome. *Ann. Intern. Med.,* 68:624–631.

81. Sawin, C. T., and Mitchell, M. L. (1970): A comparison of response of serum growth hormone to glucagon and vasopressin. *Metabolism,* 19:898–903.

82. Scott, A. P., Bloomfield, G. A., Lowry, P. J., Gilkes, J. J. H., Landon, J., and Rees, L. H. (1976): Pituitary adrenocorticotrophin and the melanocyte stimulating hormone. *Peptide Horm.,* 12:263–271.

83. Sederberg-Olsen, P., Binder, C., Kehlet, C., Neville, A. M., and Nielsen, L. M. (1973): Episodic variation in plasma corticosteroids in subjects with Cushing's syndrome of differing etiology. *J. Clin. Endocrinol. Metab.,* 36:906–910.

84. Silvestrini, F., Liuzzi, A., and Chiodini, P. G. (1978): Prolactin and pituitary tumors. In: *Current Topics in Experimental Endocrinology,* Vol. 3, edited by L. Martiniard V.H.T. James, pp. 132–172. Academic Press, New York.

85. Silvestrini, F., Liuzzi, A., Chiodini, P. G., Cattabeni, A., and Botalla, L. (1973): Comportamento del TSH plasmatico nelle neoplasie ipofisarie dopo stimolazione con TRH. *Folia Endocrinol. (Roma),* 26:398–406.

86. Takahashi, Y., Kipnis, D. M., and Daughaday, W. H. (1968): Growth hormone secretion during sleep. *J. Clin. Invest.,* 47:2079–2090.

87. Taubert, H. D., Kessler, R., Busch, G., and Werner, H. J. (1970): The effect of clomiphene and cyclofenil upon pituitary LH and hypothalamic LHRH content in female rat. *Experientia,* 26:97–99.

88. Thorner, M. O., Besser, G. M., Nagan, C., and McNeilly, A. S. (1974): Introduction of a new stimulation test for prolactin: The sulpiride test: comparison with other dynamic function tests. *J. Endocrinol.,* 43:xxxii.

89. Tyrrell, J. B., Brooks, R. M., Fitzgerald, P., Cofoid, P. B., Forsham, P. H., and Wilson, C. B. (1977): Pituitary tumors in Cushing's disease: reversal of hypercortisolism by selective transsphenoidal adenomectomy. In: *Program 59th Meet. Endocrine Soc.,* p. 142.

90. Vanderberg, G., and Yen, S. S. C. (1973): Effect of antiestrogenic action of clomiphene during the menstrual cycle: Evidence for a change in the feedback sensitivity. *J. Clin. Endocrinol. Metab.,* 37:356–365.

91. Vekemans, M., and Robyn, C. (1975): The influence of exogenous estrogen on the circadian periodicity of circulating prolactin in women. *J. Clin. Endocrinol. Metab.,* 40:886–889.

92. Verde, G., Liuzzi, A., Chiodini, P. G., Cozzi, R., Botalla, L., Rainer, E., and Horowski, H. (1978): Lisuride in acromegaly and pathological hyperprolactinemia. *Acta Endocrinol.* [*Suppl*] *(Kbh),* 225:395.

92a. Verde, G., Oppizzi, G., Cozzi, R., Favales, F., Botalla, L., Chiodini, P. G., and Liuzzi, A. (1979): Plasma prolactin after insulin hypoglycemia in patients with pituitary tumours. In: *Recent Advances in Neuroendocrinology,* edited by A. Polleri and R. MacLeod, pp. 307–302. Academic Press, New York.

93. Wall, J. A., Franklin, R. R., and Kaufman, R. H. (1964): Reversal of benign and malignant endometrial changes with clomiphene. *Am. J. Obstet. Gynecol.,* 88:107–108.

94. Weitzman, E. D., Boyar, R. M., Kapen, S., and Hellman, L. (1975): The relation of sleep and sleep stages to neuroendocrine secretion and biological rhythms in man. *Recent Prog. Horm. Res.,* 31:399–441.

95. Weitzman, E. D., Nogeire, C., Perlow, M., Fukushima, D., Sassin, J., McGregor, P., Gallagher, T. F., and Hellman, L. (1974): Effects of a prolonged 3 hour sleep wake cycle on sleep stages, plasma cortisol, growth hormone and body temperature in man. *J. Clin. Endocrinol. Metab.,* 38:1018–1030.

96. Wentz, A. C. (1977): Clinical applications of luteinizing hormone-releasing hormone. *Fertil. Steril.,* 28:901–912.

97. Winkelmann, W., Fricke, V., Hadam, W., Heesen, D., Mies, R., and Rausch, E. (1978): Influence of sulpiride on plasma prolactin in patients with pituitary tumors. *Acta Endocrinol.* [*Suppl 215*], 87:abstr. 3.

98. Woolf, P. D., Lee, L. A., Leebaw, W., Thompson, D., Lilavivathana, U., Brodows, R., and

Campbell, R. (1977): Intracellular glucopenia causes prolactin release in man. *J. Clin. Endocrinol. Metab.,* 45:377–383.

99. Wyss, R. H., Karsznia, R., Heinrichs, W. L., and Hermann, W. L. (1968): Inhibition of uterine receptors binding of estradiol by anti-estrogens (clomiphene and CL-868). *J. Clin. Endocrinol. Metab.,* 28:1824–1828.

100. Yen, S. S. C., Rebar, R., Vanderberg, G., and Judd, H. (1973): Hypothalamic amenorrhea and hypogonadotropinism: Responses to synthetic LRF. *J. Clin. Endocrinol. Metab.,* 36:811–816.

101. Yen, S. S. C., and Tsai, C. C. (1972): Acute gonadotropin release induced by exogenous estradiol during the mid-follicular phase of the menstrual cycle. *J. Clin. Endocrinol. Metab.,* 34:298–305.

102. Yen, S. S. C., Tsai, C. C., Naftolin, F., Vanderberg, G., and Ajabor, L. (1972): Pulsatile patterns of gonadotropin release in subjects with and without ovarian function. *J. Clin. Endocrinol. Metab.,* 34:671–675.

103. Youlton, R., Kaplan, S. L., and Grumbach, M. M. (1969): Growth and growth hormone. IV. Limitations of the growth hormone response to insulin and arginine and of the immunoreactive insulin response to arginine in the assessment of growth hormone deficiency in children. *Pediatrics,* 43:989–1004.

104. Young, S. R., and Jaffe, R. B. (1976): Strength-duration characteristics of estrogen effects on gonadotropin releasing hormone in women: Effects of varying concentrations of estradiol. *J. Clin. Endocrinol. Metab.,* 42:432–441.

Subject Index

Acetylcholine
  angiotensin II interaction with,373
  pituitary effects of,27
N-Acetyltransferase
  light influence on,337,341,342,347–348
  norepinephrine stimulation of,346–347
  regulation of,346–347
  rhythm of,328,337
  stress influence on,348–349
Acromegaly,433–435,452,455
Actinomycin D, melatonin suppression by,350
Adenoma, pituitary,428
Adenosine monophosphate
  ACTH stimulation by,225,226
  endorphin stimulation by,225,226
  in gonadotrophin release,208–211,213
  luteinizing hormone-releasing hormone
     stimulation of,208–209
  in prolactin regulation,212–213
  as second messenger for hormone action,235
  in somatostatin regulation,211–212
Adenylate cyclase system
  activation of,235–236
  hormone action via,209–211,235,254,255
3α-Adiol,99,103,104
3β-Adiol,99,100–101,104
Adrenocorticotropin hormone (ACTH)
  amygdala response to,308–309
  basal levels of,450
  behavioral effects of,256,258–259
  circadian rhythm of,428–429,450
  distribution of,3,159–164,202,256
  disturbance of,427–430,450,452
  glucocorticoid interaction with,223,225,227
  hippocampus response to,309–310
  hypoglycemia, response to in,457
  precursor for,176–177,186
  regulation of,34,83–84,307–308,310–311,426
  vasopressin stimulation of,397–398
Adrenogenital syndrome,128
Aggressiveness, endocrine basis for,133
Albumin, melatonin complex with,336
Alcohol, pituitary effects of,402
Aldosterone,46,61,308
Allstrom-Hallgren syndrome,440
Amenorrhea
  in anorexia nervosa,432,440,441
  in Cushing's disease,428
  in hypogonadism,431–432
  in internal hydrocephalus,423
  response to gonadotropin-releasing hormone
    in, 453

γ-Aminobutyric acid (GABA), 27
Amygdala
  ACTH regulation by,83–84,308–309
  androgen effect on fetal,131
  corticosterone binding in,60
  estrogen in,43,57
  growth hormone regulation by,312–313
  hypothalamic connections with,297–298,299
  sexual differences of,300–304
  steroid influence on,304–306
  vasopressin response to,314
Analgesia
  opioid peptide influence on,240,244
Androgen-insensitivity syndrome,129
Androgenization,68–69,78,79,131,135
Androgens
  behavioral effects of,128,129
  biological functions for,45,79
  brain distribution of,58,59,66
  cyclicity suppression by,81–82
  defeminization with,68,69
  estrogen interaction with,55,71–72,132
  follicle-stimulating hormone stimulation
    by,215
  gonadotropin response to,81–82
  hypothalamic,59,66,74,107–113
  luteinizing hormone interaction with,
    210,213–215
  metabolic conversion of,82
    age-related changes in,106–107,111
    aromatization,108–111
    enzymes involved in,101–104,108
    hormonal regulation of,104–106,
     111–112
    hydroxylative pathway for,100–101
    oxidative pathway for,95–96
    reductive pathway for,96–99
  in neonatal androgenization,69
  pituitary,59,66,74,95–106
  preoptic,66
  receptors for
    age influence on,74
    brain distribution of,58–59,66,74,79
    neonatal,61,69
    progesterone effect on,69
    sexual differences in,82
    turnover of,75–76,77
  sexual differentiation effects of,126,127,129
Androstenedione
  biological effects of,59,73
  metabolic conversion of,82,95–96,132
Anesthesia,373–374